Lifestyle Nutrition

What individuals consume in their diet has profound implications on their health. Despite overwhelming evidence that plant-based diets yield multiple health benefits, physicians often feel ill-prepared to discuss nutrition with their patients. Authored by renowned cardiologist Dr. James M. Rippe, *Lifestyle Nutrition: Eating for Good Health by Lowering the Risk of Chronic Diseases* provides physicians with an evidence-based introduction to nutrition science with a practical emphasis on how to apply this information to improve the health of their patients and enhance their own lives.

From nutrition and atherosclerosis to erectile dysfunction and chronic kidney disease to osteoporosis, this comprehensive guide covers a wide range of conditions influenced by diet. It delves into specialized areas, such as nutrition for physically active people to the elderly, ensuring relevance for diverse patient populations. The reader will find detailed analysis of the *Dietary Guidelines for Americans 2020–2025* and their applications and strategies for adopting healthy plant-based diets, such as Mediterranean, DASH, and vegan.

Each chapter begins with key points and concludes with clinical applications, making it valuable to clinicians. As part of the esteemed *Lifestyle Medicine* series, this is an indispensable resource for any healthcare provider committed to enhancing patient care through informed dietary practices.

LIFESTYLE MEDICINE

Series Editor: James M. Rippe
Professor of Medicine, University of Massachusetts Chan Medical School

Led by James M. Rippe, MD, founder of the Rippe Lifestyle Institute, this series is directed to a broad range of researchers and professionals consisting of topical books with clinical applications in nutrition and health, physical activity, obesity management, and applicable subjects in lifestyle medicine.

Increasing Physical Activity: A Practical Guide
James M. Rippe

Manual of Lifestyle Medicine
James M. Rippe

Obesity Prevention and Treatment: A Practice Guide
James M. Rippe and John P. Foreyt

Lifestyle Nursing
Gia Merlo and Kathy Berra

Integrating Lifestyle Medicine in Cardiovascular Health and Disease Prevention
James M. Rippe

Lifestyle Medicine for Prediabetes, Type 2 Diabetes, and Cardiometabolic Disease
Michael A. Via and Jeffrey Mechanick

Empowering Behavior Change in Patients: Practical Strategies for the Healthcare Professional
Beth Frates, PhD and Mark Faries, MD

Lifestyle Psychiatry: Through the Lens of Behavioral Medicine
Gia Merlo and Christopher P. Fagundes

Lifestyle Nutrition: Eating for Good Health by Lowering the Risk of Chronic Diseases
James M. Rippe

For more information, please visit: www.routledge.com/Lifestyle-Medicine/book-series/CRCLM

Lifestyle Nutrition

Eating for Good Health by Lowering the Risk of Chronic Diseases

James M. Rippe, MD

CRC Press
Taylor & Francis Group
Boca Raton London New York

CRC Press is an imprint of the
Taylor & Francis Group, an **informa** business

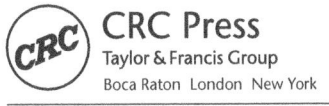

Designed cover image: Shutterstock

First edition published 2025
by CRC Press
2385 NW Executive Center Drive, Suite 320, Boca Raton FL 33431

and by CRC Press
4 Park Square, Milton Park, Abingdon, Oxon, OX14 4RN

CRC Press is an imprint of Taylor & Francis Group, LLC

ISBN: 978-1-032-59027-1 (hbk)
ISBN: 978-1-032-57637-4 (pbk)
ISBN: 978-1-003-45260-7 (ebk)

DOI: 10.1201/9781003452607

Typeset in Times
by Apex CoVantage, LLC

To my beautiful wife, Stephanie Hart Rippe, and our magnificent daughters, Hart, Jaelin, Devon, and Jamie, who inspire me and bring great joy and meaning to my life.

Contents

Preface for *Lifestyle Nutrition*

EATING FOR GOOD HEALTH BY LOWERING THE RISK OF CHRONIC DISEASES

It has been a great pleasure writing *Lifestyle Nutrition: Eating for Good Health by Lowering the Risk of Chronic Diseases.* This book is the most recent volume in the Lifestyle Medicine Series, where I have the honor of serving as the series editor.

The field of nutrition has changed dramatically over the past two decades. A number of years ago, when I started my career as a cardiologist, the mantra was to recommend to individuals, particularly those at risk for cardiovascular disease, that they consume a low-fat diet. While this was not an unreasonable recommendation, the scientific data to support dietary recommendations have subsequently undergone important changes. We now know from several major research studies that the low-fat diets do not reduce the risk of heart disease any more than placebo diets. What has emerged, however, is strong scientific evidence that diets which contain abundant fruits and vegetables and whole grains, among other healthy foods, substantially reduce the risk of cardiovascular disease and many other chronic diseases.

This new insight was demonstrated in the PREDIMED study, which provided the scientific underpinnings for the Mediterranean diet. The Dietary Approach to Stop Hypertension (DASH) also substantially reduces the risk of cardiovascular disease (CVD). In addition, the Healthy U.S.-Style Dietary Pattern contained in the *Dietary Guidelines for Americans 2020–2025* and multiple diets recommended by the American Heart Association in their most recent nutritional guidance from 2021, all have been demonstrated to substantially lower the risk of heart disease. Furthermore, all of them are very consistent with each other in recommending abundant fruits and vegetables, whole grains, and nontropical oils while minimizing red meat and processed meat, refined carbohydrates, salt, and sugar.

Unfortunately, most physicians find it daunting to keep up with the rapidly emerging field of nutrition science. Recent surveys have indicated that 93% of physicians do not feel that they are adequately trained in nutrition. Moreover, even in my subspecialty of cardiology, over 90% of cardiologists feel that they do not have adequate training to provide their patients with the most up-to-date nutritional guidance. It is reassuring, however, that 95% of cardiologists feel that recommending healthy nutrition is an imperative for our subspeciality and would welcome additional information in this area. I hope that this current book will help fill some of these gaps.

It is particularly important to link nutrition to other positive lifestyle habits and practices. Nutrition is one of the six pillars of lifestyle medicine, along with regular physical activity, weight management, avoiding risky behaviors, healthy sleep, and positive relationships with other people.

It is deeply gratifying for me to watch the field of lifestyle medicine continue to grow and prosper. I had the honor of naming the field of lifestyle medicine in the first multiauthored academic textbook that I edited in this area back in 1999 (*Lifestyle Medicine,* Blackwell Science, 1999). Even in the late 1990s it was clear that daily habits and actions powerfully impact both on short- and long-term health and quality of life. However, the academic literature in these fields is spread across many disciplines, including nutrition, exercise physiology, psychology, psychiatry, behavioral medicine, preventive medicine, public policy, and injury prevention, among others. My goal with the first edition of my first major textbook, *Lifestyle Medicine*, which has remained constant through the subsequent three editions of this large, academic textbook, has been to bring state-of-the-art, evidence-based information about the power of lifestyle habits to positively impact on health to individuals practicing in all branches of medicine.

The field of lifestyle medicine itself has grown dramatically in the past 20 years. For example, from its founding in 2004, the American College of Lifestyle Medicine has experienced phenomenal growth. This year it crossed the 11,000-member milestone, making it the most rapidly growing field of academic medicine. The reach of lifestyle medicine extends far beyond the United States into over 40 countries around the world.

The power of lifestyle medicine extends from a simple premise, namely, that the enormous literature supporting the power of lifestyle medicine's core premises has continued to grow. In fact, the World Health Organization (WHO) has launched a significant initiative to combat noncommunicable diseases (NCDs), which is based largely on helping people understand the power of their daily habits and actions. WHO has stated that over 71% of all mortality around the world each year comes from NCDs.

The time has come for physicians and other healthcare practitioners to expand their knowledge and embrace the core principles of lifestyle medicine. Given the power of daily habits and actions to improve health and lower the risk of chronic disease, it is hard to justify continuing to maintain that we are practicing evidence-based medicine without utilizing the enormous evidence that has now accumulated in the area of lifestyle and chronic disease.

While there are many aspects of lifestyle medicine, perhaps none is more important than healthy, plant-based nutrition. When it comes to plant-based nutrition, many physicians mistakenly believe that this connotes a vegetarian lifestyle. While a vegetarian lifestyle certainly is plant based, all of the healthy plant-based diets that have been demonstrated to reduce the risk of heart disease and other chronic disease, including those diets I have already mentioned, namely, the Mediterranean diet, DASH diet, and Healthy U.S.-Style Dietary Pattern—all are essentially plant-based diets that recommend increased consumption of fruits, vegetables, whole grains, and nontropical oils, while discouraging consumption of red meats, refined carbohydrates, including sugar, and saturated fats. It is also important to note that there is a clear distinction between "healthy" and "unhealthy" plant-based nutrition based on what components are included.

I hope and believe that the current book will help practicing clinicians understand the core principles and practices of recommending healthy plant-based diets to all of their patients as one of the most powerful ways of lowering the risk of chronic disease.

With the goal of providing a broad approach to healthy nutrition, I have divided *Lifestyle Nutrition: Eating for Good Health by Lowering the Risk of Chronic Diseases* into six major sections.

The first section, entitled "Perspectives in Healthy Nutrition: An Overview," focuses on the core principles of what constitutes healthy nutrition. The section starts with an overview of the linkage between healthy nutrition and other lifestyle practices, particularly as they relate to overall health.

I then move on to a detailed description of the Western diet and why it contributes to multiple chronic diseases. Next, a whole chapter is devoted to how nutritional status is measured. While I recognize that most physicians will not need to know the fine details of how nutrition professionals make measurements, it is important to understand, at least in general terms, the multiple terminologies such as nutrient density, caloric density, and the various formats that are used to measure the quality of the diet such as the Healthy Eating Index, Dietary Reference Intakes, and others.

The section then moves on to consider specific chronic diseases and how nutrition impacts on them and links this evidence to the role of physicians and other healthcare providers in recommending healthy plant-based diets to their patients. The section also contains a detailed description of the key points for the *Dietary Guidelines for Americans 2020–2025*, since these guidelines provide the most definitive, evidence-based rationale for healthy plant-based eating.

The first section concludes with a variety of other issues which are critically important and yet often ignored by practicing clinicians. These include nutrition and health equity, nutrition, hunger and malnutrition, nutrition and inflammation, and nutrition and metabolic health. All of these factors are important and should not be ignored by practicing clinicians.

The COVID-19 pandemic, in particular, underscored that major issues exist related to inequities in the current healthcare system. Many of these are based on nutritional factors. Nutrition has also been linked to the area of inflammation that is now considered to be one of the key underlying factors in virtually every chronic metabolic disease.

Another chapter is focused on metabolic health, which is also based on nutritional practices. Healthy metabolism a broad term and encompasses a variety of environmental and social factors which can impact on the overall metabolic health for each individual.

The first section concludes with a chapter on nutrition and atherosclerosis. This is a subject that is near and dear to my heart as a cardiologist. The understanding of atherosclerosis has changed dramatically during the time that I have practiced cardiology. It used to be thought that atherosclerosis was largely an issue of cholesterol and unsaturated fat combining to block coronary arteries. However, the field has now advanced to an understanding that the inciting process for atherosclerosis is based on inflammation and its effects on damaging the inner lining of the arteries. Atherosclerosis is clearly a systemic disease involving not only the arteries supplying the heart but also many other arteries throughout the body. These are handled in subsequent chapters on specific chronic diseases which are included in the second section.

The second section, "Healthy Nutrition and Chronic Diseases," focuses on various chronic diseases and the role that healthy nutrition can play in preventing and, in some instances, treating these diseases. These include coronary heart disease, hypertension, stroke, cancer, cognition and mental health, peripheral artery disease, chronic kidney disease, erectile dysfunction, prediabetes and diabetes, overweight and obesity, and osteoporosis. This section concludes with some of the modern scientific understandings in areas such as the gut microbiota. There has been a literal flood of research linking the relationship of the trillions of microbiota that inhabit our guts to various chronic diseases. Nutrition plays a key role in either promoting a healthy gut or contributing to dysbiosis.

The section concludes with a detailed description of healthy plant based diets, including the Mediterranean diet, various diets recommended by the American Heart Association (AHA) such as the DASH diet, and the Healthy U.S.-Style Dietary Pattern and vegetarian or vegan diets. While there are significant similarities among these diets, there are also some slight differences, which are emphasized in this chapter.

The third section moves on to the role of "Healthy Nutrition in Various Populations." This includes nutrition for the elderly, for children, for women, and for physically active people and athletes.

The fourth section, "Key Concepts and Components," explores specific new understandings about components of a healthy diet as well as cutting-edge research in the area of genetics, epigenetics, and precision nutrition. There has been enormous scientific ferment in these areas, and they are destined to impact on how we proceed in the area of nutritional science and nutrition recommendations for generations to come.

The fifth section focuses on topics that broaden the purview of nutrition. The first chapter in this section, "Healthy Nutrition for Planetary Health," provides an overview of how individual nutrition also impacts on the overall health of the planet. The current Western diet, which has now spread to many countries around the world, has done enormous damage to our planet. Clinicians tend to underestimate how harmful current nutritional policies are to the environment. For example, agricultural practices such as animal husbandry contribute more pollutants than any other single cause and significantly more than all automobile and other transportation effects. Agricultural practices utilize 70% of the clean water on the planet and contribute to deforestation and decreased biodiversity in ways that will not be sustainable, particularly as the population grows. It has been estimated that to generate one ounce of animal protein requires between 30 and 100 times the energy necessary to provide one ounce of fruits or vegetables.

The other chapter in this section on public policy entitled "Public Policy Support for Healthy Eating" focuses on how a wide range of public policies impact on both the provision and regulation of food. In order to make the headway toward healthier nutrition and practices that do less damage to the environment, public policy changes will be required. This will require both knowledge and the commitment of people and governments around the world.

The sixth and final section contains only one chapter. It is entitled "Healthy Nutrition to Protect the Planet." In this chapter I strongly urge physicians and other healthcare providers to focus on following healthy nutritional practices in their own lives. There are abundant data that physicians who follow positive lifestyle factors such as healthy nutrition, regular physical activity, avoiding tobacco, etc., are more likely to make these recommendations to their patients. Not only will healthy nutrition lower risk factors for chronic disease among individuals in the medical profession, but they also will increase the likelihood that these recommendations will be made throughout medical practices. This transformation is also vital to the health of our planet.

There is no longer any serious doubt that what each of us does in our daily lives profoundly impacts on short- and long-term health and quality of life. Nutrition is one of the key factors that plays a role in either lowering or increasing the risk of chronic disease.

I hope that this book will provide useful information for healthcare practitioners at all levels to increase the likelihood that they will follow healthy nutritional practices in their own lives and impart this information to every individual who they serve. My goal in writing this book remains what it has always been in the area of lifestyle medicine, namely, to provide state-of-the-art, evidence-based information that will help physicians impart knowledge to their patients about the enormous power of daily habits and actions, in this case, particularly in the area of nutrition.

As chronic diseases have continued to increase throughout the world, it is important to understand that we have the power in our hands to lower the risk of these diseases by what we do in our daily lives. Certainly, healthy nutrition is one of the leading factors that can contribute to the mandate that we as healthcare professionals have to protect and enhance the health of all the individuals that we have the honor to serve and help to protect the planet where we all live.

James M. Rippe, MD
Boston, MA

About the Author

JAMES M. RIPPE, MD

Dr. Rippe is a graduate of Harvard College and Harvard Medical School with postgraduate training at Massachusetts General Hospital and the University of Massachusetts Medical School. He is currently the founder and director of the Rippe Lifestyle Institute (RLI) and a professor of medicine at the UMass Chan Medical School.

Over the past 30 years Dr. Rippe has established and run the largest research organization in the world exploring how daily habits and actions impact short- and long-term health and quality of life. RLI has published hundreds of papers that form the scientific basis for the fields of lifestyle medicine risk factor reduction and high-performance health. RLI also conducts numerous studies every year on physical activity, nutrition, and healthy weight management. Dr. Rippe has written over 500 academic papers and abstracts and written or edited 60 books, including 33 for healthcare professionals and 27 for the general public.

A lifelong and avid athlete, Dr. Rippe maintains his personal fitness with a regular walk, jog, swimming, and weight training program. He holds a black belt in karate and is an avid windsurfer, skier, and tennis player. He lives outside of Boston with his wife, television news anchor Stephanie Hart, and their four children, Hart, Jaelin, Devon, and Jamie.

About the Author

Acknowledgments

I am grateful to many individuals who have stimulated and influenced my thinking about the interaction between lifestyle and health and the specific interactions between nutrition and the prevention and treatment of a variety of chronic diseases.

Textbook writing and editing are true collaborate efforts and involve the expertise and input from many individuals. Numerous individuals have guided my thinking in the area of nutrition and lifestyle medicine and are too many to be acknowledged by name. However, I would like to particularly thank a few individuals who have made substantial contributions to the current book and in my understanding in the field of lifestyle medicine.

First, my long-term Editorial Director, Beth Grady, who plays a critically important role in all of the major writing and editing projects that emerge from my research organization. This book is one of over 60 books that Beth has managed which have been generated through my organization. In addition to the current textbook, Beth provides editorial direction to two academic journals that I edit as well as my major *Lifestyle Medicine* textbook (*Lifestyle Medicine*, 4th ed., James M. Rippe, editor, CRC Press, 2024). My major intensive care textbook (*Irwin and Rippe's Intensive Care Medicine,* 9th ed., Wolters Kluwer, 2023). Beth has superb editorial skills and an exceptional work ethic. She remains calm and has an unfailing sense of good humor, both of which are essential to make these complex and difficult projects possible.

My office support staff also plays a critically important role in all of these publishing projects. These include my Executive Assistant, Carol Moreau, who not only seamlessly coordinates my schedule and travel plans but also word processed many of the chapters in this book. Our Editorial Office Assistant, Deb Adamonis, plays multiple and diverse roles in our organization and assists us in the numerous complex daily tasks required to execute the diverse projects in our office. In addition, Deb tracked down thousands of academic references for the current book. Our Chief Financial Officer, Wendy Graves, manages the financial processes to assure that our projects move forward smoothly.

Our research team at RLI has always contributed important insights and clarified my thinking on various aspects of healthy nutrition and lifestyle medicine. I have been pleased to employ numerous MS RDs over the course of my academic career. They have unfailingly provided not only great nutrition counseling to our various research subjects but also taught me a great deal about how nutrition can be effectively communicated to individuals.

I would like to thank the outstanding editorial team at the Taylor & Francis Group/CRC Press. Randy Brehm, Senior Editor, has been an important supporter of multiple books that I have published with CRC Press, including the second, third, and fourth editions of my major academic textbook, *Lifestyle Medicine.* Randy has also been a strong supporter of the Lifestyle Medicine Series in which the current volume resides.

Tom Connelly coordinated all aspects of the publication process and provided day-to-day assistance on multiple issues related to each chapter. Tom is a true pleasure to work with. He is conscientious, detail-oriented, and maintained a positive and helpful attitude throughout the entire arduous process of the final publication stages of this large book!

Marsha Hecht, Production Editor at the Taylor & Francis Group, oversaw all aspects of the production of this book with style and grace.

Project Manager Bryan Moloney and his team at Deanta Global have managed the day-to-day production in preparing our manuscript with great skill.

Finally, as always, I am deeply grateful to my family including my loving wife, Stephanie Hart Rippe, and our four wonderful daughters, Hart, Jaelin, Devon, and Jamie, who continue to love and support me through all of the arduous processes of writing and editing major textbooks as well as other diverse academic and professional responsibilities that I juggle along with my family life. In addition, I am blessed to live with four vegetarians and a vegan who are collectively called "The Rippe Women." While they are perhaps stricter in their diet and nutritional practices than I am, they have helped me maintain a very healthy diet, and I am proud to say that I am one of the 10% of cardiologists who actually consumes the key components of healthy plant-based diets, including the recommended servings of fruit and vegetables and whole grains. We have a great deal of fiber in our diet and consume at least two fish meals a week while largely avoiding red meat and processed meats.

If there are errors or omissions in *Lifestyle Nutrition: Eating for Good Health by Lowering the Risk of Chronic Diseases*, the responsibility is mine. If there is any credit due to the project, it belongs to the numerous people who have made and continue to make substantial contributions to my knowledge and performance along the way and bring great joy to my life.

James M. Rippe, MD
Boston, Massachusetts

1 Lifestyle Nutrition for Physicians and Other Healthcare Workers

Key Points

- An enormous amount of evidence demonstrates that healthy plant-based diets lower the risk of chronic disease.
- Modern nutrition research focuses on overall dietary patterns rather than individual nutrients and foods.
- Multiple, healthy dietary eating patterns are available, including the Dietary Approach to Stop Hypertension (DASH) diet, the Mediterranean diet, the Healthy U.S.-Style Dietary, and multiple recommended diets from the American Heart Association.
- The current Western diet is prevalent in the United States and contributes to multiple chronic diseases including coronary heart disease, type 2 diabetes, obesity, certain cancers, osteoporosis, and even certain forms of dementia.
- Guidance is available from a variety of sources to help clinicians study and recommend heart-healthy diets to all patients.
- There is an inextricable link between individual and population health and planetary health, which is a further consideration for all clinicians.

1.1 INTRODUCTION

What individuals consume in their diet has profound implications for their health. In fact, six out of the ten leading causes of death worldwide have nutritional components. For this reason, the World Health Organization (WHO) has listed improved diet as one of the six key initiatives to lower the prevalence of noncommunicable diseases (NCDs) [1].

There is overwhelming evidence that diets that are primarily plant based, including increased consumption of fruits and vegetables, more whole grains, etc., yield multiple health benefits. In fact, virtually all of the dietary recommendations from prestigious organizations such as the American Heart Association (AHA) [2], *Dietary Guidelines for Americans 2020–2025* [3], WHO, the American Diabetes Association [4], the American Cancer Association [4], and the Academy of Nutrition and Dietetics [5] share similar emphases in this area. All are similar and emphasize the importance of a primarily plant-based diet and increasing consumption of fruits and vegetables and whole grains. Numerous diets, including the AHA Prudent Diet [6], the Mediterranean diet [7], the DASH diet [8], Nordic diet [9], flexitarian diet [10], vegetarian diets, vegan

DOI: 10.1201/9781003452607-1

diets, and multiple Asian diets, including those from China, Japan, and Korea, are all based on these fundamental principles [11].

These diets, with varying degrees of rigor in the restriction of animal products and processed food, have shown varying degrees of risk factor reduction related to prevention, arrest, and even reversal of some chronic diseases. These diets not only emphasize more plant-based eating but also highlight the importance of minimizing or possibly even eliminating processed foods in favor of whole foods and a concomitant reduction of salt and refined sugar and an increase in dietary fiber.

It should be noted that not all plant-based diets can be considered "healthy." In fact, recent literature has divided plant-based diets into "healthy plant-based diets" and "unhealthy plant-based diets" [12]. The major difference between these two is that in healthy plant-based diets the emphasis is on fruits and vegetables, whole grains and fiber, while reducing tropical oils, sugar, and sodium, as well as red meat and processed meats. In contrast, unhealthy plant-based diets, while also reducing red meat and processed meats, contain more refined grains, saturated fats, and tropical oils as well as sugar and salt. Research studies have shown that healthy plant-based diets lower the risk of heart disease and other chronic diseases whereas unhealthy plant-based diets do not.

Despite the overwhelming evidence of health benefits of diets that are focused on plants, physicians in general have not advocated that their patients follow such diets. In fact, physicians often feel woefully ill-prepared to discuss nutrition with their patients. Less than 40% of physicians routinely counsel their patients on diet at all, and even if they do, much of the information is general advice, like "follow a balanced diet," without making specific recommendations [13].

Studies have indicated that only 21% of patients feel they receive adequate nutritional advice from their physicians. While the lack of dietary counseling may be somewhat due to time constraints, it is also true that many physicians lack specific knowledge about nutrition and how to prescribe healthy diets. In fact, only 20% of medical schools have a nutritional course [14], and only 14% of individuals graduating from medical school feel they have adequate nutrition knowledge [15]. Shockingly, 90% of cardiologists feel that they do not have adequate nutritional knowledge, although it is somewhat comforting to me, as a cardiologist, that 95% of cardiologists feel that nutrition counseling is important and try to do it [16]. A recent survey showed that over 93% of physicians feel that they are not adequately trained in the area of nutrition [17]. Thus, there is a significant problem and one that will be addressed by this book.

It is high time that an effort is made to enhance the nutrition education for clinicians at all levels of training. A seminal event occurred in late September 2022 with the White House Conference on Hunger, Nutrition and Health [18]. The vision of this conference was to "End hunger and increase healthy eating and physical activity by 2030, so that fewer American[s] experience diet related diseases like diabetes, coronary artery disease and hypertension."

The purpose of this book is to provide physicians evidence-based and simple motivational information on a wide variety of chronic diseases and other nutritional issues to increase their knowledge base and thereby increase the likelihood that they will recommend healthy diets to their patients.

Healthy nutrition is also one of the therapeutic cornerstones of the fastest-growing medical specialty in the United States, namely lifestyle medicine. The major academic organization in this area is the American College of Lifestyle Medicine (ACLM) [19]. Each year, over the past decade, ACLM has more than doubled its membership. There are currently more than 10,000 members. In addition, both the American College of Preventive Medicine and the American Academy of Family Practice have created lifestyle medicine tracks for individuals who wish to improve their knowledge in this area. I am proud of the fact that I introduced the concept of lifestyle medicine into the academic literature and named the field with the first edition of my *Lifestyle Medicine* textbook published in 1999 [20].

It is also comforting to me as a cardiologist that nutrition and lifestyle medicine are playing an increasing role in the recommendations for cardiologists. Included in the standards for cardiologists are the 2013 American Heart Association/American College of Cardiology (AHA/ACC) Practice Guidelines [21] which emphasize nutrition and other aspects of lifestyle medicine as fundamental components of the practice of cardiology. In addition, the recently released AHA Guidelines for Lipid Management [22] as well as Control of High Blood Pressure [23] also focus on nutrition and healthy lifestyle. The AHA's Dietary Guidance to Improve Cardiovascular Health was updated in 2021 [2] and underscores the key role of healthy nutrition to lower the risk of cardiovascular disease, diabetes, and obesity. All of these guidelines also emphasize the importance of increased physical activity and weight management, which are also areas where my research laboratory (Rippe Lifestyle Institute) has established international leadership positions.

Healthy eating is one of the most talked about and important areas of modern nutrition. It is time for physicians to take notice of this trend and its health benefits and provide specific dietary guidelines in nutrition for their patients. We know that patients are interested in the area of nutrition. When surveyed, 78% of patients indicated that they had made alterations in their eating habits following conversations with their physicians [24]. Physicians are trusted and influential figures who can play a pivotal role in helping their patients make better choices. This is an enormous opportunity given that over 70% of individuals see their primary care physician at least once a year [24].

While numerous health benefits are associated with sound nutrition, it is also important to underscore that food insecurity and hunger remain significant issues in the United States and are distributed disproportionately, impacting underserved communities including communities of color, people living in rural areas, people with disabilities, older adults, LGBTQ individuals, military families, and military veterans [18].

These individuals often have a disproportionate level of disease related to poor nutrition. The profound effects of poor nutrition on disease were dramatically underscored by responses to the COVID-19 pandemic. Individuals who were obese, had diabetes, or had high blood pressure were 3–4 times more likely to be hospitalized and/or die as a result of COVID-19, compared to individuals who did not have those conditions [25,26]. Most of the increased risk resulted from poor dietary choices, leading to chronic disease. Since physicians also see individuals in these categories, information on these issues that involve health equity are also addressed in this book.

While this book will focus on healthy eating, it also contains sections on other issues that relate to health-promoting benefits of other daily habits and actions such as regular physical activity, weight management, sleep, and stress reduction. All of these are important to improve overall health and represent cornerstones of lifestyle medicine as well as interacting with nutrition. In addition, there are chapters on public policy issues as well as why healthy eating is also important for planetary health since the Western diet makes a major contribution to global warming.

Specific chapters in this book include the importance of healthy eating in the prevention, arrest, and possible reversal of coronary artery disease, type 2 diabetes, certain adult cancers, obesity, hypertension, and stroke, as well as prediabetes and metabolic syndrome. There is also a chapter on the major, plant-based food-strong diets such as the AHA Diet (Step 2), the Mediterranean diet, the DASH diet, the vegetarian diet and its variations, the Nordic diet, the vegan diet, and some Asian diets.

This issue of better health and a longer life through the adoption of a healthier diet has broad appeal since everyone eats and most people (including physicians) experience undesirable health outcomes because of the way they eat. Many people don't seem to realize how their diet has undergone some dramatic shifts beginning in the 1970s, when we shifted from a "slow-food" to "fast-food" diet, as well as from preparing food and eating it at home to eating out, and when low-calorie potatoes turned into high-calorie potato chips or French fries, high-fiber beans turned into low-fiber burgers, and water turned into soda pop. As a result, the caloric density of our engineered food has starkly increased, as have our waistlines, while nutrient density has declined. At the same time our consumption of animal products, many of which are high in fat and cholesterol, have people everywhere on cholesterol-lowering drugs and undergoing stents and bypass surgeries trying to keep the coronary arteries open for life-sustaining blood flow. Our national diet has undergone a prodigious shift: Only 14% of our calories today are supplied in the form of nutrient-dense foods-as-grown, plant-foods such as fruits, vegetables, whole grains, and legumes. The so-called "Western diet" typically consumed in the United States not only promotes obesity but is also highly inflammatory [27].

In addition to the improved health of individuals by following a healthy eating style, a switch in this direction will also be good for the health of our planet. It is estimated that over 40% of greenhouse gases come from animal husbandry as well as ten times the amount of water use from raising domestic animals compared with growing fruits and vegetables and grain crops [28].

1.2 PERSPECTIVES ON HEALTHY NUTRITION

- **Multiple benefits of healthy plant-based nutrition**—As already indicated, multiple organizations and guidelines have been uniform in providing similar recommendations for healthy plant-based nutrition. These include the WHO, the AHA, the Dietary Guidelines for Americans (DGA) 2020–2025, the Academy of Nutrition and Dietetics, and the American Diabetes Association. These diets are very consistent with regard to recommendations. They include an emphasis on fruits and vegetables, whole grains, fish, polyunsaturated fats, oils, nuts, and legumes, while recommending decreases in saturated fats, sugar, salt, ultra-processed foods, refined grains, and tropical oils. Multiple benefits have been demonstrated from the consumption of healthy plant-based diets. These include reduction in the risk of chronic diseases such as cardiovascular disease (CVD), Type 2 Diabetes (T2DM), obesity, metabolic syndrome (MetS), and certain forms of cancer. Modern nutrition research focuses on dietary patterns rather than individual foods and nutrients, although the foods and nutrients within healthy diets play an important role in lowering the risk of chronic disease.

- **Standard American Diet: A Recipe for Chronic Diseases**—The standard American diet contains too much salt, saturated fats, and sugar [27]. It also contains too much red meat and processed foods. Numerous studies have shown that the standard American diet increases the risk of various chronic diseases. The American diet has been demonstrated to be inflammatory, which contributes to its association with various chronic diseases, all of which have an important component of inflammation. In addition, the standard American diet has been shown to adversely impact microbiota [29]. Thus, there are many reasons for clinicians to recommend individuals change their diet from the current standard American diet to one of the healthy plant-based diets indicated in the previous section.
- **The Concept of Nutritional Status and Measurements**—While most clinicians will not conduct nutrition research, familiarity with how nutrition status is determined and the various measurements involved are important in order to understand published research as well as the underpinnings for healthy diets. Various indices and recommendations such as the DGA 2020–2025, the Healthy Eating Index, and various graphics from the U.S. Department of Agriculture (USDA), such as the My Plate Program, are all important underpinnings for the type of healthy plant-based nutrition that clinicians should be recommending to all patients [30].
- **Lifestyle Medicine**—This book will focus largely on nutrition. There are multiple other components related to daily lifestyle habits and actions which also profoundly impact on both short- and long-term health and quality of life. They also interact with sound nutrition. Such components represent the core principles of the rapidly emerging field of lifestyle medicine. The pillars of lifestyle medicine include not only healthy nutrition but also increased physical activity, weight management, avoidance of tobacco products, healthy sleep, stress reduction, and positive relations with others [31]. In numerous chapters these other lifestyle measures will be emphasized as components of an overall healthy lifestyle, and their relationship to healthy nutrition will also be emphasized.
- **The Role of Physicians and Other Healthcare Workers**—Physicians and other healthcare workers are important gatekeepers for recommending various positive behaviors including nutrition, physical activity, and other pillars of lifestyle medicine. It is a fundamental goal of this book to provide the evidence base for physicians to feel comfortable in recommending healthy plant-based nutrition to the patients they see.

- **Nutrition and Health Equity**—Unfortunately, despite the fact that the United States is the wealthiest nation on the planet, there still are significant problems with health disparities and differences in health equity. These disparities were underscored in the recent COVID-19 pandemic, where individuals who had various chronic diseases that were typically nutrition related such as obesity, diabetes, and hypertension, were 3–4 times as likely to be hospitalized and, in many instances, die [26]. While disparities in healthcare and poverty are not synonymous, oftentimes these individuals come from the lower economic strata of the American population. These disparities are particularly prevalent in African Americans and Hispanics. These issues are increasingly being urgently addressed by not only the U.S. government but also various healthcare organizations such as the AHA [32], the American College of Physicians [33], and the American College of Lifestyle Medicine.
- **Nutrition, Hunger, and Malnutrition**—Unfortunately, in the United States, more than 34 million people, including 9 million children, experience food insecurity. It has been estimated that as many as 18 million children go to bed each night hungry [34]. While hunger and malnutrition are not synonymous, hunger can make a significant contribution to malnutrition. Another population that experiences malnutrition, where it is often overlooked, is the elderly population. Since physicians see individuals in all of these categories, we will devote an entire chapter to these issues.
- **Dietary Guidelines for Americans (DGA) 2020–2025**—The DGAs are released every five years by the USDA. The most recent DGAs were 2020–2025. This document provides the fundamental nutrition guidance for multiple federal programs. All clinicians should be generally familiar with the DGAs and have at least reviewed the executive summary of this important, evidence-based document.

1.3 HEALTHY NUTRITION AND CHRONIC DISEASES

Healthy dietary patterns have been demonstrated to yield a variety of health benefits for chronic disease. These include CVD, essential hypertension, other circulation-related chronic diseases including peripheral artery disease, erectile dysfunction, and chronic kidney disease. In addition, healthy nutritional patterns have been demonstrated to lower the risk of some types of cancer and play a critical role in lowering the risk of prediabetes turning into diabetes. Healthy nutrition patterns are also, by their very nature, lower in calories and play a role in helping to maintain a healthy body weight. When combined with other lifestyle measures, healthy nutritional patterns can play a key role in weight loss. A variety of other conditions and considerations also are impacted by a healthy dietary pattern. These include osteoporosis and cognition and mental health. Separate chapters will be devoted to each of these entities in this book.

A variety of other factors play into the effectiveness of healthy dietary patterns in lowering chronic disease. These include the role of healthy dietary patterns in metabolic health and their impact on gut microbiota. How nutrition interacts with other lifestyle habits will be discussed in multiple chapters throughout this book. Multiple diets are considered to be healthy plant-based diets including the Mediterranean diet, various diets from the AHA, the DASH diet, the Healthy U.S.-Style Dietary Pattern, and vegetarian and vegan diets. A key distinction has been made in recent research that not all plant-based diets can be considered healthy. In fact, some plant-based diets that contain considerable amounts of salt, sugar, and saturated fats and also refined grains and tropical oils have been shown to be "unhealthy" plant-based diets, in contrast to "healthy" plant-based diets, "unhealthy" plant-based diets do not reduce the risk of chronic disease. This will be discussed in multiple chapters in this book.

1.4 HEALTHY NUTRITION FOR VARIOUS POPULATIONS

Healthy dietary patterns should be followed by people of all ages. There are some slight differences that may be advocated for people of different ages. In this book there will be separate chapters on healthy nutrition for the elderly and for children. In addition, there will be a separate chapter on healthy nutritional patterns for women and nutrition for physically active people and athletes.

1.5 KEY CONCEPTS AND COMPONENTS

A variety of components are part of a dietary pattern. These include various foods contained in heart-healthy diets as well as concepts such as energy density, nutrient density, metabolism, fiber, protein, and epigenetics. In addition, there has been recent interest in the area of personalized nutrition, and these will be covered in multiple chapters in the book.

1.6 NUTRITION, PUBLIC POLICY, AND PLANETARY HEALTH

Healthy personal and population nutrition is inextricably linked to planetary health. The current eating patterns in the United States and other countries around the world create adverse ecological conditions, in particular, the generation of red meat and other animal products place a great strain on the planet. Currently, 70% of all fresh water on the planet is utilized in agriculture and, in particular, on raising animals for meat consumption [28]. In addition, over 30% of greenhouse gases are attributable to animal husbandry, and vast amounts of nitrogen and phosphorous are leached into fresh water and soil as a result of excessive use of fertilizers [28]. It has been estimated that producing an ounce of protein from animals generates 250 times the amount of planetary disruption compared to other protein sources such as legumes and soybeans. Moving forward, it will be incumbent upon clinicians to not only be cognizant and care about the individual health of their patients but also play a much more active role in planetary health. It will be necessary to preserve planetary health to shift to the increased fruit and vegetable consumption featured in healthy-based eating patterns. This will also involve public policy decisions on multiple levels, and physicians should play an active role in advocating healthy public policy issues in this area.

1.7 CONCLUSIONS

Healthy dietary patterns are critically important for good health for patients and for the planet. Multiple plant-based healthy dietary patterns are available, including the Dietary Approach to Stop Hypertension (DASH) diet, the Mediterranean diet, the Healthy U.S.-Style Dietary, and multiple dietary plans from the AHA. These plans are all consistent in recommending enhanced amounts of fruit and vegetable consumption, whole grains, fish, nontropical plant oils, legumes, and nuts, and they all minimize salt, sugar, saturated fats, ultra-processed foods, and refined grains. A typical Western diet contains too much salt, sugar, and saturated fats and contains a considerable amount of animal protein. This diet has been associated with increased risk of various chronic diseases including CVD, T2DM, obesity, cancer, and osteoporosis.

There is also accumulating evidence that the Western diet increases the risk of dementia, stroke, and other chronic vascular diseases such as peripheral artery disease, erectile dysfunction, and chronic kidney disease. Guidance is available for consuming healthy plant-based diets. Multiple sources of information are available. The one that all physicians should have in their toolbox is the Executive Summary of the *Dietary Guidelines for Americans 2020–2025*. This is an evidence-based document that can provide guidance for how to achieve healthy plant-based dietary patterns. Other habits and actions in daily lives including physical activity, weight management, avoidance of tobacco products, reduced stress, healthy sleep, and healthy interactions with other individuals are also key lifestyle factors and should be incorporated in an overall plan to promote healthy lifestyles. These are the key pillars of lifestyle medicine.

Clinical Applications

- Healthy dietary patterns lower the risk of various chronic diseases.
- There is a distinction between healthy plant-based diets and unhealthy plant-based diets.
- Healthy plant-based diets feature abundant fruits, vegetables, whole grains, and nontropical oils and discourage consumption of added sugar, salt, and saturated fats as well as refined grains and ultra-processed foods.
- Physician education in the area of nutrition is sadly lacking. Ninety-three percent of physicians feel that they do not have adequate nutrition knowledge to effectively counsel their patients.
- Twenty-one percent of patients feel that they do not get adequate nutritional advice from their physician.
- Making recommendations for healthy plant-based dietary patterns is a key consideration that physicians should adopt to enhance the health of their patients and lower their risk of chronic disease.

REFERENCES

1. World Health Organization. Noncommunicable diseases. (who.int) (Accessed May 23, 2023).

2. Lichtenstein A, Appel L, Vadiveloo M, et al. 2021 Dietary guidance to improve cardiovascular health: A scientific statement from the American Heart Association. Circulation. 2021;144(23):e472–e487.
3. U.S. Department of Agriculture and U.S. Department of Health and Human Services. *Dietary Guidelines for Americans, 2020–2025*, 9th edition. December 2020. DietaryGuidelines.gov. 2020. www.dietaryguidelines.gov/resources/2020-2025-dietary-guidelines-online-materials (Accessed May 23, 2023).
4. Clark A, Raine K, Raphael D. The American Cancer Society, American Diabetes Association, and American Heart Association joint statement on preventing cancer, cardiovascular disease, and diabetes: Where are the social determinants? Diabetes Care. 2004;27(12):3024.
5. Melina V, Craig W, Levin S. Position of the academy of nutrition and dietetics: Vegetarian diets. J Acad Nutr Diet. 2016;116(12):1970–1980. Epub 2016/11/26.
6. Heidemann C, Schulze M, Franco O, et al. Dietary patterns and risk of mortality from cardiovascular disease, cancer, and all causes in a prospective cohort of women. Circulation. 2008;5;118(3):230–237.
7. Estruch R, Ros E, Salas-Salvado J, et al. Primary prevention of cardiovascular disease with a Mediterranean diet. N Engl J Med. 2013;368(14):1279–1290.
8. Sacks F, Svetkey L, Vollmer W, et al. Effects on blood pressure of reduced dietary sodium and the Dietary Approaches to Stop Hypertension (DASH) diet. DASH-Sodium Collaborative Research Group. N Engl J Med. 2001;344(1):3–10.
9. Mithril C, Dragsted L, Meyer C, et al. Guidelines for the new Nordic diet. Public Health Nutr. 2012;15(10):1941–1947.
10. What is the Flexitarian diet? Food Insight. (Accessed May 23, 2023).
11. Mozaffarian D, Appel L, Van Horn L. Components of a cardioprotective diet: New insights. Circulation. 2011;123(24):2870–2891.
12. Satija A, Bhupathiraju S, Spiegelman D, et al. Healthful and unhealthful plant-based diets and the risk of coronary heart disease in U.S. adults. J Am Coll Cardiol. 2017;70(4):411–422.
13. U.S. Preventive Services Task Force. Behavioral counseling in primary care to promote a healthy diet: Recommendations and rationale. Am J Prev Med. 2003;24(1):93–100.
14. McGovern CJP. As White House conference approaches, now is the time for a national plan to address the link between hunger, nutrition education, and health. Am J Clin Nutr. 2022;116(4):841–842.
15. Nestle M, Baron R. Nutrition in medical education: From counting hours to measuring competence. JAMA Intern Med. 2014;174(6):843–844.
16. Devries S, Agatston A, Aggarwal M, et al. A deficiency of nutrition education and practice in cardiology. Am J Med. 2017;130(11):1298–1305.
17. Adams K, Kohlmeier M, Zeisel S. Nutrition education in U.S. medical schools: Latest update of national survery. Acad Med. 2010;85:1537–1542.
18. White House Conference on Hunger, Nutrition, & Health. U.S. Department of Health and Human Services. September, 2022. Ending Hunger and Reducing Diet-Related Diseases and Disparities | health.gov (Accessed May 23, 2023).
19. American College of Lifestyle Medicine. https://lifestylemedicine.org/ (Accessed May 23, 2023).
20. Rippe JM. Lifestyle Medicine. London: Blackwell Science, Inc., 1999.
21. Life's Essential 8. American Heart Association, Dallas, TX. www.heart.org/en/healthy-living/healthy-lifestyle/lifes-essential-8 (Accessed March 11, 2024).
22. Grundy S, Stone N, Bailey A, et al. 2018 AHA/ACC/AACVPR/AAPA/ABC/ACPM/ADA/AGS/APhA/ASPC/NLA/PCNA guideline on the management of blood cholesterol:

A report of the American College of Cardiology/American Heart Association task force on clinical practice guidelines. J Am Coll Cardiol. 2019;73(24):e285–e350.

23. Whelton P, Carey R, Aronow W, et al. 2017 ACC/AHA/AAPA/ABC/ACPM/AGS/APhA/ASH/ASPC/NMA/PCNA guideline for the prevention, detection, evaluation, and management of high blood pressure in adults: Executive summary: A report of the American College of Cardiology/American Heart Association task force on clinical practice guidelines. Hypertension. 2018;71(6):1269–1324.
24. Rippe J. Lifestyle medicine: The health promoting power of daily habits and practices. Am J Lifestyle Med. 2018;12(6):499–512.
25. Rippe J, Foreyt JP. COVID-19 and obesity: A pandemic wrapped in an epidemic. Am J Lifestyle Med. 2021;15(4):364–365.
26. Belanger M, Hill M, Angelidi A, et al. Covid-19 and disparities in nutrition and obesity. N Engl J Med. 2020;383:e69.
27. Cordain L, Eaton S, Sebastian A, et al. Origins and evolution of the Western diet: Health implications for the 21st century. Am J Clin Nutr. 2005;81(2):341–354.
28. Marinova D, Bogueva D. Planetary health and reduction in meat consumption. Sustain Earth. 2019;2(1):3.
29. Christ A, Lauterbach M, Latz E. Western diet and the immune system: An inflammatory connection. Immunity. 2019;51(5):794–811.
30. Dwyer J. Nutrition 101: The concept of nutritional status and guides for nutrient intakes, eating patterns, and nutrition. In Rippe J (ed). Lifestyle Medicine, 2nd edition. Boca Raton: CRC Press, 2013.
31. Rippe JM. Lifestyle Medicine, 4th edition. Boca Raton: CRC Press, 2024.
32. Angell S, McConnell M, Anderson C, et al. The American Heart Association 2030 impact goal: A presidential advisory from the American Heart Association. Circulation. 2020;141(9):e120–e138.
33. Daniel H, Bornstein S, Kane G. Health, public policy committee of the American College of P. addressing social determinants to improve patient care and promote health equity: An American College of Physicians position paper. Ann Intern Med. 2018;168(8):577–578.
34. Hunger in America Study. Feeding America. Hunger in America Study | Feeding America (Accessed May 24, 2023).

2 The Western Diet

Key Points

- The Western diet (WPD) is a relatively new phenomena in terms of epidemiologic history.
- The Western diet consists of multiple foods such as increased red meats, processed meats, saturated fatty acids, refined grains, refined sugars, and refined oils.
- The WPD also is dominated by processed foods. It is estimated that 85% of calories in WPD come from processed foods.
- The WPD contributes to inflammation, which is an underlying inciting factor in multiple chronic diseases such as CVD, obesity, diabetes, metabolic syndrome, and cancer.

2.1 INTRODUCTION

The Western pattern diet (WPD) is an eating pattern that has evolved, particularly in the United States, over the past 4–5 decades [1,2]. It is a dietary pattern that is generally characterized by high intakes of prepackaged foods, refined grains, red meat, processed meat, high-sugar drinks, candy and sweets, fried foods, conventionally raised animal products, butter and other fat dairy products, eggs, potatoes, and corn and low intakes of fruits, vegetables, whole grains, pasture-raised animal products, fish, nuts, and seeds [3]. The WPD has been largely blamed for contributing to a variety of chronic illnesses and health problems [4,5], when compared to "prudent" or other plant-based healthy diets which emphasize a higher intake of fruits and vegetables, whole grains, legumes, nuts, seeds, and low-fat dairy products. Healthier diets which have been compared to the WPD include the Healthy U.S.-Style Dietary Pattern recommended by the *Dietary Guidelines for Americans 2020–2025* [6], the Mediterranean diet [7,8], the DASH diet [9], and diets recommended by the 2021 American Heart Association Nutritional Guidelines [10]. The purpose of this chapter is to compare the WPD to the healthier diets with regard to a variety of specific dietary components as well as relationships to various chronic diseases.

2.2 COMPONENTS OF THE WESTERN DIET

The WPD is characterized by a significant amount of red meat, dairy products (including full-fat dairy products), processed and artificially sweetened foods, and salt. It has minimal intake of fruits and vegetables, fish, legumes, and whole grains. It has been characterized as having a high glycemic load, high fatty acid composition, elevated calories, low amounts of micronutrients, acidic foods, a sodium/potassium ratio emphasizing sodium, and a low fiber content [1].

DOI: 10.1201/9781003452607-2

It should also be noted that the nutritional quality of specific foods comprising the macronutrients in the Western pattern is often poor. For example, complex carbohydrates are less prominent in the WPD than are refined carbohydrates [11,12]. In addition, the energy density of the typical WPD has increased over time. In 2006, a typical WPD had approximately 2,200 calories per day. By 2015, the average daily caloric intake of the American adult was 2,390 kcals per day. It is currently estimated that the average has increased to 3,680 kcals per day [13,14]. Compounding the increased caloric consumption and promoting obesity and diabetes, American adults lead increasingly sedentary lifestyles. In fact, the Physical Activity Guidelines for Americans 2018 suggested that only 25% of American adults achieve the amount of regular physical activity that is necessary to lower their risk of various chronic diseases, including heart disease [15]. Americans currently consume over 13% of their daily calories in some form of added sugars [16], and Americans over the age of one consume more tropical oils, saturated fats, and sodium, in addition to added sugars, than are recommended by the Dietary Guidelines for Americans (DGA) 2020–2025 [6]. Almost 90% of Americans consume more sodium than recommended, while only 12% of the population consumes recommended amounts of fruit [17], and less than 10% consume the recommended amounts of vegetables [18].

While the DGA 2020–2025 recommends that whole grains should consist of over half of the total grain consumption, 85% of the grains consumed by Americans are refined, where the germ and bran are removed [19], thus decreasing nutritional quality. All of these factors show that a WPD, when compared to a healthy diet, was correlated with a variety of chronic metabolic diseases including obesity [5], cardiovascular disease (CVD), and various cancers (including breast, colon, and prostate cancer [20]. WPD also increases the risk of diabetes [21,22] and metabolic syndrome [23]. Recent data have suggested that an underlying problem with the WPD is that it contains many foods that increase inflammation and have contributed to chronic diseases which typically have an inflammatory component [24,25]. (See the further section in this chapter.)

2.3 ORIGINS OF THE WESTERN DIET AND LINK TO CHRONIC DISEASES

It has been argued that many of the chronic diseases associated with the WPD are a result of a mismatch between the human genome and the food environment currently found in many Westernized countries and increasingly around the world [1,2]. Typically, genetic traits take many thousands of years to evolve. However, food environment changes have occurred that have far outpaced the human genome to adapt.

For example, a number of profound environmental changes, which began with the introduction of large-scale agriculture and animal husbandry over the last 10,000 years, have occurred too recently in the evolutionary time frame for the human genome to adapt [26–28]. This, coupled with decreased physical activity among many Western cultures, has created what many researchers have characterized as an "obesigenic" environment and promoted diseases such as not only obesity but also diabetes, CVD, many cancers, and metabolic syndrome [29]. These chronic conditions have been called "diseases of civilization." In the United States and many other Western countries, chronic illnesses and health problems that are either wholly or partially attributable to the diet represent a serious threat to public health. For example, 73% of adults in the United States are either overweight or obese. It has been estimated that the number of deaths attributable to obesity exceeds 300,000 per year [30]. CVD is the leading cause of mortality (over 37% of all deaths in the United States), and 65 million Americans have hypertension, while over 14 million have type 2 diabetes (T2DM).

Prior to the development of large-scale agriculture and animal husbandry, human dietary choices would have been limited to minimally processed wild plants and animal foods. After the Industrial Revolution, these agricultural practices and animal husbandry were accelerated. Part of this is due to food processing procedures. Many of the foods including dairy products, refined grains and cereals, and refined vegetable oils which are now contained in the WPD would have been minimally available in the typical preagricultural diet of human beings [31,32]. In addition, the high prevalence of processed foods such as cookies, cake, crackers, snack foods, pizza, candy, and ice cream, which are highly prevalent in the U.S. diet, would not have been available to the preagricultural diet and have contributed in significant ways both to the inflammatory potential of the current WPD and the increased energy density and significant increase in calories in the diet [1,2].

2.4 NUTRITIONAL CHARACTERISTICS OF THE WESTERN DIET

- **Cereals and grains**—Cereal grains began to appear in the diet when technologies were available to grind them [31,32]. Over 85% of grains consumed in the current U.S. diet are highly processed. This is a reflection of mechanized steel roller mills that allowed removal of the germ and bran, leaving mainly the endosperm with a uniformly small particulate size. All of this took place in the last 150–200 years.
- **Dairy foods**—Utilization of milk from cows allowed the consumption of their milk by humans. This is a relatively recent event from an evolutionary point of view [33].
- **Refined sugars**—The per capita consumption of refined sugars in the United States has risen dramatically in the past 100 years, although in the past 20 years it has decreased by approximately 10% [34,35]. Starting in the 1970s, various fructose enrichment techniques allowed high fructose corn syrup (HFCS) to be utilized in a variety of foods as a potential substitute for sucrose. The increase in HFCS occurred simultaneously with a decrease in sucrose consumption. Thus, the use of HFCS also reflects advances in the food processing industry [36].
- **Refined vegetable oils**—In the past century there has been a significant increase in the use of vegetable oils in the WPD [37,38]. Once again, this was made possible by the mechanization of the oil seed industry. Also, manufacturing processes allowed vegetable oils to take on different structural characteristics. For example, margarine is made by partially solidifying vegetable oil via hydrogenation [38]. This technology was not available until approximately 1900. A similar hydrogenation process produces trans

fatty acids. Thus, in the past 100 years the quality and quantitative aspects of fatty acid intake have changed in the human diet.

- **Alcohol**—While alcohol represents a relatively minor contribution (1.4% of calories) in the human diet, alcohol has been present in the human diet for millennia [39]. The fermentation process that produces wine would not have been available to ancient human beings [40]. Thus, the increase in wine in the human diet once again involves industrial processes.
- **Salt**—The current consumption of salt in the human diet is about 3.7 grams/day. Seventy-five percent of daily salt intake comes from salt added in processed foods, and another 15% comes from either cooking or usage of table salt [41]. Abundant evidence suggests that the amount of salt in the human diet is associated with a variety of new factors for CVD, including hypertension.
- **Fatty domestic meats**—The advent of animal husbandry allowed animals to be bred and maintained such as to increase the amount of body fat. This was further stimulated by use of storage plant foods. Increased grain harvests, harvesting transportation, and technology created the practice of feeding grain (particularly corn) to cattle, which were maintained in feed lots [42,43]. The added fat in these animals is largely through excessive triglyceride accumulation in muscle and adipocytes. Thus, this meat has significant saturated fatty acid content.

2.5 HEALTH IMPLICATIONS OF FOODS IN THE WESTERN DIET

- **Fatty acid composition**—The WPD frequently contains excessive saturated fats and trans fatty acids and has too little Ω-3 PUFAs (polyunsaturated fatty acids) or Ω-6 PUFAs [28,43]. The high dietary intake of saturated fatty acids (SFAs) and trans fatty acids contributes to dyslipidemia and increases the risk of CVD. In contrast, Ω-3 PUFAs may reduce the risk of CVD. Higher intakes of Ω-3 fatty acids may also ameliorate many inflammatory and autoimmune diseases. In addition to increasing low-density lipoprotein (LDL) cholesterol, SFAs also exert multiple inflammatory effects, while trans fatty acids both increase LDL and decrease high-density lipoprotein (HDL). Furthermore, the invention of hydrogenation to allow vegetable oil to become solidified both as margarine or foods containing hydrogenated vegetable oils also introduced a new trans fatty acid (trans fat elaidics) and further increased the risk of CVD. The major sources of SFAs in the U.S. diet are fatty meats, baked goods, cheese, milk, margarine, and butter. All of these, in a sense, reflect the emergence of animal husbandry and its impact on the human diet.
- **Glycemic index/glycemic load**—The glycemic index compares the blood glucose excursion potential of various foods or combinations of foods to an equal amount of carbohydrates in their food [44]. Glycemic load simply takes glycemic index and multiplies it by the amount of carbohydrate content in a serving size [45]. Refined grains and sugar products, almost without exception, maintain higher glycemic loads than unprocessed fruits

and vegetables and may result in elevations in blood glucose concentration. Chronic elevations in insulin promote insulin resistance, which many investigators believe is the primary metabolic defect in metabolic syndrome. Insulin resistance is also thought to contribute to obesity, coronary heart disease (CHD), T2DM, hypertension, and dyslipidemia [46–48]. It should be noted that various dairy products such as milk, yogurt, and ice cream have a relatively low glycemic load, but they significantly stimulate insulin [49]. Also, fructose has a low glycemic index but has been demonstrated in multiple research trials to promote insulin resistance. Between sugars and refined grains in high glycemic loads, 39% of the total energy in a typical WPD in the United States may promote insulin resistance.

- **Macronutrient composition**—The macronutrient composition in the typical U.S. diet includes carbohydrates (52%), fat (33%), and protein (15%) [50]. Some recent research has suggested that higher levels of protein in the diet may improve blood lipid profile and may represent an effective weight loss strategy in overweight or obese individuals. Although data on this are inclusive, longer-term studies do not suggest that higher protein diets are superior to low-fat diets for long-term maintenance of weight loss.
- **Micronutrient density**—Refined sugars and grains reduce vitamin and mineral (micronutrient) density in the diet by displacing more nutrient-dense foods [51,52]. This is also true of refined vegetable oils. Between vegetable oils and refined sugars, over 36% of the energy in a typical WPD comes from these two sources and creates the potential to influence the risk of vitamin and mineral deficiencies. For example, half the U.S. population are below the recommended dietary allowance (RDA) for vitamin B_6, vitamin A, magnesium, calcium, and zinc, while one-third of the population does not meet the RDA for folate. Adequate dietary intake for both folate and vitamin B_6 prevents the accumulation of homocysteine in the bloodstream [53,54]. Elevations in homocysteine may represent an independent risk factor for developing CVD. Nutrient-dense foods such as fruits and vegetables, lean meats, and seafood help reduce the likelihood of developing vitamin deficiency diseases as well as infections and chronic diseases.
- **Acid-base balance**—Many of the foods in the WPD such as cheese, milk, cereal grains, fish, meat, poultry, and eggs are net acid producers [55]. In contrast, fruit, vegetables, tubers, roots, and nuts are net base producing. A typical Western diet yields a net acid load estimated to be 50 mEq/day. Thus, healthy adults who consume the standard WPD are subject to chronic low-grade metabolic acidosis. This worsens as kidney function declines, which is common as individuals age.
- **Sodium-potassium ratio**—As already indicated, the average sodium content in the typical WPD in the United States is 3,271 mg/day, while the average potassium content is 2,620 mg/day [56]. Most of the salt in the U.S. diet comes from manufactured sources, and vegetable oils and refined sugars do not have any potassium, while constituting 32% of total food energy. Vegetables and fruits and whole grains all contain significant amounts of potassium. The low potassium rates in the WPD are thought

to contribute to numerous diseases of civilization. Diets that are low in potassium and high in sodium may contribute to or exacerbate hypertension, stroke, kidney stones, osteoporosis, a variety of gastrointestinal tract cancers, and asthma.

- **Fiber content**—The typical fiber content of the U.S. diet is 15.1 grams/day. This is approximately one-half of the recommended amounts from the DGA 2020–2025 [6]. Many of the components of the WPD including refined sugars, vegetable oils, dairy products, and alcohol contain no fiber yet average almost half of the caloric intake in the U.S. diet. In addition, refined grains represent 85% of grains consumed in the United States and contain much less fiber than whole grains and further dilute fiber intake. Thus, displacement of fiber-rich plant food by processed foods contributes to the diminished amount of fiber in the U.S. diet. Low fiber further increases the likelihood of increased LDL and may also contribute to weight gain, given that refined grains are energy dense and create less satiety than foods containing higher levels of fiber [57]. Adequate amounts of fiber in the diet are also essential for a healthy microbiome.

2.6 WESTERN DIET AND INFLAMMATION

Inflammation is an important component of the body's ability to combat various infectious agents [24,25]. However, when there is a chronic low level of inflammation, it can create significant risk for a number of noncommunicable diseases (NCDs) including metabolic syndrome, obesity, T2DM, nonalcoholic fatty liver disease (NAFLD), CVD, neurodegenerative diseases (e.g. Alzheimer's disease), and certain cancers.

Because of the linkage between inflammation and these chronic diseases, considerable research has occurred in this area over the past 20 years. Of note, many of the components of the WPD are in and of themselves inflammatory. These include red meat, processed meats, saturated fats, refined grains, and refined sugars. Thus, the WPD contributes to adverse consequences from a low-grade inflammation by multiple mechanisms including intrinsic properties of the foods typically found in the WPD as well as increasing the likelihood of developing chronic diseases which in and of themselves present with or exhibit low-grade inflammation.

In contrast, dietary patterns that contain more natural, unprocessed ingredients, including more fruits and vegetables, whole grains, and Ω-3 fatty acids and other unsaturated fatty acids, lower the risk of inflammation. Research has shown that diets that focus on these foods such as the Mediterranean diet and other healthy diets derive other benefits from being anti-inflammatory [8].

Low-grade inflammation also adversely affects multiple components of the immune system, which further contributes to increased risk of various chronic diseases. In addition, diets that are high in fiber, which is abundantly found in vegetables, fruits, legumes, and whole grains, further reduce the inflammatory potential of the diet. An additional benefit from nondigestible fibers are that many are fermented into short-chain fatty acids (SCFAs). This can further downregulate immune responses, particularly in the microbiome.

2.7 WESTERN DIET AND THE MICROBIOME

There has been increasing interest in the role of bacteria that comprise the microbiome and their relationship to human disease. Several studies have demonstrated that the WPD can impair the bile ducts, resulting in pathogens which favor immunity-deviated inflammatory diseases like inflammatory bowel disease as well as other inflammatory chronic diseases [58]. In particular, an increase in intake of meat and animal fat and lower consumption of fruits and vegetables yield alterations in the gut microbiome that results in an imbalanced immune response and high expression of inflammatory markers. In addition, hyperglycemia associated with WPDs can further adversely affect the microbiome, which may contribute to obesity and development of other metabolic diseases. Thus, the WPD exerts a significant impact on gut microbial ecosystems and further impairs the immune system and contributes to chronic inflammatory diseases.

2.8 WESTERN DIET AND PROCESSED FOODS

As already indicated, a large percentage of foods in the typical Western diet are processed. It has been argued that the share of whole foods versus processed foods represents a dietary factor that should be independently considered as a risk for chronic disease. In fact, some investigators argue that "ultra-processed foods" are detrimental to human health. This is based on classification of foods according to the amount of processing that has occurred. This has been reviewed by Montero and coworkers in what is called the NOVA system, which groups food stuffs into categories according to the extent and purpose of the processing applied to them. The most extensively processed foods are deemed "ultra processed," which is defined as "industrial formulations made entirely or mostly from substances extracted from food (e.g. oils, fats, sugar, starch and proteins) or derived from food constituents (e.g. hydrogenated fats and modified starches) or synthesized in laboratories for food substrates or other organic sources (e.g. flavor enhancers, colors) and several food additives used to make products hyper palatable" [59].

Whether or not the NOVA classification carries any benefit is subject to debate. Some experts have argued that any evidence that ultra-processed foods contribute to chronic disease can be accounted for by nutrient composition, energy density, and food matrices. In this argument, adverse consequences for processed foods can be explained by more conventional and quantifiable dietary factors including energy density, intrinsic fiber, glycemic load, and added sugar.

Nonetheless, the NOVA classification has been at least acknowledged in several reports from the United Nations (UN) and World Health Organization as well as in some scientific journals. Whether or not this NOVA classification provides any new beneficial understandings, it is clear that foods that undergo a great deal of processing are a major hallmark of the WPD. Such foods now dominate the food supply, including an increased targeting of low-income countries at the expense of traditional foods. It is clear that individuals consuming large amounts of these types of foods are at greater risk of being obese than people who consume relatively few processed foods. Furthermore, the dietary share of ultra-processed food determines the nutritional quality of diets in several populations.

2.9 WESTERN DIET AND CHRONIC DISEASE

There is strong evidence to underscore that the WPD is related to a variety of increases in chronic diseases. These include CVD, obesity, diabetes, metabolic syndrome, and cancer [60–63]. Many of these diseases have a component of inflammation as an underlying etiology. However, in the area of CVD, abnormal lipids and lack of physical activity also contribute in significant ways to the likelihood of developing CVD. In the area of obesity, not only the inflammatory components of foods in the WPD but also the increased energy density and the likelihood of overconsuming calories are important. The dramatic increase in diabetes around the world is associated not only with the increased levels of obesity but also body fat distribution and inflammatory components of the diet, as well as the inflammatory nature of increased levels of insulin resistance. These factors are combined in metabolic syndrome [63]. In fact, it has been argued that the relationship between CVD, obesity, and diabetes should be actually considered one entity, which investigators have called "cardiodiabesity."

There is also strong evidence that the Western diet contributes significantly to multiple cancers [60,61]. In particular, breast cancer, prostate cancer, and multiple cancers of the gastrointestinal system have all been linked to nutritional factors resulting from WPD. Multiple cohort studies support the concept that the WPD is associated with all-cause mortality for cancers and other chronic diseases.

2.10 WESTERN DIET AND COVID-19

The response of various populations to COVID-19 infection clearly underscores the relationship between WPD and infection. Individuals who followed the WPD and, in particular, were obese, had hypertension, or had type 2 diabetes were 3–4 times as likely to die in this pandemic than individuals who followed a plant-based diet and maintained a healthy body weight and were free of any of these chronic diseases [64].

2.11 WESTERN DIET AND OTHER LIFESTYLE FACTORS

While considering the WPD and its clear association with the development of chronic diseases, it should also be emphasized that other lifestyle factors also contribute in significant ways to adverse health consequences. In particular, it has been clearly shown that increased levels of physical activity lower the risk of various chronic diseases [15]. It has also been shown that increased levels of physical activity lower the risk of infections such as COVID-19. This is not to say that physical activity is a panacea. However, those individuals who led sedentary lifestyles were more susceptible to morbidity and mortality from COVID-19. Response to COVID-19 adds to an ever-growing list of chronic conditions that can be somewhat ameliorated by increased levels of physical activity [65]. Other lifestyle factors such as levels of stress, healthy sleep, weight management, and relationships with other people also carry profound linkages to lowering the risk of chronic disease. Thus, while it is important to emphasize the inherent number of consequences of following the WPD, it is also important for clinicians to emphasize multiple other factors which comprise the core principles of healthy lifestyle habits and practices.

2.12 CONCLUSIONS

The WPD is clearly associated with increased risk of chronic diseases. The mechanisms for this include the increased inflammatory nature of components of the WPD as well as increased caloric consumption in individuals who follow a WPD. When WPD is compared to healthy diets, such as the Mediterranean diet, the Healthy U.S.-Style Dietary Pattern, or DASH diet, the WPD is clearly associated with increased risk of multiple chronic diseases including CVD, obesity, T2DM, metabolic syndrome, and cancer. The adverse health consequences of WPD are clearly in evidence in response to the COVID-19 pandemic. Individuals who followed WPD and also were obese, had hypertension, or had T2DM were 3–4 times more likely to die from this novel virus than were individuals who ate a plant-based diet, maintained a healthy weight, and did not suffer from any of these chronic diseases.

Clinical Applications

- It is incumbent upon physicians to assess in general terms the nutritional patterns of all patients.
- Those patients who are following a typical WPD should be counseled that this diet is associated with multiple chronic diseases including CVD, obesity, diabetes, metabolic syndrome, and cancers.
- Physicians should counsel patients to follow a healthy plant-based diet such as the Mediterranean diet, Healthy U.S.-Style Dietary Patterns, or DASH diet.
- These healthy diets can lower the risk of chronic diseases, largely through reducing inflammation not only from the foods consumed but also from the risk of various chronic diseases which may further exacerbate inflammation.

REFERENCES

1. Cordain L, Eaton S, Sebastian A, et al. Origins and evolution of the Western diet: Health implications for the 21st century. Am J Clin Nutri. 2005;81(2):341–354.
2. Boaz NT. Evolving Health: The Origins of Illness and How the Modern World Is Making Us Sick. New York: Wiley & Sons, Inc., 2002.
3. Carrera-Bastos P, Fontes O, Lindeberg S, Cordain L. The Western diet and lifestyle and diseases of civilization. Res Rep Clin Cardiol. 2011;2:15–35.
4. Halton T, Willett W, Liu S, Manson J, et al. Potato and French fry consumption and risk of type 2 diabetes in women. Am J Clin Nutri. 2006;83(2):284–290.
5. Fung T, Rimm E, Spiegelman D, et al. Association between dietary patterns and plasma biomarkers of obesity and cardiovascular disease risk. Am J Clin Nutri. 2006;73(1):61–67.
6. U.S. Department of Health and Human Services and U.S. Department of Agriculture. 2020–2025 Dietary Guidelines for Americans. www.dietaryguidelines.gov/sites/default/files/2020-12/Dietary_Guidelines_for_Americans_2020-2025.pdf (Accessed May 24, 2023).
7. Bloomfield HE, Kane R, Koeller E, et al. Benefits and Harms of the Mediterranean Diet Compared to Other Diets. Washington, DC: Department of Veterans Affairs, 2015 Nov.
8. Ruiz-Canela M, Estruch R, Corella D, Salas-Salvadó J, Martínez-González MA. Association of Mediterranean diet with peripheral artery disease: The PREDIMED randomized trial. JAMA. 2014;311(4):415–417.

9. Sacks F, Svetkey L, Vollmer W, et al. Effects on blood pressure of reduced dietary sodium and the Dietary Approaches to Stop Hypertension (DASH) Diet. DASH-Sodium Collaborative Research Group. N Engl J Med. 2001;344(1):3–10.
10. Lichtenstein AH, Appel LJ, Vadiveloo M, et al. 2021 Dietary guidance to improve cardiovascular health: A scientific statement from the American Heart Association. Circulation. 2021;144(23):e472–e487.
11. Taubes G. Is sugar toxic? The New York Times, April 13, 2011. www.nytimes.com/2011/04/17/magazine/mag-17Sugar-t.html.
12. Murtagh M, Reiser K, Harris R, et al. Source of dietary carbohydrate affects life span of Fischer 344 rats independent of caloric restriction. J Gerontol Series A: Biol Sci Med Sci. 1995;50(3):B148–B154.
13. Bentley J. U.S. Trends in Food Availability and a Dietary Assessment of Loss-Adjusted Food Availability, 1970–2014. USDA Economic Research Service. Economic Information Bulletin No. (EIB-166), 2017, 38 pp.
14. Gould S. 6 charts that show how much more Americans eat than they used to. Business Insider. May 10, 2017. (Accessed May 24, 2023).
15. Physical Activity Guidelines Advisory Committee. 2016 Physical Activity Guidelines Advisory Committee Scientific Report. Washington, DC: U.S. Department of Health and Human Services, 2016.
16. Philpoff T. The American diet in one chart, with lost of fats and sugars. Industrial Agriculture. Grist. https://grist.org/industrial-agriculture/2011-04-05-american-diet-one-chart-lots-of-fats-sugars/ (Accessed June 5, 2023).
17. Current Eating Patterns in the United States. US. Department of Health and Human Services and U.S. Department of Agriculture. 2020–2025 Dietary Guidelines for Americans. www.dietaryguidelines.gov/sites/default/files/2020-12/Dietary_Guidelines_for_Americans_2020-2025.pdf (Accessed May 24, 2023).
18. A Closer Look at Current Intakes and Recommended Shifts 2015–2020 Dietary Guidelines. U.S. Department of Health and Human Services and U.S. Department of Agriculture. 2015–2020 Dietary Guidelines for Americans, 8th edition. December 2015. https://health.gov/our-work/food-nutrition/previous-dietary-guidelines/2015.
19. Lobb A. Eating habits: A look at the average US diet. The Wall Street Journal. September 17, 2005. (Accessed June 12, 2023).
20. Kesse E, Clavel-Chapelon F, Boutron-Rault M. Dietary patterns and risk of colorectal tumors: A cohort of French women of the national education system. Am J Epidemiol. 2006;164(11):1085–1093.
21. Kant A. Dietary patterns and health outcomes. J Am Diet Assoc. 2004;104(4):615–635.
22. Hu F. Globalization of diabetes: The role of diet, lifestyle, and genes. Diabetes Care. 2011;34(6):1249–1257.
23. Drake I, Sonestedt E, Ericson U, et al. A Western dietary pattern is prospectively associated with cardio-metabolic traits and incidence of the metabolic syndrome. Br J Nutr. 2018;119(10):1168–1176.
24. Christ A, Lauterbach M, Latz E. Western diet and the immune system: An inflammatory connection. Immunity. 2019;51(5):794–811.
25. Christ A, Latz E. The Western lifestyle has lasting effects on metaflammation. Nat Rev Immunol. 2019;19:267–268.
26. Nesse R, Williams G. Why We Get Sick: The New Science of Darwinian Medicine. Vintage, 1996.
27. Eaton S, Konner M. Paleolithic nutrition: A consideration of its nature and current implications. N Engl J Med. 1985;312(5):283–289.

28. Cordain L, Watkins B, Florant G, et al. Fatty acid analysis of wild ruminant tissues: Evolutionary implications for reducing diet-related chronic disease. Eur J Clin Nutr. 2002;56(3):181–191.
29. Frassetto L, Morris R. Sellmeyer D, et al. Diet, evolution and aging: The pathophysiologic effects of the post-agricultural inversion of the potassium-to-sodium and base-to-chloride ratios in the human diet. Eur J Nutri. 2002;40:200–213.
30. Rippe J, Foreyt JP. Obesity Prevention and Treatment: A Practical Guide. Boca Raton: CRC Press, 2022.
31. Wright K. The origins and development of ground stone assemblages in Late Pleistocene Southwest Asia. Paléorient. 1991:19–45.
32. Nelson J. Wheat: It's processing and utilization. Am J Clin Nutri. 1985;41:1070–1076.
33. Loftus R, Ertugrul O, Harba A, et al. A microsatellite survey of cattle from a centre of origin: The Near East. Mol Ecol. 1999;8:2015–2022.
34. Galloway J, Sugar. In Kiple K, and Ornelas K (eds). The Cambridge World History of Food. Cambridge: The Cambridge University Press, 2000: 437–449.
35. Cleave T. The Saccharine Disease. Bristol, UK: John Wright & Sons. Ltd., 1974, 6–27.
36. Hanover M, White J. Manufacturing, composition, and applications of fructose. Am J Clin Nutri. 1993;58(5):724S–732S.
37. O'Keefe S. An overview of oils and fats, with a special emphasis on olive oil. In Kiple K, and Ornelas KC (eds). The Cambridge World History of Food. Cambridge: Cambridge University Press, 2008: 375–397.
38. Emken E. Nutrition and biochemistry of trans and positional fatty acid isomers in hydrogenated oils. Annu Rev Nutri. 1984;4:339–376.
39. Comer J. Distilled beverages. In Kiple K, and Ornelas KC (eds). The Cambridge World History of Food. Cambridge: Cambridge University Press, 2008: 653–664.
40. Newman J. Wine. In Kiple K, and Ornelas KC (eds). The Cambridge World History of Food. Cambridge: Cambridge University Press, 2008: 730–738.
41. James P, Ralph A, Sanchez-Castillo C. The dominance of salt in manufactured food in the sodium intake of affluent societies. Lancet. 1987;329:426–429.
42. Whitaker J. Feedlot empire: Beef cattle feeding in Illinois and Iowa 1840–1900. Ann Iowa. 1976;43(3):233–234.
43. Rule D, Broughton K, Shellito S, Maiorano G. Comparison of muscle fatty acid profiles and cholesterol concentrations of bison, beef cattle, elk, and chicken. J Anim Sci. 2022;80(5):1202–1211.
44. Jenkins D, Wolever T, Taylor R, et al. Glycemic index of foods: A physiological basis for carbohydrate exchange. Am J Clin Nutri. 1981;34(3):362–366.
45. Liu S, Willett W. Dietary glycemic load and atherothrombotic risk. Curr Atheroscler Rep. 2002;4(6):454–461.
46. Thorburn A, Brand J, Truswell A. Slowly digested and absorbed carbohydrate in traditional bushfoods: A protective factor against diabetes. Am J Clin Nutri. 1987;45(1):98–106.
47. Jenkins D, Wolever J, Collier G, et al. The metabolic effects of a low-glycemic-index diet. Am J Clin Nutri. 1987;46(6):968–975.
48. Miller J. Importance of glycemic index in diabetes. Am J Clin Nutri. 1994;59(3):747S–7 52S.
49. Reaven G. Pathophysiology of insulin resistance in human disease. Physiol Rev. 1995;75(3):473–486.
50. Krauss, RM, et al. AHA dietary guidelines: Revision 2000: A statement for healthcare professionals from the Nutrition Committee of the American Heart Association. Circulation. 2000;102(18):2284–2299.

51. Kurtzweil P. Nutritional info available for raw fruits, vegetables, fish. FDA Consumer Magazine. May 1993. US Health and Human Services, Food and Drug Administration, Rockville, MD.
52. US Department of Agriculture, Economic Research Service. 1999. America's eating habits: Changes and consequences. In Frazao E (ed). Washington, DC. (Agriculture Information Bulletin No. 750).
53. Wald D, Law M, Morris J. Homocysteine and cardiovascular disease: Evidence on causality from a meta-analysis. BMJ. 2002;325:1202–1208.
54. Meleady R, Graham I. Plasma homocysteine as a cardiovascular risk factor: Causal, consequential, or of no consequence? Nutr Rev. 1999;57:299–305.
55. Frassetto L, Todd K, Morris R, Sebastian A. Estimation of net endogenous noncarbonic acid production in humans from diet potassium and protein contents. Am J Clin Nutr. 1998;68:576–583.
56. US Department of Agriculture, Agricultural Research Service. Data tables: Results from USDA's 1994–96 Continuing Survey of Food Intakes by Individuals and 1994–96 Diet and Health Knowledge Survey. ARS Food Surveys Research Group, 1997.
57. Carrera-Bastos P, Fontes M, O'Keefe J, et al. The Western diet and lifestyle disease and diseases of civilization. Res Rep Clin Cardiol. 2011;2:15–35.
58. Zinöcker M, Lindseth I. The Western diet-microbiome-host interaction and its role in metabolic disease. Nutrients. 2018;10(3):365.
59. Montero C, Fraile-Martínez O, Gómez-Lahoz A, et al. Nutritional components in Western diet versus Mediterranean diet at the Gut Microbiota—immune system interplay. Implications for health and disease. Nutrients. 2021;13(2):699.
60. Entwistle M. Schweizer D, Cisneros R. Dietary patterns related to total mortality and cancer mortality in the United States. Cancer Causes Control. 2021;32(11):1279–1288.
61. Heidemann C, Schulze M, Franco O, et al. Dietary patterns and risk of mortality from cardiovascular disease, cancer, and all causes in a prospective cohort of women. Circulation. 2008;118(3):230–237.
62. Fung T, Rimm E, Spiegelman D, et al. Association between dietary patterns and plasma biomarkers of obesity and cardiovascular disease risk. Am J Clin Nutri. 2001;73(1):61–67.
63. Pomerleau J, McKee M, Lobstein T, et al. The burden of disease attributable to nutrition in Europe. Public Health Nutri. 2003;6:453–461.
64. Belanger M, Hill M, Angelidi A, et al. COVID-19 and disparities in nutrition and obesity. N Engl J Med. 2020;383:e69.
65. Hasson R, Sallis J, Coleman N, et al. COVID-19: Implications for physical activity, health disparities, and health equity. Am J Lifestyle Med. 2022;16(4):420–433. Epub 2022/07/21.ent

3 Measuring Nutritional Status

Key Points

- Various criteria and frameworks have been developed to measure nutritional status.
- While most physicians will not need detailed knowledge in this area unless they are performing nutritional research, it is still useful to know the various measurement techniques that are available and some of the terminology that is utilized.
- This concept of nutritional status and dietary status are two separate terms, although they have considerable overlap.
- Nutritional status is the broader term and includes dietary status.
- Various useful indices are available such as the Healthy Eating Index. This index should be understood by clinicians, at least in general terms.
- Modern nutrition research focuses on dietary patterns, rather than individual nutrients or foods. This is the strategy that is used throughout this book.

3.1 INTRODUCTION

Diet and nutrition play enormous roles in virtually every aspect of human health as well as human growth development and a wide range of bodily functions. This chapter will focus on some of the issues related to how nutritional status is measured. While most physicians will not engage in nutritional research, it is still valuable to understand the terminology and techniques used in evaluating nutritional status. This understanding will enable physicians to have a clearer grasp of how nutritional science works and how it can be applied to various health conditions. This chapter will also describe the various guidelines that are available for diet and nutrition and discuss some of the terms that are used to describe nutritional status.

3.2 THE CONCEPT OF NUTRITIONAL STATUS

It should be noted that nutritional status is a much broader term than dietary status. Nutritional status represents the bodily state resulting from the intake, absorption, utilization, and metabolism of the foods consumed by the individual. Nutritional status can be measured at both the individual and group levels. Disordered nutritional status runs the gamut from undernutrition (malnutrition), to nutritional deficiency, to overnutrition—excess in energy or nutrient intake, which may result in overweight or obesity. Collectively these deviations from normal are referred to as malnutrition.

DOI: 10.1201/9781003452607-3

- **Nutrient requirements**—Nutrients are substances that are not synthesized in sufficient amounts in the body and, therefore, must be supplied by the diet. Their absence leads to growth impairment, organ dysfunction, and failure to maintain nitrogen balance or adequate status of protein and other nutrients. Human beings require energy-providing nutrients, which are typically classed as macronutrients including protein, fat and carbohydrates, vitamins, minerals, and water. Requirements for organic nutrients include nine essential amino acids, several fatty acids, glucose, four fat-soluble vitamins, ten water-soluble vitamins, dietary fiber, and choline.

  The amounts of essential nutrients required by individuals differ by age and physiologic state such as growth, pregnancy, lactation, inflammation, and certain disease states. Human beings all need the same nutrients, but they differ somewhat from one another in the amounts needed. In addition, some individuals have "special nutritional requirements" because they may have certain genetic, epigenetic, or other causes that lead to much higher or lower amounts of one or more nutrients in their diet.
- **Bioactive food components**—Foods may contain many constituents other than nutrients such as pesticides, contaminants, phytochemicals, and zoochemical and microbial products and may also have health effects. These constituents are collectively referred to as bioactive. Examples of some bioactive foods include the polyphenols, flavonoids, lutein, and omega-3 fatty acids. These bioactives may have beneficial functions in particular organs or organ systems, even though they are not considered essential nutrients.

3.3 MEASUREMENT OF NUTRITIONAL STATUS

Nutritional status includes multiple components such as anthropometric, biochemical, clinical, and dietary measures as well as food-related quality of life. As indicated in Table 3.1, the full nutrition indicators may be necessary to describe nutritional status. Much more detail concerning malnutrition in its various forms and how to diagnose it is found in Chapter 6.

- **Evaluating the diet**—One aspect of nutritional status is dietary status. This refers to an individual's consumption of nutrients, foods, food groups, or food patterns. Dietary status can be altered to affect nutritional status, while many other determinants of malnutrition cannot. Dietary status and nutritional status are not synonymous, since food consumption is only one of many factors that influence whether food intake will suffice to maintain health. Dietary assessment is a proxy for nutritional status because it is less expensive and easier to maintain than a full-fledged nutritional status assessment and will often provide enough useful information to remedy problems [1].
- **Dietary assessment methods**—Characteristics of diet measurement include the amount of food eaten, what nutrients are contained in the foods, the forms that they are present in (e.g. foods, beverages, or supplements), and the presence of other bioactives in food known to have beneficial or

TABLE 3.1
Forms of Malnutrition and Clinical Terms Used to Describe Them

Form and Cause of Malnutrition	Clinical Terms to Describe It	Comments
Dehydration: Inadequate fluid intake to meet bodily needs	Dehydration	Often occurs secondary to fever, exertion, very warm and dry climate, or because of diets with high solute loads or drugs that have diuretic effects.
Starvation: Virtually totally inadequate intake of all nutrients	Marasmus, emaciation, cachexia	Occurs with prolonged fasting; withholding of fluids worsens its effects.
Protein-Calorie Malnutrition	Kwashiorkor, protein-calorie malnutrition.	Often occurs secondary to disease and infection, probably via cytokine-mediated responses to acute infection or trauma; examples include HIV/AIDS. Sarcopenia due to inadequate intake of protein and/or cytokine-mediated responses to insults.
Vitamin, mineral, or other specific nutrient deficiencies	Pellagra (niacin/tryptophan), scurvy (ascorbic acid deficiency), rickets and osteomalacia (vitamin D deficiency in children and adults, respectively), iron deficiency anemia (iron deficiency), nutritional anemia (iron, vitamin B_6, folic acid or vitamin B_{12} deficiency), essential fatty acid deficiency	These deficiencies often occur secondarily to inadequate food intake or inadequate dietary quality. May also occur as conditioned deficiencies secondary to disease.
Imbalances: Increased diet-related chronic disease risk factors due to imbalances of nutrients	Excess of saturated fat, cholesterol, and other atherogenic and thrombogenic dietary lipids (hyperlipidemias and perhaps altered clotting factors), excess of salt and/or sodium (blood pressure risk factors)	Imbalances or excesses of energy-yielding nutrients or related substances may give rise to metabolic aberrations and increase risks of ill health, especially in those with certain genetic profiles.
Obesity: Excess food energy intake and/or insufficient energy output	Excess food energy regardless of source gives rise to obesity and overweight	Physical inactivity may increase likelihood of excess energy intakes.
Alcohol excess	Alcoholism, problem drinking	At very high levels of alcohol intake, all persons develop physical signs of chronic disease; at lower levels of intake, some individuals are particularly susceptible.

(*Continued*)

TABLE 3.1 (*Continued*)
Forms of Malnutrition and Clinical Terms Used to Describe Them

Form and Cause of Malnutrition	Clinical Terms to Describe It	Comments
Excess of other specific nutrients (vitamins, minerals, others)	Specific toxicities vary: hypervitaminosis A (vitamin A), hypervitaminosis D (vitamin D), fluorosis (fluoride), etc.	Intakes that exceed the upper level of the Dietary Reference Intakes generally increase risk of compromising one or more functions. The possible functions vary from nutrient to nutrient.
Toxicity: Excesses of other constituents in food, drink, or supplements	Names vary depending on substance; lead poisoning, lathyrism, etc.	Many substances other than nutrients in food and supplements may cause illness.
Food-borne disease	Food poisoning or food intoxication: salmonellosis, botulism, staphylococcal food poisoning, others. Parasites such as beef tapeworm may cause problems. Prions or viruses as in bovine spongiform encephalopathy (BSE).	Food is the carrier for a microorganism, virus, or parasite.

Source: Dwyer J. Nutrition 101: The Concept of Nutritional Status and Guides for Nutrient Intakes, Eating Patterns, and Nutrition. IN: Rippe JM. Lifestyle Medicine (3rd edition). CRC Press (Boca Raton), 2019. (Used with Permission.)

harmful effects. Dietary assessment can be done on a short- or long-term basis [2]. For example, a food record is a detailed list of all foods and beverages consumed within a specified period of time. Usually, these are measured for three to four days, including a weekend day. A 24-hour recall is used to assess an individual's intake over the previous 24 hours. Multiple 24-hour recalls are recommended based on day-to-day variability and intake. The 24-hour recall methodology is used in multiple cohort studies including the Nurses' Health Trial and Physicians' Health Study.

The Food Frequency Questionnaire (FFQ) is also often used in large cohort or case-controlled studies [3]. FFQs are a cost-effective alternative to the 24-hour recall since they can be self-administered [4]. It should be noted, however, that the 24-hour recall administered on multiple occasions has been shown to be less biased than FFQs. As technology has advanced, web-based 24-hour dietary recalls are available for research purposes from the National Cancer Institute at no cost.

All dietary assessments are subject to error, and research clearly recognizes that the error in self-reported dietary assessments must be considered in the analysis and interpretation of findings. A major problem with self-reported dietary data is that people may not recall or remember every unit that was consumed or fail to accurately estimate the portion sizes that were consumed. This may also be respondent biased because of the social desirability to overreport foods that are healthy and underreport less healthy foods. Various research organizations that utilize self-reported data have found ways to try to minimize or account for the errors that are inherent to self-reporting of food [5–7].

- **Biomarkers of nutritional status**—If precise estimates of food intake are necessary, surrogate biomarkers of intake are often used [8,9]. Dietary biomarkers are used to assess dietary intake for exposures without having to rely on the bias or errors involved in self-reported dietary intakes [10,11]. Some dietary markers such as 25-OHD and blood measures of folate and iron status are routinely connected in the National Health and Nutrition Examination Survey (NHANES). Some typical biomarkers are listed in Table 3.2.

3.4 GUIDELINES FOR ENERGY AND NUTRIENT INTAKES

The Dietary Reference Intakes are the authoritative energy and nutrient standards for the United States and Canada. The World Health Organization and many other groups also make dietary recommendations that are used in other countries.

- **Dietary Reference Intakes (DRI)**—The DRI are a group of quantitative standards for nutrient reference intakes that are used for planning and assessment of diets of healthy individuals [12–20]. The various criteria and recommendations are outlined in Table 3.3. The DRIs are based on the best evidence available for intake of levels of nutrients that are compatible with good health. The DRIs are the basis for other recommendations such as the Dietary Guidelines for Americans (DGA) to provide food-based dietary guidelines and for food labels. The DRIs are periodically updated when new data are available to allow the commission of a report.

  Although the DRIs are designed as recommendations for healthy individuals, over half of Americans have one or more chronic conditions, and the number is growing as the population ages. The association between nutrient intake and the risk of most chronic diseases has proven more difficult to establish and remains an area of controversy and research. The major challenge is how to assess the links between dietary constituents and chronic disease endpoints as outcomes.

  In the existing DRIs only five nutrients have been assigned reference values based on chronic disease endpoints. They are calcium and vitamin D for osteoporosis and fractures; fluoride and dental carries; dietary fiber and coronary heart disease; and potassium and a combination of endpoints including salt sensitivity (a risk factor for hypertension, kidney stones, and blood pressure). These endpoints do not fit well into the existing DRI paradigm since they are multifactorial and many dietary and nondietary factors

TABLE 3.2
Some Biochemical Biomarkers of Intake (Exposure) and/or Nutritional Status

Nutrient	Biomarker	Comments
Iron	Hemoglobin	Low specificity (many different causes of anemia decrease hemoglobin, not just iron). Cutoffs vary by age, sex, and ethnicity. This is a good indicator for monitoring improvement in iron status if the individual is iron deficient.
	Serum plasma ferritin	This is an acute-phase protein, and it is nonspecific; it increases independently due to acute or chronic inflammation, infection, malignancy, hyperthyroidism, liver disease, or heavy alcohol use.
	Serum transferrin receptor	A specific indicator of iron deficient erythropoiesis that is not affected by inflammation.
	TIBC (total iron binding capacity)	Nonspecific and varies over the day.
	ZnPP erythrocyte (zinc protoporphyrin)	A sensitive indicator for diagnosis of the deficiency. However, the specificity is limited since it is affected by lead poisoning, the anemia of chronic disease, chronic infection, inflammation, hemoglobinopathy, and hemolytic anemias.
Zinc	Serum plasma zinc	Responds to zinc supplementation, but it is easily affected by contamination and is also affected by inflammation, fasting, estrogen use, hemolysis, and chronic illness.
B_{12}	Serum/plasma total zinc	Measures total biologically active B_{12}. Poor correlation with dietary zinc. Also, cutoffs are uncertain and kits for the test vary.
	Serum/plasma methylmalonic acid (MMA)	Cutoffs are uncertain. Test is sensitive.
	Serum/plasma holotranscobalamin (HoloTC)	
Folate	Serum/plasma folate	Varies with recent intake, and kits to test vary.
	Erythrocyte folate	Kits vary. Samples are difficult to prepare and cannot be stored.
	Serum/plasma total homocysteine (Hcys)	Depends on B_2 status, B_{12} status, B_6 status, and MTHR polymorphism state.
Vitamin A	Serum retinol	Sensitive to intake, but only if stores are low. It is not very sensitive because it is under homeostatic control.

Source: Dwyer J. Nutrition 101: The Concept of Nutritional Status and Guides for Nutrient Intakes, Eating Patterns, and Nutrition. IN: Rippe JM (ed) Lifestyle Medicine (3rd edition). CRC Press (Boca Raton), 2019.

TABLE 3.3
The Dietary Reference Intakes and Their Description and Uses

EAR	The EAR is the amount of a nutrient that is estimated to meet the requirement of half of the healthy individuals in a specific life stage and sex group. The EAR is used to assess the adequacy of intakes of population groups and, along with knowledge of the distribution of requirements, to develop Recommended Dietary Allowances.
RDA	The RDA is the average daily dietary intake level that is sufficient to meet the nutrient requirements of nearly all (e.g. 97%–98%) healthy persons of a specific sex at a particular stage of life or physiological condition, such as pregnancy or lactation. The only use of the RDA is to serve as a goal for individuals. The RDA is the value that should be used for planning individual intakes. The RDA is not appropriate for assessing the diets of either individuals or groups or for planning diets for groups.
AI	The adequate intake (AI) is a recommended daily intake level based on observed or experimentally determined estimates of nutrient intake in a group of healthy people. The main use of the AI is as a goal for the nutrient intake of individuals. It is used when an RDA cannot be determined. The AI is usually based on observed levels of intake that appear to maintain an acceptable level of health or growth.
UL	The tolerable (or safe) upper intake level (UL) is the highest level of chronic and usual daily nutrient intake that is likely to pose no risks of adverse health effects to almost all individuals in the general population. The UL is not an intended level of a nutrient to be consumed. Moreover, the UL is not a level at which there is a beneficial effect. Rather, it describes the intake level at which there is a high probability that the dose of the nutrient can be tolerated biologically.
EER	The Estimated Energy Requirement (EER) is the average energy intake needed to maintain energy balance in an adult, for growth in infants and children, to sustain fetal development in pregnancy, and to produce milk in lactating women. For adults, the EER is estimated using equations that consider the person's sex, age, weight, height, and level of physical activity. The EER can be used at the individual level to appropriately plan energy intakes to maintain, lose, or gain body weight.
AMDR	The Acceptable Macronutrient Distribution Range (AMDR) is the recommended range of the percentage of total energy intake from five macronutrients: total fat, Ω-6 polyunsaturated fatty acids (linoleic acid), Ω-3 polyunsaturated fatty acids (alpha-linolenic acid), carbohydrate, and protein. The AMDRs represent intakes that minimize the risk of chronic disease and permit an adequate intake of essential nutrients.

Source: Dwyer J. Nutrition 101: The Concept of Nutritional Status and Guides for Nutrient Intakes, Eating Patterns, and Nutrition. IN: Rippe JM. Lifestyle Medicine (3rd edition). CRC Press (Boca Raton), 2019.

contribute to them. For example, in heart disease, dietary factors are only one of many risk factors.

- **Dietary risk assessment and excessive intake**—The DRIs are also utilized for risk assessment, which entails the relationships between exposure of a nutrient and the likelihood of adverse health effects that occur in the exposed population. The measurement of risk assessment is called the upper limit (UL). A variety of scientific principles for risk assessment are used to assess the UL [21]. For many nutrients UL data are not available or are sparse based on anecdotal experience. Lack of an established UL does not mean that there is no risk for high intake of a nutrient. It should be noted that concerns about excessive energy intake leading to overweight or obesity or alcohol intake have been present for many years, and more research is currently going into these areas.

Furthermore, DRIs are limited for the very old and very young. For example, DRIs for infants less than 32 weeks gestation or people over 80 years are derived largely by extrapolation. It can be very challenging to update the DRI. Many of the DRI recommendations are more than 20 years old, and most were arrived at by deliberation and consensus of volunteer expert committees. As systematic reviews have become more common, it will be useful to further update the DRIs. However, the process of conducting these systematic reviews requires considerable money and time and cannot be accomplished by a staff of volunteer experts.

3.5 GUIDELINES FOR DIETARY INTAKE

As will be discussed and utilized throughout this book, modern nutrition research focuses on dietary patterns rather than individual foods and nutrients. It is the overall diet and quality of this diet, rather than the content of individual foods, that determine associations with health [22,23]. This does not mean that recommendations cannot include individual foods and how they can be incorporated into various dietary patterns. In addition, portion sizes should be determined to elucidate what constitutes a serving. Finally, individuals who have a diet-related disease may require a therapeutic diet where food exchange lists may be useful. For example, the American Diabetes Association Food Exchange List for Diabetes and the Academy of Nutrition and Dietetic Food Exchange List for Weight Management are both very useful [24,25].

- **Food groups versus nutrients**—Foods can be categorized into similar groups on the basis of the content of nutrients and other bioactives. This can be very useful since it can help identify foods that are high or low in specific nutrients and make it easier for consumers to choose wisely. Food groups are also the basis for dietary eating patterns. In addition, certain nutrients may be singled out because of the risk of low (i.e. calcium) or high intake (i.e. saturated [not total] fat) and added (not total) sugar.
- **Dietary patterns**—Dietary guidelines for consumers in the United States are based on the DGAs. These focus on food groups and dietary patterns. The Nutrition Evidence Library Technical Expert Collaborative Study on Dietary Patterns defines them as "the quantities, proportions, varieties and combinations of different foods, drinks and nutrients in a diet and the frequency with which they are habitually consumed" [26].

  As will be emphasized throughout this book, an enormous literature exists on what constitutes a healthy dietary pattern. Healthy dietary patterns, which are emphasized in the DGA, include the Dietary Approaches to Stop Hypertension (DASH) diet [27], Mediterranean diet [28], Healthy

U.S.-Style Dietary, and various [29] diets from the American Heart Association [30]. The DGA are issued every five years by the federal government. They are guided by a panel of independent research scientists called the Dietary Guidelines for Americans Advisory Committee. The DGA are recommendations that help individuals make healthy dietary choices including balance, variety, moderation, and consumption patterns that have been shown to decrease dietary risks of chronic diseases. Historically, the DGA have been targeted to people over the age of two years, because of a lack of data for those under two years. However, the DGA 2020–2025 now include infants from the time of birth. Examples of different healthy meal plans are provided in Table 3.4 (from DGA 2020–2025).

- **The Healthy Eating Index**—The Healthy Eating Index (HEI) is an instrument used to assess compliance with dietary guidelines [31–33]. It is also updated every five years. The most recent one available, however, is the HEI 2015 [34], which is derived from intakes based on criteria derived

TABLE 3.4
Healthy Dietary Patterns in the 2015–2020 Dietary Guidelines Advisory Committee Report

Component	Healthy U.S.	Healthy Mediterranean-Style	DASH	Healthy Vegetarian
Total fruit (whole not juice)	2	2.5	4	2
Total vegetables (cups)	2.5	2.5	4.0	2.D5
Dark green	1.5/wk	2.5/wk		1.5/wk
Red/orange	5.5	5.5		5.5
Starchy	5.0	5.0		5.0
Legumes	1.5	1.5		3.0
Total grains (oz equivalent) 50%	6	6	6	6
Whole grain				
Dairy, cups	3	2	3	3
Protein foods (oz equivalent)	5.5	6.5	-	3.5
Nuts/seeds	4/wk	4/wk	4–5/wk	7/wk
Red and processed meats	12.5/wk	12.5/wk	_<6/wk	-
Poultry	10.5	10.5	-	-
Seafood	8/wk	15/wk	=	=
Eggs	3/wk	3/2k	=	3/wk
Processed soy (tofu)	0.5/wk	0.5/wk	=	8/wk
Fats				
Solid fats, g (tsp)	18 (2)	17 (0.9)	2–3	21(2.3)
Oils g (tsp)	27 (3)	27 (3)	-	27 (3)

Source: U.S. Department of Agriculture and U.S. Department of Health and Human Services. *Dietary Guidelines for Americans, 2020–2025*. 9th Edition.

from the DRIs and the DGA. The HEI does not focus on energy needs or calorie contributions of food directly. It is, instead, a combination system based on points, taking into consideration a certain food group, and also assesses nutrients to avoid and nutrients to limit, which are based on the DGA. Figure 3.1 lists components of the HEI 2015 scoring system.

The perfect score is 100. Previous dietary intakes for the HEI rarely scored above 70 and often much lower than this [32–34]. It has been argued that the present availability of food supplies are insufficient to meet these dietary recommendations [34] and that the cost of meeting the recommendations in the HEI is relatively high. More research is clearly needed on these points [35].

Component	Maximum points	Standard for maximum score	Standard for minimum score of zero
Adequacy:			
Total Fruits[2]	5	≥0.8 cup equiv. per 1,000 kcal	No Fruit
Whole Fruits[3]	5	≥0.4 cup equiv. per 1,000 kcal	No Whole Fruit
Total Vegetables[4]	5	≥1.1 cup equiv. per 1,000 kcal	No Vegetables
Greens and Beans[4]	5	≥0.2 cup equiv. per 1,000 kcal	No Dark Green Vegetables or Legumes
Whole Grains	10	≥1.5 oz equiv. per 1,000 kcal	No Whole Grains
Dairy[5]	10	≥1.3 cup equiv. per 1,000 kcal	No Dairy
Total Protein Foods[6]	5	≥2.5 oz equiv. per 1,000 kcal	No Protein Foods
Seafood and Plant Proteins[6,7]	5	≥0.8 oz equiv. per 1,000 kcal	No Seafood or Plant Proteins
Fatty Acids[8]	10	(PUFAs + MUFAs)/SFAs ≥2.5	(PUFAs + MUFAs)/SFAs ≤1.2
Moderation:			
Refined Grains	10	≤1.8 oz equiv. per 1,000 kcal	≥4.3 oz equiv. per 1,000 kcal
Sodium	10	≤1.1 gram per 1,000 kcal	≥2.0 grams per 1,000 kcal
Added Sugars	10	≤6.5% of energy	≥26% of energy
Saturated Fats	10	≤8% of energy	≥16% of energy

1: Intakes between the minimum and maximum standards are scored proportionately.
2: Includes 100% fruit juice.
3: Includes all forms except juice.
4: Includes legumes (beans and peas).
5: Includes all milk products, such as fluid milk, yogurt, and cheese, and fortified soy beverages.
6: Includes legumes (beans and peas).
7: Includes seafood, nuts, seeds, soy products (other than beverages), and legumes (beans and peas).
8: Ratio of poly- and monounsaturated fatty acids (PUFAs and MUFAs) to saturated fatty acids (SFAs).

FIGURE 3.1 Healthy Eating Index (HEI—2015) 2015: Components and scoring standards.

Source: www.epi.grants.cancer.gov **(public domain)**.

- **USDA Food Group Patterns**—The U.S. Department of Agriculture (USDA) has designed food group patterns that conform with recommendations both from the DGAs and the Recommended Daily Allowances (RDA) and the DRIs. These are available on the USDA website for consumers to tailor for their age, sex, and physical activity level. The food patterns identify recommended foods from five major groups (fruits, vegetables, grains, protein foods, and dairy foods) as well as subgroups such as dark green vegetables, orange and red vegetables, starchy vegetables, other vegetables, beans and peas, whole grains, enriched and refined grains, meat, poultry, eggs, nuts, seeds, soy products, and seafood. The recommended amounts to consume for each food group differ depending on an individual's energy and nutrient needs. These patterns are consistent with the 2020–2025 DGA also with regard to sodium, saturated fat, and added sugar.
- **My Plate**—The USDA has developed a graphic entitled Choose My Plate, which provides a pictorial representation intended to emphasize the balance between calories and nutritional needs and to encourage increased intakes of fruits and vegetables, whole grains, and low-fat milk and reduced intake of sodium and high-calorie sugar drinks. An example of the Choose My Plate graphic is shown in Figure 3.2.

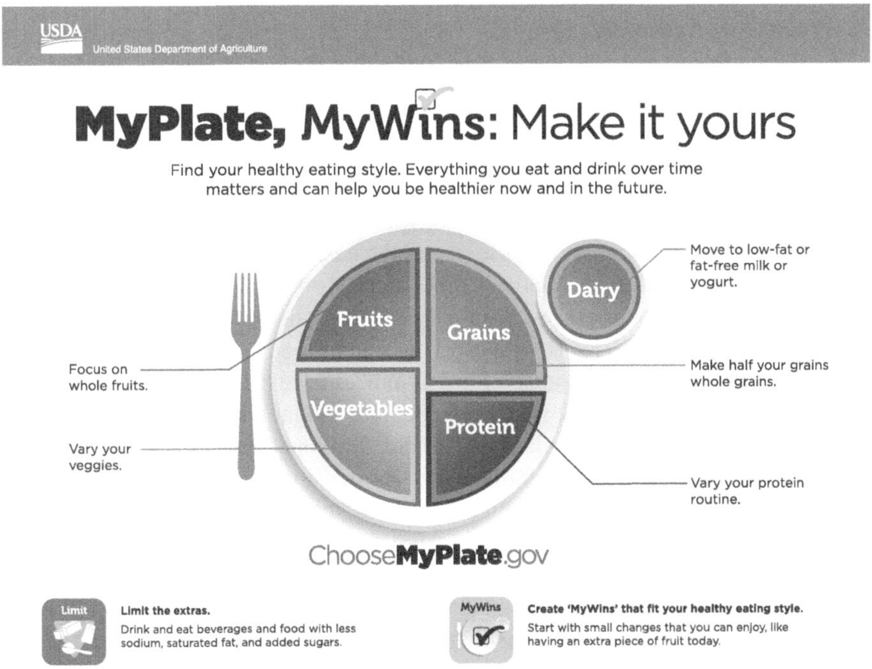

FIGURE 3.2 This is a graphic developed by the USDA to emphasize various aspects of healthy eating.

Source: MyPlate I U.S. Department of Agriculture (public domain).

3.6 OTHER TERMS USED IN DESCRIBING DIETS AND FOODS

A number of terms are described in diets and foods relative to a health standpoint. Here are a few selected common descriptors beyond the dietary eating patterns:

- **Energy density and nutrient density**—Both energy density and nutrient density will be utilized throughout this book. Energy density and nutrient density are two characteristics of foods that are associated with nutritional health. Energy density is defined in a number of different ways [36,37]. Most commonly, it is defined as calories per gram of foods and beverages in the diet. Some calculations do not include beverages. Energy density has been linked to overall energy intake because it is easier to consume too much of high-energy dense foods like alcohol and fatty/sugary foods than foods that are lower energy density and higher in bulk and water, like fruits and vegetables.

  Nutrient density, in contrast, is another term commonly used. It refers to nutrients per unit. The units may differ, but most commonly it is either nutrients per calorie or nutrients per gram. Nutrient density is relevant to health since nutrient-dense foods are more likely to assure that nutrient as well as energy needs are met. There is good evidence that nutrient density in the usual American diet is much lower than recommended in the DGA and other frameworks [38].
- **Determining nutrient quality of foods and diets**—A variety of indices and scores for dietary quality exist. Typically, nutrient quality of foods is discouraged since it can be difficult without demonizing certain foods and elevating others [39–44]. Measures of overall dietary quality are more relevant. A leading researcher in the area of maximizing nutrients per gram or per serving is Adam Drewnowski, who states: "nutrient profile is a technique of rating or classifying foods on the basis of their nutritional value" [44]. Foods that supply relatively more nutrients than calories are defined as nutrient dense. Nutrient profile models calculate the content of key nutrients per 100 grams, 100 kcals, or preserving size of food.
- **Nutrient Rich Foods Index**—Several indices have been developed that are used to identify nutrient-rich foods. Perhaps the most commonly used one is the Nutrient Rich Foods (NRF) Index developed by Drewnowski from the 2005 DGA, which identified nutrient density as a key component of dietary quality [45]. This is underscored by the phrase that "every calorie should count." The NRF Index successfully ranks foods based on a nutritional value and can be applied to individual foods, meals, menus, and even the daily diet.
- **Nutrient information on food labels**—Food labels that assess nutrient content on individual food products are used to assist consumers in making better food choices when they are shopping [46]. The nutrient facts label and packaging on other foods in the United States provide information on various nutrients, and similar labels are provided on supplement facts

panels on dietary supplements. These nutrient composition data determine whether a particular food product can be claimed to be low fat, high calcium, etc.

Nutrition information on the nutrient facts label is important for helping consumers choose foods wisely. Food labels that are regulated by the Federal Food, Drug, and Cosmetic Act are required on all packaging and prepared foods and beverages and are voluntary for produce. Front-of-pack labels provide scores or logos to help consumers make food choices by identifying healthier foods at a glance. The nutrition facts panel provides information about energy and contents of certain macro- and micronutrients to emphasize those to limit and those to include by their amounts in standardized portion sizes for almost all processed foods.

Figure 3.3 presents an example of the new nutrition fact label. Two changes on this label compared to previous labels involve bolded values for calories, and also total fat, saturated fat, and trans fats were called out since they are consumed in excess by many Americans. "Sugars" was

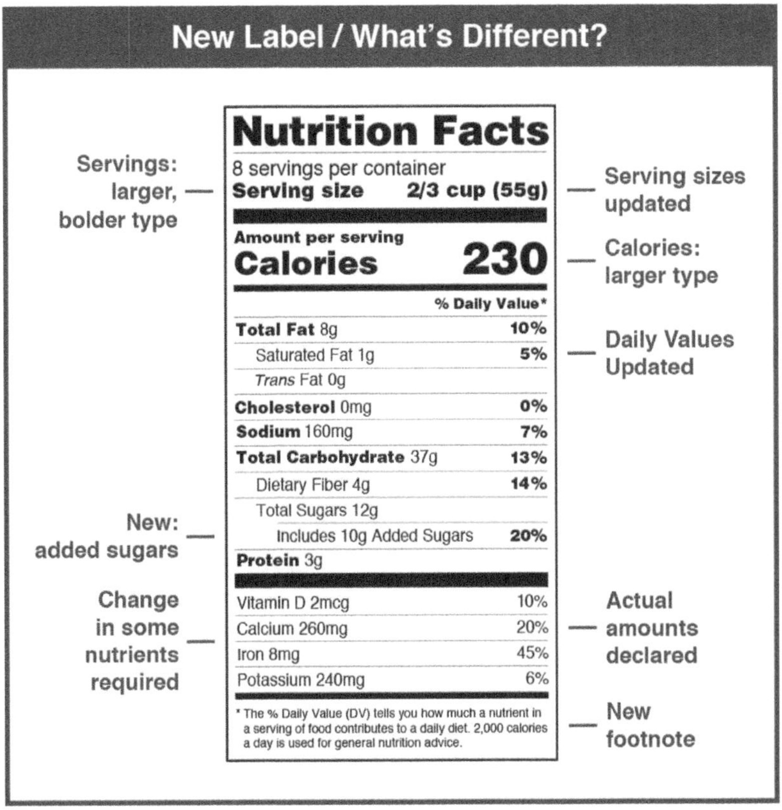

FIGURE 3.3 The new nutrition label

Source: www.fda.gov/food/food-labeling-nutrition/changes-nutrition-facts-label (**Public domain**).

updated to include "added sugars" and sugars naturally occurring in the food. Even though both types of sugars are identical from a nutritional standpoint, many major sources of added sugars may contribute to obesity and lower micronutrient density. The most recent revision of the food label also includes serving sizes updated to reflect the amounts of food people are actually eating today and displaying calories more prominently than in years past.

- **Label claims**—In addition to nutrient facts, other information in the form of claims can be made on packaged foods and dietary supplements. Three types of claims are regulated by the Food and Drug Administration (FDA) [47]. They are nutrient content claims, health claims, and structure/function claims.
- **Nutrient claims**—Nutrient claims are regulated by the Nutrition Labeling and Education Act of 1990, which allows the amount of energy or nutrients in a product to be in the label. Words that describe nutrient content include "good source," "high," "low," "free," "reduced," and "light." Each of these descriptors has a defined regulatory definition.
- **Health claims**—Two types of health claims exist. Health claims are met with "significant scientific agreement" for "qualified health claims." There are currently only 12 approved health claims that meet the standard of significant scientific agreement. These include claims about the role of nutrients and foods in health and disease. A good example regarding folic acid is as follows: "Healthful diets with adequate folate may reduce a woman's risk of having a child with a brain or spinal cord birth defect."

  Qualified health claims indicate that the evidence stating a connection is less certain than the unqualified claim. These claims require statements that they are not endorsed by the FDA. For example, the claim for walnuts and coronary heart disease must state "supportive, but not conclusive research shows that eating 1.5 ounces per day of walnuts as part of a low, saturated fat or low cholesterol diet and not resulting in increased caloric intake may reduce the risk of coronary heart disease."
- **Structure/function claims**—These claims describe an association of a particular nutrient or food component with the body's structure or function. An example of a claim referring to "structure" is: "The protein in [name of food] helps maintain strong muscles." An example of a claim referring to "function" is: "The vitamin A in [name of food] helps to promote normal vision" (e.g. function). The FDA recommends that the manufacturer voluntarily list the amount and percentage of the daily value.
- **Voluntary and front-of-pack labels**—There are some voluntary systems that are defined to help consumers make choices or determine if a food is a healthy option. Front-of-pack labeling (FOP) allows some of this information to be on the front of the packaged goods [48,49].
- **Facts up front**—The "facts up front" label was developed in 2010 by the Grocery Manufacturers Association at the request of then-First Lady Michele Obama to develop an FOP system to enable shoppers to make decisions. Nutrients are presented in standard formats: calories, saturated fats,

sodium, and sugar. Manufacturers can add up to two additional "nutrients" to encourage that the food is a "good" source," meaning that it contains at least 10% of the desired nutrient per serving.

- **Heart Check**—The Heart Check Program from the American Heart Association was designed to help consumers find and choose "heart-healthy" foods both in grocery stores and meals in restaurants. Products with the heart check must meet mandatory requirements for the heart-healthy claim. The cost to manufacturers for obtaining this label was considerable, and many companies have ceased to use it, particularly since the advent of the new nutrition facts label.
- **Other labeling systems**—A number of other voluntary labeling systems have been developed and have been subject to discussion and debate. Some supermarkets have also developed scoring systems, including, for example, Walmart's "Great for You" Program. There are also private groups that rate products. Criteria for these may vary and are not regulated by the FDA. Since multiple systems are available and one has not dominated the field, consumers may be confused by multiple different offerings.

3.7 PERSONALIZED NUTRITION

There are differences between nutritional responses between healthy people related to age, diet, and genetics [50]. These have led to an expanding field that is called "personalized nutrition." Researchers working on it hope to use various molecular profiling technologies to assess DNA, RNA, and protein and tailor metabolic responses to be more individualized [51]. While there is great potential for this, this field is still in its infancy. Despite there being a number of options in this area, there is very little evidence that medicalizing diets with elaborate food plans is effective and, in addition, may promote needless worries. The National Institutes of Health (NIH) has allocated $170 million for research on personalized nutrition [52].

3.8 TECHNOLOGICAL ADVANCES

Technological advances offer great promise in the area of increasing accuracy and ease of application toward nutritional assessment. For example, multiple applications such as MyFitnessPal allow individuals to scan a barcode of their food using their smartphone camera, which automatically identifies food and quantifies food volume through artificial intelligence [53,54]. Wearable sensor devices such as eyeglasses containing a mounted camera utilizing automatic ingestion monitoring (AIM) are also now being developed for automatically identifying and quantifying food intake [55]. There are also technologies such as the Portion Size app that allows an individual to capture images of their food so they can identify it and estimate the amount of volume [56]. All of these images can be sent to a trained reviewer for further analysis utilizing a validated method. The Automated Self-Administered 24-Hour (ASA24) Dietary Assessment Tool is another technology-assisted food record application that is available online and is a web-based tool [57].

While these technological advances are welcome, they still have significant limitations. One limitation is that they require access to technology (e.g. access to smartphone) and they may exhibit technical challenges such as reliance on internet connectivity and, in addition, privacy concerns related to collecting sensitive dietary information [58,59]. Nonetheless, these technological advancements offer additional opportunities to advance the field of measuring nutritional status.

3.9 CONCLUSIONS

A variety of tools are available for measuring nutritional status and for evaluating the diet. Nutritional status is a broad term that includes anthropometric, biochemical, clinical, and dietary measures, as well as food-related quality of life. Dietary intake is an important component of nutritional status, but the two are not synonymous. A number of useful indices are available to help determine how healthful a dietary pattern is. Perhaps the most useful one is the HEI, which is explained in this chapter. Every five years the USDA lists the DGA. The executive summary of this should be in the toolbox of every clinician.

Clinical Applications

- All clinicians should have a general familiarity with nutritional status and how it is measured.
- As clinicians are counseling patients, utilizing information that is available from the DGA can play an important role.
- Healthy dietary patterns include the DASH diet, the Mediterranean diet, the Healthy U.S.-Style Dietary, and various diets recommended by the American Heart Association.
- Clinicians should discuss the difference between healthy dietary practices and the typical Western diet in all patient encounters.

REFERENCES

1. Subar A, Freedman LS, Tooze JA, et al. Addressing current criticism regarding the value of self-report dietary data. J Nutr. 2015;145(12):2639–2645.
2. Thompson F, Kirkpatrick SI, Subar AF, et al. The National Cancer Institute's dietary assessment primer: A resource for diet research. J Acad Nutr Diet. 2015;115(12):1986–1995.
3. Thompson F, Byers T. Dietary assessment resource manual. J Nutri. 1994;124(Suppl 11):2245S–2317S.
4. Heady J. Diets of bank clerks. Development of a method of classifying the diets of individuals for use in epidemiologic studies. J R Statist Soc. 1961;124:336–361.
5. Bailey R, Miller PE, Mitchell DC, et al. Dietary screening tool identifies nutritional risk in older adults. Am J Clin Nutr. 2009;90(1):177–183.
6. Bailey R, Mitchell DC, Miller CK, et al. A dietary screening questionnaire identifies dietary patterns in older adults. J Nutr. 2007;137(2):421–426.
7. Yaroch A, Tooze J, Thompson FE, et al. Evaluation of three short dietary instruments to assess fruit and vegetable intake: The National Cancer Institute's food attitudes and behaviors survey. J Acad Nutr Diet. 2012;112(10):1570–1577.

8. Strimbu K, Tavel J. What are biomarkers? Curr Opin HIV AIDS. 2010;5(6):463–466.
9. Raiten D, Namasté S, Brabin B, et al. Executive summary—Biomarkers of Nutrition for Development: Building a Consensus. Am J Clin Nutr. 2011;94(2):633S–650S.
10. Combs G Jr, Trumbo PR, McKinley MC, et al. Biomarkers in nutrition: New frontiers in research and application. Ann N Y Acad Sci. 2013;1278:1–10.
11. Potischman N, Freudenheim J. Biomarkers of nutritional exposure and nutritional status: An overview. J Nutr. 2003;133(Suppl 3):873S–874S.
12. Food and Nutrition Board. Dietary Reference Intakes for Calcium, Phosphorus, Magnesium, Vitamin D and Floride. Washington, DC: National Academy Press, 1997.
13. Food and Nutrition Board. Dietary Reference Intakes for Thiamin, Riboflavin, Niacin, Vitamin $B_{6,}$ Folate, Vitamin $B_{12,}$ Pantothenic Acid, Biotin, and Choline. Washington, DC: National Academy Press, 1998.
14. Food and Nutrition Board. Dietary Reference Intakes for Vitamin C, Vitamin E, Selenium, and Carotenoids. Washington, DC: National Academy Press, 2000.
15. Food and Nutrition Board. Dietary Reference Intakes for Vitamin A, Vitamin K, Arsenic, Boron, Chromium, Copper, Iodine, Iron, Molybdenum, Nickel, Silicon, Vanadium and Zinc. Washington, DC: National Academy Press, 2001.
16. Food and Nutrition Board. Dietary Reference Intakes for Energy, Carbohydrate, Fiber, Fat, Fatty Acids, Cholesterol, Protein, and Amino Acids (Macronutrients). Washington, DC: Institute of Medicine, 2002/2005.
17. Food and Nutrition Board. Dietary Reference Intakes: Applications in Dietary Planning. Washington, DC: Institute of Medicine, 2003.
18. Food and Nutrition Board. Dietary Reference Intakes for Water, Potassium, Sodium, Chloride, and Sulfate. Washington, DC: Institute of Medicine, 2004.
19. Food and Nutrition Board. Dietary Reference Intakes: The Essential Guide to Nutrient Requirements. Washington, DC: Institute of Medicine, 2006.
20. Food and Nutrition Board. Dietary Reference Intakes for Calcium and Vitamin D. Washington, DC: National Academy Press, 2011.
21. World Health Organization. A Model for Establishing Upper Levels of Intake for Nutrients and Related Substances: A Report of a Joint FAO/WHO Technical Workshop on Food Nutrient Risk Assessment. Geneva, Switzerland: World Health Organization, 2006.
22. Patterson RP, Haines PS, Popkin BM. Diet quality index: Capturing a multidimensional behavior. J Am Diet Assoc. 1994;94(1):57–64.
23. Ioannidis J. We need more randomized trials in nutrition-preferably large, long-term, and with negative results. Am J Clin Nutr. 2016;103(6):1385–1386.
24. Geil P. American Diabetes Association and American Dietetic Association. Choose Your Foods: Exchange Lists for Diabetes: The 2008 Revision of Exchange Lists for Meal Planning. October 2008.
25. Academy of Nutrition and Dietetics and American Diabetes Association. Choose Your Foods: Food Lists for Weight Management. Chicago, IL: American Diabetes Association, American Dietetic Association. Academy of Nutrition and Dietetics, 2019.
26. Nutrition Evidence Library. A Series of Systematic Reviews on the Relationship between Dietary Patterns and Health Outcomes. 2014 US Department of Agriculture, Center for Policy and Promotion. Alexandra, VA.
27. Sacks F, Svetkey L, Vollmer W, et al. Effects on blood pressure of reduced dietary sodium and the Dietary Approaches to Stop Hypertension (DASH) diet. DASH-Sodium Collaborative Research Group. N Engl J Med. 2001;344(1):3–10.
28. Estruch R, Ros E, Salas-Salvado J, et al. Primary prevention of cardiovascular disease with a Mediterranean diet. N Engl J Med. 2013;368(14):1279–1290.

29. U.S. Department of Agriculture and U.S. Department of Health and Human Services. *Dietary Guidelines for Americans, 2020–2025*, 9th edition. December 2020. Dietary Guidelines.gov.
20. www.dietaryguidelines.gov/resources/2020-2025-dietary-guidelines-online-materials
30. Lichtenstein A, Appel L, Vadiveloo M, et al. 2021 Dietary guidance to improve cardiovascular health: A scientific statement from the American Heart Association. Circulation. 2021;144(23):e472–e487. Epub 2021/11/03.
31. Kennedy E, Ohls J, Carlson S, et al. The healthy eating index: Design and applications. J Am Diet Assoc. 1995;95(10):1103–1108.
32. Krebs-Smith SM, Guenther PM, Subar AF, et al. Americans do not meet federal dietary recommendations. J Nutr. 2010;140(10):1832–1838.
33. Guenther P, Casavale KO, Reedy J, et al. Update of the healthy eating index: HEI-2010. J Acad Nutr Diet. 2013;113(4):569–580.
34. Guenther P, Kirkpatrick SI, Reedy J, et al. The healthy eating index-2010 is a valid and reliable measure of diet quality according to the 2010 dietary guidelines for Americans. J Nutr. 2014;144(3):399–407.
35. Miller P, Reedy J, Kirkpatrick SI, et al. The United States food supply is not consistent with dietary guidance: Evidence from an evaluation using the healthy eating index-2010. J Acad Nutr Diet. 2015;115(1):95–100.
36. Rehm CP, Monsivais P, Drewnowski A. Relation between diet cost and healthy eating index 2010 scores among adults in the United States 2007–2010. Prev Med. 2015;73:70–75.
37. Kant A, Graubard B. Energy density of diets reported by American adults: Association with food group intake, nutrient intake, and body weight. Int J Obes (Lond). 2005;29(8):950–956.
38. Ledikwe J, Blanck HM, Khan LK, et al. Dietary energy density determined by eight calculation methods in a nationally representative United States population. J Nutr. 2005;135(2):273–278.
39. Britten P, Cleveland LE, Koegel KL, et al. Impact of typical rather than nutrient-dense food choices in the US Department of Agriculture Food Patterns. J Acad Nutr Diet. 2012;112(10):1560–1569.
40. Drewnowski A. Concept of a nutritious food: Toward a nutrient density score. Am J Clin Nutr. 2005;82(4):721–732.
41. Drewnowski A, Fulgoni V. 3rd. Nutrient profiling of foods: Creating a nutrient-rich food index. Nutr Rev. 2008;66(1):23–39.
42. Drewnowski A, Fulgoni V. 3rd. Comparing the nutrient rich foods index with "Go," "Slow," and "Whoa," foods. J Am Diet Assoc. 2011;111(2):280–284.
43. Drewnowski A, Fulgoni V. 3rd. Nutrient density: Principles and evaluation tools. Am J Clin Nutr. 2014;99(Suppl 5):1223S–1228S.
44. Drewnowski A, Fulgoni VL, Young MK, et al. Nutrient-rich foods: Applying nutrient navigation systems to improve public health. J Food Sci. 2008;73(9):H222–H228.
45. Fulgoni V. 3rd, Keast D, Drewnowski A. Development and validation of the nutrient-rich foods index: A tool to measure nutritional quality of foods. J Nutr. 2009;139(8):1549–1554.
46. Food and Drug Administration, HHS. Food labeling: Revision of the nutrition and supplement facts labels. Final rule. Fed Regist. 2016;27;81(103):33741–33999.
47. Food and Drug Administration. Label Claims for Conventional Foods and Dietary Supplements. www.fda.gov/Food/IngredientsPackagingLabeling/LabelingNutrition/ucm111447.htm

48. Institute of Medicine. Purpose and Merits of Front-of-Package Nutrition Rating Systems, in Front-of-Package Nutrition Rating Systems and Symbols: Phase I Report. Wartella EA, Lichtenstein AH, and Boon CS (ed). Washington, DC: National Academies Press, 2010.
49. Miller LM, Cassady DL, Beckett LA, et al. Misunderstanding of front-of-package nutrition information on US food products. PLoS One. 2015;29;10(4):e0125306.
50. Celis-Morales C, Livingstone KM, Marsaux CF, et al. Effect of personalized nutrition on health-related behaviour change: Evidence from the Food4Me European randomized controlled trial. Int J Epidemiol. 2017;46(2):578–588.
51. Tucker K, Smith CE, Lai CQ, et al. Quantifying diet for nutrigenomic studies. Annu Rev Nutr. 2013;33:349–371.
52. The CUNY Graduate School of Public Health and Health Policy (CUNY SPH). January 20, 2020. https://sph.cuny.edu/ (Accessed March 12, 2024).
53. MyFitnessPal | MyFitnessPal. Published April 3, 2023. www.myfitnesspal.com (Accessed March 12, 2024).
54. Lozano CP, Canty EN, Saha S, et al. Validity of an artificial intelligence-based application to identify foods and estimate energy intake among adults: A pilot study. Curr Dev Nutr. 2023;29;7(11):1020.
55. Fontana JM, Farooq M, Sazonov E. Automatic ingestion monitor: A novel wearable device for monitoring of ingestive behavior. IEEE Trans Biomed Eng. 2014;61(6):1772–1779.
56. Saha S, Lozano CP, Broyles S, Martin CK, Apolzan JW. Assessing the initial validity of the portion size app to estimate dietary intake among adults: Pilot and feasibility app validation study. JMIR Form Res. 2022;6(6):e38283.
57. ASA24® Dietary Assessment Tool | EGRP/DCCPS/NCI/NIH. https://epi.grants.cancer.gov/asa24/ (Accessed March 12, 2024).
58. Boushey CJ, Spoden M, Zhu FM, Delp EJ, Kerr DA. New mobile methods for dietary assessment: Review of image-assisted and image-based dietary assessment methods. Proc Nutr Soc. 2017;76(3):283–294.
59. Amoutzopoulos B, Steer T, Roberts C, et al. Traditional methods v. new technologies: Dilemmas for dietary assessment in large-scale nutrition surveys and studies: A report following an international panel discussion at the 9th International Conference on Diet and Activity Methods (ICDAM9), Brisbane, 3 September 2015. J Nutr Sci. 2018;7:e11.

4 Nutrition, Lifestyle Medicine, and Chronic Disease

Key Points

- Healthy nutrition should be placed in the context of other positive lifestyle habits and actions to lower the risk of chronic disease.
- Multiple lifestyle habits and actions can lower the risk of multiple chronic diseases such as cardiovascular disease (CVD), type 2 diabetes mellitus (T2DM) and prediabetes, obesity, cancer, and dementia/reduction of cognitive function.
- Clinicians should emphasize an overall approach to a healthy lifestyle that encompasses not only healthy nutrition but the other lifestyle factors in an overall, integrated approach to lowering the risk of chronic disease and improving short-term health and quality of life.

4.1 INTRODUCTION

While this book focuses throughout on the powerful area of healthy nutrition and its multiple impacts on lowering the risk of chronic disease and improving health and quality of life, this powerful modality should also be recommended in the context of other lifestyle medicine modalities.

In Chapter 25, we list the key lifestyle medicine modalities that should be utilized in addition to nutrition. These include physical activity, weight management, avoiding tobacco products, stress reduction, weight management, developing positive relationships with others, and healthy sleep. In this chapter, we focus on the specific ways that these lifestyle medicine modalities, used in conjunction with each other and, of course, with proper nutrition being one of the keys, to specifically lower the risk of chronic disease and/or assist in its treatment.

4.2 CARDIOVASCULAR DISEASE

CVD remains the single leading cause of death in the United States, representing over 37% of annual mortality. Multiple different lifestyle activities significantly impact on lowering the risk of heart disease [1–6]. Physical activity is one of the major, and most powerful, risk factor reducers for CVD [7]. Some studies have suggested that regular physical activity is more powerful than either cigarette smoking or hypertension for its association with CVD. Unfortunately, less than half of adults in the United States

DOI: 10.1201/9781003452607-4

meet the minimum requirements for physical activity and only 25% meet the recommended criteria issued in the Centers for Disease Control and Prevention (CDC) and the Physical Activity Guidelines for Americans (PAGA) 2018. Unfortunately, young people are even less likely to meet recommended standards, with less than 20% of adolescents performing 60 minutes or more daily physical activity as recommended by the PAGA 2018 [7].

Of note, a sedentary lifestyle also is a significant risk factor for CVD [8]. Sedentary individuals carry a 150–240% higher risk of CVD than those who achieve physical activity levels as recommended by the CDC and the PAGA 2018 [9–11]. The PAGA 2018 Scientific Report recommends 150 minutes of moderate-intensity physical activity or 75 minutes of vigorous physical activity per week as well as muscle strengthening activities at least two days per week.

Even levels of physical activity significantly lower than those recommended by the PAGA 2018 yield substantial benefits. This is illustrated in Figure 4.1. As can be seen from this figure, individuals who engage in 150–300 minutes per week of moderate-intensity physical activity achieve the greatest benefits. However, as clearly identified in the figure, there is essentially no lower threshold for individuals who begin to engage in physical activity. Even individuals who obtain only 30 minutes of regular physical activity every week significantly lower their risk of all-cause mortality by approximately 20%. Also noted, is that the American Heart Association (AHA) [12] and CDC [13] guidelines as well as PAGA 2018 emphasize that more physical activity significantly lowers the risk of adult weight gain and helps control blood pressure. While the relationship between physical activity and lipids is modest, regular physical activity has been shown to increase high-density lipoprotein (HDL).

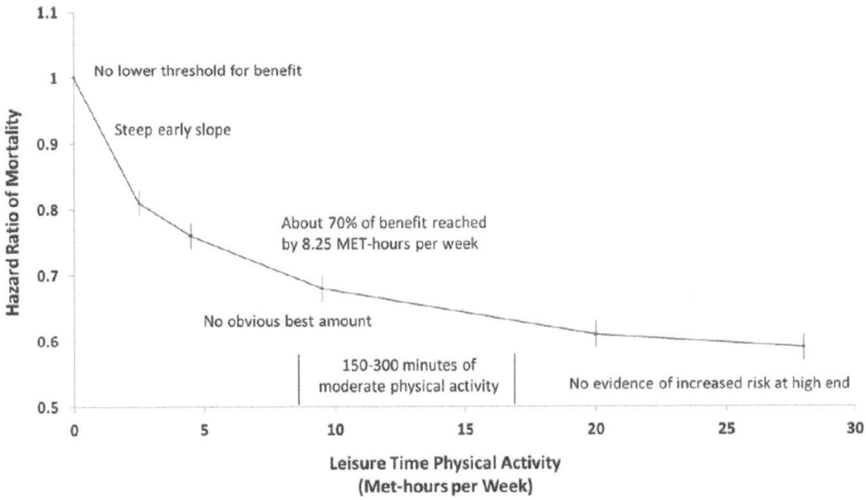

FIGURE 4.1 Relationships of moderate-to-vigorous physical activity.

- **Nutrition**—As emphasized in multiple chapters throughout this book, dietary factors play a critical role in multiple ways for lowering the risk of chronic disease (2,12,14,15). This is certainly true of CVD and coronary heart disease (CHD). Multiple recommendations from the AHA and American College of Cardiology (ACC) as well as Dietary Guidelines for Americans (DGA) 2020–2025 [16] recommend various dietary interventions to lower the risk of CVD [17,18]. These are handled in multiple places in this book. It should be noted, however, that all of these guidelines invariably place nutrition in the context of other lifestyle factors such as regular physical activity and weight management.
- **Weight management and obesity**—Both overweight and obesity are significant risk factors for CVD. Unfortunately, over 70% of the adult population in the United States is either overweight (body mass index [BMI] >25 and <30 kg/m^2) or obese (BMI>30 kg/m^2) [19]. Obesity is also a significant risk factor for diabetes, dyslipidemias, and hypertension. Distribution of body fat adds another risk since abdominal obesity is an independent and strong risk factor for CVD. The AHA and the ACC as well as The Obesity Society (TOS) issued guidelines in 2013 for treating overweight and obesity [20]. These can be found under the references indicated in this chapter. It is important to recognize that all five of the recommendations from the AHA/ACC/TOS carry a significant lifestyle component.
- **Smoking and tobacco products**—Overwhelming evidence from multiple sources exists demonstrating that cigarette smoking significantly increases the risk of heart disease and stroke [21]. Cigarette smoking in men remains high at approximately 18% and in women more than 15% [22,23]. The benefits of cigarette smoking cessation occur over a very brief period of time [21]. Smokers lose at least one decade of life expectancy compared to never smokers. Smokers who quit reduce the risk of a coronary event by 50% within the first two years after cessation [21,24]. Most of this benefit occurs within the first three months. CHD risk falls substantially with one to two years of cessation, and the risk of former smokers approaches that of never smokers after three to five years. The U.S. Healthy People 2020 Initiative recommended reducing the national problem of cigarette smoking among adults to a target of 12% [25]. Unfortunately, the consumption of tobacco products is increasing globally. Almost 80% of the world's 1 billion smokers live in low- or middle-income countries. It should also be noted that secondhand smoke substantially increases the risk of CVD [26].
- **Psychological factors and stress**—Psychological factors may impact on the risk of CVD. Anxiety, which has a prevalence of over 31%, increases the risk of CVD [27]. Depression may also increase the risk of heart disease by making individuals less likely to adhere to programs for risk reduction [28].
- **Blood pressure**—Elevated blood pressure remains a significant risk factor for CVD and the leading risk factor for stroke. The Joint National Commission VII (JNC VII) defines normal blood pressure as <120 mm/Hg systolic and <80 mm/Hg diastolic, 120–139 mm/Hg systolic and 89 mm/

Hg diastolic were considered prehypertension, and >140 mm/Hg systolic and >90 mm/Hg were defined as hypertension [29]. Multiple lifestyle medicine modalities can positively impact on lowering the risk of high blood pressure.

- **Elevated blood lipids**—It is important to control blood lipids to lower the risk of heart disease. Most of the modalities to reduce low-density lipoprotein (LDL) have to do with nutrition, although physical activity may also impact on raising HDL [17]. There is some debate about the role of elevated triglycerides and their increased risk of CVD [30]. Triglycerides typically vary inversely with HDL.
- **Blood glucose, prediabetes, and diabetes**—T2DM is a significant risk factor for CHD. In fact, over two-thirds of all individuals with T2DM will die of CHD. Lifestyle therapies, most prominently nutrition, although other factors such as physical activity and weight management, are all important for lowering the risk of T2DM and also lowering the risk of prediabetes progressing to diabetes [31]. Metabolic syndrome is a clustering of risk factors including blood pressure >130/85 mm/Hg, triglycerides >150 mg/dL fasting glucose >100 mg/dL, abdominal circumference >40 inches in men and >35 inches in women, and an HDL less than <40 mg/dL [32]. All of these factors constitute a significant risk factor for heart disease. The good news is that lifestyle medicine modalities can impact on all of these risk factors.

4.3 DIABETES AND PREDIABETES

Substantial increases in diabetes have occurred around the world in the last two decades. In the United States, the current estimated prevalence of diabetes is approximately 12% [33]. Nutrition therapy (also called medical nutrition therapy [MNT]) is the cornerstone treatment for diabetes [34]. In addition, physical activity, education, counseling, and support are all of considerable importance for the vast majority of individuals who have either diabetes or prediabetes.

The International Diabetes Federation estimates that over 400 million individuals in the world live with type 1 or type 2 diabetes [35]. Tragically, almost half of these individuals do not know they have the disease. It is estimated that the number of individuals living with this condition will increase to 420 million by 2035.

There is a higher prevalence of adults with diabetes who are non-Hispanic Black, non-Hispanic Asian, or Hispanic. There is some good news that the portion of people who have undiagnosed diabetes has decreased between 3.5% and 5.2% during this period of time [33].

Unfortunately, the prevalence of prediabetes has remained stationary between 37% and 38% of the overall U.S. population [33]. Consequently, over half of the U.S. population has either diabetes or prediabetes. Lifestyle modalities are very important in both of these conditions. The strongest evidence of the benefits of lifestyle modalities in prediabetes comes from the Diabetes Prevention Program (DPP), which demonstrated that intensive lifestyle intervention in individuals with prediabetes could reduce the incidence of this progressing to type 2 diabetes by over 58% over three years [36]. Other studies have also supported this, including the Da Qing

Study [37] and the Finnish Diabetes Prevention Study [38], both of which showed similar reductions in the risk of prediabetes turning into T2DM following multicomponent lifestyle interventions.

The major goals of DPP in the lifestyle intervention arm established the goal to achieve a minimum of 7% weight loss and 150 minutes of physical activity of moderate intensity each week based on brisk walking [36]. A heart-healthy diet with mild caloric restriction was essential for the weight loss portion of this intervention. This diet in DPP was consistent with both the Mediterranean diet [39] and DASH diet [40] eating patterns. Red meat and sugar-sweetened beverages were also minimized because of their association both with CVD and T2DM. Education and support in the DPP was provided with an individual model of treatment. This was conducted in a 16-session core curriculum completed in the first 24 weeks of intervention.

As already indicated, MNT is the cornerstone of diabetes care [33]. Also included are other lifestyle modalities including physical activity, smoking cessation, counseling, psychosocial care, and diabetes self-management education support.

MNT promotes healthy eating patterns by emphasizing a variety of nutrient-dense foods at appropriate levels for the goal of achieving and maintaining healthy body weight; maintaining individual glycemia, blood pressure, and lipid goals; and delaying or preventing the complications of diabetes. Weight management is necessary and is also an important component, particularly for overweight and obesity, for people with diabetes. Regular physical activity is also vitally important in the management of diabetes. The recommendation for physical activity for people with T2DM is consistent with the overall 150 minutes of moderate physical activity per week advocated for all adults by the PAGA 2018 [7]. The American Diabetes Association (ADA) Consensus Report recommends that prior to starting an exercise program, a medical provider should perform a careful history and be aware of atypical presentations of CHD in patients with diabetes [33,41,42]. Healthcare providers should also customize exercise regimens based on individual needs.

4.4 OBESITY

Obesity is the result of energy imbalance, since both energy expenditure and energy intake are key factors in the energy balance equation [42,43]. Nutritional and physical activity components of lifestyle intervention are critically important both for short-term weight loss and also long-term maintenance of healthy body weight. Dietary treatments for obesity have also employed MNT. This therapeutic approach has been used in a variety of medical conditions, but there is particularly strong proof that MNT improves waist circumference, waist-to-hip ratio, fasting blood sugar, LDL cholesterol, HDL cholesterol, and blood pressure.

Typical nutritional interventions for weight loss in obese individuals involve sustaining an average daily caloric deficit of 500 kcals. Energy recommendations also include that total intake should not be <1,200 calories/day in order to maintain adequate nutrient intake.

A variety of evidence-based guidelines have been demonstrated to assist in healthy weight loss. These include the Mediterranean diet [39], DASH diet, and the Healthy U.S.-Style Dietary Plan [16]. Numerous studies have shown that macronutrient composition of weight loss plans (e.g. low fat versus low carb, etc.) do not achieve different results in studies lasting longer than one year [44].

It has been argued that physical activity alone is not a powerful tool for initial weight loss. It should be noted, however, that abundant evidence supports the concept that regular physical activity is a key component of long-term maintenance of weight loss [45]. In addition, regular physical activity can result in preservation of lean body mass, which is a key component of maintaining adequate metabolism to support maintenance of weight loss. As will be discussed in multiple chapters in this book, regular physical activity also conveys a host of health-enhancing benefits in addition to its role in weight loss and weight management.

4.5 CANCER

Multiple lifestyle measures play critically important roles in the prevention of cancer and treatment of individuals who already have established cancer. In addition, lifestyle measures play a very important role in the ongoing health of cancer survivors. These facts were underscored by the joint statement issued by the American Cancer Society and the ADA and the AHA in their Statement on Preventing Cancer, CVD and Diabetes [5]. The importance of nutrition has been emphasized both in prevention and treatment of cancer. An important article by Doll and Peto emphasized that approximately 35% of cancers in the United States can be attributable to dietary factors [46]. This was corroborated in 2007 by research from the World Cancer Research Fund and the American Institute for Cancer Research (WCRF/AICR), who evaluated 7,000 studies and concluded that diet and physical activity are major determinants of cancer risk [47]. An additional role for healthy nutrition relates to the association of obesity with cancer. Adipocytes, which are the predominant cells in body fat, secrete a variety of metabolically reactive substances that promote inflammation, insulin resistance, and a variety of other factors which may promote cancer growth.

General nutrition guidelines for cancer prevention and treatment are similar to those generally recommended for healthy eating. It may, however, be necessary for some modifications to be made in certain cancers or treatments for various side effects of cancer therapy such as excessive weight loss. Recommendations for healthy eating are similar in cancer to other metabolic conditions and health in general. Individuals should decrease consumption of processed foods (including ham and bacon and red meat) and should follow diets that emphasize whole grains, vegetables, fruits, and legumes. These are cornerstones of healthy diets which have been emphasized throughout this book including the Mediterranean diet, DASH diet, and the Healthy U.S.-Style Dietary [48,49]. Physical activity also plays a key role in the association of lifestyle risk with cancer. Regular physical activity has been shown in multiple large cohort studies to be associated with a lower risk of cancer [50,51].

4.6 DEMENTIA, COGNITION, AND BRAIN HEALTH

Brain health and the maintenance of cognitive function are vital for maintaining quality of life and functional independence and are particularly important components of the aging process. There is a strong link between brain health and cardiovascular health. This fact was underscored by the Presidential Advisory from the AHA and the American Stroke Association (ASA) on "Defining Optimal Brain Health in Adults" [6].

Multiple lifestyle measures play a central role in the recommendations from the AHA/ASA in maintaining healthy cognition throughout a lifetime. The same factors that have been discussed earlier in this chapter related to CVD also apply to brain health and cognition. Factors such as maintenance of a healthy body weight, regular physical activity at the levels recommended by the PAGA 2018, and healthy dietary patterns all play a role in lowering the risk of dementia and maintaining cognitive health. As in other chronic diseases and, in particular, in CVD, a healthy diet such as Mediterranean diet and the DASH diet as well as the Healthy U.S.-Style Dietary Pattern all are appropriate for lowering the risk of dementia and increasing and maintaining cognitive function. A combination of the Mediterranean and DASH diets has been called the "MIND" diet and also has been shown to decrease the risk of dementia [52]. This diet maintains similar recommendations for healthy, nutrient-dense components of the healthy diets that are emphasized throughout this book.

4.7 LIFESTYLE MEDICINE AND PEDIATRICS

While a detailed discussion of lifestyle medicine in children is beyond the scope of this book, it should be noted that many of the conditions that manifest themselves in adults have their roots in childhood. In particular, there has been a dramatic increase in the prevalence of overweight and obesity in children [53] and a corresponding increase in the presence of T2DM, dyslipidemia, and hypertension [54,55].

The same lifestyle medicine modalities that apply to adults also apply to children. It is particularly important to note that eating and physical activity habits of children often reflect those of their parents. Thus, it is never too early to institute heart-healthy nutrition, physical activity, and weight management. Good information on physical activity in children can be found in the PAGA 2018, whereas nutritional guidance may be found in the 2020–2025 DGA. It has been recommended by the American Academy of Pediatrics and others that issues of nutrition, physical activity, and weight management be discussed in the family setting.

4.8 CONCLUSIONS

While this book focuses on the critically important area of nutrition and health, it is important to place nutrition in the context of an overall healthy lifestyle. In Chapter 25 the specific components of lifestyle modalities including physical activity, weight management, stress reduction, sleep, avoiding tobacco products, and positive interrelations with other people are all discussed. In this chapter we close the loop by discussing how those modalities specifically relate to the risk factors for major metabolic diseases including CVD, T2DM, obesity, cancer, and dementia or decreased brain health. Thus, a comprehensive approach to lowering risk factors of various metabolic disease includes not only the prominent role of nutrition but also nutrition placed in the context of other positive lifestyle habits and actions.

Clinical Applications

- Multiple lifestyle factors, in addition to nutrition, significantly impact on various metabolic diseases.
- Clinicians should discuss the importance of an overall healthy approach to lifestyle habits and actions in every patient encounter.
- Positive lifestyle habits and practices can help reduce the risk of major metabolic diseases including CVD, T2DM and prediabetes, obesity, cancer, and dementia.

REFERENCES

1. Rippe J. Lifestyle Medicine, 3rd edition. Boca Raton: CRC Press, 2019.
2. US Department of Health and Human Service. National Heart Lung and Blood Institute, National Institutes of Health. Third Report of the Expert Panel on Detection, Evaluation, and Treatment of High Blood Cholesterol in Adults (Adult Treatment Panel III). Washington, DC: National Academic Press, 2004.
3. Gidding S, Lichtenstein A, Faith M, et al. Implementing American Heart Association pediatric and adult nutrition guidelines: A scientific statement from the American Heart Association Nutrition Committee of the Council on Nutrition, Physical Activity and Metabolism, Council on Cardiovascular Disease in the Young, Council on Arteriosclerosis, Thrombosis and Vascular Biology, Council on Cardiovascular Nursing, Council on Epidemiology and Prevention, and Council for High Blood Pressure Research. Circulation. 2009;119:1161–1175.
4. Lloyd-Jones D, Hong Y, Labarthe D, et al. Defining and setting national goals for cardiovascular health promotion and disease reduction: The American Heart Association's strategic impact goal through 2020 and beyond. Circulation. 2010;121:586–613.
5. Eyre H, Kahn R, Robertson R, et al. Preventing cancer, cardiovascular disease, and diabetes: A common agenda for the American Cancer Society, the American Diabetes Association, and the American Heart Association. Circulation. 2004;109:3244–3255.
6. Gorelick P, Furie K, Iadecola C, et al. Defining optimal brain health in adults: A presidential advisory from the American Heart Association/American Stroke Association. Stroke. 2017;48:e284–e303.
7. Physical Activity Guidelines Advisory Committee. 2018 Physical Activity Guidelines Advisory Committee Scientific Report. Washington, DC: U.S. Department of Health and Human Services, 2018.
8. Thorp A, Owen N, Neuhaus M, et al. Sedentary behaviors and subsequent health outcomes in adults a systematic review of longitudinal studies, 1996–2011. Am J Prev Med. 2011;41(2):207–215.
9. Proper K, Singh A, van Mechelen W, et al. Sedentary behaviors and health outcomes among adults: A systematic review of prospective studies. Am J Prev Med. 2011;40(2):174–182.
10. Wilmot E, Edwardson C, Achana F, et al. Sedentary time in adults and the association with diabetes, cardiovascular disease and death: Systematic review and meta-analysis. Diabetologia. 2012;55(11):2895–2905.
11. Chau J, Grunseit A, Chey T, et al. Daily sitting time and all-cause mortality: A meta-analysis. PLoS One. 2013;8(11):e80000.
12. Lichtenstein A, Appel L, Vadiveloo M, et al. 2021 Dietary guidance to improve cardiovascular health: A scientific statement From the American Heart Association. Circulation. 2021;144(23):e472–e487.

13. Centers for Disease Control and Prevention. Physical activity. Guidelines and Recommendations. www.cdc.gov/physicalactivity/index.html (Accessed October 27, 2023).
14. Stone N, Robinson J, Lichtenstein A, et al. 2013 ACC/AHA guideline on the treatment of blood cholesterol to reduce atherosclerotic cardiovascular risk in adults: A report of the American College of Cardiology/American Heart Association Task Force on Practice Guidelines. Circulation. 2014;129(25 Suppl 2):S1–S45.
15. American Diabetes Association. Classification and diagnosis of diabetes: Standards of medical care in diabetes—2018. Diabetes Care. 2018;41(Suppl 1):S13–S27.
16. U.S. Department of Agriculture and U.S. Department of Health and Human Services. *Dietary Guidelines for Americans, 2020–2025*, 9th edition. December 2020. DietaryGuidelines.gov. 2020; www.dietaryguidelines.gov/resources/2020-2025-dietary-guidelines-online-materials
17. Writing Group M, Mozaffarian D, Benjamin EJ, Go AS, Arnett DK, Blaha MJ, et al. Heart disease and stroke statistics-2016 update: A report from the American Heart Association. Circulation. 2016;133(4):e38–e360. Epub 2015/12/18.
18. Whelton PK, Carey RM, Aronow WS, et al. 2017 ACC/AHA/AAPA/ABC/ACPM/AGS/APhA/ASH/ASPC/NMA/PCNA guideline for the prevention, detection, evaluation, and management of high blood pressure in adults: A report of the American College of Cardiology/American Heart Association Task Force on Clinical Practice Guidelines. J Am Coll Cardiol. 2018;71:e127–e248.
19. National Center for Health Statistics. Health, United States, 2016: With Chartbook on Long-Term Trends in Healthy. Hyattsville, MD: National Center for Health Statistics, 2017.
20. Jensen M, Ryan D, Apovian C, et al. 2013 AHA/ACC/TOS guideline for the management of overweight and obesity in adults: A report of the American College of Cardiology/American Heart Association Task Force on Practice Guidelines and The Obesity Society. J Am Coll Cardiol. 2014;63(25 Pt B):2985–3023.
21. Jha P, Ramasundarahettig C, Landsman V, et al. 21st-century hazards of smoking and benefits of cessation in the United States. N Engl J Med. 2013;368:341–350.
22. Adams P, Kirzinger W, Martinez M. Summary health statistics for the US population: National Health Interview Survey, 2012. Vital Health Stat 10. 2013;259:1–95.
23. Centers for Disease Control and Prevention. Smoking and Tobacco Use: Data and Statistics. www.cdc.gov/tobacco/data_statistics/index.htm (Accessed October 19, 2023).
24. US Department of Health and Human Services. The Health Consequences of Smoking: 50 Years of Progress. A Report of the Surgeon General. Atlanta, GA: US Department of Health and Human Services, Centers for Disease Control and Prevention, National Center for Chronic Disease Prevention and Health Promotion, Office of Smoking and Health, 2014.
25. Centers for Disease Control and Prevention. National Center for Health Statistics. Healthy People 2020. Healthy People—Healthy People 2020 (cdc.gov) (Accessed October 19, 2023).
26. Halligan K, Campagna A. Indoor air quality. In Rippe JM (ed). Lifestyle Medicine, 4th edition. Boca Raton: CRC Press, 2024.
27. Gaulditz K, von Lindenberger B, Strohle A. A physical activity and anxiety. In Rippe JM (ed). Lifestyle Medicine, 3rd edition. Boca Raton: CRC Press, 2019.
28. Fair K, Rethorst C. Physical activity and depression. In Rippe JM (ed). Lifestyle Medicine, 3rd edition. Boca Raton: CRC Press, 2019.
29. Chobanian A, Bakris G, Black H, et al. The seventh report of the joint national committee on prevention, detection, evaluation, and treatment of high blood pressure: The JNC 7 report. JAMA. 2003;289(19):2560–2572.

30. Miller M, Stone N, Ballantye C, et al. Triglycerides and cardiovascular disease: A Scientific Statement from the American Heart Association. Circulation. 2011; 123:2292–2333.
31. Franz MJ. Lifestyle therapies for the management of diabetes. In: Rippe JM (ed). Lifestyle Medicine, 3rd edition. Boca Raton: CRC Press, 2019.
32. National Cholesterol Education Program Expert Panel on Detection Evaluation. Treatment of High Blood Cholesterol in Adults. Third Report of the National Cholesterol Education Program (NCEP) Expert Panel on Detection, Evaluation, and Treatment of High Blood Cholesterol in Adults (Adult Treatment Panel III) final report. Circulation. 2002;106(25):3143–3421.
33. American Diabetes Association. Professional Practice Committee: Standards of medical care in diabetes—2018. Diabetes Care. 2018;41(Suppl 1):S3.
34. Guthrie G. Implementing nutritional lifestyle treatment programs in type 2 diabetes. In Rippe JM (ed). Lifestyle Medicine, 3rd edition. Boca Raton: CRC Press, 2019.
35. Alberti K, Zimmet P, Shaw J. Metabolic syndrome—a new world-wide definition: A Consensus statement from the international diabetes federation. Diabet Med. 2006;23(5):469–480.
36. The Diabetes Prevention Program (DPP) Research Group. The Diabetes Prevention Program (DPP): Description of lifestyle intervention. Diabetes Care. 2002;25:2165–2171.
37. Pan X, Li G, Hu Y, et al. Effects of diet and exercise in preventing NIDDM in people with impaired glucose tolerance: The Da Qing IGT and Diabetes Study. Diabetes Care. 1997;20:537–544.
38. Lindström J, Louheranta A, Mannelin M, et al. Finnish diabetes prevention study group. The Finnish Diabetes Prevention Study (DPS): Lifestyle intervention and 3-year results on diet and physical activity. Diabetes Care. 2003;26:3230–3236.
39. Ruiz-Canela M, Estruch R, Corella D, et al. Association of Mediterranean diet with peripheral artery disease: The PREDIMED randomized trial. JAMA. 2014;311(4):415–417.
40. Sacks F, Svetkey L, Vollmer W, et al. Effects on blood pressure of reduced dietary sodium and the Dietary Approaches to Stop Hypertension (DASH) diet. DASH-Sodium Collaborative Research Group. N Engl J Med. 2001;344(1):3–10.
41. Inzucchi SE, Bergenstal RM, et al. Management of hyperglycemia in type 2 diabetes, 2015: A patient-centered approach: Update to a position statement of the American Diabetes Association and the European Association for the Study of Diabetes. Diabetes Care. 2015;38(1):140–149.
42. Colberg S, Sigal R, Yardley J, et al. Physical activity/exercise and diabetes: A position statement of the American Diabetes Association. Diabetes Care. 2016;39:2065–2079.
43. Hall K, Heymsfield S, Kemnitz J, et al. Energy balance and its components: Implications for body weight regulation. Am J Clin Nutr. 2012;95:989–994.
44. Heymsfield S, Wadden T. Mechanisms, pathophysiology, and management of obesity. N Engl J Med. 2017;376(3):254–266.
45. Jakicic J, Rogers R, Collins K. Exercise management for the obese patient. Chapter 37 In Rippe JM (ed). Lifestyle Medicine, 3rd edition. Boca Raton: CRC Press, 2019.
46. Doll R, Peto R. The causes of cancer: Quantitative estimates of avoidable risks of cancer in the United States today. J Natl Cancer Inst. 1981;66:1191–1308.
47. World Cancer Research Fund; American Institute for Cancer Research. Food, Nutrition, Physical Activity and the Prevention of Cancer: A Global Perspective. Washington, DC: American Institute for Cancer Research, 2007.
48. Keltner C, Bowles H. Physical activity and the prevention and treatment of cancer. In Rippe JM (ed). Lifestyle Medicine, 3rd edition. Boca Raton: CRC Press, 2019.

49. National Cancer Institute. About Cancer: Physical Activity and Cancer. www.cancer.gov/about-cancer/causesprevention-causes/prevention/risk/obesity/physical-activityfact-sheet (Accessed October 27, 2023).
50. Gonçalves A, Dantas Florencio G, Maisonnette de Atayde Silva M, et al. Effects of physical activity on breast cancer prevention: A systematic review. J Phys Act Health. 2014;11:445–454.
51. Monninkhof E, Elias S, Vlems F, et al. Physical activity and breast cancer: A systematic review. Epidemiology. 2007;18:137–157.
52. Morris M, Tangney C, Wang Y, et al. MIND diet associated with reduced incidence of Alzheimer's disease. Alzheimer Dement: J Alzheimer Assoc. 2015;11(9):1007–1014.
53. Kaar J, Simon S. Sleep and obesity prevention in children and adolescents. In Rippe JM (ed). Lifestyle Medicine, 3rd edition. Boca Raton: CRC Press, 2019.
54. Brothers J, Daniels S. Identification and management of children with dyslipidemia. In Rippe JM (ed). Lifestyle Medicine, 3rd edition. Boca Raton: CRC Press, 2019.
55. Baker-Smith C, Gidding S. Diagnosis, management, and treatment of systemic hypertension in youth, updates from the 2017 American Academy of Pediatrics Clinical Practice guideline. In Rippe JM (ed). Lifestyle Medicine, 3rd edition. Boca Raton: CRC Press, 2019.

5 The Role of Physicians and Other Healthcare Workers in Incorporating Healthy Nutrition and Other Lifestyle Medicine Concepts

Key Points

- Poor diet is a key factor in virtually every metabolically based chronic disease including cardiovascular disease, type 2 diabetes, obesity, metabolic syndrome, and cancer.
- National guidelines from multiple prestigious organizations including the American Heart Association, World Health Organization, *Dietary Guidelines for Americans 2020–2025*, and the Academy of Nutrition and Dietetics all consistently recommend healthy diets as a way of lowering the risk of chronic disease.
- Physician education in nutrition is currently at extremely low levels.
- Multiple initiatives are underway to help physicians achieve higher levels of nutritional knowledge.
- Clinicians should counsel patients at every clinical encounter on the high importance of healthy nutrition for good health.

5.1 INTRODUCTION

There is no longer any serious doubt that nutrition significantly impacts chronic diseases [1,2]. In fact, seven out of the ten leading causes of death around the world have a nutrition- or alcohol-related component [3]. Poor nutrition is associated with leading causes of death including cardiovascular disease (CVD), type 2 diabetes mellitus (T2DM), obesity, metabolic syndrome (MetS), and many cancers.

For this reason, healthy nutrition, as discussed in multiple chapters in this book, serves as the cornerstone for both prevention and treatment guidelines from virtually every major medical and healthcare association that deals with metabolic disease including the World Health Organization (WHO) [3], American Heart Association (AHA) [4], American Diabetes Association (ADA) [5], and many others.

DOI: 10.1201/9781003452607-5

Among the top 17 risk factors identified by the U.S. Burden of Disease Collaborators, poor diet is listed as the leading cause of premature death and disabilities in the United States [6]. Multiple cohort studies and randomized control trials have shown that poor nutrition increases the risk of chronic disease, while healthy nutrition lowers the risk. For this reason, healthy diets that are high in fruits and vegetables and whole grains and low in saturated fats, red meats, processed meats, salt, and sugar are recommended by virtually every prestigious medical organization including the Dietary Guidelines for Americans (DGA) 2020–2025, 2021 [7] and nutrition recommendations from the AHA [4] and the Centers for Disease Control and Prevention (CDC) [8].

Despite overwhelming evidence that diet impacts on chronic disease, the likelihood that physicians will be educated in this area at any point in their training is woefully low. In fact, only 20% of medical schools have any nutritional courses [9], and 93% of graduates of medical schools in the United States feel that they do not have adequate training in nutrition [10].

Even in the area of cardiovascular medicine, which has been a leader in the area of the relationship between nutrition and health, over 90% of cardiologists report receiving minimal education during fellowship training, and only 8% describe themselves as having "expert" nutrition knowledge [11]. This, despite the fact that over 95% of cardiologists believe that their role includes providing patients with at least basic nutrition information [11]. Furthermore, both the 2013 Practice Guidelines from the AHA and the American College of Cardiology (ACC) recommend nutrition counseling as a key component of the practice of cardiology [12].

In addition, the recently released Guidelines for Lipid Management [13] as well as Detection and Management of High Blood Pressure [14] from the AHA and ACC both strongly recommend dietary intervention as a key component of managing these CVD risk factors.

While some progress has been made in the last five years, there still is a dearth of effective education in the area of nutrition for physicians at all levels of training. This is unfortunate, given that over 70% of individuals see their primary care physician at least once a year and over 60% of patients feel that they do not receive adequate nutritional counseling from their physician [15]. This is particularly disheartening, given that physician recommendation in multiple surveys has been shown to be the leading prompt for behavior change in multiple areas including nutrition.

The purpose of this chapter is to discuss the current state of nutrition education for physicians and recommend some potential changes to improve this important issue.

5.2 THE ROLE OF NUTRITION IN EVIDENCE-BASED GUIDELINES

Multiple organizations have released evidence-based guidelines for what constitutes either "healthy" or "unhealthy" nutrition [16]. The DGA 2020–2025, 2021 AHA diet recommendations, and recommendations from the Academy of Nutrition and Dietetics [17] all call for diets that are high in fruits and vegetables and whole grains, fiber, oily fish, polyunsaturated fatty acids (PUFAs), and monounsaturated fatty acids (MUFAs), while decreasing red meat, processed meats, saturated fats, added sugars, and salt. All of these guidelines also recommend consuming calories at a level to maintain a healthy weight and also include other lifestyle-related recommendations including regular physical activity.

Nutrition research now focuses on overall healthy dietary patterns. Dietary patterns that have been shown to be healthy include the Dietary Approach to Stop Hypertension (DASH) [18], Mediterranean diet [19], the Healthy U.S.-Style Dietary Plans recommended by the AHA, the Nordic diet [20], and many vegetarian diets.

5.3 CURRENT LEVELS OF PHYSICIAN KNOWLEDGE IN NUTRITION

A recent survey of over 1,000 physicians revealed that only 13.5% agreed or strongly agreed that they were adequately trained to discuss nutrition with their patients [20]. A significant majority (78.4%) thought additional training in nutrition would help them provide better clinical care in the prevention of CVD. When physicians were asked to rate the importance of different therapies in CVD on a scale of 1–10 (with 10 being the most important), respondents rated nutrition at 8.1 ± 2.05 and physical activity at 8.2 ± 1.56, which were both higher than statins (7.8 ± 2.11).

It is interesting and somewhat disconcerting that physicians' views of the importance of nutrition counseling diminished significantly during the course of training. In one survey 72% of the students reported nutritional counseling to be highly relevant in their first year, but only 46% did in their final year of training [21]. The lack of training and declining interest in nutrition are further complicated by the fact that there are no nutrition requirements in internal medicine residency or CVD fellowships. This leaves students, residents, and fellows with minimal motivation to seek additional nutritional training.

When it comes to specific dietary plans, in one survey physicians commonly reported that they recommended the Mediterranean diet (55.1%), followed closely by the low-fat diet (40.4%), the DASH diet (38.2%), low glycemic index diet (18.2%), and low-carbohydrate diet (16.4%) [22]. It is interesting that 16% of physicians did not recommend a specific diet for their patients.

The majority of physicians (57.7%) spent three minutes or less counseling patients about diet and lifestyle to prevent CVD during a routine appointment. Of note, less than half of physicians understood that a low-fat diet was not demonstrated to lower the risk of CVD. In contrast, it is encouraging to know that almost 90% of physicians (89.7%) knew the Mediterranean diet reduced CVD events in randomized control trials. Knowledge regarding blood pressure–lowering effects of fruits and vegetables and low-density lipoprotein cholesterol–lowering effects of soluble fiber was good (81.7% and 87.6%, respectively). However, only 69.5% could identify foods high in soluble fiber and only 30.8% could identify omega-3–rich fish.

5.4 NUTRITION EDUCATION FOR PHYSICIANS

There are missed opportunities to train physicians in the area of nutrition, which is evident at every stage of medical education [23]:

- **Medical School**—Medical school, which is formally referred to as "undergraduate medical education" (UME), is the first stage in medical education. U.S. medical schools offer an average of 19 hours total nutritional education over four years. However, much of this is devoted to nonclinical topics such as biochemistry. The primary accrediting body for medical education in the United States, the Liaison Committee on Medical Education (LCME), does not mention nutrition education in its medical school accreditation standards, which sends the message that nutrition education is not regarded by this committee as important to the overall educational experience in medical schools.
- **Residency/Fellowship**—Residency/fellowship trainings are known as "graduate medical education" (GME). This is the stage of medical education that includes both clinical and didactic training requirements for physicians in their chosen specialty area such as internal medicine, pediatrics, and surgery, as well as subspecialty trainings (e.g. cardiology, gastroenterology, etc.). The national accrediting body for GME programs, the American Council of Graduate Medical Education (ACGME), does not require competency in diet and nutrition for accreditation of GME programs. In fact, ACGME has no reference to "food" or "diet" or "nutrition" in the common program requirements which apply to all GME programs or most specialty requirements for residents or fellows.
- **Step and Board Exams**—Prospective physicians must take three medical licensing "step" exams to become licensed physicians. Two occur during UME and the third during GME. Medical students must pass all three step exams to continue their medical education. These exams are cosponsored by the National Board of Medical Examiners (NBME) and the Federation of State Medical Boards (FSMB). In addition, physicians who opt to pursue specialty training must take a specialty-specific board exam in order to achieve board certification. This process is managed by the American Board of Medical Specialties (ABMS). Both the step and board exams do not contain questions to test whether or not a physician understands and can advise on general prevention of diet-related diseases and promotion of a healthy diet.
- **Continuing Medical Education**—Continuing medical education (CME) requirements are generally set by each state, which define the number of hours and topic areas that physicians and other healthcare professionals must take in CME courses in order to maintain licensure. The only state or district that has any requirements in the area that encompasses nutrition is the District of Columbia, which requires that 10% of total CME hours must be in topics identified as "public health priorities." One of these topics is nutrition and obesity prevention.

5.5 PUBLIC POLICY TOOLS TO ENHANCE NUTRITION EDUCATION FOR PHYSICIANS

The lack of knowledge and education in the area of nutrition for physicians has drawn considerable interest in whether or not public policy tools might be available to enhance nutrition education for physicians. While a variety of remedial efforts have been proposed, most involve such efforts as amending educational requirements at all levels of medical education to require nutrition education. In addition, there has been some suggestion that grant funding should involve the requirement of inclusion of nutrition education [24].

Other suggestions include such initiatives as conditioning Medicare/Medicaid and other funding on inclusion of nutrition in medical education. This could be a powerful mechanism, since the federal government provides the lion's share of funding for GME programs. In fact, training hospitals that support GME residents rely almost exclusively on federal funds. Given that Medicare patients, who are typically individuals over the age of 65, are at increased risk of suffering from diseases caused by diet, this could be a powerful incentive to include nutrition education as a component of GME education [25]. In fact, in one recent study a very modest shift in American diets on this population could result in savings of between 16.7 and 31.5 billion dollars per year in healthcare costs. Thus, an investment in nutrition education could result in substantial savings due to an improved diet yielding better health outcomes as evidence that this money would be well-spent.

5.6 CASE STUDY: NUTRITION EDUCATION AND THE PRACTICE OF CARDIOLOGY

As indicated in multiple other chapters in this book, nutrition is a key foundation of multiple guidelines for CVD risk reduction and treatment. However, even cardiologists whose professional organizations strongly support the importance of nutrition are often not adequately educated in this area.

A recent survey showed that 31% of cardiologists and 21% of cardiology fellows in training did not recall receiving any nutrition education during medical school. During internal medicine residency training, 60% of cardiologists did not recall receiving any nutritional lectures, while 9% recalled only a single lecture and 6% reported a series of nutritional lectures.

During cardiology fellowship training, 90% of cardiologists reported receiving no or minimum nutrition education, only 8% had a "solid" nutrition education, and only 1% reported a "high level" of nutrition education gave them excellent skills for counseling patients [11]. Following cardiovascular fellowship, 56% of cardiologists described receiving no formal education in nutrition, and 20% received two hours or more per year. On the positive side, 53% of cardiologists reported that they were likely to participate in an online series of webinars discussing nutrition and lifestyle if offered.

This surprising lack of nutrition education contrasts with attitudes that most cardiologists display. In this same survey a total of 89% of cardiologists and 87% of fellows in training believed that "dietary interventions are likely to provide substantial benefits to patients with cardiovascular disease who adhere to guideline based therapy" [11]. Moreover, 95% of cardiologists believe their role includes personally providing patients with at least basic nutrition intervention. As already indicated, however, 90% of cardiologists reported they do not have adequate training to provide this.

With regard to personal health habits, 74% of cardiologists who ate five servings or more of fruits and vegetables per day felt that their role personally included delivering detailed dietary information [26], whereas only 51% of those who ate one to two servings of fruits and vegetables agreed with that statement. With regard to nutrition counseling in patients, 4% of cardiologists reported not discussing nutrition, 18% reported spending a minute or less on nutrition, and 40% spent two to three minutes per visit.

The lack of nutrition education for cardiologists is all the more surprising, given the 2013 ACC/AHA Guidelines for the Treatment of Blood Cholesterol to Reduce Atherosclerotic Cardiovascular Risk in Adults and Cardiovascular Guidelines also issued that year include nutritional counseling as an important component of CVD risk reduction.

5.7 CURRENT INITIATIVES

Given the paucity of nutrition education for physicians, there is at least some encouraging news that a number of initiatives are now in progress to try to help ameliorate this significant problem. These include the following:

- **White House Conference on Hunger, Nutrition and Health**—This conference, which was held in late September 2022, announced over $8 billion as part of a call to action to the White House Conference on Hunger, Nutrition and Health [27]. The leading elected official behind this initiative is Congressman James McGovern. In an editorial in the *American Journal of Clinical Nutrition* he stated that "the key outcome of the conference must be amelioration of the dismal state of medical education in the area of nutrition" [28].
- **CDC Foundation**—Following the previously referenced White House Conference on Hunger, Nutrition and Health, the CDC Foundation dedicated several staff members to specifically look at the areas of hunger, nutrition, and physician education [29].
- **AAMC and ACGME**—In response to the conference, the AAMC and ACGME committed to organizing and hosting a Medical Education Summit on Nutritional Practices in March 2023. This initiative was intended to convene 150 medical education leaders from across medical schools, residency training, and continuing education programs with the goal of determining the best strategies for integrating nutrition and food insecurity into medical education curriculum with a focus on interprofessional care and health equity [29].
- **American College of Lifestyle Medicine (ACLM)**—In response to the White House Conference on Hunger, Nutrition and Health, the ACLM made an in-kind contribution of $24.1 million to improve nutrition training for medical professionals. This included donating 5.5 hours of CME course credits on nutrition and "food is medicine" topics for 100,000 healthcare providers in areas with high rates of diet-related disease [30].

- **Various Curricula**—Various curricula on lifestyle medicine in general and nutrition in particular have been developed and are available free of charge on the internet. One of these curricula from the University of South Carolina deals with the general area of lifestyle medicine [31]. The other curricula developed by a team at the Gable Institute offers nutrition education for physicians free of charge [32].
- **Food Is Medicine Movement** [33]—The Coalition of Nonprofit Organizations offers nutrition education for all healthcare providers, including physicians.

5.8 OPPORTUNITIES FOR IMPROVEMENT

Given the low level of nutrition education currently available for physicians at all levels of training, it is imperative that further efforts be undertaken to address this problem. The good news is that there is a high level of interest among physicians and commensurate enthusiasm for participating in more nutrition education.

It is hoped that this level of interest as well as the multiple initiatives that have been stimulated by the White House Conference on Hunger, Nutrition and Health will address the issue of nutrition counseling by physicians. The physician community has a history of responding positively to major health problems. For example, the physician community was very instrumental in helping to reduce the prevalence of cigarette smoking.

There seems to be more interest and knowledge of physical activity among physicians at the current time. In fact, in one survey 89% of residents were familiar with the importance of physical activity and were willing to recommend it to their patients.

The opportunities in this area are great. At the current time less than 40% of physicians counsel their patients in areas of physical activity, obesity management, and nutrition. This is a wasted opportunity because 70% of individuals see their primary care physician on at least an annual basis [34]. Moreover, in multiple surveys physician recommendation has been shown to be the most powerful motivator to elicit behavioral change [34].

5.9 CONCLUSIONS

There is a strong linkage between dietary habits and the likelihood of developing chronic disease. This spans virtually every metabolic disease including CVD, T2DM, obesity, MetS, cancers, and even dementia. Given the power and importance of nutrition in these areas, it is unfortunate that physician education to deliver nutrition counseling is woefully small. There is some hope, however, given the high level of interest that physicians have in this area and the multiple initiatives that are currently being undertaken to help address this problem.

Clinical Applications

- Clinicians should counsel all patients in the area of the importance of healthy nutrition to lower the risk of chronic metabolically based disease.
- Multiple opportunities exist for physicians to enhance their knowledge in the area of nutrition.
- It is imperative that physicians play a more active role in this area, given the importance of nutrition to combat various chronic diseases.

REFERENCES

1. Rippe J , Angelopoulos TJ. Obesity and health. In Rippe JM (ed). Lifestyle Medicine, 3rd edition. Boca Raton: CRC Press, 2019.
2. Rippe J. Lifestyle medicine: The health promoting power of daily habits and practices. Am J Lifestyle Med. 2018;12(6):499–512.
3. World Health Organization. Noncommunicable Diseases. (who.int) (Accessed June 9, 2023).
4. Lichtenstein A, Appel L, Vadiveloo M, et al. 2021 Dietary guidance to improve cardiovascular health: A scientific statement from the American Heart Association. Circulation. 2021;144(23):e472–e487.
5. Clark A, Raine K, Raphael D. The American Cancer Society, American Diabetes Association, and American Heart Association Joint Statement on Preventing Cancer, Cardiovascular Disease, and Diabetes: Where are the social determinants? Diabetes Care. 2004;27(12):3024.
6. Murray C, Atkinson C, Bhalla K, et al. The state of US health, 1990–2010: Burden of diseases, injuries, and risk factors. JAMA. 2013;310(6):591–608.
7. U.S. Department of Agriculture and U.S. Department of Health and Human Services. *Dietary Guidelines for Americans, 2020–2025*, 9th edition. December 2020. DietaryGuidelines.gov. 2020; www.dietaryguidelines.gov/resources/2020-2025-dietary-guidelines-online-materials (Accessed June 9, 2023).
8. Centers for Disease Control and Prevention. Nutrition. www.cdc.gov/nutrition/index.html (Accessed June 9, 2023).
9. Touger-Decker R, Barracato JM, O'Sullivan-Maillet J. Nutrition education in health professions programs: A survey of dental, physician assistant, nurse practitioner, and nurse midwifery programs. J Am Diet Assoc. 2001;101(1):63–69.
10. Kris-Etherton PM, Akabas SR, Bales CW, et al. The need to advance nutrition education in the training of health care professionals and recommended research to evaluate implementation and effectiveness. Am J Clin Nutri. 2014;99(Suppl 5):1153S–1166S.
11. Devries S, Agatston A, Aggarwal M, et al. A deficiency of nutrition education and practice in cardiology. Am J Med. 2017;130(11):1298–1305.
12. O'Gara P, Kushner F, Ascheim D, et al. 2013 ACCF/AHA guideline for the management of ST-elevation myocardial infarction: A report of the American College of Cardiology Foundation/American Heart Association task force on practice guidelines. Circulation. 2013;127(4):e362–e425.
13. Grundy S, Stone N, Bailey A, et al. 2018 AHA/ACC/AACVPR/AAPA/ABC/ACPM/ADA/AGS/APhA/ASPC/NLA/PCNA Guideline on the management of blood cholesterol: A report of the American College of Cardiology/American Heart Association Task Force on clinical practice guidelines. J Am Coll Cardiol. 2019;73(24):e285–e350. Epub 2018/11/14.
14. Whelton P, Carey R, Aronow W, et al. 2017 ACC/AHA/AAPA/ABC/ACPM/AGS/APhA/ASH/ASPC/NMA/PCNA guideline for the prevention, detection, evaluation, and management of high blood pressure in adults: Executive summary: A report of the American College of Cardiology/American Heart Association Task Force on clinical practice guidelines. Hypertension. 2018;71(6):1269–1324. Epub 2017/11/15.
15. Ha J, Longnecker N. Doctor-patient communication: A review. Ochsner J. 2010;10(1): 38–43.
16. Cordola Hsu AR, Xie B, Peterson D, et al. Metabolically healthy/unhealthy overweight/obesity associations with incident heart failure in postmenopausal women: The women's health initiative. Circ Heart Fail. 2021;14(4):e007297.
17. Melina V, Craig W, Levin S. Position of the academy of nutrition and dietetics: Vegetarian diets. J Acad Nutr Diet. 2016;116(12):1970–1980.

18. Sacks F, Svetkey L, Vollmer W, et al. Effects on blood pressure of reduced dietary sodium and the Dietary Approaches to Stop Hypertension (DASH) diet. DASH-Sodium Collaborative Research Group. N Engl J Med. 2001;344(1):3–10.
19. Estruch R, Ros E, Salas-Salvado J, et al. Primary prevention of cardiovascular disease with a Mediterranean diet. N Engl J Med. 2013;368(14):1279–1290.
20. Kushner R. Barriers to providing nutrition counseling by physicians: A survey of primary care practitioners. Prev Med. 1995;24(6):546–552.
21. Kushner R, Van Horn L, Rock C, et al. Nutrition education in medical school: A time of opportunity. Am J Clin Nutri. 2014;99(Suppl 5):1167S–1173S.
22. Russell NK, Roter DL. Health promotion counseling of chronic-disease patients during primary care visits. Am J Public Health. 1993;83(7):979–982.
23. Aspry K, Van Horn L, Carson J, et al. Medical nutrition education, training, and competencies to advance guideline-based diet counseling by physicians: A science advisory from the American Heart Association. Circulation. 2018;137(23):e821–e841.
24. Broad Leib E. Doctoring our Diet: Policy Tools to Include Nutrition in U.S. Medical Training. Harvard Law School Food Law and Policy Clinic, 2019. https://chlpi.org/wp-content/uploads/2013/12/Doctoring-Our-Diet_-September-2019-V2.pdf (Accessed June 9, 2023).
25. US National Research Council Committee on Nutrition in Medical Education. Nutrition Education in U.S. Medical Schools. Washington, DC: National Academy Press, 1985.
26. Frank E, Segura C, Shen H, et al. Predictors of Canadian physicians' prevention counseling practices. Can J Public Health = Revue Canadienne de Sante Publique. 2010;101(5):390–395.
27. White House Conference on Hunger, Nutrition, & Health. U.S. Department of Health and Human Services. September, 2022. Ending Hunger and Reducing Diet-Related Diseases and Disparities | health.gov (Accessed June 9, 2023).
28. McGovern C. As White House conference approaches, now is the time for a national plan to address the link between hunger, nutrition education, and health. Am J Clin Nutri. 2022;116(4):841–842.
29. McGovern Resolution on Nutrition Education in Medical Schools Passes House. Press Release. Washington, DC, May 17, 2022. https://mcgovern.house.gov/news/documentsingle.aspx?DocumentID=398867 (Accessed July 5, 2023).
30. American College of Lifestyle Medicine. https://lifestylemedicine.org/ (Accessed June 9, 2023).
31. South Carolina Curriculum Standards. Columbia, SC. https://ed.sc.gov/instruction/standards/ (Accessed June 9, 2023).
32. Gaples Institute. www.gaplesinstitute.org/ (Accessed June 9, 2023).
33. Food is Medicine. A collaboration of the American Heart Association and the Rockefeller Foundation. www.heart.org/en/professional/food-is-medicine-initiative/ (Accessed June 9, 2023).
34. Kennedy M. What physicians need to know, do and say to promote physical activity. In Rippe JM (ed). Lifestyle Medicine, 3rd edition. Boca Raton: CRC Press, 2019.

6 Nutrition and Health Equity

Key Points

- Social determinations of health (SDOH) are responsible for most health inequalities.
- SDOH issues can result in overall inequities in both physical and mental health.
- Nutrition inequalities play a significant role in SDOH and may be particularly amenable to both individual and government action.

6.1 INTRODUCTION

Multiple diverse factors impact on health, perhaps none more so than SDOH, which have been clearly demonstrated to impact on health equity [1–4]. These issues were brought into stark focus during the COVID-19 pandemic when individuals from some disadvantaged groups were found to be three to four times as likely to have severe infections and die from COVID-19 compared to more affluent, advantaged individuals [5]. In particular, individuals in lower socioeconomic status (SES) groups were found to be more at risk for serious complications from COVID-19 than individuals of higher SES [5–7]. Both Black and Hispanic populations were more susceptible to severe adverse responses to COVID-19 compared to more affluent Caucasians.

SDOH are defined as "the conditions in which people are born, grow, work, live, age and the wider set of forces and systems shaping the conditions of daily lives," as articulated in 2018 by the World Health Organization (WHO) [8]. These SDOH are responsible for most health inequalities and also impacted by resource allocation that influences factors at the local, national, and global levels [9]. Abundant evidence gathered over the last 30 years supports the substantial effect that SDOH exerts on both physical and mental health. While many factors impact on SDOH, nutrition is one of the major factors that plays a prominent role [10–15]. Studies measuring adult deaths attributable to SDOH in 2000 found that approximately 240,000 deaths were attributable to low education, 176,000 were due to racial segregation, 162,000 were due to low social support, 133,000 were due to individual-level poverty, and 119,000 were to due income inequality [1,16].

In the United States, health equity has become a critically important issue, and it is imperative that it be addressed not only by the medical profession but also by public policy makers. Despite high affluence in the United States, sizable disparities exist that are related to social, economic, and environmental factors. Shockingly, on average, there is a 15-year difference in life expectancy between the most advantaged

DOI: 10.1201/9781003452607-6

and disadvantaged citizens [17]. This difference correlated with a variety of lifestyle-related factors as well as geographic characteristics.

It has been estimated that population-level inequalities in healthcare result in 309 billion dollars in losses to the economy annually and disproportionately affect disadvantaged populations [18]. Conversely, investment in interventions to address SDOH have been shown to yield positive outcomes. Perhaps there is no more single factor in SDOH that is potentially amendable to amelioration than nutrition [19]. For this reason, multiple public policy initiatives have focused on nutrition and health equity. These will be highlighted in this chapter.

6.2 WHAT IS MEANT BY HEALTH EQUITY?

There has been a great deal of research and discussion about health equity in medicine and public health and research from over the past two decades. The field has been made more complex and perhaps hindered by a variety of definitions of what is meant by the term "health equity."

The Robert Wood Johnson Foundation published a report in 2017 that sought to clarify various definitions of health equity. In general terms, health equity connotes that everyone has a fair and just opportunity to be as healthy as possible [20]. To accomplish this, it is essential to remove obstacles to help, such as poverty and discrimination and their consequences. Also, lack of access to a good-paying job, quality education, housing, healthcare, and safe environments are other factors.

In the area of research, health equity has been defined as reducing and ultimately eliminating disparities in health and determinations of health that adversely affect excluded or marginalized groups. As indicated in this definition, the terms "fairness" and "justice" are employed on a population basis as a means to achieving widely held standards of fairness as well as broader ethical concerns related to human rights, laws, and principles. Rights include not only civil and political rights, such as freedom of speech, assembly, and religion but also social, economic, and cultural rights including rights to education, decent living standards, and freedom of avoidable obstacles to good health.

The concept of being healthy is typically measured by assessing SDOH such as income, wealth, education, neighborhood, characteristics, or social inclusion that people experience across their lives [21–26]. While individual responsibility is important, these concepts recognize that some people lack access to opportunities and resources needed to make healthy choices and that societal action is needed to address these obstacles. Certainly, nutrition fits into this category.

It should be noted that health equity and health disparities are strongly related to each other [2]. Health equity is a human rights principle and motivates people to eliminate health disparities that typically are related to avoidable differences in health that adversely affect marginalized or excluded groups. It should be noted that health equity involves being as healthy as possible but does not include issues such as genetic endowment, which may limit an individual's health potential.

Health equity is based on the concept that an individual can achieve the best health possible for himself or herself [27,28]. Health disparity, in contrast, is considered avoidable if current scientific understandings suggest that better health is possible or could be provided if the adequate political will is present. It is clear that health equity in the broadest sense involves not only healthcare but other social determinants such as poverty, discrimination, and their consequences. These broader issues will also be explored in this chapter through the lens of nutrition and health equity.

6.3 SOCIAL DETERMINATIONS OF HEALTH AND HEALTH EQUITY

While nutrition plays a central role in many of the aspects of SDOH, the field and concept of SDOH are much broader. A recent position paper from the American College of Physicians lists six separate areas that contribute to SDOH. These include socioeconomic status, housing, transportation, food and agriculture, the digital divide, and racial and ethnic health disparities [1].

- Socioeconomic Status
  The primary nonmedical factor affecting health is socioeconomic status. This may be assessed by wealth, education, and occupation. Inequality in the United States has increased markedly since 1980 [29]. The top 1% of earners in the United States earn three times as much as they did in the 1980s, whereas the bottom 50% earn the same average income as they did in 1980. Interestingly, individuals born between 1981 and 1987 have only a 50% chance of earning more than their parents. SES is also linked to racial and ethnic disparities. Excess mortality among African American adults compared to White non-Latino adults is estimated at 38% [30]. In 2016, 14% of the U.S. population had a household income below the federal poverty threshold. African Americans have the highest poverty rate both in metropolitan and non-metropolitan areas (23% and 33%, respectively) [31].

  To compound this problem in the areas of nutrition, neighborhoods with concentrated poverty often lack grocery stores with fresh food (food deserts), adequate public transportation, access to public spaces, adequate employment prospects and access to health care services. Education and employment status also contribute to socioeconomic status. For example, the unemployment rate among persons who have not completed high school is more than 50% [32].
- Housing
  Adequate housing is essential for the basic needs of humans. Not only does adequate housing protect from the elements, but dilapidated housing is associated with exposure to lead as well as asthma triggers such as dust, mold, moisture, and rodents [33]. As was clearly reflected in COVID-19 pandemic, overcrowded living conditions contribute to the spread of airborne diseases. Families or individuals who spend more than 30% of their income on housing are considered to be "cost burdened," and this may contribute to difficulties affording necessities such as food, transportation, and medical care [34]. Individuals are also at higher risk for possible homelessness following eviction. Multiple adverse health consequences and psychological consequences are found in the homeless population [35]. For example, 80% of the homeless population have a marked decline in

cognitive function. The prevalence of tuberculosis is 46 times higher in the homeless population than in the general population. In addition, hepatitis C is four times higher than in the general population when considering the homeless population [36].

- Transportation
Automobiles are the primary source of transportation in the United States. Lack of transportation options significantly increases barriers to healthcare access [37]. This is true particularly for low-income, uninsured, or underinsured persons. Low-income persons and persons of color are more likely to rely on "active transportation" such as walking, bicycling, or public transportation to get to work. Poor, disadvantaged communities also have poorer infrastructure for walking or biking such as sidewalks, street lighting, etc.
- Food and Agriculture
Nutrition and an adequate supply of food are necessary to live a healthy and productive life. This will be dealt with in multiple sections of this chapter. Approximately 11% of households in the United States (25.8 million adults and 12.4 million children) are food insecure [38]. The concept of food insecurity fuels both feelings of hunger and the anxiety of access to food. This may result in unhealthy food behaviors such as skipping meals or consuming low-cost but calorie-dense foods or highly processed foods that have little nutritional value. Food insecurity is also strongly associated with poverty. A significant hurdle for improving access to fresh produce and nutritious food is hindered because of a lack of groceries or supermarkets in areas where there is poverty. These have been called "food deserts." Data from the U.S. Department of Agriculture show that adults who live in food deserts are at increased risk of obesity and diabetes [39].
- The Digital Divide
The digital divide is defined as the gap between those who have access to technology or the internet and those who do not [40]. This is typically based on SES. There has been an increased emphasis in integrating technology into medical care. Thus, the lack of reliable internet access can hinder a person's ability to access medical portals and electronic health records [41]. Thirty-nine percent of rural areas lack reliable access to broadband technologies. Of note, a 2012 survey showed that 21% of uninsured persons do not use the internet, and 59% of uninsured persons do not report seeking health information online.
- Racial and Ethnic Health Disparities
Addressing SDOH also includes increasing health equity among racial and ethnic populations [42,43]. Racial and ethnic issues are interconnected to a variety of other SDOH considerations that may impact a person's health. For example, Latino women are more likely to lack health insurance than White, non-Latino women [44]. African Americans have the highest incidence of cancer burden of any racial or ethnic group for all types of cancer. Furthermore, racism and ethnic discrimination cause unavoidable and unfair inequalities with regard to power and resources as well as opportunities.

6.4 NUTRITION AND HEALTH EQUITY

As already indicated, the term "health equity" according to the WHO involves giving all people the opportunity to reach their full potential regardless of race, education, gender identity, sexual orientation, job, neighborhood location, or disability [8]. Health equity identifies barriers and allocates resources to remove them. A classic example of disparities that harm health equity relates to nutrition. For example, one school in Bibb County in Georgia implemented a standard menu to ensure all students received nutritious meals. Inadequacies, however, existed because some schools did not have either the equipment or staff necessary to prepare this food. To solve this problem and create a more equitable access to a healthy menu, the nutrition program built a centralized kitchen to prepare and cook foods.

It is clear that people with less money, less education, and poor living conditions are more likely to experience food insecurity and have a less healthy eating pattern and higher level of diet-related diseases such as obesity and diabetes [45,46]. Another example relates to food deserts where there are no accessible supermarkets that allow ready access to fresh produce [47]. People have also added the term "food swamps" indicating areas where there is a high ratio of fast food outlets and convenience stores. These convenience stores usually offer significant proportion of high-fat, high-calorie, sugary, salty, and ultra-processed foods which are low in nutritional value. If healthy options are available at convenience stores, prices are typically high, variety is poor, and quality is low. Individuals who are already struggling to make ends meet may not be able to afford more expensive, healthier options. It should also be noted that even when a full service grocery store is placed in a community, there may be difficulties in people changing eating habits since these supermarkets continue to market snacks, sweets, and other nutrient-poor, heavily processed package foods. Thus, it is important to not only have a supermarket available but also teach fundamental skills such as cooking and meal planning as a means of promoting behavior change.

As a strategy to help reduce food disparities and lessen the health equity gap, healthcare, food, and nutritional professionals must recognize that health and illness result from broad social, political, and economic structures. Thus, physicians and other healthcare professionals need to advocate for social justice. For example, as an individual practitioner, the healthcare professional must first acknowledge the presence of structural racism and recognize the impact of poverty and other factors that have already been outlined in this chapter that impact on SDOH. It is important that healthcare professionals also acknowledge that their client's culture can have an impact on food choices as well as their health behavior. Thus, nutrition care plans should be individualized, rather than offering "one size fits all" perspectives such as what a "healthy plate" might look like. Interventions should include nutritious foods that are compatible with the person's culture and are acceptable to them.

Healthcare professionals' interactions with clients and patients must start with screening for food insecurity and other determinants of health. Thus, medical practices and hospitals and clinics should routinely screen patients for food insecurity and partner with local food banks and farmers' markets to offer quality produce and groceries to underserved communities at affordable costs. Multiple stakeholders can be employed in this area including community gardens and social organizations as well as beauty salons and barbershops. With regard to policy, food assistance programs such as the National School Lunch Program, Supplemental Nutrition Assistance Program (SNAP), and the Supplemental Nutrition for Women, Infants and Children (WIC) can improve food security and improve healthy eating patterns by promoting purchases of nutritious fruits and beverages [48].

For example, in 2009, when WIC introduced the requirements for the purchases of fruits and vegetables, the participants bought 29% more fruits and 18% more vegetables. In addition, an important initiative involves nutrition education at all levels of healthcare. An example of this was the Medical Nutrition Therapy Act of 2020, which expanded access to medical nutrition therapy (MNT) to conditions such as obesity, hypertension, cancer, and unintentional weight loss in addition to diabetes and renal disease, which are currently covered for Medicare beneficiaries.

It is also important that professional organizations work to establish a diverse work force. For example, the Academy of Nutrition and Dietetics currently has less than 4% Asian members, 3% Hispanic or Latino, and 0.3% American Indians or Alaskan Natives and only 2.6% Black or African Americans [11]. Similar findings are true of physicians, where a distinct minority are Black or Hispanic. Only 5.8% of physicians are Hispanic and 5.0% are Black or African American.

6.5 NUTRITION AND HEALTH EQUITY IN CHILDREN

Significant inequities exist in nutrition in other health parameters when it comes to children. Current estimates suggest that between 12% and 14% of families in the United States face food insecurity. That means that as many as 9 million children in the United States live in "food insecure" environments. This suggests that in these households there is not enough food for every family member to lead a healthy life. While the number of children living with hunger has fallen steadily over the past decade, the COVID-19 pandemic significantly exacerbated the problem of food insecurity in children.

Hunger tracks closely with poverty, so hunger in children mostly affects children from low-income families. In fact, 37 million Americans live under the poverty line, and 12 million of those are children [45]. Federal school programs have tried to help families and children overcome food insecurities [49]. These programs include SNAP, WIC, and the National School Lunch Program [50,51,52]. Other programs that can help with this issue include the School Breakfast Program, the National Summer Meals Program, and the After School Meals Program [53]. These programs reflect the fact that many children do not have an adequate breakfast at home, and since many children rely on school for regular meals, in the summer these meals disappear. The After School Meals Program also helps children get nutritious meals in a safe, supervised location as the school day ends.

The Healthy Hunger Free Kids Act of 2010 also authorized the U.S. Department of Agriculture to revise nutrition standards for school meals and smart snacks in school [54]. These standards were the first revisions of school nutrition standards in several decades and highlight federal attention to improving nutrition environments. Some research, however, has now suggested that a considerable inequity exists in these programs, with more affluent schools able to supply more health-related foods compared to less affluent school environments. These programs were also accompanied by nutrition education initiatives. Once again, however, there are disparities between more affluent and less affluent school systems. This underscores the issue that nutrition and health equity for children is complicated and emphasizes that it's not just providing food to children, but healthy food to children, that will make a difference in their long-term health.

6.6 NUTRITION-RELATED BURDENS IN THE HEALTHCARE SYSTEM

Multiple nutrition-related deficiencies create problems for the healthcare system and are an additional basis for health inequalities in the U.S. population. While many factors influence this problem, the following appear to the be most significant issues:

- Poor food availability and access, which may lead to disparities and dietary quality in malnutrition and also contribute to the obesity epidemic.
- Insufficient nutrition knowledge from the healthcare provider, which contributes to insufficient ability to identify and treat poor nutrition.
- Insufficient knowledge among the public, which may include limited knowledge of nutritious food and the impact of diet on health and/or lack of cooking skills.

These deficiencies can contribute to multiple adverse effects including increasing the financial and personal burdens of chronic illnesses which are more prevalent among older adults, contributing to adverse medical research outcomes based on underlying nutrition status. These deficiencies also exacerbate poor health conditions particularly among disadvantaged populations.

6.7 MALNUTRITION AND FOOD INSECURITY

Multiple definitions of malnutrition have been developed. The concept of malnutrition basically encompasses the lack of proper nutrition, which may be caused by not having enough to eat, not eating enough of the right things, or being unable to utilize the food that one does eat [55]. The underlying principle is that malnutrition is a serious condition that happens when diet does not contain the right amount of nutrients. Malnutrition means "poor nutrition." It can be referred to as undernutrition, meaning not getting enough nutrition, or overnutrition, meaning getting more nutrients than needed.

The connection between malnutrition and food insecurity or food equity can have significant implications for the management of chronic diseases and anticipated health outcomes. The relationship between malnutrition and chronic disease is often not understood completely by healthcare professionals, particularly those lacking in nutritional training. While some aspect of malnutrition can be ameliorated by alleviating food insecurity, the concept of malnutrition also results in lack of adequate affordable nutritious foods. Of note, malnutrition may be underrecognized in the United States since it may be perceived as an issue in the developing countries where it is associated with starvation and inadequate food supplies. In many neighborhoods food insecurity and malnutrition do not necessarily stem from scarce food, but instead from the lack of fresh, high-quality, nutritious food. Unless healthcare providers understand the link between malnutrition and food insecurity, unsuccessful malnutrition interventions may result.

Malnutrition may result from inequitable access to nutritious food, which may be caused by high food costs, neighborhood limitations (such as safety and walkability), limited personal or public transportation, limited food literacy, and/or traditional living patterns not conducive to chronic conditions or limited access to an understanding of technology. Inequitable access to nutrition care may be further exacerbated by the inability of such care (MNT from registered dietitians) or lack of knowledge of nutrition by physicians. Furthermore, equitable access may be limited by patients' social risk factors (see the section on SDOH) and perceptions or concerns about the healthcare system.

To address these issues, healthcare professionals including physicians, nurses, registered dietitian nutritionists (RDNs), and others providing healthcare should strive to become more knowledgeable about nutrition and health equity. In addition, social workers and community agencies should address the larger social needs that relate to food insecurity, while hospital leadership and administrators should implement policy and practices that prioritize nutrition management. It should be emphasized that health outcome and cost savings data showed substantial differences and outcomes between those who have and those who lack adequate access to high-quality nutritious foods. It is imperative that initiatives and policy proposals recognize and address nutrition as a key component of health equity.

6.8 FOOD INSECURITY, NUTRITION, AND OBESITY

Strong links exist between food insecurity and obesity. Both elevated body mass index and dietary risk factors are central to driving the global noncommunicable diseases (NCDs) burden which includes cardiovascular disease, type 2 diabetes mellitus (T2DM), and some cancers [56]. Diet and NCD-related health outcomes are not equitably distributed. Those in lower SES circumstances often experience worse health outcomes compared to higher SES counterparts. While there are many contributing factors to this, the social and commercial determinants of food choice and access play important roles. Therefore, equity-oriented social policies that target these upstream determinants, including daily living conditions, are likely to improve population nutrition. One framework that provides a conceptual overview of actions to equitably improve population nutrition and weight involves population policies that emphasize structural changes to the food system, including environments across such diverse settings such as food and meal programs and early education in schools. Education and awareness-raising initiatives should also be significant and must be designed using equity principles. These actions must be grounded on inclusive governance to foster participation of all social groups.

Despite recognizing the importance of policies to promote healthy eating and reduce diet- and health-related inequalities, social and economic differences in obesity are widening, particularly among children. In particular, studies have been identified that obesity is frequently framed by governments, the media, and food industries as a problem of individual choice, with few actions established to regulate the food environment.

6.9 IMPROVING FRUIT AND VEGETABLE ACCESSIBILITY TO ADVANCE NUTRITION SECURITY AND HEALTH EQUITY

National and local efforts to improve diet and health in the United States have stressed the importance of nutrition security. These efforts emphasize consistent access to foods and beverages that promote health and prevent disease. Fruits and vegetables (FV) consumption are central to attaining and sustaining a healthy diet [13]. Unfortunately, there are currently significant inequities of FV accessibility, purchasing, and consumption, particularly among populations that are socially and economically disadvantaged. In order to achieve nutrition and health equity, nutrition security initiatives should aim to increase FV consumption. According to the Dietary Guidelines for Americans (DGA) 2020–2025, Americans should consume an adequate amount and variety of FVs to prevent diet-related chronic disease. This includes a minimum of 1.5–2 cups a day of fruit and 2.5–3 cups per day of vegetables as components of a healthy diet. The Centers for Disease Control and Prevention, however, estimates that less than 12% of adults meet the fruit requirement and 9% of adults meet the vegetable requirement. Furthermore, FV consumption has been documented to show inequalities by sex, race, ethnicity, and SES. A number of government initiatives are now in progress to try to increase FV consumption. These include the Gus Schumacher Nutrition Incentive Program (GusNIP), which was included in the 2018 Farm Bill, and changes in the U.S. Department of Agriculture (USDA) WIC program in 2009 to better align with the DGAs 2020–2025 by increasing supplemental dollars for households to purchase FVs. These resulted in substantial increases in these purchases [13]. While these represent important first steps, further initiatives to emphasize FV purchase in SNAP, GusNIP, and WIC should be undertaken to attempt to improve dietary quality, particularly in disadvantaged groups.

6.10 NUTRITION, COVID-19, AND HEALTH EQUITY

Problems of nutrition and health equity were exacerbated by the COVID-19 pandemic [6,7]. Recommendations for people to shelter indoors and avoid unnecessary contact with other people further limited access to healthy nutrition. The impact of poor nutrition and health equity was clearly demonstrated in the fact that people who had poor nutrition and were obese experienced three to four times the morbidity and mortality from COVID-19 compared to individuals who had better nutrition and maintained a healthy weight [5]. A component of this disparity may have been from increased purchases of calorie-dense but nutrient-poor foods, particularly for individuals who were economically disadvantaged.

6.11 FOOD INSECURITY AND FOOD ADDICTION SYMPTOMS

Several studies have documented that there is an association between food insecurity and food addiction symptoms [12]. Individuals who experience food insecurity may also be subject to disordered eating. One particularly troublesome aspect may be that individuals who experience food insecurity may choose less expensive, highly processed foods, which may, in turn, activate neural reward responses associated with behavioral patterns that mirror substance abuse disorders. While these are preliminary data, they suggest further complications of food insecurity.

6.12 HEALTH EQUITY IN THE HEALTHY PEOPLE 2030

The issue of health equity is reflected in one of the overarching goals of Healthy People 2030, where it is stated "reduce health disparities, achieve health equity and attain health literacy to improve the health and wellbeing of all" [57]. While multiple issues related to SDOH are included in Healthy People 2030, nutritional strategies and initiatives will play a central role in many of the actions that are recommended.

6.13 NIH NUTRITION HEALTH DISPARITIES FRAMEWORK: A MODEL TO ADVANCE HEALTH EQUITY

A significant initiative on the part of the National Institutes of Health (NIH) reflects the understanding that nutrition such as poor diet quality and inadequate nutrient intake rises from multiple factors. These factors are related to multiple adverse health outcomes such as obesity, T2DM, cardiovascular disease, and diet-related cancers. The goal of the NIH is to develop a nutrition-centric, socioeconomic framework that helps determine ways that diet-related disparities are perpetuated among disadvantaged populations. The goal of this framework is to provide an important resource for nutrition professionals to help in the development of multi-level nutrition interventions to improve health outcomes and increase health equity in diverse populations.

6.14 UNITED NATIONS INITIATIVE ON SUSTAINABLE DEVELOPMENT GOALS AND HEALTH EQUITY

In 2012, the United Nations launched an unprecedented global consultation on Sustainable Development Goals (SDGs) under the rubric "the world we want" [58]. Three years later, the UN General Assembly agreed to 17 sustainability goals with the overarching principle of "leaving no one behind." Goals #1 and #2 are directly related to nutrition and equity. Goal #1 is to end poverty in all forms everywhere, and goal #2 is to end hunger, achieve food security, improve nutrition, and promote sustainable agriculture.

6.15 NUTRITIONAL SECURITY, HEALTH EQUITY, AND QUALITY CARE

Improving the health and nutrition security of Americans will require both affordable healthcare and a strong emphasis on preventive care. Such prevention requires comprehensive nutrition care and services. The COVID-19 pandemic enforced the understanding that the SDOH, including access to nutritious food, can have a major impact on people's health [6]. This understanding further emphasizes that SDOHs are intrinsically linked to health equity. This is particularly true of older adults (age 65 years or older). We know, for example, that an unhealthy diet is a significant contributor to poor health and that disparities of dietary quality reflect SES, which contributes to health disparities.

A number of national initiatives have sought to address nutritional security. Many of these are incorporated in the Healthy People 2030 initiative [59]. The Healthy People 2030 objectives also emphasize the importance of impacting on upstream factors such as access to transportation, food deserts, etc., all of which impact on nutrition security. The Healthy People 2030 objectives are focused not only on reducing food insecurity and hunger but also increasing FV consumption in the general population. These issues are particularly important for addressing nutrition security and malnutrition in older adults.

6.16 NATIONAL NUTRITION POLICIES AND HEALTH EQUITY

It is clear that equity-oriented policy actions represent a key public health principle [11]. While multiple approaches have been undertaken, several principles clearly stand out and bear more emphasis. First, many of the issues related to health equity relate to upstream problems such as daily living conditions, lack of transportation, food prices, and the school food environment. These issues ultimately reflect on reduced nutritional equity and health equity, particularly for underserved or less affluent populations.

A secondary issue that must be emphasized is that health equity issues have often been framed as a behavioral problem that requires an individual response. This is particularly prominent in the area of obesity. This type of problem framing reduces the impetus for governments to act on the important upstream problems that lead to inequities and contribute to health problems. Moving forward, national policy must reflect equitable nutrition and obesity prevention policies and focus on population-wide, behavioral based issues related to diet and health.

6.17 RELATIONSHIP OF NUTRITION AND HEALTH EQUITY TO OTHER LIFESTYLE MODALITIES

Clearly, nutrition equity relates to other important lifestyle-related issues. For example, many of the recommendations in the area of physical activity strategies to combat COVID-19 resulted in decreased physical activity, as well as poor nutrition—both of which impacted adversely on health equity. In addition, both nutrition and physical activity relate to sleep [6]. Disordered eating can adversely impact on sleep, as can a sedentary lifestyle. Thus, practitioners of lifestyle medicine should focus on the interrelationship between these factors and health equity. Of course, issues related to stress and interpersonal relationships also intersect with nutrition and can further exacerbate adverse consequences related to health equity [60].

6.18 CONCLUSIONS

SDOH, which relate to a wide variety of circumstances and forces shaping the conditions of daily life, are responsible for most health inequities. Nutrition plays a prominent role in many of the adverse consequences of health inequity. In the United States an estimated 10–11% of households live below the poverty line. These disadvantaged individuals often suffer multiple health consequences related to health equity. Nutrition often plays a major role in health equity. Disadvantaged populations often either do not have enough food to eat or consume more energy-dense, nutrient-poor diets, which further exacerbate adverse health consequences. These problems were underscored recently in the COVID-19 pandemic where individuals who were in lower socioeconomic classes were three to four times as likely to suffer morbidity and mortality from COVID-19. These problems were particularly marked in Hispanic and African American populations, especially those who lived in urban environments. It is incumbent upon all physicians to focus on SDOH. Nutrition represents a significant area where both individuals and public policy strategies can help to reduce problems with health equity.

Clinical Applications

- All physicians should assess SDOH.
- Physicians should be particularly cognizant of the ways nutrition may create health inequities.
- Malnutrition is common in the United States, particularly for people over the age of 65.
- Various factors related to nutrition and health equity should be assessed in all patient encounters, but particularly for people over the age of 65, who should be queried concerning the adequacy of their food environment and whether or not they have access to and are consuming healthful diets that include increased consumption of FV.
- School-aged children are also particularly vulnerable, so physicians should become knowledgeable about the entire family when it comes to nutrition and health equity.

REFERENCES

1. Daniel H, Bornstein S, et al. Health public policy committee of the American College of Physicians. Addressing social determinants to improve patient care and promote health equity: An American College of Physicians Position Paper. Ann Inter Med. 2018;168(8):577–578.
2. Braveman P, Arkin E, Orleans T, et al. What is health equity? Behav Sci Policy. 2018;4(1):1–14.
3. Braveman P, Egerter S, Williams D. The social determinants of health: Coming of age. Annu Rev Public Health. 2011;32:381–398.
4. Healthy People 2030. Heath Equity in Healthy People 2030. Health Equity in Healthy People 2030—Healthy People 2030 | health.gov (Accessed January 12, 2024).
5. Belanger M, Hill M, Angelidi A, et al. Covid-19 and disparities in nutrition and obesity. N Engl J Med. 2020;383(11):e69.

6. Hasson R, Sallis J, Coleman N, et al. COVID-19: Implications for physical activity, health disparities, and health equity. Am J Lifestyle Med. 2022;16(4):420–433.
7. McLoughlin G, McCarthy J, McGuirt J, et al. Addressing food insecurity through a health equity lens: A case study of large urban school districts during the COVID-19 pandemic. J Urban Health: Bull N Y Acad Med. 2020;97(6):759–775.
8. Daniel H, Bornstein S, Kane G. Health public policy committee of the American College of Physicians. Addressing Social Determinants to Improve Patient Care and Promote Health Equity: An American College of Physicians Position Paper. Ann Intern Med. 2018;168(8):577–578.
9. Marmot M, Bell R. The sustainable development goals and health equity. Epidemiology. 2018;29(1):5–7.
10. Zorbas C, Browne J, Chung A, et al. National nutrition policy in high-income countries: Is health equity on the agenda? Nutr Rev. 2021;79(10):1100–1113.
11. Blankenship J, Blancato R. Nutrition security at the intersection of health equity and quality care. J Acad Nutr Diet. 2022;122(10S):S12–S19.
12. Parnarouskis L, Gearhardt A, Mason A, et al. Association of food insecurity and food addiction symptoms: A secondary analysis of two samples of low-income female adults. J Acad Nutr Diet. 2022;122(10):1885–1892.
13. Houghtaling B, Greene M, Parab K, et al. Improving fruit and vegetable accessibility, purchasing, and consumption to advance nutrition security and health equity in the United States. Int J Environ Res Public Health. 2022;19(18):11220.
14. Harris J, Tan W, Mitchell B, et al. Equity in agriculture-nutrition-health research: A scoping review. Nutr Rev. 2021;80(1):78–90.
15. Leung CW, Parnarouskis L, Slotnick MJ, et al. Food insecurity and food addiction in a large, national sample of lower-income adults. Curr Dev Nutr. 2023 Nov 20;7(12):102036.
16. Galea S, Tracy M, Hoggatt KJ, et al. Estimated deaths attributable to social factors in the United States. Am J Public Health. 2011;101(8):1456–1465.
17. Chetty R, Stepner M, Abraham S, et al. The association between income and life expectancy in the United States, 2001–2014. JAMA. 2016;26;315(16):1750–1766.
18. Ubri P, Artiga A. Disparities in Health and Health Care: Five Key Questions. The Henry J. Kaiser Family Foundation. August 2016. https://collections.nlm.nih.gov/catalog/nlm:nlmuid-101694257-pdf (Accessed January 16, 2024).
19. Taylor LA, Tan AX, Coyle CE, et al. Leveraging the social determinants of health: What works? PLoS One. 2016 Aug 17;11(8):e0160217.
20. Braveman P, Arkin E, Orleans T, et al. What is health equity? And what difference does a definition make? Robert Wood Johnson Foundation, 2017. www.rwjf.org/content/dam/farm/reports/issue_briefs/2017/rwjf437393 (Accessed January 30, 2024).
21. Isaacs SL, Schroeder SA. Class: The ignored determinant of the nation's. N Engl J Med. 2004;351:1137–1142.
22. Cutler DM, Lleras-Muney A. Education and Health: Evaluating Theories and Evidence (NBER Working Paper No. 12352). Cambridge, MA: National Bureau of Economic Research, 2006.
23. Evans GW. The environment of childhood poverty. Am Psychol. 2004;59:77–92.
24. Diez-Roux AV, Mair C. Neighborhoods and health. In Adler NE, and Stewert J (eds.). Annals of the New York Academy of Sciences: Vol. 1186. The biology of disadvantage: Socioeconomic status and health. New York, NY, 2010: 125–145.
25. Acevedo-Garcia D, Osypuk TL, McArdle N, et al. Toward a policy-relevant analysis of geographic and racial/ethnic disparities in child health. Health Aff. 2008;27:321–333.
26. Williams DR, Mohammed SA. Racism and health I: Pathways and scientific evidence. Am Behav Sci. 2013;57:1152–1173.

27. Whitehead M. The concepts and principles of equity and health. Health Promot Int. 1991;6:217–228.
28. Braveman P, Gruskin S. Defining equity in health. J Epidemiol Comm Health. 2003;57:254–258.
29. Chetty R, Grusky D, Hell M, et al. The fading American dream: Trends in absolute income mobility since 1940. Science. 2017;28;356(6336):398–406.
30. Braveman PA, Cubbin C, Egerter S, Chideya S, Marchi KS, Metzler M, Posner S. Socioeconomic status in health research: One size does not fit all. JAMA. 2005;14;294(22): 2879–2888.
31. Bishaw A. Changes in areas with concentrated poverty: 2000–2010. American Community Survey Reports. United States Census Bureau, June 2014. www.census.gov/library/publications/2014/acs/acs-27.html (Accessed January 16, 2024).
32. National Center for Education Statistics. Employment and Unemployment Rates by Educational Attainment. Condition of Education. U.S. Department of Education, Institute of Education Sciences, 2023. https://nces.ed.gov/programs/coe/indicator/cbc (Accessed January 16, 2024).
33. Hood E. Dwelling disparities: How poor housing leads to poor health. Environ Health Perspect. 2005;113(5):A310–A317.
34. US Department of House and Urban Development. Affordable Housing, 2017. www.huduser.gov/portal/datasets/cp.html (Accessed January 17, 2024).
35. National Health Care for the Homeless Council. What Is the Official Definition of Homelessness? 2024. https://nhchc.org/understanding-homelessness/ (Accessed January 17, 2024).
36. The Commonwealth Fund. In Focus: Using Housing to Improve Health and Reduce the Costs of Caring for the Homeless, 2014. www.commonwealthfund.org/publications/newsletter-article/2014/oct/focus-using-housing-improve-health-and-reduce-costs-caring (Accessed January 17, 2024).
37. Syed ST, Gerber BS, Sharp LK. Traveling towards disease: Transportation barriers to health care access. J Community Health. 2013;38(5):976–993.
38. Seligman HK. Food Insecurity and Diabetes Prevention and Control in California. 2016. UCLA Center for Health Policy Research. https://cvp.ucsf.edu/sites/cvp.ucsf.edu/files/images/seligman_food.pdf (Accessed January 17, 2024).
39. Safe Routes to School National Partnership. Fighting for Equitable Transportation. Why it Matters. American Public Health Association. 2015. www.saferoutespartnership.org/sites/default/files/resource_files/fighting-for-equitable-transportation-why-it-matters_0.pdf (Accessed January 17, 2024).
40. Stanford University. Digital Divide 2017. https://cs.stanford.edu/people/eroberts/cs201/projects/digital-divide/start.html (Accessed January 17, 2024).
41. Pai A. Letter Regarding Request for Comment—Actions to Accelerate Adoption and Accessibility of Broadband-Enabled Health Care Solutions and Advanced Technologies, 2017. www.federalregister.gov/documents/2017/05/10/2017-09309/fcc-seeks-comment-and-data-on-actions-to-accelerate-adoption-and-accessibility-of-broadband-enabled (Accessed January 17, 2024).
42. American College of Physicians. Racial and Ethnic Disparities in Health Care, Updated 2010. Philadelphia: American College of Physicians, 2010.
43. Williams DR, Priest N, Anderson NB. Understanding associations among race, socioeconomic status, and health: Patterns and prospects. Health Psychol. 2016;35(4):407–411.
44. Mann L, Foley KL, Tanner AE, et al. Increasing cervical cancer screening among US hispanics/latinas: A qualitative systematic review. J Cancer Educ. 2015;30(2):374–387.

45. Coleman-Jensen A, Rabbit M, Gregory C. Household Food Security in the United States in 2021. Economic Research Service. US Department of Agriculture. Economic Research Report No. (ERR-309), September 2022, 51 pp.
46. Bailey ZD, Krieger N, Agénor M, et al. Structural racism and health inequities in the USA: Evidence and interventions. Lancet. 2017;8;389(10077):1453–1463.
47. Larson NI, Story MT, Nelson MC. Neighborhood environments: Disparities in access to healthy foods in the U.S. Am J Prev Med. 2009;36(1):74–81.e10.
48. US Department of Health and Human Services. Healthy People 2020 Leading Health Indicators: Progress Update. www.cdc.gov/nchs/healthy_people/hp2020.htm (Accessed February 5, 2024).
49. National Academies of Sciences, Engineering, and Medicine; Health and Medicine Division; Board on Population Health and Public Health Practice. Committee on applying neurobiological and socio-behavioral sciences from prenatal through early childhood development: A health equity approach. In Negussie Y, Geller A, DeVoe JE (eds). Vibrant and Healthy Kids: Aligning Science, Practice, and Policy to Advance Health Equity. Washington, DC: National Academies Press (US), 25 July 2019. PMID: 31855338.
50. Asada Y, Hughes A, Chriqui J. Insights on the intersection of health equity and school nutrition policy implementation: An exploratory qualitative secondary analysis. Health Educ Behav. 2017 Oct;44(5):685–695.
51. Zhang F, Liu J, Rehm CD, et al. Trends and disparities in diet quality among US adults by supplemental nutrition assistance program participation status. JAMA Network Open. 2018;1(2):e180237.
52. Leung CW, Ding EL, Catalano PJ, et al. Dietary intake and dietary quality of low-income adults in the Supplemental Nutrition Assistance Program. Am J Clin Nutr. 2012;96(5):977–988.
53. Mozaffarian D, Angell SY, Lang T, et al. Role of government policy in nutrition-barriers to and opportunities for healthier eating. BMJ. 2018;13;361:k2426.
54. Healthy, Hunger Free Kids Act of 2010. www.govinfo.gov/content/pkg/COMPS-10332/pdf/COMPS-10332.pdf (Accessed January 17, 2024).
55. World Health Organization. Social Determinants of Health. 2018. www.who.int/health-topics/social-determinants-of-health (Accessed January 30, 2024).
56. Kumanyika SK. A framework for increasing equity impact in obesity prevention. Am J Public Health. 2019;109(10):1350–1357.
57. Social Determinants of Health at CDC. Centers for Disease Control and Prevention. December 8, 2022. Washington, DC.
58. Baker P, Hawkes C, Wingrove K, et al. What drives political commitment for nutrition? A review and framework synthesis to inform the United Nations Decade of Action on Nutrition. BMJ Glob Health. 2018;10;3(1):e000485.
59. Social Determinants of Health. World Health Organization. www.who.int/health-topics/social-determinants-of-health (Accessed January 17, 2024).
60. Cassoobhoy A, Sardana JJ, Benigas S, et al. Building health equity: Action steps from the American College of Lifestyle Medicine's Health Disparities Solutions Summit (HDSS) 2020. Am J Lifestyle Med. 2021;5;16(1):61–75.

7 Hunger, Food Insecurity, and Malnutrition

Key Points

- Hunger, food insecurity, and malnutrition are interrelated.
- Malnutrition is the broadest concept of these three, representing all manifestations of poor nutrition including all forms of undernutrition, overweight, and obesity.
- Hunger, food insecurity, and malnutrition are a worldwide problem. In the United States, despite being the most affluent country in the world, over 10% of all households experience food insecurity, meaning that they do not have an adequate amount to eat.
- The COVID-19 pandemic underscored health disparities in nutrition. Over 21% of Black families and 17% of Latinx families experienced food insecurity. This was double that of White households (7.1%).
- The poor nutritional habits and food insecurity are related to obesity, diabetes, hypertension, and heart failure. These were underscored in the disparate responses to COVID-19, where two-thirds of COVID-19 hospitalizations were related to these conditions.
- Clinicians have an important role to play in assessing whether or not their patients are experiencing hunger or food insecurity or any of the manifestations of malnutrition.

7.1 INTRODUCTION

Hunger, food insecurity, and malnutrition are significant problems in the United States and an enormous burden around the world, particularly in third world countries.

There are many definitions of hunger, which will be discussed in this chapter. Hunger has been a significant and unfortunate condition in the United States, which is the world's most affluent country [1–5]. Food insecurity has also been a major issue in the United States and tracks, to some degree [6–9], with poverty, although the two are not synonymous. Malnutrition is a much broader concept and has components of both hunger and food insecurity. Malnutrition also has other components that make it particularly dangerous and associated with ongoing chronic illness, particularly in the most vulnerable populations, including children and individuals over the age of 65 [1,10,11].

While this chapter will focus mostly on issues related to hunger, food insecurity, and malnutrition in the United States, around the world these are enormous and often deadly problems. For this reason, issues related to hunger, food insecurity, and malnutrition are high on the list of the World Health Organization (WHO) in their

DOI: 10.1201/9781003452607-7

initiative to reduce the prevalence of noncommunicable diseases (NCDs). According to the WHO, NCDs comprise 71% of all mortality, more than all communicable diseases combined [12]. There is no question that hunger, food insecurity, and malnutrition all contribute to a variety of chronic illnesses including diabetes, cardiovascular disease (CVD), obesity, and metabolic syndrome [9–11]. Nutrition plays a very substantial role in all of these conditions. The relationship of nutrition to hunger, food insecurity, and malnutrition will be highlighted in this chapter.

7.2 HUNGER, FOOD INSECURITY, AND MALNUTRITION

These three concepts are interrelated. For example, hunger and food insecurity, while related, have distinct definitions. There are also multiple definitions of hunger. One definition of hunger is that it is the "uneasy or painful sensation caused by lack of food." We are all familiar with hunger [1–5]. In very mild forms, it is a sensation that can last only a few hours without food but often disappears when an individual fasts in a prolonged way.

In a sense, hunger is characterized not only by an individual sensation and behavioral responses but also food scarcity (actual or feared). The National Food Balance Sheet focuses on supply of energy (kilocalories) in an overall country relative to the minimum threshold for need [13]. This Food Balance Sheet is the only standard of measurement of food availability used globally. It is based on data collected by the Food and Agricultural Organization of the United Nations. In fact, this organization has replaced previous use of the word "hunger" to describe this condition with "chronic undernourishment." This concept is further defined as a "person's inability to acquire enough food to meet daily minimum energy requirements during one year."

Food insecurity is a broader concept that incorporates the physical sensation of hunger and also the anxiety that not enough food is available [6–8], the experience of running out of food without money to buy more, perceptions that food is inadequate in quality or quantity, adjustments in normal food intake, and reduced food intake.

These elements of food insecurity encompass sensory strategies used in adults who are food insecure to prevent the physical sensation of hunger. For example, this might rely on using a few low-cost, energy-dense foods for much of the calorie intake. Of course, these low-cost, energy-dense foods are often highly processed and offer little nutritional value.

In 1990, one organization defined food insecurity as the limited or uncertain "availability of nutritionally adequate and safe foods" or "the ability to acquire acceptable foods" [14] without resorting to soup kitchens, food banks, scavenging, or other coping strategies. It should be noted that some organizations draw the distinction between low and very low food secure environments, both of which are considered food insecure.

In the United States, increasingly severe levels of food insecurity result in a predictable progression of responses. Households that are categorized as reporting "low food security" display a variety of compensatory behaviors, while households categorized as having "very low food security" adopt additional behaviors. More than 70% of low food secure households report anxiety about running out of food, the experience of running out of food, or the inability to afford balanced meals. In response, many adults in low food security households cut down the size of their meals or skip meals and eat less than they feel they should and, in fact, experience the physical sensation of hunger. These compensatory strategies are further experienced by adults and only affect children as household food insecurity becomes more severe [15].

Malnutrition is an inclusive term that represents all manifestations of poor nutrition. It can include any or all forms of undernutrition, overweight, and obesity [16]. Undernutrition refers to any form of nutritional deficiency, which may manifest as maternal underweight, child stunting, child wasting, or micronutrient deficiencies. Undernutrition does not include reference to overweight or obesity [16]. Maternal underweight is defined as a body mass index (BMI) of <18.5 kg/m^2 among women of reproductive age. It often is coupled with a lack of key macronutrients or micronutrients. Child stunting is defined as height for age more than two standard deviations below the median for children under the age of five utilizing WHO child growth charts.

Overweight and obesity for nonpregnant adults are defined by BMI criteria. A BMI of ≥ 25 kg/m^2 is categorized as being overweight. In most countries, thresholds for obesity are defined as BMI ≥ 30 kg/m^2. There is increasing concern about childhood obesity to the degree that the latest Global Nutrition Goals for 2030 include "no increase in childhood obesity" [17]. It should be noted that many public health officials now make the distinction between food insecurity and nutrition security. (See Section 7.4.)

7.3 FACTS ABOUT HUNGER IN THE UNITED STATES

In the United States, it is estimated that 11.2% of households are food insecure [5,15]. These households encompass 36.2 million people, of which 12.4 million are children and adolescents. Of these 33.8 million households, 1 in 26 (3.8%) in the United States experiences very low food insecurity, where households report regularly skipping meals or reducing intake because they cannot afford more food.

Food insecurity was greatly exacerbated during the COVID-19 pandemic. (See the subsequent section.) It should be noted that the number of children in households where adults could not buy enough food for their families is 12.5%, which is much higher than the rate of households without children (9.4%) who could not afford to buy adequate amounts of food. It should also be noted that households in rural areas experienced deeper struggles with hunger compared to those in metro areas (10.8% in rural areas compared to 10.1% in metro areas).

Black and Latinx households are disproportionately impacted by food insecurity [15]. Black households with food insecurity are 19.8% and Latinx 15.2%; this is compared to White households of 7.0%.

It should be noted that both low and very low food security are strongly related to, although not synonymous, with poverty. About one-third of households with incomes less than 130% of the Federal Poverty Level are food insecure [15]. However, more than half the food-insecure households had incomes greater than 130% of the Federal Poverty Level, which makes them generally ineligible for the Supplemental Nutrition Assistance Program (SNAP) (formerly called food stamps) benefits. The fact that the prevalence of food insecurity in Black and Latinx families is more than double that of White families relates to the broader issue of socioeconomic, racial, and ethnic inequalities in health. This is particularly true for diseases that are sensitive to dietary intake, such as diabetes.

7.4 FOOD INSECURITY VERSUS NUTRITION SECURITY

As already indicated, there is a strong association between food insecurity and poor nutrition. This results from most food-insecure individuals carrying a higher risk of developing diet-related diseases such as obesity, diabetes, and hypertension. In contrast, food security focuses on ensuring that everyone in the family has enough to eat, and nutrition security ensures that everyone receives and consumes calories that contribute to their overall health. For example, estimates suggest that as many as one-third of cancer cases could be prevented with diet and nutrition alone. The U.S. Department of Agriculture (USDA) is playing an active role in the area of nutrition security [18].

7.5 THE IMPACT OF POOR NUTRITION ON HEALTH

The USDA estimates that poor nutrition is the leading cause of illness in the United States and is responsible for more than 600,000 deaths per year [19]. This represents over 50,000 deaths per month from poor nutrition. For example, seven in ten American adults have either overweight or obesity, with 40% of adults having obesity. One in two adults has either diabetes or prediabetes. Unfortunately, obesity [20], diabetes, and prediabetes are rising in children. It has been estimated that most American children will have obesity by the time they are 35 years old [21].

Poor nutrition is widespread across all social and geographical sections of America. The overall diet quality score for Americans is 59 out of 100 [22], indicating the average American diet does not align with federal dietary guidelines found in the *Dietary Guidelines for Americans 2020–2025* [23]. The resulting health burden is not equally shared. For example, Black and Indigenous children are more likely to have obesity than White children [24]. Those who face food insecurity are also at greater risk.

In addition to the adverse effects on health, poor nutrition has other far-reaching impacts including decreased academic performance and increased financial stress [25]. These other impacts result in lower productivity, weakened military readiness, widening health disparities, and rapidly increasing healthcare costs. For example, it is estimated that now approximately 85% of current healthcare spending is related to management of diet-related chronic disease.

It is clearly mandated, based on these nutritionally related issues, that major effort needs to be undertaken to assure that Americans across all geographical areas and social classes and races and genders have equal access to healthy foods that promote well-being in an equitable way.

While the adverse impact of poor nutrition is prevalent for many chronic diseases, perhaps its most dramatic impact is in the areas of diabetes and obesity. Among non-elderly adults living in U.S. households with incomes less than 300% of the Federal Poverty Line, diabetes is about 7.1% in food-secure households and nearly double at

16.6% in very low food-secure households [26]. If one accounts for the differences in obesity, the risk of diabetes is almost three times higher in low food-secure environments. Thus, diabetes in very low food-secure households is not only related to increased risk of poverty or obesity.

In the area of obesity there is a well-established connection between low food security and overweight/obesity, particularly in women. In nonelderly women in the United States with incomes less than 300% of the Federal Poverty Level, the average BMI is 29 kg/m^2 [27]. There are multiple hypotheses for why this association exists. One potential explanation is the association between food insecurity and dietary substitutions, as well as geographic lack of access to healthy food alternatives.

It should be noted that in the United States food with the highest energy density also tends to cost the least. For example, cookies, butter, sugar, bread, pasta, and rice all cost far less per calorie of energy than fruits, vegetables, meats, and most dairy products. Between 1985 and 2000, increases in the price of fruits, vegetables, and dairy products far outstripped the increases in the price of sugars and sweets, fats and oils, and carbonated soft drinks.

The increased consumption of these energy-dense foods has also resulted in reduced consumption of nutrient-rich foods. In a typical week, U.S. adults living in a food-secure household consume an average of 11 servings of fruits, 19 servings of vegetables, and 13 servings of milk/dairy, compared to 8, 17, and 11 servings, respectively, in food-insecure households. This results not only in differences in macronutrients but also a wide variety of micronutrients including B vitamins, magnesium, iron, zinc, and calcium, which are lower in food-insecure households [11].

7.6 MALNUTRITION

As already indicated, malnutrition is a broad term representing all manifestations of poor nutrition, which can include any or all forms of undernutrition, overweight, or obesity [28]. All of these can represent different forms of nutritional deficiency, which result from an individual getting either low or too many nutrients, resulting in health problems. In essence, malnutrition reflects not receiving the correct amount of nutrition.

Malnutrition also includes diseases that are categorized as either undernutrition or overnutrition. These can result in either underweight or overweight, but both can be manifestations of not getting appropriate nutrition. While most clinical studies use the term "malnutrition" to refer to undernutrition, the 2019 report by the Lancet Commission suggests expanding the definition of malnutrition to include all forms, including obesity, undernutrition, and dietary risk [29,30]. This has also been characterized by the WHO as the "double burden of malnutrition" indicating the "coexistence of over-nutrition alongside of undernutrition" [30,31].

7.7 INTERACTION BETWEEN MALNUTRITION, FOOD INSECURITY, AND HUNGER

Multiple interactions exist between malnutrition, food insecurity, and hunger. While malnutrition is the broadest of these three terms, all of them are related to increased risk of a variety of significant chronic diseases. A recent report from the World Committee on Food Security argues that malnutrition in all its forms—not only hunger but also micronutrient deficiencies as well as overweight and obesity—is a critical challenge not only for developing countries but also developed countries [32]. Clearly, resolving these issues requires a better understanding of the multiple factors that influence diet.

Malnutrition is found in all countries, irrespective of their economic development, where people lack high-quality diets. Thus, solutions to hunger and all forms of malnutrition need to focus on ensuring adequate supply of not just food but equally the quality of the diet. As the World Committee on Food Security argued, risk factors for ill health associated with poor-quality diets are the main causes of global chronic disease [33]. Low-quality diets lack key vitamins, minerals, and fiber or contain too many calories, saturated fat, salt, and sugar.

By 2015, 6 of the top 11 global risk factors were related to diet including undernutrition, high BMI, and high cholesterol. Thus, issues related to the interaction between malnutrition, food security, and hunger are strongly related to each other, and mechanisms to ameliorate these conditions all relate to the complex interactions related to nutrition.

7.8 MALNUTRITION IN CHILDREN

Around the world the highest prevalence of undernutrition is among children under the age of five. In 2020, 149 million children under five years old experienced stunted growth, 45 million were wasted, and 38.9 million were overweight or obese. It has been estimated that 45% of deaths in children worldwide are linked to undernutrition [11]. This is a particular problem in underdeveloped countries in Africa, where the prevalence of undernutrition ranges from 29.9% in Kenya to 53% in Burundi [34]. In one particular area, vitamin A deficiency affects one-third of children under the age of five around the world and leads to 670,000 deaths and 250,000–500,000 cases of blindness [16]. In the United States, over 54,000 pediatric patients admitted to hospitals were diagnosed with malnutrition [35].

Patients with malnutrition experience worse clinical outcomes, longer times of stay, and increased cost of medical care. There is still a significant lack of comprehensive information related to childhood malnutrition and serious illness. An attempt to ameliorate this problem was published by a study from the Academy of Nutrition and Dietetics and the American Society for Parenteral and Enteral Nutrition (ASPEN) [36]. In the general population of the United States food insecurity among households with children actually fell slightly from 2020 to 2021. This was thought to be largely from government intervention related to the COVID-19 pandemic and, in particular, the Supplemental Poverty Measure (SPM) [37]. Nonetheless, food insecurity among households with children remains alarmingly high at 12.5% [5]. Schools also played an important role by offering meals to all students as they returned to in-person schooling. Unfortunately, disparities in food insecurities still persist by race and ethnicity. As already indicated, Black and Hispanic households had over twice the level of food insecurity compared to Caucasian families.

7.9 MALNUTRITION IN OLDER ADULTS

As of June 2021, 1.9 billion adults around the world were overweight or obese, while 462 million adults were underweight. Certain adult groups have higher rates of undernutrition, including elderly people and women. Undernutrition is particularly prevalent and a problem among people over the age of 65, even in developed countries [38]. In the elderly population, undernutrition is more commonly due to physical, psychological, and social factors, not a lack of food. Age-related reduced dietary intake due to chewing and swallowing problems, sensory decline, deprivation, poverty, and loneliness were major contributors to undernutrition in the elderly population.

Individuals over the age of 65 accounted for approximately 9% of all food-insecure homes in the United States. As the response to the COVID-19 pandemic illustrated, elderly individuals may employ various strategies to ensure adequate food during times of reduced food access. They may restrict personal intake of food, overeat when food is available, and consume primarily low-cost foods or eat the same foods regularly, all of which may contribute to overall decline in essential nutrient intake. In addition to financial barriers to achieving food security, issues in the elderly population that can restrict access to food include inadequate transportation, physical limitations, and cognitive decline. Thus, interventions ensuring adequate nutritional intake in elderly individuals should begin by assessing the affordability and accessibility and individuals' ability to prepare their food.

Malnutrition is a leading cause of morbidity and mortality, particularly in older patients. However, the diagnosis and treatment of malnutrition in a hospital setting are often overlooked. To help address this issue, the Academy of Nutrition and Dietetics and multiple other stakeholders developed a malnutrition toolkit for hospitals called the "MQii Toolkit," which is now in use in over 50 hospitals around the United States [39].

7.10 TREATMENT AND PUBLIC POLICY

Public policy in the future must stem from the fundamental understanding that food is a basic human right, much like air and water. It remains unacceptable that in the world's most affluent country, the United States, hunger and food insecurity are widespread. Not only does 10% of the population in the United States not have enough food to meet their needs but, in addition, food insecurity travels along racial and ethnic lines, as already indicated. Numerous policy interventions are in place planned to help reduce issues related to hunger and food insecurity. Several key pieces of food and nutrition legislation are coming up in the current session of Congress for reauthorization. The recent White House Conference on Hunger, Nutrition, and Health held in September 2022 argued that the United States has a once-in-a-generation opportunity to reform in a collective way systems to address domestic hunger and food insecurity by adopting a whole-government cross-sectional process of eliminating hunger. The report issued from this conference indicated, in general terms, strategies necessary to end hunger in the United States [40], namely:

- Reduce poverty as an integral step of reducing hunger.
- Create more accessible and affordable food production and distribution systems.
- Address the impact of climate change and improve market competition to ensure long-term food stability for all.

While a number of programs are available that attack hunger and food insecurity from various perspectives, these programs are typically designed to reduce hunger by supplementing incomes or enlisting new criteria for eligibility. One goal coming out of the White House Conference on Hunger, Nutrition, and Health relates to legislative opportunities to take meaningful action to build a food system that is more affordable, accessible, and equitable. Congress needs to reauthorize the Special Supplemental Nutrition Program for Women, Infants, and Children (WIC), which authorizes all the federal child nutrition programs that reach millions of children and families every day. In 2023, Congress had the opportunity to reauthorize the Farm Bill, which includes funding for SNAP, which is the nation's largest antihunger program, to allow vulnerable families to purchase healthy food and move toward self-sufficiency.

7.11 CLIMATE CHANGE AND MALNUTRITION

Climate change and malnutrition constitute two of the greatest threats to planetary and human health [41]. The cost of obesity represents almost 3% of the world's gross domestic product (GDP), and the cost of undernutrition in Asia and Africa ranges from 4% to 11% of GDP [42]. The cost of climate change, which will disproportionately affect low-income communities, may exceed 7% of the world GDP and 10% of the U.S. GDP by 2100 [43]. The pandemics of obesity, undernutrition, and climate change interact in time and place [44]. These three pandemics are all connected by underlying systems of agriculture and food production. For example, methane produced by cattle to meet the demands of meat consumption is associated with 9% of increased greenhouse gases (GHG) in the United States [45]. Furthermore, GHG production reduces micronutrients in crops, which contributes to food insecurity and undernutrition in many low- and middle-income countries.

Compared to the average U.S. diet, nutritional plans lower in meats, such as the Mediterranean diet and other healthy diets, have been estimated to decrease GHGs by 72%, land use by 58%, and energy consumption by 52% [46,47]. These observations are incorporated in both the 2015–2020 Dietary Guidelines for Americans Advisory Committee Report [48] and the 2020–2025 Advisory Report. Of note, both the Mediterranean [49] and DASH diets are not only better for the planet but also improve health [50]. Both of these diets have been demonstrated to reduce the risk of cardiovascular disease (CVD), type 2 diabetes mellitus (T2DM), and cancer by

6–10%. While there was an attempt to include this issue in several of the most recent DGAs, ultimately, it did not survive into the final document due to opposition from various commercial entities in the food industry in the United States, including the beef industry [51].

As indicated in multiple chapters in this book, plant-based diets have many positive attributes going for them, not the least of which is significantly reduced risk of various metabolic diseases. As a result, the healthcare sector, including the American Medical Association and over 100 other organizations, issued a call to action to address climate change and health.

It is important to note that the 2018 Gallup Poll showed that 70% of respondents age 18–34 were worried "a great deal" or "fair amount" about global warming [52]. It is important that these groups mobilize to take action in this area. We live in a world where climate change, health, malnutrition, nutritional practices, and food insecurity can no longer be placed into separate silos.

7.12 HUNGER, FOOD INSECURITY AND MALNUTRITION, AND THE COVID-19 PANDEMIC

The COVID-19 pandemic clearly underscored health disparities and the vital need to bring healthy food to the forefront [53]. One study estimated that two-thirds of the COVID-19 hospitalizations in the United States were related to obesity, diabetes, hypertension, and heart failure [54,55], all of which are chronic diseases associated with lack of access and consumption of healthy food. Given that 10% of all households and 21.7% of Black households and 17% of Latinx households experience food insecurity, the issue of food insecurity, hunger, malnutrition, and health disparities can no longer be ignored. Promoting food and nutrition security is key to improving health outcomes and addressing health disparities to give all Americans a chance for a healthy future.

7.13 CONCLUSIONS

Hunger, food insecurity, and malnutrition are ultimately related to each other. While malnutrition is a broader concept, hunger and food insecurity interact with each other in very important ways. In the United States, in particular—the world's most affluent country—the fact that over 10% of households experience food insecurity is not acceptable. Moreover, poor nutrition has been found to be the leading cause of illness in the United States and is responsible for more than 600,000 deaths per year. Poor nutrition is an underlying cause and contributor to CVD, T2DM, obesity, metabolic syndrome, and many cancers. Poor nutrition is also strongly related to health disparities experienced by Black and Hispanic households in the United States. For all these reasons, it is important that clinicians be alert to issues related to the combined issues of hunger, food insecurity, and malnutrition. Nutrition plays a very important role in all of these and is a key determinant of health in the United States and around the world.

Clinical Applications

- Hunger, food insecurity, and malnutrition are significant problems around the world. It has been estimated that poor nutrition, which underlies all three of these conditions, is the leading cause of illness in the United States, responsible for more than 600,000 deaths per year.
- Poor nutrition underlies chronic diseases such as obesity, T2DM, hypertension, and heart failure.
- It has been estimated that two-thirds of all hospitalizations during the COVID-19 pandemic were related to these conditions.
- There is a difference between food insecurity and nutritional security. Nutritional security involves not only adequate supply of calories but also focuses on ensuring everyone has not only enough to eat, but that everyone receives and consumes quality calories that contribute to their overall health.

REFERENCES

1. Webb P, Stordalen G, Singh S, et al. Hunger and malnutrition in the 21st century. BMJ. 2018;361:k2238.
2. High level and emerging issues for food security and nutrition. Panel of experts. Second note on critical high level panel of experts on food security and nutrition of the Committee on World Food Security. Rome, Italy. 2017. Nutrition and Food Systems. A Report by the High Level Panel of Experts on Food Security and Nutrition of the Committee on World Food Security. September 2017. HLPE Report 12 |Policy Support and Governance| Food and Agriculture Organization of the United Nations (fao.org). (Accessed November 2, 2023).
3. Food and Agriculture Organization of the United Nations. International fund for agricultural development. World Food Programme. The State of Food Security and Nutrition in the World. Rome, Italy. 2017. docs.wfp.org/api/documents/WFP-0000022419/download/?ga=2.91393434.1221853846.1698945941-1391691674.1698945941 (Accessed November 2, 2023).
4. Pangaribowo E, Evita H, Gerber N, et al. Food and Nutrition Security Indicators: A Review (February 1, 2013). SSRN. 2013(ZEF Working Paper No 108). Food and Nutrition Security Indicators: A Review by Evita Hanie Pangaribowo, Nicolas Gerber, Maximo Torero: SSRN. (Accessed November 2, 2023).
5. Feeding American. U.S. Hunger Relief Organization | Feeding America. (Accessed November 2, 2023).
6. U.S. Department of Agriculture Economic Research Service. Trends in Food Insecurity and Very Low Food Security by Race and Ethnicity, 2000–2014. 2016.
7. Berkowitz S, Seligman H, Meigs J, et al. Food insecurity, healthcare utilization, and high cost: A longitudinal cohort study. Am J Manag Care. 2018;24(9):399–404.
8. No Kid Hungry. End Child Hunger in America | No Kid Hungry. (Accessed December 4, 2023).
9. Friel S, Hattersley L, Ford L, et al. Addressing inequities in healthy eating. Health Promot Int. 2015;30(Suppl 2):ii77–ii88.
10. USDA. Economic Research Service. U.S. Department of Agriculture. USDA ERS—Key Statistics & Graphics. (Accessed December 4, 2023).
11. World Health Organization. Malnutrition—Facts Sheets—Fact sheets—Malnutrition (who.int). (Accessed November 2, 2023).

12. World Health Organization. Noncommunicable diseases. (who.int). (Accessed November 3, 2023).
13. Food and Agriculture Organization of the United States. Home | Food and Agriculture Organization of the United Nations (fao.org). (Accessed November 2, 2023).
14. Anderson S. The 1990 Life Sciences Research Office (LSRO) report on nutritional assessment defined terms associated with food access. Core Indicators of Nutritional State for Difficult to Sample Populations. 1990.
15. Nord M, Andrews M, Carlson S. Household food security in the United States, 2007. Economic Research Report 66. www.ers.usda.gov/webdocs/publications/46084/11227_err66.pdf?v=41056
16. Black R, Allen L, Bhutta Z, et al. Maternal and child undernutrition: Global and regional exposures and health consequences. Lancet. 2008;371(9608):243–260.
17. World Health Organization. Global Nutrition Targets 2025: Policy Brief Series (who.int). (Accessed November 3, 2023).
18. USDA. U.S. Department of Agriculture. Food and nutrition service. USDA Actions on Nutrition Security | Food and Nutrition Service. (Accessed November 3, 2023).
19. Centers for Disease Control and Prevention. National center for health statistics. Leading causes of death. FastStats—Leading Causes of Death (cdc.gov). (Accessed November 3, 2023).
20. Centers for Disease Control and Prevention. National center for health statistics. Prevalence of Obesity and Severe Obesity among Adults: United States, 2017–2018 Products—Data Briefs—Number 360—February 2020 (cdc.gov). (Accessed November 3, 2023).
21. Ward Z, Long M, Resch S, et al. Simulation of growth trajectories of childhood obesity into adulthood. N Eng J Med. 2017;377(22):2145–2153.
22. USDA. Food and Nutrition Service. HEI scores for Americans. HEI Scores for Americans | Food and Nutrition Service (usda.gov). (Accessed November 3, 2023).
23. U.S. Department of Agriculture and U.S. Department of Health and Human Services. *Dietary Guidelines for Americans, 2020–2025*, 9th edition. December 2020. DietaryGuidelines.gov.www.dietaryguidelines.gov/resources/2020-2025-dietary-guidelines-online-materials
24. Institute of Medicine (US). Hunger and Obesity: Understanding a Food Insecurity Paradigm: Workshop Summary. Washington, DC: National Academies Press (US), 2011. 2, Setting the Stage for the Coexistence of Food Insecurity and Obesity. www.ncbi.nlm.nih.gov/books/NBK209359/.
25. Dieleman J, Cao J, Chapin A, et al. US health care spending by payer and health condition, 1996–2016. JAMA. 2020;323(9):863–884.
26. USDA. U.S. Department of Agriculture. Economic research service. Household Food Security in the United States in 2020. USDA ERS—Household Food Security in the United States in 2020. (Accessed November 3, 2023).
27. Kvamme J, Olsen J, Florholmen J, et al. Risk of malnutrition and health-related quality of life in community-living elderly men and women: The Tromso study. Qual Life Res. 2011;20(4):575–582.
28. Wellman N, Weddle D, Kranz S, et al. Elder insecurities: Poverty, hunger, and malnutrition. J Am Diet Assoc. 1997;97(10 Suppl 2):S120–S122.
29. Swinburn B, Kraak V, Allender S, et al. The global syndemic of obesity, undernutrition, and climate change: The lancet commission report. Lancet. 2019;393(10173):791–846.
30. The Double Burden of Malnutrition. The double burden of malnutrition (thelancet.com). The Lancet. (Accessed December 4, 2023).
31. Ghattas H, Acharya Y, Jamaluddine Z, et al. Child-level double burden of malnutrition in the MENA and LAC regions: Prevalence and social determinants. Matern Child Nutr. 2020;16(2):e12923.

32. Min J, Zhao Y, Slivka L, et al. Double burden of diseases worldwide: Coexistence of undernutrition and overnutrition-related non-communicable chronic diseases. Obes Rev. 2018;19(1):49–61.
33. Committee on World Food Security. CFS: Making a Difference in Food Security and Nutrition (fao.org). (Accessed November 17, 2023).
34. Tesema G, Yeshaw Y, Worku M, et al. Pooled prevalence and associated factors of chronic undernutrition among under-five children in East Africa: A multilevel analysis. PLoS One. 2021;16(3):e0248637.
35. Carvalho-Salemi J, Salemi J, Wong-Vega M, et al. Malnutrition among hospitalized children in the United States: Changing prevalence, clinical correlates, and practice patterns between 2002 and 2011. J Acad Nutr Diet. 2018;118(1):40–51.e7.
36. Becker P, Nieman Carney L, Corkins MR, et al. Consensus statement of the Academy of Nutrition and Dietetics/American Society for Parenteral and Enteral Nutrition: Indicators recommended for the identification and documentation of pediatric malnutrition (undernutrition). J Acad Nutr Diet. 2014;114(12):1988–2000.
37. Handu D, Moloney L, Rozga M, et al. Malnutrition care during the COVID-19 pandemic: Considerations for registered dietitian nutritionists. J Acad Nutr Diet. 2021;121 (5):979–987.
38. Fitall E, Pratt K, McCauley S, et al. Improving malnutrition in hospitalized older adults: The development, optimization, and use of a supportive toolkit. J Acad Nutr Diet. 2019;119(9 Suppl 2):S25–S31.
39. Malnutrition Quality Improvement Initiative. Malnutrition quality improvement initiative complete toolkit. MQii Toolkit—MQii (malnutritionquality.org). (Accessed December 4, 2023).
40. White House Announces Conference on Hunger, Nutrition and Health in September. The White House. 2022. www.whitehouse.gov/briefing-room/statements-releases/2022/05/04/white-house-announces-conference-on-hunger-nutrition-and-health-in-september/
41. Dietz W. Climate change and malnutrition: We need to act now. J Clin Invest. 2020;130 (2):556–558.
42. Kumanyika S. A framework for increasing equity impact in obesity prevention. Am J Public Health. 2019;109(10):1350–1357.
43. Kahn M, Mohaddes K, Ng RNC, et al. Long-term macroeconomic effects of climate change: A cross-country analysis. National Bureau of Economic Research. August, 2019. www.nber.org/papers/w26167. (Accessed November 20, 2019).
44. Singer M, Bulled N, Ostrach B, et al. Syndemics and the biosocial conception of health. Lancet. 2017;389(10072):941–950.
45. Environmental Protection Agency. Sources of Green House Emissions. www.epa.gov/ghgemissions/sources-greenhouse-gasemissions. (Accessed November 20, 2019).
46. Sáez-Almendros S, Obrador B, Bach-Faig A, et al. Environmental footprints of Mediterranean versus Western dietary patterns: Beyond the health benefits of the Mediterranean diet. Environ Health. 2013;12:118.
47. Aleksandrowicz L, Green R, Joy E, et al. The impacts of dietary change on greenhouse gas emissions, land use, water use, and health: A systematic review. PLoS One. 2016;11 (11):e0165797.
48. U.S. Department of Health and Human Services and U.S. Department of Agriculture. 2015–2020 Dietary Guidelines for Americans, 8th edition. December 2015. http://health.gov/dietaryguidelines/2015/guidelines/
49. Martínez-González M, Corella D, Salas-Salvadó J, et al. Cohort profile: Design and methods of the PREDIMED study. Int J Epidemiol. 2012;41:377–385.

50. Appel L, Moore T, Obarzanek E, et al. A clinical trial of the effects of dietary patterns on blood pressure. DASH Collaborative Research Group. N Engl J Med. 1997;336(16):1117–1124.
51. Vilsack T, Burwell S. Dietary guidelines: Giving you the tools you need to make healthy choices. US Department of Agriculture. 2015. www.usda.gov/media/blog/2015/10/06/2015-dietary-guidelines-giving-you-tools-you-needmake-healthy-choices. Posted February 21, 2017. (Accessed November 21, 2023).
52. Reinhart R. Global warming age gap: Younger Americans most worried. Gallup. https://news.gallup.com/poll/234314/globalwarming-age-gap-younger-americans-worried.aspx. May 11, 2018. (Accessed November 21, 2023).
53. Kurtz A, Grant K, Marano R, et al. Long-term effects of malnutrition on severity of COVID-19. Sci Rep. 2021;11(1):14974.
54. Barazzoni R, et al. ESPEN expert statements and practical guidance for nutritional management of individuals with SARS-CoV-2 infection. Clin Nutr. 2020;39:1631–1638.
55. Bedock D, et al. Prevalence and severity of malnutrition in hospitalized COVID-19 patients. Clin Nutr ESPEN. 2020;40:214–219.

8 Dietary Guidelines for Americans 2020–2025

Key Points

- The Dietary Guidelines for Americans (DGAs) are issued every five years. The current version is 2020–2025.
- The DGAs are based on the concept of dietary patterns, which is an approach that is also taken in this book.
- The information in the DGAs 2020–2025 forms the evidence-based underpinnings for multiple federal nutrition programs as well as recommendations from a variety of professional organizations.
- Clinicians should be familiar with the DGAs 2020–2025 and use it as an evidence base for making nutritional recommendations to every patient.

8.1 INTRODUCTION

The DGAs are issued every five years [1]. They represent the definitive, evidence-based summary of up-to-date nutritional information, which serves the important role of providing the basis for many government programs and recommendations in the area of nutrition and health. The scientific connection between food and health has been well documented for many decades. Substantial evidence exists that leading a generally healthy lifestyle, including following a healthy dietary pattern, can help people achieve and maintain good health as well as reduce the risk of chronic diseases throughout the phases of the lifespan.

The first edition of the DGAs was published in 1980 [2]. As mentioned, they are published every five years and provide scientific-based advice on what to eat and drink to promote health and reduce the risk of chronic disease while meeting nutrient needs. The DGAs also serve as a basis for policy makers in nutrition and health professionals to help individuals consume healthy nutrition and an adequate diet. The DGAs should be in the tool kit of every clinician.

The DGAs are not intended to be clinical guidelines for treating chronic diseases; rather, the goal is to promote health and prevent disease. Chronic diseases, of course, result from a variety of different considerations ranging from biological and behavioral to socioeconomic, environmental, and genetic factors. DGAs represent the U.S. population and include people who are healthy as well as those at risk for diet-related chronic conditions and diseases such as cardiovascular disease (CVD), type 2 diabetes mellitus (T2DM), and obesity. The DGAs are based on the recognition that CVD, T2DM, and obesity, as well as some types of cancer, are prevalent among Americans and pose major public health issues. The DGAs 2020–2025 also are based on the understanding that over half of the adults in the United States have

 DOI: 10.1201/9781003452607-8

one or more diet-related chronic conditions. The DGAs 2020–2025 are also based on the understanding that just about everyone, irrespective of health status, can benefit from making food and beverage choices that better support healthy dietary patterns.

The DGAs also focus on dietary patterns, rather than individual foods or nutrients. This strategy is consistent with modern understandings of nutritional science and is the same approach that is adopted throughout this book.

In addition, the most recent DGAs focus on a lifespan approach. This highlights the importance of encouraging healthy dietary patterns at every stage of life from infancy to older adulthood and involves identifying needs specific to each life stage.

8.2 TERMS TO KNOW

Several nutritional terms are used in the DGAs that are vital to put them into action. These are the same terms that are utilized throughout this book. They are the following:

- **Dietary pattern**—This is the combination of foods and beverages that constitute an individual's complete dietary intake over time. This term may be used to describe a customary eating pattern or a description of a combination of foods recommended for consumption.
- **Nutrient dense**—Nutrient-dense foods and beverages are defined as those that provide vitamins, minerals, and other health-promoting components and have little added sugars, saturated fat, and sodium [3]. Included among nutrient-dense foods are vegetables, fruits, whole grains, seafood, eggs, beans, peas, and lentils, as well as unsalted nuts and seeds, fat-free and low-fat dairy products, and lean meats and poultry. Nutrient-dense foods are prepared with little or no added sugar, saturated fat, or sodium.

8.3 HISTORICAL BACKGROUND

The DGAs 2020–2025 represent a key part of the complex and multifaceted approach to promote health and reduce chronic disease risk. The DGAs are a foundation for federal food, nutrition, and health policies and programs. They are also a key body of information for health professionals and other healthcare and nutrition professionals who work with and advise the general public on how to consume a healthy and nutritionally adequate diet. A fundamental premise of the DGAs is that everyone, no matter their age or race, ethnicity or economic circumstances, or current health status, can benefit from making healthy food and beverage choices that support overall healthy dietary patterns. Over time, eating patterns in the United States have remained far below the DGA recommendations. (See Figure 8.1—this is page 4 of the DGA.) As depicted in this figure, the U.S. population is far below recommendations set by the Healthy Eating Index-2015 (HEI-2015). The HEI-2015 health score is based on 100 possible points [4]. A score of 100 indicates that all recommendations on average were met or exceeded. The higher the total score, the higher the dietary quality. An important goal for the DGAs remains to increase the average score based on HEI-2015 scales.

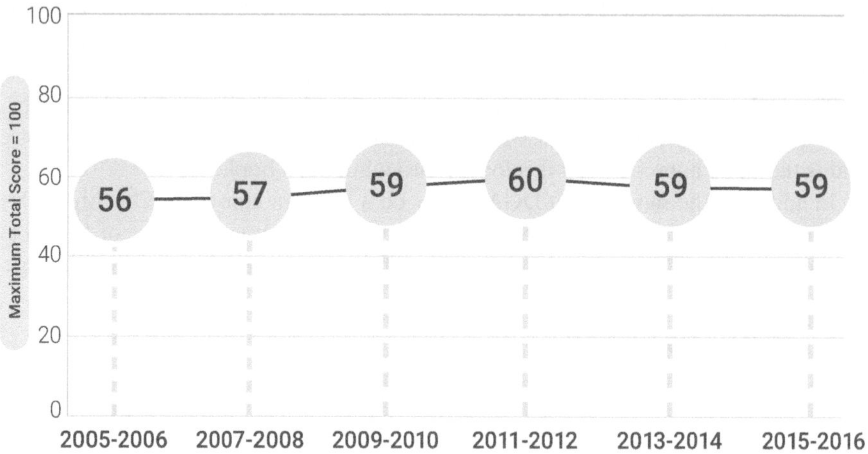

FIGURE 8.1 Adherence of the U.S. population to the dietary guidelines over time.

Source: U.S. Department of Agriculture and U.S. Department of Health and Human Services. U.S. Department of Agriculture and U.S. Department of Health and Human Services. *Dietary Guidelines for Americans, 2020–2025*. 9th Edition. December 2020. Available at DietaryGuidelines.gov.

8.4 NUTRITION-RELATED HEALTH CONDITIONS

Nutrition-related health conditions in the United States are extremely prevalent. The DGAs provide a useful and important table that provides current statistics on health conditions and the likelihood of individuals having them. These conditions are outlined in the DGAs 2020–2025 and are found on Figure 8.2.

8.5 DIETARY PATTERNS

The DGAs have evolved to the point that they now recommend overall dietary patterns. This is consistent with modern scientific understandings. The DGAs were at the forefront of making this determination based on scientific studies. Prior DGAs had focused on individual nutrients and foods. However, multiple experts have now recognized that nutrients and foods are not consumed in isolation. People consume them in various combinations over time; hence, dietary patterns. These foods also appear to act synergistically to influence health. The 2025 DGAs carried this underlying understanding forward by recommending an overall healthy dietary pattern. This also allows flexibility so that people can personalize their food and beverage choices to accommodate their wants and ethnic backgrounds and meet food preferences and budgetary considerations.

8.6 HEALTHY DIETARY PATTERNS AT EVERY LIFE STAGE

The 2020–2025 DGAs also focus on encouraging healthy dietary patterns at every stage of life from birth to older adulthood. This allows incorporating recommendations specific to each life stage and also allows a healthy dietary pattern to be

HEALTH CONDITIONS	STATISTICS
Overweight and Obesity	• About 74% of adults are overweight or have obesity. • Adults ages 40 to 59 have the highest rate of obesity (43%) of any age group with adults 60 years and older having a 41% rate of obesity. • About 40% of children and adolescents are overweight or have obesity; the rate of obesity increases throughout childhood and teen years.
Cardiovascular Disease (CVD) and Risk Factors: • Coronary artery disease • Hypertension • High LDL and total blood cholesterol • Stroke	• Heart disease is the leading cause of death. • About 18.2 million adults have coronary artery disease, the most common type of heart disease. • Stroke is the fifth leading cause of death. • Hypertension, high LDL cholesterol, and high total cholesterol are major risk factors in heart disease and stroke. • Rates of hypertension and high total cholesterol are higher in adults with obesity than those who are at a healthy weight. • About 45% of adults have hypertension.[a] • More Black adults (54%) than White adults (46%) have hypertension. • More adults ages 60 and older (75%) than adults ages 40 to 59 (55%) have hypertension. • Nearly 4% of adolescents have hypertension.[b] • More than 11% of adults have high total cholesterol, ≥240 mg/dL. • More women (12%) than men (10%) have high total cholesterol, ≥240 mg/dL. • 7% of children and adolescents have high total cholesterol, ≥200 mg/dL.
Diabetes	• Almost 11% of Americans have type 1 or type 2 diabetes. • Almost 35% of American adults have prediabetes, and people 65 years and older have the highest rate (48%) compared to other age groups. • Almost 90% of adults with diabetes also are overweight or have obesity. • About 210,000 children and adolescents have diabetes, including 187,000 with type 1 diabetes. • About 6-9% of pregnant women develop gestational diabetes.
Cancer[c] • Breast Cancer • Colorectal Cancer	• Colorectal cancer in men and breast cancer in women are among the most common types of cancer. • About 250,520 women will be diagnosed with breast cancer this year. • Close to 5% of men and women will be diagnosed with colorectal cancer at some point during their lifetime. • More than 1.3 million people are living with colorectal cancer. • The incidence and mortality rates are highest among those ages 65 and older for every cancer type.
Bone Health and Muscle Strength	• More women (17%) than men (5%) have osteoporosis. • 20% of older adults have reduced muscle strength. • Adults over 80 years, non-Hispanic Asians, and women are at the highest risk for reduced bone mass and muscle strength.

FIGURE 8.2 Facts About Nutrition

Source: U.S. Department of Agriculture and U.S. Department of Health and Human Services. U.S. Department of Agriculture and U.S. Department of Health and Human Services. *Dietary Guidelines for Americans, 2020–2025*. 9th Edition. December 2020. Available at DietaryGuidelines.gov.

carried forward in the next stage of life. This approach also recognizes that each life stage is distinct and that nutrient needs may vary over the course of a lifespan, while each life stage has unique implications and demands for food and beverage choices to minimize chronic disease risk. This approach also recognizes the importance of continuity, emphasizing that a healthy dietary pattern established in early life may have beneficial impacts on disease prevention and health promotion over the course of many decades.

8.7 QUANTITATIVE GUIDANCE FROM FOODS, NOT NUTRIENT REQUIREMENTS

Nutrient requirements are a separate issue compared to the dietary guidance found in the DGAs. Nutrient requirements are established by the National Academies of Science, which are known as Dietary Reference Intakes (DRI) on nutrients [5]. These include macronutrients (e.g. protein, carbohydrates, and fat) as well as vitamins and minerals (e.g. vitamin C, iron, and sodium) and food components (e.g. dietary fiber). The DGAs translate the National Academies of Science recommendations into food and beverage recommendations. The DGAs also recognize that occasionally fortified foods and dietary supplements may be useful, although the core recommendation remains to achieve nutrients through food and beverage choices.

8.8 HEALTH PROMOTION, NOT DISEASE TREATMENT

The fundamental mission of the DGAs is health promotion and disease prevention. It should be noted, however, that the DGAs represent the U.S. population, which includes healthy individuals and also individuals who are either at risk of or have already developed diet-related chronic conditions and diseases. The DGAs are not intended as a clinical guideline for treating chronic diseases, but may serve as a reference for various organizations such as medical, federal, voluntary, or patient organizations as these organizations develop clinical nutrition guidance specifically related to people living with a particular medical condition. In the area of chronic diseases, of course, nutrition is only one of many variables and includes multiple other lifestyle medicine modalities as well as genetic, socioeconomic, and environmental factors.

8.9 THE PROCESS FOR DEVELOPING THE DIETARY GUIDELINES FOR AMERICANS

The cornerstone of the development process for the DGAs is to survey and employ the best scientific evidence available. As already indicated, this process occurs every five years. It starts with the appointment of the DGAs Advisory Committee to review current scientific evidence [5]. These experts typically provide scientific reviews of research projects and also, particularly in the current DGAs, utilize the process of food pattern modeling. This type of modeling analysis relates to how changes in the amount or types of foods and beverages in a dietary pattern might affect meeting nutrient needs across the U.S. population. A variety of different approaches are used in the modeling process. This includes both profiles of nutrient-dense foods and current U.S. population dietary data.

8.10 FOUR OVERARCHING GUIDELINES

The DGAs 2020–2025 emphasizes the tagline "Make every bite count" and is enlivened by four overarching guidelines. These guidelines are as follows:

- **<u>Guideline #1: Follow a healthy dietary pattern at every life stage</u>**—The DGAs are based on the fundamental premise that almost everyone, irrespective of their age, race, ethnicity, or health status, can benefit from making food and beverage choices to support a healthy dietary pattern.

  The concept and practice of healthy eating start at birth and carry on through older adulthood. The fundamental guide for healthy eating is supplied by the Healthy U.S.-Style Dietary Pattern. An example of this for the 2,000 calorie level, given in either daily or weekly amounts, is found in Figure 8.3 (page 20 of the DGA). The Healthy U.S.-Style Dietary Pattern is based on an enormous body of scientific information that is applicable to every life stage. Common characteristics of multiple healthy dietary patterns include higher intake of vegetables, fruits, legumes, whole grains, low and nonfat dairy, lean meats and poultry, seafood, nuts, and unsaturated vegetable oils, as well as a relatively lower consumption of red and processed meats, sugar-sweetened foods and beverages, and refined grains.

FOOD GROUP OR SUBGROUP[a]	Daily Amount[b] of Food From Each Group (Vegetable and protein foods subgroup amounts are per week.)
Vegetables (cup eq/day)	**2 ½**
	Vegetable Subgroups in Weekly Amounts
Dark-Green Vegetables (cup eq/wk)	1 ½
Red and Orange Vegetables (cup eq/wk)	5 ½
Beans, Peas, Lentils (cup eq/wk)	1 ½
Starchy Vegetables (cup eq/wk)	5
Other Vegetables (cup eq/wk)	4
Fruits (cup eq/day)	**2**
Grains (ounce eq/day)	**6**
Whole Grains (ounce eq/day)	≥ 3
Refined Grains (ounce eq/day)	< 3
Dairy (cup eq/day)	**3**
Protein Foods (ounce eq/day)	**5 ½**
	Protein Foods Subgroups in Weekly Amounts
Meats, Poultry, Eggs (ounce eq/wk)	26
Seafood (ounce eq/wk)	8
Nuts, Seeds, Soy Products (ounce eq/wk)	5
Oils (grams/day)	**27**
Limit on Calories for Other Uses (kcal/day)[c]	**240**
Limit on Calories for Other Uses (%/day)	12%

FIGURE 8.3 Healthy U.S.-Style Dietary Pattern

Source: U.S. Department of Agriculture and U.S. Department of Health and Human Services. U.S. Department of Agriculture and U.S. Department of Health and Human Services. *Dietary Guidelines for Americans, 2020–2025. 9th Edition*. December 2020. Available at DietaryGuidelines.gov.

The premise that these patterns yield health benefits has been demonstrated in multiple different population groups. In addition, the healthy dietary pattern supports appropriate caloric levels. These may vary considerably depending on the person's level of physical activity, age, sex, height and weight, and pregnancy or lactation status. It should be noted that calorie needs for older adults decrease somewhat, as does the basal metabolic rate. The best general rule for regulating caloric intake is by measuring body weight status.

- **Guideline #2: Customize and enjoy food and beverage choices to reflect personal preferences, cultural traditions, and budgetary considerations**—At every life stage, the dietary pattern should be enjoyable. While there are many different aspects of the American population, including different ages, life stages, racial and ethnic backgrounds, and socioeconomic status, a healthy dietary pattern can benefit all of these individuals. The fundamental premise of this guideline is to start with personal preferences and incorporate cultural traditions while considering budgetary implications. Exposure to different types of foods will allow children to enjoy a variety of foods. Cultural background can also significantly influence food and beverage choices. Customizing the DGAs to reflect specific cultures and traditions is an important strategy for helping diverse communities enjoy a healthy dietary pattern.

  It is a common misconception that eating healthily is expensive. However, a variety of strategies exist to help individuals and families follow healthy dietary patterns. Multiple documents are available from the U.S. Department of Agriculture (USDA) to help individuals take simple steps to make a healthy dietary pattern fit within budgetary constrictions. Tables are available both from the DGA 2020–2025 and various documents through the USDA to provide a wide variety of components that meet nutrient-dense criteria and will help individuals customize and enjoy a healthy diet.
- **Guideline #3: Focus on meeting food group needs with nutrient-dense foods and beverages and stay within calorie limits**—The DGA recommendations for food groups, including vegetables, fruit, grains, dairy, and protein foods, should be eaten at the appropriate calorie level, and limited amounts of added sugars, saturated fats, and sodium should be incorporated into the diet. (See Guideline #4.) Unfortunately, at the current time, 80% of Americans have dietary patterns that are low in vegetables, fruits, and dairy. More than half the population is meeting or exceeding total grain and protein food recommendations but not meeting recommendations for subgroups in each of these groups. For example, within the total grain group many more Americans are consuming refined grains than whole grains. In the protein group more Americans are consuming meat, poultry, and eggs than are consuming either seafood or nuts, seeds, and soy products. Over 90% of the U.S. population does not meet the recommendations for vegetables, while 80% of the U.S. population does not meet the fruit recommendations. Almost three-quarters of the adult population meets or exceeds

the recommendations for meat, poultry, and eggs, but 90% do not meet the recommendation for seafood, and more than half do not meet the recommendation for nuts, seeds, and soy products.

- **Guideline #4: Limit foods and beverages higher in added sugars, saturated fats, and sodium and limit alcoholic beverages**—Most of the calories that a person needs to meet each day, approximately 85%, are needed to meet food group recommendations in nutrient-dense forms. The remaining calories, representing about 15%, are available for other uses. (These used to be called discretionary calories, although it was determined that many people did not understand this concept. Thus, it was changed to "calories from other sources.") For most Americans, the 15% of calories that "are for other uses" equates to 250–350 calories per day. The DGAs 2020–2025 recommends added sugars at less than 10% of calories per day. If added sugars in foods and beverages exceed 10% of calories in a healthy dietary pattern within calorie limits, this is very difficult to achieve.

  Current average intakes of saturated fat in the United States are 11% of calories. Only 22% of individuals consume amounts of saturated fat consistent with a limit of less than 10% of calories. It should be noted that both the DGAs and the National Academies of Science recommend trans fat and dietary cholesterol intake be as low as possible without compromising nutritional adequacy in the diet. The recommendation to limit cholesterol in foods is somewhat controversial since some data suggest that dietary cholesterol has minimal impact on blood levels of cholesterol.

  Sodium is found in a variety of foods, which results in Americans consuming more sodium than is recommended by the DGAs. In fact, the average intake of sodium for individuals above the age of one is 3,400 milligrams/day. Most of the salt consumed in the United States comes from salt added during commercial food processing and preparation, including food prepared at restaurants. The DGAs 2020–2025 do not recommend that individuals who do not drink alcohol start drinking for any reason. For adults age 21 or older who chose to drink alcoholic beverages, drinking less is better for health than drinking more. The DGAs recommend that for those who consume alcohol do so in moderation by limiting intake to two or fewer drinks per day for men and one drink per day or less for women on days when alcohol is consumed. One alcoholic drink is equivalent to 12 ounces of regular beer (5% alcohol), 5 fluid ounces of wine (12% alcohol), or 1.5 fluid ounces of 80 proof distilled spirits (40% alcohol). Approximately 60% of adults report alcoholic beverage consumption in the past month. Approximately 30% binge drink, sometimes multiple times per month. Alcoholic beverages translate to approximately 9% of calories per month. Thus, for those who drink, alcoholic beverages alone account for most of the calories that remain after meeting the food group recommendations in nutrient-dense form, leaving very few calories for added sugars or saturated fats.

8.11 OVERVIEW OF THE *DIETARY GUIDELINES FOR AMERICANS 2020–2025*

The current DGA guidelines contain six chapters and the appendices. They are the following:

- Chapter 1: **Nutrition and Healthy Across the Lifespan: Guidelines and Key Recommendations**—This chapter discusses health benefits for lifelong healthy dietary choices.
- Chapter 2: **Infants and Toddlers**—This chapter provides key recommendations for this age group, along with guidance for how to put these recommendations into action.
- Chapter 3: **Children and Adolescents**—This chapter describes nutrition issues specific for children and adolescents ages 2–18. This chapter also has recommendations containing specific dietary guideline considerations for this life stage and concludes with a discussion of ways to support healthy dietary patterns for this age group and looks forward to the next life stage—adult.
- Chapter 4: **Adult**—This chapter contains a discussion of nutrition issues that characterize the adult life stage (ages 19–59) and discusses how current intakes compare with these recommendations. This chapter also has suggestions for supporting healthy dietary patterns related to two important lifestyle changes in the next two chapters, namely women who are pregnant or lactating and older adults.
- Chapter 5: **Women Who Are Pregnant and Lactating**—This chapter contains a discussion of selected nutrition issues important to this stage in adult life and also contains suggestions for how to support healthy eating dietary patterns for this population group.
- Chapter 6: **Older Adults**—This chapter includes a discussion of selected nutrition issues important to older adults ages 60 and older. It also contains information related to how current intakes compare to these recommendations and provides specific dietary guidelines related to considerations of this group.
- **Appendices**—The appendices contain a variety of tables summarizing various nutritional goals for age or sex groups as well as estimated caloric needs for all ages at three different physical activity levels.

8.12 IMPLEMENTING THE DIETARY GUIDELINES

The DGAs are used for a wide variety of federal programs including food assistance and meal programs, nutrition education efforts, and assistance about national health objectives. The DGAs form the basis for the National School Lunch Program [6] and also the Older Americans Act: Nutrition Services Program [7]. In addition, the Supplemental Nutrition Assistance Program (SNAP) [8] and the Healthy People Objectives for the Nation [9] are based on DGA guidelines. Thus, multiple mechanisms rely on the DGAs. Implementation of the guidelines relies on the work of a variety of organizations. It is also important to emphasize that despite decades of recommendations that are generally consistent with each other, dietary guidelines are still not met by a large number of individuals. It is important for clinicians to know the DGAs and recommend principles based on them for their patients, as well as address potential barriers that might exist for incorporating the healthy recommendations from the DGAs to improve each individual patient's life. While the DGAs were geared toward the professional audience, it is important to translate these guidelines into actionable consumer messages to help individuals achieve healthy dietary patterns. One example of this is the MyPlate Program [10]. Details about this program are available at www.myplate.gov/. A graphic is available to share with patients to illustrate how the MyPlate Program works. This is found in Figure 8.4 (page 13 of the DGA). Different guidelines exist that are slight modifications of this graphic for specific population groups such as older Americans.

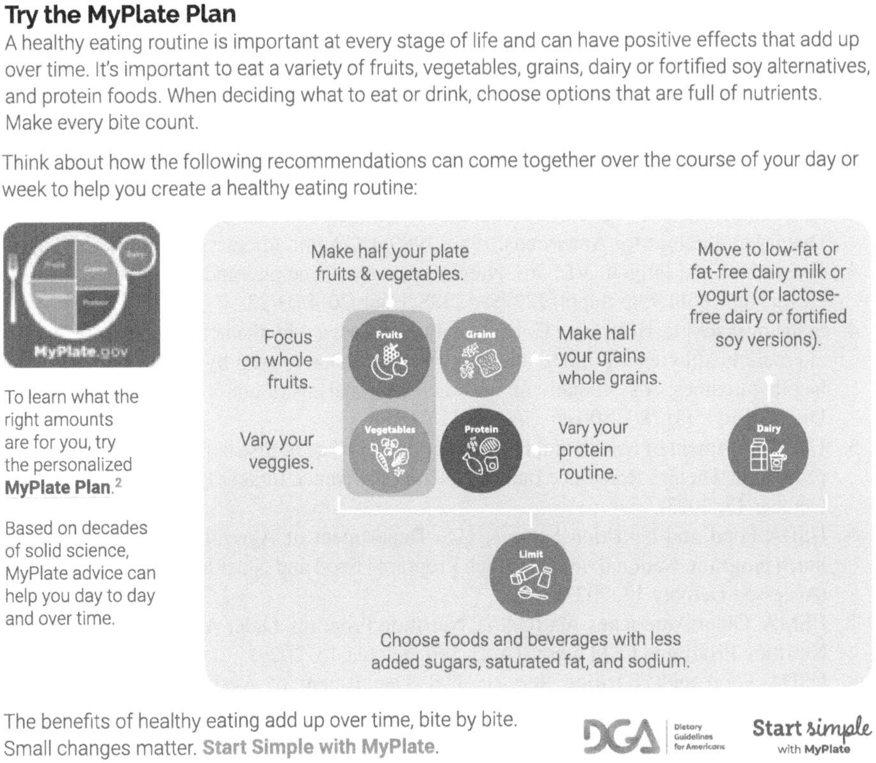
Try the MyPlate Plan
A healthy eating routine is important at every stage of life and can have positive effects that add up over time. It's important to eat a variety of fruits, vegetables, grains, dairy or fortified soy alternatives, and protein foods. When deciding what to eat or drink, choose options that are full of nutrients. Make every bite count.
Think about how the following recommendations can come together over the course of your day or week to help you create a healthy eating routine:
MyPlate.gov
To learn what the right amounts are for you, try the personalized MyPlate Plan.2
Based on decades of solid science, MyPlate advice can help you day to day and over time.
Make half your plate fruits & vegetables.
Focus on whole fruits.
Vary your veggies.
Fruits
Grains
Vegetables
Protein
Make half your grains whole grains.
Vary your protein routine.
Move to low-fat or fat-free dairy milk or yogurt (or lactose-free dairy or fortified soy versions).
Dairy
Limit
Choose foods and beverages with less added sugars, saturated fat, and sodium.
The benefits of healthy eating add up over time, bite by bite. Small changes matter. Start Simple with MyPlate.
DGA Dietary Guidelines for Americans
Start simple with MyPlate

FIGURE 8.4 MyPlate plan.

Source: U.S. Department of Agriculture and U.S. Department of Health and Human Services. U.S. Department of Agriculture and U.S. Department of Health and Human Services. *Dietary Guidelines for Americans, 2020–2025*. 9th Edition. December 2020. Available at DietaryGuidelines.gov.

8.13 CONCLUSIONS

The DGAs 2020–2025 are an indispensable summary of scientific information relating to food and beverage choices and how they fit into dietary patterns to achieve improved health for all Americans. The DGA document should be in the tool kit of all clinicians to help to guide them in their counseling of patients to meet healthy nutritional guidelines.

Clinical Applications

- The DGAs are a science-based approach to nutrition.
- Every clinician should be familiar with the content of the DGAs 2020–2025 as the basis for making recommendations to their patients for healthy nutritional patterns.
- The DGAs 2020–2025 are based on a lifespan approach providing information at every stage of life from birth to older adulthood.
- The DGAs 2020–2025 should be an important component of the toolbox of every practicing clinician in order to provide evidence-based nutritional guidance to improve the health of all patients.

REFERENCES

1. U.S. Department of Agriculture and U.S. Department of Health and Human Services. *Dietary Guidelines for Americans, 2020–2025*, 9th edition. December 2020. DietaryGuidelines.gov. 2020. www.dietaryguidelines.gov/resources/2020-2025-dietary-guidelines-online-materials
2. U.S. Department of Agriculture and U.S. Department of Health and Human Services. Dietary Guidelines for Americans, 1980. 1980. DGA.pdf. (dietaryguidelines.gov)
3. Drewnowski A, Fulgoni VL, 3rd. Nutrient density: Principles and evaluation tools. Am J Clin Nutr. 2014;99(5 Suppl):1223S–1228S. Epub 2014/03/22.
4. Schwingshackl L, Hoffmann G. Diet quality as assessed by the healthy eating index, the alternate healthy eating index, the dietary approaches to stop hypertension score, and health outcomes: A systematic review and meta-analysis of cohort studies. J Acad Nutr Diet. 2015;115(5):780–800.e5. Epub 2015/02/15.
5. U.S. Department of Health and Human Services. Office of disease prevention and health promotion. Dietary Reference Intakes. Dietary Reference Intakes | health.gov. (Accessed October 13, 2023).
6. USDA Food and Nutrition Service. U.S. Department of Agriculture. National school lunch program. National School Lunch Program | Food and Nutrition Service (usda.gov). (Accessed October 13, 2023).
7. FEMA. Older Americans Act (OAA): Nutrition Program. Older Americans Act (OAA): Nutrition Program | FEMA.gov. (Accessed October 13, 2023).
8. USDA Food and Nutrition Service. U.S. Department of Agriculture. Supplemental Nutrition Assistance Program (SNAP). Supplemental Nutrition Assistance Program (SNAP) | Food and Nutrition Service (usda.gov). (Accessed October 13, 2023).
9. Centers for Disease Control and Prevention. National Center for Health Statistics. Healthy people 2020. Healthy People—Healthy People 2020 (cdc.gov). (Accessed October 13, 2023).
10. USDA. U.S. Department of Agriculture. MyPlate. MyPlate | U.S. Department of Agriculture. (Accessed October 13, 2023).

9 Nutrition and Inflammation

Key Points

- Inflammation is considered to be an important and often inciting event in contributing to multiple chronic diseases including cardiovascular disease (CVD), diabetes, obesity, cancer, dementia, and cognitive decline.
- The recent COVID-19 pandemic showed that underlying inflammation can often lead to hyperinflammation and cause morbidity and mortality in people who have underlying chronic conditions.
- Nutrition can play a significant role in either reducing underlying inflammation or contributing to it.
- Multiple healthy diets that include increased fruits and vegetable consumption and whole grains and reduction in red meat, processed meat, saturated fat, salt, and sugar can lower inflammation.
- The typical Western diet, which is high in saturated fat and processed foods, is considered an inflammatory diet.
- For all of these reasons, healthy nutrition to reduce inflammation should be a highlight in the counseling of individuals by physicians.

9.1 INTRODUCTION

There is an increasing understanding that inflammatory processes underly many of the chronic diseases suffered throughout the world [1–6]. These include CVD, diabetes, obesity, cancer, and dementia. The linkages between inflammation and the immune system have become prominent, particularly in the last few years, underscored by the relationship between the COVID-19 pandemic and significant inflammatory response [7–10]. Many other factors can impact on the inflammatory response. Multiple lifestyle factors play a particularly prominent role in either lowering or increasing inflammation. The chief among these are nutritional factors. Other lifestyle-related factors that impact on inflammation include level of physical activity [11–14], body weight [15–17], underlying chronic disease, sleep [18,19], and stress. The purpose of the current chapter is to focus attention particularly on the relationship between nutrition and inflammation, although some discussion will occur related to other significant lifestyle factors.

It has long been known that a low-protein status such as found in malnutrition increases the likelihood of infection and decreases the immune response [20–22]. Optimal nutritional status is also fundamental to modulate inflammatory and oxidative stress processes, which are all interrelated with the immune system. Recent research has demonstrated the strong relationship between dietary constituents,

DOI: 10.1201/9781003452607-9

nutrition, inflammation, and oxidative stress and has even led to instruments such as a population-based dietary inflammatory index [23–25].

9.2 THE IMMUNE SYSTEM, INFLAMMATION, AND DISEASE RISK

The inflammatory response is a cornerstone for defending against infections in the human body, with circulating phagocytes (neutrophils, monocytes, and eosinophils) and lymphocytes playing critical roles in generating an inflammatory response to infections [26]. These phagocytes respond to chemical signals initiated by an infective agent. A complicated sequence occurs that has a variety of humeral mediators. Once the phagocyte arrives at the focus of an infection, it can adhere to a microorganism, ingest it, and digest it. A wide variety of bacteria and fungi are killed by phagocytes in this manner. The immune response includes cellular components such as T lymphocytes and B lymphocytes to create a multitude of cytokines, which also serve to provide an important immunologic defense in the body [27–31].

When there is a chronic level of inflammation, this response may become pathological. It is now recognized that a number of metabolic conditions such as atherosclerotic CVD [32], responses to insulin in diabetes, and generation of a variety of inflammatory responders in obesity, cancer, and even dementia contribute to the ongoing consequences observed in these conditions. Recently, it became clear that inflammation was one of the key underlying main effects of the COVID-19 pandemic. In some individuals, an exuberant inflammatory response damaged a variety of human tissues, particularly pulmonary tissues.

In contrast, at the first exposure of pathogens, a strong response from the innate defense system occurs at the beginning of infection. Thus, a certain level of inflammation is physiologic and required for optimal triggering of the immune response. However, low-grade, systemic inflammation may harm the human body and, as already indicated, is common in a variety of conditions including CVD, inflammatory bowel disease, type 2 diabetes mellitus (T2DM), arthritis, cancer, and obesity.

Individuals who have this type of low-grade inflammation may present with a dysregulated innate immune system, which may result in an increased risk of infection. This appears to be one of the underlying factors in complications resulting in the severe acute respiratory syndrome caused by COVID-19, which appears to be due to pronounced inflammation caused by viral replication. Patients with severe COVID-19 have been demonstrated to produce a variety of inflammatory cytokines including interleukin (IL)-6 and IL-8, as well as a variety of other cytokines. This suggests a cytokine storm resulting in hyperinflammation and potentially life-threatening organ failure [33–38]. In addition to the inflammatory response, a high level of oxidative stress may also be provoked by viral replication, further hindering the immune response [9].

There is now increasing evidence that various nutritional factors can play a role in helping to reduce low levels of inflammation further and also protect against hyperinflammation [9,10]. Thus, consideration of nutritional factors can serve as an important adjunct to the immune system of preventing acute infection and also helping to mitigate the chronic inflammation that is found in multiple diseases.

9.3 NUTRITION AND INFLAMMATION

Multiple avenues of evidence exist suggesting that nutrition can play an important role in lessening inflammation [9,10]. For example, when the World Health Organization issued guidelines for reducing noncommunicable diseases (NCDs), underlying inflammation was thought to play a major role in chronic conditions such as CVD, diabetes, and obesity [39–43]. In addition, the link between viral illness, infection, and NCDs has been observed in a variety of infections such as influenza and now also COVID-19.

Chronic and unresolved inflammation is implicated in the onset, progression, and development of NCDs. Underlying inflammation may have exacerbated COVID-19 infection in a variety of chronic conditions such as obesity, hypertension, and diabetes, where mortality from COVID-19 was two to four times greater in individuals who did not have one of these underlying conditions than in individuals who did not [44]. One goal to reduce an individual's risk of developing an NCD is to help mitigate inflammatory mediators and modifiable risk factors such as diet, exercise, and other healthy lifestyle choices.

A consistent healthy dietary pattern is particularly important in this area. Conversely, an unhealthy diet and lifestyle are associated with low-grade inflammation and increased oxidative stress [41]. Considerable evidence exists that food and nutrients consumed affect how the immune system functions. Nutritional status carries a significant impact for overall health and reduction of NCDs as well as a reduced susceptibility to developing infections. It is important to emphasize that this is not a panacea. There is no single food or nutritional remedy that has been proven to prevent COVID-19 infection. Based on evidence from other viral infections, however, it is clear that nutritional status can play a significant role in patient outcomes [9,10].

Given the safety and ease of application, nutrition is a highly appropriate target to play a key role in "keeping healthy people healthy." This issue is particularly important as the population around the world continues to age, since elderly individuals are most at risk for NCDs as well as for developing significant COVID-19. The functional decline of the immune system is called immunosenescence, which may be based to some degree on nutritional deficiencies in the elderly population and perhaps even malnutrition.

9.4 DIETARY COMPONENTS, INFLAMMATION, AND IMMUNITY

- **Proteins**—Low protein status contributes to inflammation and increases the risk of infection. Therefore, intake of protein from sources of high biologic value such as eggs, fish, lean meat (e.g. poultry), and whey protein or other nonfat dietary protein may lower inflammation [20,45]. Thus, these high-quality proteins are an essential component of an anti-inflammatory diet. Consumption of proteins of high biological value is known to be crucial for optimal production of antibodies.
- **Lipids**—Fatty acids (FAs) may impact on anti-inflammatory responses. For example, high sensitive C-reactive protein (hs-CRP) has been linked to

saturated FA consumption [46–48]. Lower hs-CRP levels have been linked to polyunsaturated fats. Omega-3 FAs appear to have potent anti-inflammatory capability, while trans fatty acid intake, particularly from processed foods such as fries and chips, appears to be pro-inflammatory and associated with increased tumor necrosis factor (TNF)-alpha, IL-6, and hs-CRP levels. Two essential FA classes, omega-6 and omega-3, must be consumed within the diet, since the human body is unable to produce them. Intake of omega-3 FAs from fish and seafood triggers anti-inflammatory reactions. It should be noted, however, that high intake ratio of omega-6 to omega-3 FAs, which may be in the range of 10:1 in Westernized diets, may actually foster pro-inflammatory responses.

- **Carbohydrates and Dietary Fiber**—A diet that is high in processed carbohydrates (white flour, refined sugar) may cause increased production of oxidative stress through free radicals, which can provoke the release of inflammatory cytokines [49–51]. Thus, choosing higher-quality carbohydrates such as whole grains, vegetables, fruits, and nuts has been recommended in multiple healthful diets. One of the reasons is that these types of higher-quality carbohydrates do not trigger adverse pro-inflammatory effects. Dietary fibers, in particular, help to lower inflammation. In addition, dietary fibers positively influence gut health. Fiber may have a significant effect on short-chain fatty acid (SCFA) production, which is considered anti-inflammatory. The area of modulating gut microbiota through nutrition is an emerging and important area of research.
- **Micronutrients**—Micronutrients include multiple vitamins, several minerals, and trace elements, all of which are defined as essential. These include vitamin A [52–54], vitamin D [55], vitamin E [56,57], vitamin C [58–60], and the B vitamins. Vitamin A has been associated with decreased inflammation and enhanced resistance to infection. Vitamin D, which is taken up in the diet from fish, eggs, fortified milk, and mushrooms, can also be synthesized in the skin in the presence of ultraviolet (UV) light and cholesterol. There is some suggestion that vitamin D may lower inflammatory responses. Vitamin E seems to improve T-cell function and immune system function [61]. Vitamin C has been associated as a classical antioxidant directly quenching free radicals. The B vitamins are directly involved in many energy regulating and enzymatic processes. Some evidence exists that they can lead to decreased inflammation. However, definitive information is needed about the role of B vitamins immune system functioning and the anti-inflammatory response.

9.5 MEASURING DIETARY QUALITY WITH THE HEALTHY EATING INDEX, ALTERNATIVE HEALTHY EATING INDEX, AND DIETARY APPROACHES TO STOP HYPERTENSION

As discussed in multiple chapters throughout this book, most modern nutrition research is done evaluating dietary quality and overall dietary patterns rather than individual foods or nutrients. For this reason, one way of evaluating dietary quality, particularly as it relates to inflammation and association with chronic disease, is to assess eating patterns based on well-established, evidence-based frameworks. Three of these are the Healthy Eating Index (HEI), the Alternative Healthy Eating Index (AHEI), and the Dietary Approach to Stop Hypertension (DASH) score, as they relate to health outcomes as analyzed through cohort studies [62].

The HEI was developed to measure how well diets conformed to the federal dietary guidelines, which are released every five years in the Dietary Guidelines for Americans. Most recently this was the *Dietary Guidelines for Americans 2020–2025*. The HEI-2010 involved 12 components: total fruit (5 points), total vegetables (5 points), greens and beans (5 points), whole grains (10 points), dairy (10 points), total protein foods (5 points), seafood and plant proteins (5 points), and fatty acids (polyunsaturated fatty acids, plus monounsaturated fatty acids to saturated fats ratio) (10 points); negative point values were assigned to refined grains (10 points), sodium (10 points), and empty calories from solid fats and alcoholic beverages such as wine and distilled spirits and added sugars (20 points). The overall scoring range was 0–100. The AHEI has 11 components (vegetables, fruits, nuts and soy, protein, ratio of white to red meat, cereal, fiber, trans fats, polyunsaturated to saturated fat ratio, duration of multivitamin use, and alcohol). For alcohol, the maximum score was awarded for 1.5–2.5 servings per day for men and 0.5–1.5 servings per day for women. The AHEI was updated in 2010 and has 14 components: vegetables, fruits, whole grains, sugar-sweetened beverages and fruit juice, nuts and legumes, red/processed meats, trans fats, long-chain (omega-3) fatty acids, octanoic acid, diclofenac acid, phenylacetic acid, polyunsaturated fat, sodium, and alcohol. The overall scoring range is 0–110.

The DASH diet score has two versions of eight components (fruit, vegetables, nuts and legumes, whole grains, low-fat dairy, sodium, red and processed meats, and sweetened beverages). These are scored differently, either minimal or maximal component scores 1 and 5 or minimal and maximum component scores of 0–10. Thus, the overall scoring range initially was 8–40, 0–80, or 0–11 using these different scoring scales. The goal in assessing dietary patterns with these three overall strategies was to develop guidelines for nutrition that are likely to reduce the incidence of CVD, cancer, type 2 diabetes mellitus (T2DM), and neurodegenerative diseases, which remain the most common causes of death in the Western world ever since 1970.

In a meta-analysis performed of these three frameworks, the highest scores on HEI, AHEI, and DASH were all associated with significant reduction of all-cause mortality risk of CVD by 22%, risk of cancer by 15%, and risk of diabetes by 22%, respectively. All of these diets feature increased fruits and vegetables, whole grains, and fish (particularly oily fish) and limit the amount of red meat, sugar-sweetened products, and salt. These findings support that the HEI, AHEI, and DASH dietary approaches, which all favorably improve health by lowering the risk of chronic disease. All three of these diets are essentially anti-inflammatory diets.

This type of work has been extended through the development and validation of an Empirical Dietary Inflammatory Index [23–25]. This work associated various components of the diet with either high plasma inflammatory markers (as measured by hs-CRP), IL-6, and IL-9 or lower or inverse inflammatory markers. Not surprisingly, components of dietary patterns that were associated with high inflammatory markers included processed meat, red meat, organ meat, refined grains, and high-energy beverages. Those that were associated with anti-inflammatory effects included dark yellow vegetables, leafy green vegetables, beer, wine, tea, and coffee.

A recent study evaluated healthy eating patterns and the risk of total and cause-specific mortality. In this study investigators utilized the HEI-2015 or the Alternative Mediterranean Diet (AMED) score, the Healthful Plant Based Diet Index (HPBDI) and AHEI. The study was conducted on 75,230 women from the Nurses Health Study and 44,085 men from the Health Professionals Follow Up Study [63]. These findings showed in this large sample that following healthy eating patterns as assessed by the previous four frameworks, individuals lowered their risk of chronic disease by 25% both for total and disease-specific mortality. Specifically, the healthy dietary scores were significantly and inversely associated with death from CVD, cancer, and respiratory disease, while the AMED score and the AHEI score were inversely associated with mortality from neurodegenerative diseases.

Other investigators have utilized diverse populations across multiple articles published from 2010 to 2014 and developed the Dietary Inflammatory Index. Not surprisingly, total fat as well as red meat and processed meat scored highly with regard to inflammatory markers.

9.6 DIETARY PATTERNS AND INFLAMMATION

As discussed in multiple other chapters in this book, the modern approach to nutrition involves looking at dietary patterns rather than single foods or nutrients. This is the approach that is adopted by the *Dietary Guidelines for Americans 2020–2025* as well as the 2021 nutrition guidance from the American Heart Association. A number of dietary patterns have been associated with decreased inflammation. These include the Mediterranean diet, the DASH diet, the Healthy U.S.-Style Dietary Plan, and vegetarian diets.

Perhaps the most studied of these dietary patterns is the Mediterranean diet. This pattern has been demonstrated to have strong anti-inflammatory properties and is characterized by relatively high dietary intake of minimally processed fruit, vegetables, legumes, olive oils, whole grains, nuts, and monounsaturated fats; low to moderate consumption of fermented dairy products, fish, poultry, and wine; and lower consumptions of processed and red meat. A diet that is rich in these foods is associated with anti-inflammatory and immunomodulatory compounds, including essential vitamins C, D, and E and minerals (zinc, copper, calcium, etc.) [64–67]. The PREDIMED study showed that these diets lower the risk of CVD [68]. This finding is postulated to have been achieved because of the lower inflammatory potential of this diet.

A subsequent study showed that individuals who followed the Mediterranean diet had a 25% decrease in risk factors for CVD events. Of this reduction, the highest amount of underlying etiology of the reduction came from reduced impact of inflammation.

There are other patterns that follow relatively closely in the dietary composition of the Mediterranean diet. These include the DASH diet, the Healthy U.S.-Style

Dietary Plan found in the *Dietary Guidelines for Americans 2020–2025*, and multiple vegetarian diets. All of these diets feature higher consumption of fruits and vegetables, whole grains, fish (preferably oily fish), and legumes. All of them recommend limited consumption of red meat, processed meat, sugar-containing foods and beverages, and salt. These diets have been assessed by the HEI and the AHEI and have been shown to be largely anti-inflammatory [62].

In contrast, the "Western" dietary (WD) pattern, which is prevalent in many developed countries, is characterized by high consumption of processed foods such as refined grains, cured and red meats, desserts and sweets, deep fried foods, and high-fat products. The WD also has a high intake of sugars, saturated fats, and refined carbohydrates and may be associated with lipid abnormalities. There is also a high prevalence of T2DM and obesity. The WD is also highly associated with hyperglycemia and linked strongly to inflammation, metabolic complications, and chronic disease [69–71]. Of note, individuals with resulting conditions of diabetes, obesity, and heart disease were at three to four times the risk of mortality from COVID-19 compared to individuals who followed lower inflammatory diets. Thus, inflammation has now become recognized as an even more vital component of health.

9.7 INFLAMMATION AND CHRONIC DISEASE

Multiple chronic metabolic diseases share an underlying component of inflammation. These include CVD, T2DM, and obesity [72–74]. The process of atherosclerosis, which underlies much of CVD including coronary heart disease and peripheral artery disease, is thought to be incited initially through inflammatory processes and their impact on the endothelium of arterial walls. Diabetes, which also comprises insulin resistance, has been shown to have an underlying etiology that presumably impacts on the likelihood that individuals with diabetes will also have concomitant CVD. It has been demonstrated in multiple studies that between two-thirds and three-quarters of people who have diabetes will ultimately die of heart disease. Obesity used to be thought as a condition with excess storage of fat, which was thought to be relatively inert. However, research now has shown clearly that adipocytes generate multiple inflammatory markers. Thus, obesity is considered to be a condition with an underlying chronic low-grade inflammation [74].

Recent cancer research has also shown that inflammation plays a role in the etiology of many cancers [73]. It is hypothesized that one of the linkages between obesity and cancer (obesity is the second leading cause of cancers) may come from manifestations of underlying inflammation.

Recent research into dementia of all kinds and particularly Alzheimer's disease has also now linked cognitive decline to inflammation.

Perhaps most prominently, the COVID-19 pandemic, which ultimately increased hyperinflammation in many individuals, was much more serious in people who had underlying, low-grade inflammatory diseases such as obesity, diabetes, and CVD. The good news is that proper nutrition can help mitigate some of the issues related to inflammation and should be strongly considered by all practitioners of lifestyle medicine in their counseling with individuals who have any of the multiple chronic diseases outlined in this chapter.

9.8 NUTRITION AND WEIGHT LOSS

As noted in multiple chapters in this book, weight loss results in significant reduction in risk factors for a variety of conditions including CVD, diabetes, and cancer. In both the DPP and the Look AHEAD Trial, individuals who lost 5–7% of their body weight lowered the risk of various chronic diseases, including heart disease and diabetes [75]. It has been hypothesized that reductions in inflammation played a significant role in reduction in the risk of these chronic diseases. Both DPP and Look AHEAD employed nutritional strategies that involved reducing the amount of fat in the diet, while restricting calories. Individuals were encouraged to increase the amounts of fruits and vegetables and whole grains, while lowering the fat in their diets. Thus, the nutrition intervention was key to both DPP and Look AHEAD and, it is hypothesized, reduced chronic disease in part by reducing inflammation.

9.9 INTERACTION WITH OTHER LIFESTYLE MODALITIES

While nutrition plays a key role in helping to modulate inflammation, multiple other lifestyle modalities also play significant roles. Chief among these are increased physical activity, avoiding cigarette smoking, and obtaining adequate sleep. Thus, when clinicians encourage people to reduce the amount of inflammation in their lives to lower their risk of chronic disease, all of these lifestyle-related modalities should play a central role. These various lifestyle modalities should be emphasized as ways of reducing inflammation, which is an underlying component for many of the chronic diseases suffered in the modern world, particularly the NCDs outlined in this chapter.

9.10 NUTRITION AND HEALTH EQUITY

In the area of nutrition and inflammation, it is important to also address the issue of health equity [76–78]. Consumption of increased fruits and vegetables and whole grains is clearly associated with health equity. In fact, many people have argued that more affluent individuals are able to reduce inflammation in their diet because they are more able to afford fruits and vegetables and whole grains compared to individuals of lower socioeconomic status. Individuals of lower socioeconomic status typically are more susceptible to consuming energy-dense but nutrient-poor diets including sugar-sweetened beverages, fast food, red meats, and other processed foods that are high in salt. Thus, addressing issues related to inflammation must also take into consideration issues related to health equity. This is such an important topic it will be dealt with in a separate chapter in this book.

9.11 CONCLUSIONS

Inflammation has been increasingly demonstrated to play a significant role in multiple chronic diseases including CVD, T2DM, obesity, cancer, and even cognitive decline and dementia. Nutrition can play a very significant role in the area of inflammation. Diets that are high in fruits and vegetables and whole grains and low in saturated fats, sugar, and salt have been repeatedly demonstrated to lower inflammation and reduce the risk of chronic disease. For this reason, it is important for all clinicians to counsel patients about nutrition with a particular emphasis on how the well-established healthy nutritional plans such as the DASH diet, the Mediterranean diet, and the Healthy U.S.-Style Dietary can significantly lower the risk of chronic disease by reducing inflammation.

Clinical Applications

- Abundant data are now available on the types of diet that can lower inflammation in the body.
- Inflammation is considered to be an underlying cause of multiple chronic diseases including CVD, T2DM, obesity, cancer, and dementia.
- Multiple health studies have now shown that healthy nutrition can play a role in lowering inflammation in the body and reduce the risk of chronic diseases to which inflammation contributes.

REFERENCES

1. Dudgeon W, Nieman D, Kelley E. Exercise, inflammation, and respiratory infection. In Rippe JM (ed). Lifestyle Medicine, 3rd edition. Boca Raton: CRC Press, 2019.
2. Libby P, Bornfeldt KE, Tall AR. Atherosclerosis: Successes, surprises, and future challenges. Circ Res. 2016;19;118(4):531–534.
3. Khansari N, Shakiba Y, Mahmoudi M. Chronic inflammation and oxidative stress as a major cause of age-related diseases and cancer. Recent Pat Inflamm Allergy Drug Discov. 2009;3(1):73–80.
4. Moran AE, Forouzanfar MH, Roth GA, et al. Temporal trends in ischemic heart disease mortality in 21 world regions, 1980 to 2010: The Global Burden of Disease 2010 study. Circulation. 2014;8;129(14):1483–1492.
5. GBD 2019 Stroke Collaborators. Global, regional, and national burden of stroke and its risk factors, 1990–2019: A systematic analysis for the Global Burden of Disease study 2019. Lancet Neurol. 2021;20(10):795–820.
6. Anuurad E, Semrad A, Berglund L. Human immunodeficiency virus and highly active antiretroviral therapy-associated metabolic disorders and risk factors for cardiovascular disease. Metable Syndr Relat Disord. 2009;7(5):401–410.
7. Devaraj S, Valleggi S, Siegel D, et al. Role of C-reactive protein in contributing to increased cardiovascular risk in metabolic syndrome. Curr Atheroscler Rep. 2010 Mar;12(2):110–118. Erratum in: Curr Atheroscler Rep. 2019;25;21(1):4.
8. Shapiro MD, Fazio S. From lipids to inflammation: New approaches to reducing atherosclerotic risk. Circ Res. 2016;19;118(4):732–749.
9. Iddir M, Brito A, Dingeo G, et al. Strengthening the immune system and reducing inflammation and oxidative stress through diet and nutrition: Considerations during the COVID-19 crisis. Nutrients. 2020;12(6):E1562.
10. Zabetakis I, Lordan R, Norton C, et al. COVID-19: The inflammation link and the role of nutrition in potential mitigation. Nutrients. 2020;19;12(5):1466.
11. Beavers KM, Brinkley TE, Nicklas BJ. Effect of exercise training on chronic inflammation. Clin Chim Acta. 2010;3;411(11–12):785–793.
12. Matthews CE, Ockene IS, Freedson PS, et al. Moderate to vigorous physical activity and risk of upper-respiratory tract infection. Med Sci Sports Exerc. 2002;34(8):1242–1248.

13. Markofski N, Coen P, Flynn M. Chronic exercise and immunity. In Rippe JM (ed). Lifestyle Medicine, 3rd edition. Boca Raton: CRC Press, 2019.
14. Moro-García MA, Fernández-García B, Echeverría A, et al. Frequent participation in high volume exercise throughout life is associated with a more differentiated adaptive immune response. Brain Behav Immun. 2014;39:61–74.
15. Rippe JM, Angelopoulos T. Obesity: Prevention and Treatment. Boca Raton: CRC Press, 2012.
16. Via M. Adiposity-based chronic disease: A new diagnostic term. In Lifestyle Medicine, 3rd edition. Boca Raton: CRC Press, 2019.
17. Guideline for the Management of Overweight and Obesity in Adults. A report of the American College of Cardiology/American Heart Association Task Force on Practice Guidelines and the Obesity Society. Circulation. 2014;129(25 Suppl 2):S102–S138.
18. Van Cauter E. Sleep disturbances and insulin resistance. Diabet Med. 2011;28(12): 1455–1462.
19. Gupta K, Nagalli S, Kalra R, et al. Sleep duration, baseline cardiovascular risk, inflammation and incident cardiovascular mortality in ambulatory U.S. adults: National health and nutrition examination survey. Am J Prev Cardiol. 2021;17;8:100246.
20. Amaral JF, Foschetti DA, Assis FA, et al. Immunoglobulin production is impaired in protein-deprived mice and can be restored by dietary protein supplementation. Braz J Med Biol Res. 2006;39:1581–1586.
21. Hruby A, Jacques PF. Dietary protein and changes in biomarkers of inflammation and oxidative stress in the Framingham heart study offspring cohort. Curr Dev Nutr. 2019;28;3(5):nzz019.
22. Li P, Yin YL, Li D, et al. Amino acids and immune function. Br J Nutr. 2007;98:237–252.
23. Shivappa N, Steck SE, Hurley TG, et al. Designing and developing a literature-derived, population-based dietary inflammatory index. Public Health Nutr. 2014;17(8):1689–1696.
24. Hébert JR, Shivappa N, Wirth MD, et al. Perspective: The Dietary Inflammatory Index (DII)-lessons learned, improvements made, and future directions. Adv Nutr. 2019;1;10(2):185–195.
25. Tabung FK, Smith-Warner SA, Chavarro JE, et al. Development and validation of an empirical dietary inflammatory index. J Nutr. 2016;146(8):1560–1570.
26. Porcelli SA. Innate immunity. In Firestein GS, Budd RC, Gabriel SE, McInnes IB, and O'Dell JR (eds). Kelley and Firestein's Textbook of Rheumatology, 10th edition. Amsterdam, The Netherlands: Elsevier, 2017: 247–287.
27. Spiering MJ. Primer on the immune system. Alcohol Res. 2015;37:171–175.
28. Lee JH, Jung JY, Jeong YJ, et al. Involvement of both mitochondrial- and death receptor-dependent apoptotic pathways regulated by Bcl-2 family in sodium fluoride-induced apoptosis of the human gingival fibroblasts. Toxicology. 2008;243:340–347.
29. Park J, Min JS, Kim B, et al. Mitochondrial ROS govern the LPS-induced pro-inflammatory response in microglia cells by regulating MAPK and NF-kappaB pathways. Neurosci Lett. 2015;584:191–196.
30. Perez GI, Acton BM, Jurisicova A, et al. Genetic variance modifies apoptosis susceptibility in mature oocytes via alterations in DNA repair capacity and mitochondrial ultrastructure. Cell Death Differ. 2007;14:524–533.
31. Pohanka M. Role of oxidative stress in infectious diseases. A review. Folia Microbiol. 2013;58(6):503–513.
32. Libby P. Mechanisms of acute coronary syndromes and their implications for therapy. N Engl J Med. 2013;23;368(21):2004–2013.
33. Li G, Fan Y, Lai Y, et al. Coronavirus infections and immune responses. J Med Virol. 2020;92:424–432.

34. Zhang W, Zhao Y, Zhang F, et al. The use of anti-inflammatory drugs in the treatment of people with severe coronavirus disease 2019 (COVID-19): The perspectives of clinical immunologists from China. Clin Immunol. 2020;214:108393.
35. Conti P, Ronconi G, Caraffa A, et al. Induction of pro-inflammatory cytokines (IL-1 and IL-6) and lung inflammation by coronavirus-19 (COVID-19 or SARS-CoV-2): Anti-inflammatory strategies. J Biol Regul Homeost Agents. 2020;34:1.
36. Zhou F, Yu T, Du R, et al. Clinical course and risk factors for mortality of adult inpatients with COVID-19 in Wuhan, China: A retrospective cohort study. Lancet. 2020;395: 1054–1062.
37. Kritas SK, Ronconi G, Caraffa A, et al. Mast cells contribute to coronavirus-induced inflammation: New anti-inflammatory strategy. J Biol Regul Homeost Agents. 2020;34:34.
38. Mehta P, McAuley DF, Brown M, et al. COVID-19: Consider cytokine storm syndromes and immunosuppression. Lancet. 2020;395:1033–1034.
39. World Health Organization. Global Noncommunicable Diseases Compact 2020–2030. www.who.int/initiatives/global-noncommunicable-diseases-compact-2020-2030 (Accessed January 31, 2024).
40. Yang J, Zheng Y, Gou X, et al. Prevalence of comorbidities in the novel Wuhan coronavirus (COVID-19) infection: A systematic review and meta-analysis. Int J Infect Dis. 2020;94:91–95.
41. Van Kerkhove MD, Vandemaele KAH, Shinde V, et al. Risk factors for severe outcomes following 2009 influenza a (H1N1) infection: A global pooled analysis. PLoS Med. 2011;8:e1001053.
42. Tsoupras A, Lordan R, Zabetakis I. Inflammation, not cholesterol, is a cause of chronic disease. Nutrients. 2018;10:604.
43. Hotamisligil GS. Inflammation, metaflammation and immunometabolic disorders. Nature. 2017;542:177–185.
44. Yue Y, Ma W, Accorsi EK, et al. Long-term diet and risk of Severe Acute Respiratory Syndrome Coronavirus 2 (SARS-CoV-2) infection and Coronavirus Disease 2019 (COVID-19) severity. Am J Clin Nutr. 2022;19;116(6):1672–1681.
45. Trumbo P, Schlicker S, Yates AA, et al. Food and Nutrition Board of the Institute of Medicine, The National Academies. Dietary reference intakes for energy, carbohydrate, fiber, fat, fatty acids, cholesterol, protein and amino acids. J Am Diet Assoc. 2002;102(11):1621–1630.
46. Harbige LS. Fatty acids, the immune response, and autoimmunity: A question of Ω-6 essentiality and the balance between Ω-6 and Ω-3. Lipids. 2003;38(4):323–341.
47. The Institute of Medicine. Dietary Reference Intakes for Energy, Carbohydrate, Fiber, Fat, Fatty Acids, Cholesterol, Protein and Amino Aacids. Washington, DC: The National Academies Press, 2005.
48. Innes JK, Calder PC. Omega-6 fatty acids and inflammation. Prostaglandins Leukot Essent Fatty Acids. 2018;132:41–48.
49. Liu S, Manson JE, Buring JE, et al. Relation between a diet with a high glycemic load and plasma concentrations of high-sensitivity C-reactive protein in middle-aged women. Am J Clin Nutr. 2002;75(3):492–498.
50. Monnier L, Mas E, Ginet C, et al. Activation of oxidative stress by acute glucose fluctuations compared with sustained chronic hyperglycemia in patients with type 2 diabetes. JAMA. 2006;12;295(14):1681–1687.
51. Neuhouser ML, Schwarz Y, Wang C, et al. A low-glycemic load diet reduces serum C-reactive protein and modestly increases adiponectin in overweight and obese adults. J Nutr. 2012;42(2):369–374.

52. McCullough FS, Northrop-Clewes CA, Thurnham DI. The effect of vitamin A on epithelial integrity. Proc Nutr Soc. 1999;58:289–293.
53. Shrestha S, Kim SY, Yun YJ, et al. Retinoic acid induces hypersegmentation and enhances cytotoxicity of neutrophils against cancer cells. Immunol Lett. 2017;182:24–29.
54. Stephensen CB. Vitamin A, infection, and immune function. Annu Rev Nutr. 2001;21:167–192.
55. Aranow C. Vitamin D and the immune system. J Investig Med. 2011;59:881–886.
56. Xuan NT, Trang PT, Van Phong N, et al. Klotho sensitive regulation of dendritic cell functions by vitamin E. Biol Res. 2016;49:45.
57. Tan PH, Sagoo P, Chan C, et al. Inhibition of NF-kappa B and oxidative pathways in human dendritic cells by antioxidative vitamins generates regulatory T cells. J Immunol. 2005;174:7633–7644.
58. Carr AC, Shaw GM, Fowler AA, et al. Ascorbate-dependent vasopressor synthesis: A rationale for vitamin C administration in severe sepsis and septic shock? Crit Care. 2015;19:418.
59. Englard S, Seifter S. The biochemical functions of ascorbic acid. Annu Rev Nutr. 1986;6:365–406.
60. Duarte TL, Cooke MS, Jones GD. Gene expression profiling reveals new protective roles for vitamin C in human skin cells. Free Radic Biol Med. 2009;46:78–87.
61. Meydani SN, Meydani M, Blumberg JB, et al. Vitamin E supplementation and in vivo immune response in healthy elderly subjects. A randomized controlled trial. JAMA. 1997;7;277(17):1380–1386.
62. Schwingshackl L, Bogensberger B, Hoffmann G. Diet quality as assessed by the healthy eating index, alternate healthy eating index, dietary approaches to stop hypertension score, and health outcomes: An updated systematic review and meta-analysis of cohort studies. J Acad Nutr Diet. 2018;118(1):74–100.
63. Chiuve SE, Fung TT, Rimm EB, et al. Alternative dietary indices both strongly predict risk of chronic disease. J Nutr. 2012;142(6):1009–1018.
64. Chrysohoou C, Panagiotakos DB, Pitsavos C, et al. Adherence to the Mediterranean diet attenuates inflammation and coagulation process in healthy adults: The ATTICA study. J Am Coll Cardiol. 2004;7;44(1):152–158.
65. Casas R, Sacanella E, Estruch R. The immune protective effect of the Mediterranean diet against chronic low-grade inflammatory diseases. Endocr Metable Immune Disord Drug Targets. 2014;14(4):245–254.
66. Shah R, Makarem N, Emin M, et al. Mediterranean diet components are linked to greater endothelial function and lower inflammation in a pilot study of ethnically diverse women. Nutr Res. 2020;75:77–84.
67. Willett WC, Sacks F, Trichopoulou A, et al. Mediterranean diet pyramid: A cultural model for healthy eating. Am J Clin Nutr. 1995;61:1402s–1406s.
68. Estruch R, Ros E, Salas-Salvado J, et al. Primary prevention of cardiovascular disease with a Mediterranean diet. N Engl J Med. 2013;368(14):1279–1290.
69. Varraso R, Fung TT, Barr RG, et al. Prospective study of dietary patterns and chronic obstructive pulmonary disease among us women. Am J Clin Nutr. 2007;86:488–495.
70. Carey OJ, Cookson JB, Britton J, et al. The effect of lifestyle on wheeze, atopy, and bronchial hyperreactivity in Asian and white children. Am J Respir Crit Care Med. 1996;154:537–540.
71. Christ A, Lauterbach M, Latz E. Western diet and the immune system: An inflammatory connection. Immunity. 2019;19;51(5):794–811.
72. Shan Z, Wang F, Li Y, et al. Healthy eating patterns and risk of total and cause-specific mortality. JAMA Intern Med. 2023;1;183(2):142–153.

73. Tabung FK, Wang W, Fung TT, et al. Association of dietary insulinemic potential and colorectal cancer risk in men and women. Am J Clin Nutr. 2018;1;108(2):363–370.
74. Dietz W, Santos-Burgoa C. Obesity and its implications for COVID-19 mortality. Obesity (Silver Spring). 2020;28(6):1005.
75. Berger SE, Huggins GS, McCaffery JM, et al. Comparison among criteria to define successful weight-loss maintainers and regainers in the Action for Health in Diabetes (Look AHEAD) and diabetes prevention program trials. Am J Clin Nutr. 2017;106(6):1337–1346.
76. American Heart Association. 2024 Health Equity Impact Goal. www.heart.org/en/about-us/2024-health-equity-impact-goal (Accessed January 23, 2024).
77. American College of Physicians. Advance Equity in Health Care. www.acponline.org/advocacy/where-we-stand/acps-advocacy-priorities-2023/advance-equity-in-health-care (Accessed January 23, 2024).
78. Davis M-G, Shurney D, Stone T, et al. HEALing Our Nation—health equity achieved through lifestyle medicine capturing highlights from the "HEALing Our Nation" session at LM2023 and outlining the important work of the HEAL initiative. Am J Lifestyle Med. 2023;17(5):694–703.

10 Nutrition and Metabolic Health

Key Points

- Metabolism, which is the basic process by which the body converts food into energy, is essential to maintaining the balance of what physicians call homeostasis.
- Abnormalities in metabolism can create an increased risk of chronic disease.
- Healthy nutrition, as recommended by the DASH diet, Mediterranean diet, *Dietary Guidelines for Americans 2020–2025*, and multiple American Heart Association diets, can contribute to metabolic health. These diets consistently emphasize abundant fruits and vegetables and whole grains, while reducing red meat, sugar, and salt.
- Unhealthy diets that feature energy-dense products are often deficient in nutrients.
- Physicians should counsel their patients on the relationship between nutrition and healthy metabolism to lower the risk of developing chronic diseases.

10.1 INTRODUCTION

Metabolism is a fundamental process in every human body that provides energy for central bodily functions such as breathing and digestion [1]. Many factors impact on metabolism including age, sex, muscle mass, and physical activity. At the most fundamental level, metabolism refers to the chemical (metabolic) processes that take place as the body converts foods and drinks consumed into energy. Metabolism is a complex process that combines the calories from the foods we eat to the oxygen we breath to create and release energy. This energy, in turn, fuels bodily functions. While eating is essential to life, it is not only a necessity but also a pleasure. It is the process of metabolism that allows us to absorb a range of nutrients so that our cells have building blocks for metabolic processes that release energy and also manufacture new proteins, cells, and body parts as well as recycling materials in the cell.

There have been many recommendations for how to eat related to basic mechanisms of metabolism. For example, there is a mantra that a good breakfast gives people energy to get through most of the day. It is also a common recommendation to eat a balanced diet, but particularly one with plenty of fruits and vegetables.

Many different factors impact on metabolism. For example, depending on age, gender, activity level, fuel consumption, and lean body mass, metabolism may vary from individual to individual and may fluctuate throughout life. By modifying the diet and increasing physical activity or decreasing it, an individual can increase or

 DOI: 10.1201/9781003452607-10

decrease lean body mass and metabolic rate. This is a potentially important issue for individuals over the age of 50, since aging is known to decrease muscle mass and slow the metabolic rate by as much as 5% per year [2]. Research has also demonstrated that metabolic rate is impacted by proteins and enzymes, which are derived by each individual from their genetic background. Thus, genetic background also plays a significant role in metabolism. However, every person's body engages in fundamentally the same metabolic processes.

Metabolism is further divided into two, general categories: catabolism and anabolism. The reactions that determine the breakdown of food to obtain energy are called catabolic reactions. Conversely, anabolic reactions use the energy produced by catabolic reactions to synthesize large molecules such as proteins. Both anabolic and catabolic reactions are critical to maintaining life and fostering growth.

Metabolism is the centerpiece for maintaining the body in balance, which in medicine is referred to as homeostasis. It is only when metabolism becomes disordered that it can lead to a variety of chronic diseases. Nutrition plays a very important role both in normal and abnormal metabolism. For this reason, we will focus a great deal of attention in this chapter on the interaction between nutrition and metabolism as well as chronic disease.

10.2 METABOLIC HEALTH IN NORMAL-WEIGHT AND OBESE INDIVIDUALS

One area where the issue of healthy metabolism versus unhealthy metabolism has achieved considerable prominence is in the area of obesity. For example, cardiovascular complications are commonly associated with obesity. There is a subset of obese individuals, however, who do not seem to be at increased risk for cardiovascular complications [3]. These individuals are said to have "metabolically healthy obesity" (MHO). In contrast, "metabolically unhealthy" individuals are at much higher risk for cardiovascular disease, for instance, coronary heart disease (CHD), irrespective of their body mass index (BMI). This latter group can also include individuals who are within the normal weight category (BMI 18.5–24.9 kg/m^2).

Distinguishing between MHO individuals and metabolically unhealthy individuals carries significant implications. It should be noted, however, that MHO has been subject to a great deal of debate since it lacks a uniform definition and does not take into account other chronic risks associated with obesity other than CVD. Individuals in the normal weight category of BMI 18.5–24.9 kg/m^2 may not receive as much attention in the area of prevention of diseases that are more commonly associated with obesity such as CVD.

The term "MHO" applies to obese individuals in whom increased cardiometabolic risk factors are largely absent. These individuals do not appear to have elevated cardiometabolic risk compared to individuals of normal weight. Additional categorizations of MHO may also include absence of metabolic syndrome and normal insulin sensitivity [3]. An example of how MHO may be confusing could be based on different criteria utilized in the definition. For example, the prevalence of MHO when based on the absence of metabolic syndrome, as defined by the National Cholesterol Education Program Panel III, was found to be 47% of individuals [4].

However, if the distinction is based on all of the components of metabolic syndrome being simultaneously absent, it dropped to 10%.

In contrast to studies of MHO, individuals with metabolically unhealthy normal health weight (MUNHW) have a higher risk of cardiovascular complications irrespective of BMI. It should also be noted that there is limited evidence that risk factors are overall different from those with normal weight compared to those who are in overweight or obese BMI subgroups if MUNHW is present. It should also be noted that BMI does not reflect body fat distribution and waist circumference, which reflect abdominal fat accumulation and better predict cardiovascular events than BMI.

Major concern about the use of MHO relates to the potential conversion of individuals with MHO into an unhealthy genotype over time. Cohort studies, for example, have found higher CVD risk for MHO subgroups when a longer duration of follow-up has been utilized. Thus, the phenotype of MHO may be transient. Indeed, the conversion from MHO to MUNHW has been demonstrated to be related to higher baseline BMI and waist circumference as well as the longer duration of obesity.

Importantly, metabolic risk factors are not only markers of body fat but also lifestyle choices (specifically, nutritional practices). One study of the Dietary Approaches to Stop Hypertension (DASH) diet has shown that risk factors for CVD can be reduced by following a diet containing more fruits and vegetables [5]. Similar findings occurred in the PREDIMED (Prevención con Dieta Mediterránea), which showed a marked decrease in risk factors for CVD with the Mediterranean diet supplemented with olive oil or nuts [6]. Thus, nutrition plays a very significant role, as we have discussed in multiple chapters in this book, with respect to either metabolically healthy individuals or metabolically unhealthy individuals.

10.3 HEALTHY NUTRITION FOR METABOLIC HEALTHY AND UNHEALTHY PHENOTYPES

When viewed through the lens of risk factors for chronic disease, comparing metabolically healthy individuals to metabolically unhealthy individuals, healthy nutrition, particularly featuring abundant fruits and vegetables and whole grains as well as weight management, plays a very central role.

One study that utilized DASH diet scores in obese individuals showed that individuals who followed the DASH diet had significantly lower risk for MUNHW [5]. Similar findings have been demonstrated for the Mediterranean diet, particularly when supplemented with olive oil or nuts [6].

One of the hallmarks of metabolically unhealthy individuals is that their risks of chronic disease such as cardiovascular disease (CVD), type 2 diabetes mellitus (T2DM), obesity, metabolic syndrome, and even cancer are all significantly elevated. Part of this increased risk undoubtedly results from the fact that diets that are followed by many Americans are likely to promote inflammation. In turn, these diets are associated with chronic conditions such as CVD, T2DM, obesity, and metabolic syndrome, which in and of themselves are inflammatory. While the research trials, as noted earlier, were typically in obese individuals, there is no question that similar advantages of healthy nutrition apply also to MHO and MUHO subjects who are not obese.

10.4 METABOLIC HEALTH AND COVID-19

The COVID-19 pandemic has created multiple challenges around the world. Many of these challenges are based on how this virus has disrupted metabolic patterns including nutrition, physical activity, sleep, and diurnal rhythms [7, 8].

Many metabolic and physiologic processes are controlled by 24-hour biologic oscillations under the control of a central circadian clock located in the superchiasmatic nucleus of the hypothalamus [9–11]. These circadian rhythms are governed not only by the light and dark cycle but also by patterns of sleep, eating, and physical activity.

Nutritional practices, including timing, quantity, and choice, are governed by complex interactions between factors that change when individuals disrupt their normal patterns and experience isolation. One likely result of individuals being advised to self-quarantine if they have been exposed to or have COVID-19 is that they are likely to experience a positive energy balance, where energy intake exceeds energy expenditure and subsequent weight gain ensues. Moreover, if individuals who are facing isolation also experience decreases in sleep or disturbed sleep, these factors can also yield increase in appetite, changes in energy regulating hormones, and binge eating.

Individuals who are obese, have high blood pressure, or T2DM were three to four times as likely to experience hospitalization and mortality compared to individuals who did not have these conditions. It is likely that changes in metabolism underlie many of these discrepancies. Furthermore, unfortunately, many of these discrepancies also further exacerbate health disparities and inequities in modern healthcare.

10.5 THERE ARE MULTIPLE IMPORTANT INTERACTIONS BETWEEN NUTRITION AND METABOLIC HEALTH

Factors such as the energy density of the diet, sleep/wake cycle, level of physical activity, and timing of meals can all significantly impact metabolic health. When individuals feel excessive stress due to concerns about such issues as the COVID-19 virus, they are likely to overeat, particularly "discretionary" or "comfort" foods, and often late at night [7,8]. The normal eating pattern followed by most individuals, where three or more meals are eaten on a regular basis, with regular timing is deeply ingrained in the United States and many other societies. This typically takes place within a 12-hour window. During the COVID-19 pandemic, however, many individuals, particularly those who were overweight or obese, expanded the hours during which food was consumed and also adopted irregular eating patterns, which adversely impacted on circadian control of metabolism [7,8].

10.6 METABOLIC HEALTH AND PHYSICAL ACTIVITY

The role of regular physical activity as a key component of metabolic health has been demonstrated in multiple studies. Many of these are summarized in the Physical Activity Guidelines for Americans 2018 (PAGA 2018) [12]. Not only does physical activity burn calories, but it also has many other effects that can enhance healthy metabolism. For example, maintaining or increasing skeletal muscle mass depends on either aerobic physical activity and/or resistance strength training. Regular physical activity also promotes muscle health and increases metabolism in the muscle.

A recent review of physical activity during the COVID-19 pandemic demonstrated that opportunities to exercise significantly decreased during the pandemic, largely because of the recommendations for individuals with COVID to self-isolate [13]. This caused significant decreases in physical activity and undoubtedly increased the likelihood of individuals experiencing adverse metabolic consequences. In general, regular physical activity plays multiple beneficial effects in metabolic health and is advocated by not only organizations such as the PAGA 2018 but also nutritional guidelines from numerous authoritative organizations including the American Heart Association (AHA) [14], the Guidelines for Americans 2020–2025 Advisory Committee Report [15], and multiple recommendations from the American College of Cardiology and AHA, including recent recommendations for controlling lipids [16] and blood pressure [17].

10.7 METABOLISM AND THE CIRCADIAN CLOCK

Many of the metabolic and hormonal processes in the body are controlled by diurnal rhythms. Nutrition, including the timing of meals, affects a wide variety of these functions, including the sleep/wake cycle, core body temperature, athletic performance, and mental alertness. In addition, the timing of meals has a profound effect on skeletal muscle insulin sensitivity and whole-body metabolic health. Multiple components of human nutrition are impacted by circadian rhythms [9–11]. For example, insulin sensitivity and the thermic effect of food are all higher in the morning than in the afternoon or evening, which suggests that human metabolism is geared more toward greater food intake in the morning than in the evening.

A number of human studies have shown that eating that is in alignment with circadian rhythms (increased food time at breakfast and reduced at dinnertime) improves glycemic control, weight loss, and lipid levels [9–11]. In contrast, irregular daily eating patterns have adverse effects on circadian biology. This overall concept suggests that eating in coordination with the body's daily rhythms, in addition to the content of food and the timing of meals, is critical for metabolic health.

Circadian rhythm is controlled by what has been called the "circadian clock." The controlling clock appears to be in the small region of the hypothalamus located just above the optic chiasm. There are also other clocks throughout the body, particularly in the gastrointestinal tract [9–11]. The circadian rhythm involved in eating is not just a function of the output of the clock, but the clock receives input from a variety of peripheral tissues, which communicate back to the brain via ghrelin, leptin, glucose, insulin, etc., which allows circadian feeding to interact with the clock and the metabolism that appears to be crucial for metabolic homeostasis. It is interesting to note that types of foods that humans consume are often aligned closely to the same times of the day. For example, alcohol typically is consumed at the end of the day, as are sweets (refined sugar) and foods such as ice cream. This suggests that perhaps a reduction of food intake later in the day may not only reduce total energy intake but also curtail discretionary food intake and improve overall dietary quality.

10.8 METABOLISM, SLEEP, AND CHRONIC DISEASES

Sleep is an underestimated component of overall good health and is one of the pillars of lifestyle medicine. Any significant alteration in life may result in changes in sleep quality, quantity, and timing. Sleep also influences obesity, insulin resistance, and risk of type 2 diabetes. Disordered sleep increases the risk of CVD by 30–40% [18–20].

Circadian rhythm is influenced primarily by light/dark cycles and is "fine-tuned" by timing of meals and levels of activity and inactivity, all of which exert profound influences on the sleep/wake cycle. Light synchronizes the circadian rhythm to the external environment. Any interruption of the external light/dark cycle negatively impacts on sleep [21].

Physical activity has always been recognized as a safe and inexpensive accessible way to improve sleep. The potential mechanism for this is likely to be the influence of light exposure to the circadian rhythm as well as an increase in energy and body temperature, as well as antianxiety and antidepressant effects of physical activity. Much less is known about the negative influence of sedentary behavior on sleep.

The interaction between nutrition and meal timing with sleep is an area that has emerged as important in research, since this is likely to influence sleep quality and quantity [21]. The alignment of sleep and mealtimes may also influence food choices, since shortened sleep has been shown to increase the likelihood of consuming energy-dense and nutrient poor-food [22]. Sleep quality and quantity also influence hormonal actions. For example, overnight leptin concentrations have been shown to be higher under normal meal conditions than when a late meal is consumed. Thus, it is not surprising that overeating right before going to bed might increase the amount of calories consumed, since leptin plays a role in satiety [23]. For all of these reasons, optimizing sleep is likely to play a very significant role in the maintenance of metabolic health.

10.9 METABOLISM AND SEDENTARY BEHAVIOR

Sedentary behavior has become a topic of considerable interest and research over the past decade. Sedentary behavior has clearly been associated with increased risk of various metabolic diseases [24]. For example, there is a clear association between metabolic syndrome risk factors and type 2 diabetes and indices of sedentary time. Studies have shown that the classification of people with metabolic syndrome and related metabolic risk factors, including excessive adiposity and weight gain, poor glucose management, and T2DM risk, have been directly related to sitting time and/or to low or no exercise activity.

One of the problems with research in sedentary behavior is to define what exactly is meant by this term [12]. Most definitions of sedentary behavior now coalesce around the time that is either spent sitting or lying, where energy expenditure is no more than would be expected at rest. There is also a correlation between the number of hours spent watching screens or TV and sedentary behavior [25,26]. Research published in the PAGA 2018 showed that individuals who complemented their relatively high levels of sedentary time with the recommended amounts of physical activity (150 minutes of moderate-intensity physical activity per week) largely mitigate the risk of sedentary behavior. It has also been suggested that taking periodic breaks every 30–45 minutes by getting up and standing and walking around for 5 minutes, so-called "exercise snacks," may also somewhat mitigate the amount of sedentary behavior and its risk factors.

The average adult in the United States spends between seven and nine hours in sedentary behavior each day [27]. Thus, this is an important area to understand. It should also be noted that the recommendations for healthy eating and healthy nutrition are similar for individuals who are sedentary as for people who are more physically active. However, it must be underscored that the number of calories consumed should be less in individuals who are truly sedentary.

It is important for clinicians to underscore to their patients, particularly office workers or individuals who spend a great deal of time on their computer, that there are inherent metabolic and health risks related to this type of sedentary behavior. It should also be noted that sedentary behavior is strongly correlated with sleep problems, which further creates a scenario for adverse health consequences. Finally, there are studies now that suggest that even relatively short periods of decreased physical activity may increase metabolic risk. For example, in one study of young men who were asked to decrease the number of daily steps from 12,000 to 2,000, within two weeks insulin sensitivity was reduced, as was cardiovascular fitness and lean leg muscle mass [28].

10.10 NUTRITION, METABOLISM, AND THE MICROBIOTA

An area of dramatic increase in research in the past decade has been on the metabolic effects of the microbiota. In particular, some studies have shown that dietary fat quantity and quality negatively influence the gut microbiota composition, which may, in turn, adversely affect metabolic health [29]. In particular, high intake of saturated fatty acids (SFAs) may negatively impact microbiota richness and diversity, whereas polyunsaturated fatty acids (PUFAs) have no effect on richness and diversity. Thus, diets that are high in SFA unfavorably impact gut microbiota and are associated with unhealthy metabolic states. Work in this area is at a preliminary stage, but the impact of nutritional practices on gut microbiota can play a very important role in adverse metabolic states and increased risk of chronic disease.

The microbiota in a number of different populations has been studied, including overweight and obese pregnant women, postmenopausal obese women, and Filipino children. In these settings, certain types of Bacteroides which are thought to have negative health effects, were increased based on high-fat diets. Other groups that have been studied are healthy men aged 23–45 and adults that are at increased risk for metabolic syndrome. In healthy young men there were no significant changes in the fecal microbiota or changes in blood lipid profile, insulin, or glucose concentration, despite a high-fat diet. However, in individuals with increased risk of metabolic syndrome, a variety of negative microbiota findings were discovered. Microbiota play a very important role in overall chronic disease development or risk reduction. These issues are handled in much more detail in Chapter 24.

10.11 NUTRITION, HOME PREPARATION OF FOOD, AND INDICATORS OF HEALTHY EATING

Some research suggests that the amount of time spent on food preparation and cooking may have positive implications for dietary quality and health. In the busy world that most people live in, it may be difficult to find the amount of time for food preparation, while a high priority is placed on convenience [30]. However, research suggests that a greater amount of time spent on food preparation results in higher dietary quality, including significantly more frequent intake of vegetables, salads, fruits, and fruit juices. In addition, individuals who spend less than one hour a day on food preparation spend more money on food away from home and more frequently use fast food restaurants compared to those who spend more time on food preparation.

One area that has been of concern related to food preparation is the relative lack of cooking skills. Even a survey of members of the Academy of Nutrition and Dietetics found that a high percentage did not feel confident in their culinary skills [31]. Thus, it is important to spend more time understanding and implementing education in the area of food preparation.

In various medical schools culinary medicine has taken a rightful place, and some medical schools have even established teaching kitchens to help train medical students and residents in food preparation with the thought that doctors who are comfortable with food preparation in their own lives are more likely to discuss this with their patients.

10.12 NUTRITION, METABOLIC RESPONSES, AND THE POTENTIAL FOR PRECISION NUTRITION

Emerging research relates to specifically how metabolic responses to food influence the risk of cardiometabolic disease [32]. This can vary considerably between individuals. There are a number of different directions that the field of precision nutrition is pursuing. One intriguing study is called the PREDICT study, which recruited 1,002 twins and unrelated healthy adults in the United Kingdom to assess postprandial metabolic responses in a clinical setting and at home [33]. This study showed large interindividual variability in postprandial responses to blood triglycerides (102%), glucose (68%), and insulin (59%) following identical meals. A number of factors impacted on these responses. Specific factors such as the gut microbiome had a greater influence (7.1% of variance) than did meal macronutrients (3.6%) for postprandial glycemia, but not for postprandial glycemia (6.0% and 15.4%, respectively). Genetic variants had a modest impact on prediction (9.5% for glucose and 0.8% for triglycerides and 0.2% for high-sensitivity C-reactive protein [hs-CRP]).

This type of study is time consuming and expensive to conduct. However, such studies offer an intriguing insight into the future of nutrition. The investigators in the PREDICT Study have developed a learning model to predict both triglycerides ($R = 0.47$) and glycemic responses ($R = .77$) to food intake. It is hoped this type of research will eventually lead to developing personalized diet strategies.

10.13 METABOLIC HEALTH, EQUITY, AND PUBLIC POLICY

An emerging area of considerable interest and concern in the United States and around the world is the issue of health equity, particularly as it relates to food, nutrition, and metabolic health. These issues were dramatically underscored by responses to the COVID-19 pandemic, where individuals who had obesity, diabetes, or hypertension were three to four times as likely to be hospitalized and experience mortality compared to individuals who did not have these conditions [34]. These chronic conditions are particularly prevalent in Black and Hispanic populations, which have been traditionally underserved [35].

The sad fact is that over 11% of households in the United States do not have adequate food, and this is disproportionately found in individuals who are at or below the poverty line [36]. It is important to note, however, that food insecurity and poverty are not synonymous. Individuals who are facing food insecurity often compensate by eating energy-dense, less expensive foods that have poor nutritional value. This contributes to the increased likelihood of unhealthy metabolism and sets the stage for an increased risk of various metabolic diseases including obesity, T2DM, CVD, and metabolic syndrome. Some cancers may also be attributed to this.

A number of public policy initiatives are currently in progress to deal with health equity. Some of these policies are already in place such as the Women and Children's Program (WIC) and the Supplemental Nutrition Assistance Program (SNAP). The recently completed White House Conference on Nutrition, Hunger and Health advocated a wide variety of additional initiatives [37]. It is also hoped that the bills in front of Congress to reauthorize a broader SNAP and also the FON bill will include significant initiatives to help address nutrition and health equity.

10.14 CONCLUSIONS

Metabolism is the basic process by which the body converts food that is consumed to maintain various bodily functions, including providing energy, growing and replenishing cells, managing hormone levels, regulating body temperature, and digesting food. The goal of healthy metabolism is to maintain the body's balance in what clinicians call homeostasis. Disturbances in metabolism, however, can increase the risk of a variety of unhealthy responses and set the stage for multiple chronic diseases.

Nutrition is the key determinant for metabolism, although physical activity and other factors also play roles. There are also components that have to do with genetics and the environment. Healthy nutrition has been shown to increase the likelihood of metabolic health, whereas unhealthy nutrition can contribute to unhealthy metabolism. Thus, healthy diets such as the DASH diet, Mediterranean diet, Healthy U.S.-Style Dietary Pattern, and multiple diets recommended by the American Heart Association are all appropriate to maintain a healthy metabolism. Clinicians should routinely talk to their patients about the importance of healthy metabolism and lowering their risk of chronic disease.

Clinical Applications

- The relationship between nutrition and metabolism is well established.
- Healthy metabolism is essential for maintaining a body in balance in what physicians call homeostasis.

- Unhealthy nutrition can result in unhealthy phenotypes, which create an increased risk of chronic disease.
- The COVID-19 pandemic showed that individuals who followed unhealthy diets often resulted in obesity, T2DM, and hypertension, which significantly increased the risk of hospitalization and mortality.
- Clinicians should speak to all of their patients about the linkage between nutrition and metabolic health.

REFERENCES

1. Cleveland Clinic—Metabolism. https://my.clevelandclinic.org/health/body/21893-metabolism#:~:text=Metabolism%20refers%20to%20the%20chemical%20%28metabolic%29%20processes%20that,Cleveland%20Clinic%20is%20a%20non-profit%20academic%20medical%20center (Accessed July 3, 2023).
2. Leon A. Reducing aging-associated risk of sarcopenia. In Rippe JM (ed). Lifestyle Medicine, 3rd edition. Boca Raton: CRC Press, 2019.
3. Schulze M. Metabolic health in normal-weight and obese individuals. Diabetologia. 2019;62(4):558–566.
4. Third Report of the National Cholesterol Education Program (NCEP). Expert Panel on Detection, Evaluation and Treatment of High Blood Cholesterol in Adults (Adult Treatment Panel III), Executive Summary. www.nhlbi.nih.gov/files/docs/guidelines/atglance.pdf (Accessed July 3, 2023).
5. Farhadnejad H, Darand M, Teymoori F, et al. The association of Dietary Approach to Stop Hypertension (DASH) diet with metabolic healthy and metabolic unhealthy obesity phenotypes. Sci Rep. 2019;9(1):18690.
6. Guasch-Ferré M, Salas-Salvadó J, Ros E, et al. PREDIMED Investigators. The PREDIMED trial, Mediterranean diet and health outcomes: How strong is the evidence? Nutr Metab Cardiovasc Dis. 2017;27(7):624–632.
7. King A, Burke L, Halson S, et al. The challenge of maintaining metabolic health during a global pandemic. Sports Med (Auckland, N.Z.). 2020 Jul;50(7):1233–1241.
8. Stefan N, Birkenfeld A, Schulze M. Global pandemics interconnected—obesity, impaired metabolic health and COVID-19. Nat Rev Endocrinol. 2021;17:135–149.
9. Asher G, Sassone-Corsi P. Time for food: The intimate interplay between nutrition, metabolism, and the circadian clock. Cell. 2015;161(1):84–92.
10. Eckel-Mahan K, Sassone-Corsi P. Metabolism and the circadian clock converge. Physiol Rev. 2013;93(1):107–135.
11. Delezie J, Challet E. Interactions between metabolism and circadian clocks: Reciprocal disturbances. Ann New York Acad Sci. 2011;1243:30–46.
12. Physical Activity Guidelines for Americans 2018 (PAGA 2018). https://health.gov/our-work/nutrition-physical-activity/physical-activity-guidelines (Accessed July 3, 2023).
13. Hasson R, Sallis JF, Coleman N, et al. COVID-19: Implications for physical activity, health disparities, and health equity. Am J Lifestyle Med. 2022;16(4):420–423.
14. Lichtenstein A, Appel L, Vadiveloo M, et al. 2021 dietary guidance to improve cardiovascular health: A scientific statement from the American Heart Association. Circulation. 2021;144(23):e472–e487.
15. *Dietary Guidelines for Americans 2020–2025.* www.dietaryguidelines.gov/resources/2020-2025-dietary-guidelines-online-materials. (Accessed July 3, 2023).
16. Grundy S, Stone N, Bailey A, et al. 2018 AHA/ACC/AACVPR/AAPA/ABC/ACPM/ADA/AGS/APhA/ASPC/NLA/PCNA guideline on the management of blood cholesterol:

A report of the American College of Cardiology/American Heart Association task force on clinical practice guidelines. J Am Coll Cardiol. 2019;73(24):e285–e350.
17. Whelton P, Carey R, Aronow W, et al. 2017 ACC/AHA/AAPA/ABC/ACPM/AGS/APhA/ASH/ASPC/NMA/PCNA guideline for the prevention, detection, evaluation, and management of high blood pressure in adults: Executive summary: A report of the American College of Cardiology/American Heart Association task force on clinical practice guidelines. Hypertension. 2018;71(6):1269–1324. Epub 2017/11/15.
18. Rod N, Vahtera J, Westerlund H, et al. Sleep disturbances and cause-specific mortality: Results from the GAZEL cohort study. Am J Epidemiol. 2011;173(3):300–309.
19. Meisinger C, Heier M, Lowel H, et al. Sleep duration and sleep complaints and risk of myocardial infarction in middle-aged men and women from the general population: The MONICA/KORA Augsburg cohort study. Sleep. 2007;30(9):1121–1127. Epub 2007/10/04.
20. Javaheri S, Barbe F, Campos-Rodriguez F, et al. Sleep apnea: Types, mechanisms, and clinical cardiovascular consequences. J Am Coll Cardiol. 2017;69(7):841–858.
21. St-Onge M, Pizinger T, Kovtun K, et al. Sleep and meal timing influence food intake and its hormonal regulation in healthy adults with overweight/obesity. Eur J Clin Nutr. 2019;72(Suppl 1):76–82.
22. Reutrakul S, Van Cauter E. Sleep influences on obesity, insulin resistance, and risk of type 2 diabetes. Metabolism. 2018;84:56–66.
23. Kant A, Graubard B. Association of self-reported sleep duration with eating behaviors of American adults: NHANES 2005–2010. Am J Clin Nutr. 2014;100(3):938–947.
24. Yang Y, Shin J, Li D, et al. Sedentary behavior and sleep problems: A systematic review and meta-analysis. Int J Behav Med. 2017;24(4):481–492.
25. Grøntved A, Hu F. Television viewing and risk of type 2 diabetes, cardiovascular disease, and all-cause mortality: A meta-analysis. JAMA. 2011;15;305(23):2448–2455.
26. Sun J, Zhao L, Yang Y, et al. Association between television viewing time and all-cause mortality: A meta-analysis of cohort studies. Am J Epidemiol. 2015;182(11):908–916.
27. Matthews C, Chen K, Freedson P, et al. Amount of time spent in sedentary behaviors in the United States, 2003–2004. Am J Epidemiol. 2008;167(7):875–881.
28. Krogh-Madsen R, Thyfault J, Broholm C, et al. A 2-wk reduction of ambulatory activity attenuates peripheral insulin sensitivity. J Appl Physiol. 2010;108(5):1034–1040.
29. Wolters M, Ahrens J, Romaní-Pérez M, et al. Dietary fat, the gut microbiota, and metabolic health—a systematic review conducted within the MyNewGut Project. Clin Nutr. 2019;38(6):2504–2520.
30. Monsivais P, Aggarwal A, Drewnowski A. Time spent on home food preparation and indicators of healthy eating. Am J Prev Med. 2014;47(6):796–802.
31. McWhorter J, LaRue D, Almohamad M, et al. Training of registered dietitian nutritionists to improve culinary skills and food literacy. J Nutr Educ Behav. 2022;54(8):784–793.
32. Berry S, Valdes A, Drew D, et al. Human postprandial responses to food and potential for precision nutrition. Nat Med. 2020;26(6):964–973.
33. The PREDICT Program. https://joinzoe.com/whitepapers/the-predict-program (Accessed July 3, 2023).
34. Belanger M, Hill M, Angelidi A, et al. Covid-19 and disparities in nutrition and obesity. N Engl J Med. 2020;383(11):e69.
35. Chowkwanyun M, Reed A, Jr. Racial health disparities and Covid-19—caution and context. N Engl J Med. 2020;383(3):201–203.
36. Feeding America. www.feedingamerica.org (Accessed July 3, 2023).
37. The White House Conference on Hunger, Nutrition and Health. https://health.gov/our-work/nutrition-physical-activity/white-house-conference-hunger-nutrition-and-health/conference-details (Accessed July 3, 2023).

11 Nutrition and Atherosclerosis

Key Points

- Atherosclerosis is the common underlying condition that plays a significant role in multiple chronic diseases including coronary heart disease (CHD), stroke, kidney disease, peripheral artery disease, and erectile dysfunction.
- Modern nutrition understandings emphasize the complex etiology of atherosclerosis, including the role of oxidation and inflammation as well as various fats.
- Healthy dietary patterns that include abundant fruits and vegetables and whole grains are thought to lower the likelihood of atherosclerosis through multiple mechanisms.
- Multiple foods in healthy diets include abundant fruits and vegetables, whole grains, and healthy fats, which all contribute in overlapping and diverse ways to lowering the risk of atherosclerosis.

11.1 INTRODUCTION

Atherosclerosis is a common systemic disease and is the fundamental pathology that underlies a variety of chronic vascular diseases [1,2]. These diseases include CHD, stroke, chronic kidney disease (CKD), peripheral artery disease (PAD), and erectile dysfunction (ED) [3–5]. Each of these entities will be handled in separate sections of this chapter as well as in other chapters in this book.

Nutrition plays a critically important role in both the initiation and progression of atherosclerosis [6–11]. Over the past two decades, understandings about how nutrition in general and various components of nutrition interact with atherosclerosis has undergone significant change [1–2]. In the 1970s and 1980s, it was thought that plaque in the arteries, which is the cardinal finding of atherosclerosis, was caused by fat in the diet. Hence, for several decades, individuals were counseled to consume diets that were low in fat (particularly saturated fat). In addition, levels of dietary cholesterol were thought to also play a critically important role in atherosclerosis, and individuals were advised to lower the amount of cholesterol in their diets.

Modern understandings of atherosclerosis indicate a much more complicated picture. Research has now demonstrated that atherosclerosis has a significant inflammatory component. Thus, healthy diets include a number of foods that lower the risk of inflammation [12]. In addition, oxidative stress is now thought to play a significant role in the progression of atherosclerosis. For that reason, diets that contain high levels of antioxidants have also been demonstrated to lower the risk of atherosclerosis. All of the key healthy diets that are emphasized throughout this book contain multiple fruits and vegetables, whole grains, etc., which contribute to lowering the risk of

DOI: 10.1201/9781003452607-11

atherosclerosis and the various vascular diseases that it causes [12–14]. Conversely, the Western diet and many of its components, including red meat, processed meats, salt, refined carbohydrates, and ultra-processed foods, have all been shown to be inflammatory and to increase the risk of total body inflammation. This chapter will focus on modern understandings of healthy dietary patterns with particular emphasis on the various components that contribute to lowering the risk of atherosclerosis.

11.2 THE PATHOPHYSIOLOGY OF ATHEROSCLEROSIS

Atherosclerosis is an inflammatory disease that involves the arterial wall. It is characterized by progressive accumulation of lipids and inflammatory cells within the intima of large arteries [15–22]. Atherosclerosis is the fundamental process that underlies multiple diseases of the vasculature including CHD, stroke, CKD, and PAD.

In the last 20 years a substantial revision has occurred about how we understand the process of atherosclerosis. While nutritional factors are still central to our understanding of atherosclerosis, other lifestyle-related factors such as decreased physical activity, increased prevalence of obesity, cigarette smoking, and high blood pressure all contribute to atherosclerosis.

The view of arteries has undergone significant changes in the past 20 years. A clear link exists between atherosclerosis and the lining of the arteries. In the early 20th century, experiments done initially in rabbits showed that a diet high in fat would result in fatty deposition in the arteries, and cholesterol was initially identified as the culprit. As a more sophisticated view of lipoprotein particles in the 20th century arose, understandings became available regarding lipoprotein particles, and a more sophisticated view of atherosclerosis emerged [15–23].

A great deal of emphasis was placed initially on lowering low-density lipoprotein (LDL) cholesterol. It was felt that this would represent a significant reduction in atherosclerosis; unfortunately, this has not completely occurred. The more sophisticated view of atherosclerosis involves the interaction between the inner lining of the arteries (endothelium), lipids within the lumina of the artery, and inflammatory cells that invade the epithelium. Nutritional modalities are now increasingly being understood as important not only for lowering lipids within the arteries but also substantially reducing inflammation. This complex process has increasingly become a hallmark of the modern understanding of atherosclerosis.

Low-fat diets, in fact, have been shown to not reduce the risk of CHD in and of themselves over and above usual diets. Healthy nutritional plans, however, such as the Mediterranean diet (MedDiet), the U.S. Department of Agriculture (USDA) recommendations, Dietary Approaches to Stop Hypertension (DASH) [13] diet, and other healthy nutritional plans have all been shown to lower the risk of atherosclerosis [14]. There are multiple components of these plans that may contribute to the health benefits. Research has demonstrated that they significantly lower the risk of atherosclerosis and its manifestations.

Multiple authoritative organizations such as the American Heart Association (AHA), American College of Cardiology (ACC) [24], and the *Dietary Guidelines for Americans 2020–2025* have provided guidance based on foods and nutrients known to lower the risk of atherosclerosis. In addition, the 2013 ACC Lifestyle Guidance to Reduce Cardiovascular Risk stated that there is strong evidence for a dietary pattern that emphasizes vegetables, fruits, and whole grains and includes low-fat dairy products, poultry, fish, legumes, nontropical vegetable oils, and nuts and limits the intake of sweets, sugar-sweetened beverages, and red meats, which in turn lowers the risk of atherosclerosis [25].

11.3 DIETARY PATTERNS

The two most studied dietary patterns that have been demonstrated to lower the risk of atherosclerotic disease are the Mediterranean diet and the DASH diet. It should be noted that other healthy dietary patterns that emphasize similar nutrient composition are likely to also significantly lower the risk of atherosclerotic vascular disease, but less research has been conducted on them.

- The Mediterranean diet [12]

  The Mediterranean diet, which contains 35% fat; 22% monounsaturated fatty acids; less than 50% carbohydrates; and abundant fruits and vegetables, complex carbohydrates, fish, and daily consumption of a glass of wine (in non-Islamic countries) has been shown in multiple trials to significantly lower the risk of atherosclerotic heart disease. The MedDiet has been shown to improve blood pressure (BP), lipid profile, glucose metabolism, arrhythmia risk, and the gut microbiome.

  It has also been suggested that the components of the Mediterranean diet exert anti-inflammatory effects as well as improvements in the gut microbiome. There are some data to suggest that the MedDiet reduces expression of pro-atherogenic genes as well as LDL receptor–related proteins. This further lowers the likelihood of plaque rupture. Within the Mediterranean diet various vitamins, omega-3 fatty acids, monounsaturated fats (particularly from olive oil), fiber, polyphenols, and lycopene all are thought to reduce the risk of atherosclerosis (more on some of these individual nutrients will be discussed in subsequent sections of this chapter).

When the MedDiet was supplemented with extra-virgin olive oil (EVOO) or nuts, in the PREDIMED study, these additions further reduced the risk of atherosclerosis in comparison to a low-fat diet after five years of intervention [26]. It is thought that the EVOO or nuts may influence methylation of white blood cell genes and thus reduce genetic and epigenetic factors, which may increase the risk of atherosclerosis.

- The DASH diet [13]

  Significant evidence supports that adherence to the DASH dietary pattern lowers the risk of atherosclerosis and improves BP, body weight, glucose-insulin homeostasis, blood lipids, and lipoproteins. The DASH pattern also reduces inflammation grade and improves endothelial function and improves the microbiome composition resulting in decreased cardiovascular disease (CVD) risk and decreased total mortality. Similar to the MedDiet, the DASH diet is characterized by high intake of fruits and vegetables, legumes, low-fat dairy, whole grain products, nuts, fish, and poultry while reducing saturated fat, red meat, processed meats, and sweetened beverages and lowering the intake of sodium and refined grains. Studies of the DASH diet have shown that it lowers inflammatory markers and oxidative stress. A second research study further reduced sodium (the DASH Sodium diet), which resulted in further reductions in BP and further reductions in risk of atherosclerosis.

- Low-fat diet
  As already indicated in the PREDIMED study, the MedDiet substantially lowered risk more than the control diet, which was a low-fat diet. This finding is also consistent with multiple randomized controlled trials which have demonstrated that a low-fat diet by itself does not lower the risk of CHD when compared to usual care [27].
- Western diet
  As indicated in Chapter 2, the Western diet, which contains considerable amounts of red meat, saturated fat, processed foods, and refined grains, has been shown to exert inflammatory effects and increase the risk of atherosclerosis.
- Keto diet
  Low-carbohydrate, high-protein diets (which may also be high in saturated fats) in recent studies have been shown to increase the risk of CVD.

11.4 NONSTARCHY FRUITS AND VEGETABLES

The AHA and the European Society of Cardiology (ESC) both strongly endorse the daily consumption of multiple servings of fruits and vegetables to reduce atherosclerosis risk. Multiple studies support this recommendation.

- Starchy vegetables
  Potatoes are a widely consumed starchy vegetable. They contain fiber, potassium, vitamin C and B_6, and other trace minerals; however, potatoes predominantly contain starch. Based on this high starch content and increased risk of type 2 diabetes mellitus (T2DM) and weight gain, intake of potatoes is not advisable for reduction of atherosclerosis; however, when consumed in small portion sizes and including the nutrient-rich skin as part of mixed meals, they are not associated with any harm [28–30].
- Olive oil
  A number of studies have demonstrated anti-inflammatory effects of olive oil–rich diets [31–33]. EVOO, which is a major component of the MedDiet, has resulted in improvements in inflammatory status, oxidative stress, and endothelial function. The added EVOO in the PREDIMED study has been suggested as one of the major reasons for its significant reduction in risk of CVD.
- Nuts and seeds
  Nuts, particularly peanuts and walnuts, have been demonstrated to reduce CVD morbidity and mortality in numerous large-cohort studies, presumably because of their positive effects on reducing atherosclerosis [34].

- Wine
  Wine contains multiple phenolic compounds, which decrease oxidation of LDL-C and oxidative stress. Consumption of wine also increases nitric oxide, which is a potent vasodilator in the arteries [35–38]. In addition, the ethanol in wine increases high-density lipoprotein cholesterol (HDL-C) levels, inhibits platelet aggregation, and reduces systemic inflammation—all of which are important in reducing atherosclerosis. It is important to emphasize that these health benefits of wine come from moderate consumption (no more than one 5-ounce glass of wine per day for women and no more than two glasses per day for men).
- Meat and processed meats
  Initial concerns concerning meat in general and particularly lean cuts of red meat were initially based on nutrient contents such as saturated fat and dietary cholesterol. Modern nutrition research has demonstrated, however, relatively neutral cardiovascular effects of saturated fat and dietary cholesterol, while other compounds in meats such as heme iron, sodium, and other components also appear to have relatively neutral effects on atherosclerosis [39–41].

  In contrast, there are consistent findings that stronger adverse effects result from processed meats. These findings may be explained on the basis of high levels of sodium (greater than 400% higher in processed meats) on BP levels and subsequent effects of elevated BP on clinical endpoints [42]. In addition, processed meats may adversely affect the microbiome. Of note, both red and processed meats are linked to higher incidence of diabetes, where they [39–41] approximately double the risk, although the mechanism of increased risk is not known. Of note, feeding practices for cattle may significantly impact on risk of atherosclerosis. Grass-fed beef in particular that is well-trimmed may be a reasonable source of omega-3 fatty acids.
- Poultry and eggs
  Relatively little research-based evidence exists related to poultry as a risk factor for atherosclerosis [42]. In several studies there was no significant association between poultry and atherosclerosis, and in some cohorts, a modestly lower risk for CVD, although less benefit observed than for fish, nuts, and legumes [42–46]. Egg consumption is not significantly associated with atherosclerosis in population studies [42,43,47,48]. There is, however, some suggestion that consumers of eggs have higher evidence of diabetes [48]. Thus, it appears that occasional consumption of poultry and eggs is relatively neutral with regard to atherosclerosis.
- Fish
  Fish is a potent source of omega-3 fatty acids. The cardiovascular effects of omega-3 fatty acids have been studied for several decades [49–52]. Research findings in this area are the basis of the recommendation from the AHA to serve two plus servings of fish (preferably oily fish) per week to obtain long-chain omega-3 fatty acids to lower the risk of atherosclerosis. Omega-3 fatty acids also reduce inflammatory biomarkers and improve risk

factors for atherosclerosis, including BP and endothelial function as well as triglycerides and adiponectin.

- Dairy products
  The effect of a variety of dairy products on atherosclerosis is the subject of considerable debate, although many unanswered questions remain. Typical dietary guidelines group dairy products according to the amount of dietary fat, recommending selection of low-fat products [53–57]. These recommendations, however, are also subject to considerable debate. Most of the research in this area has been done on milk. Some evidence exists, however, on cheese consumption and yogurt largely in the area of their effects on weight gain. Both cheese and yogurt have been shown in some studies to lower the risk of long-term weight gain when consumed in modest quantities.

  Of note, some studies have suggested that fat from dairy products may actually promote cardiometabolic health. This finding is presumed to be through its effects on atherosclerosis. It is not clear whether these findings related to dietary fat are related to specific dairy fatty acids. When all of these findings are taken together, there is little support for the recommendation of consuming only low-fat dairy products with regard to atherosclerosis. There are significant other benefits of consuming dairy products, however, particularly milk as a major source of calcium and vitamin D for bone health.
- Butter
  A large research project on a European cohort showed that butter did not increase the risk of atherosclerosis [58,59]. Consumption of butter, however, appears to be associated with an increased risk of both diabetes and weight gain. The fact that butter has not been demonstrated to increase the risk of atherosclerosis is consistent with the emerging evidence that total saturated fat is less likely to increase atherosclerosis than previously thought [54,55].
- Vegetable oils
  The relationship between atherosclerosis and vegetable oils has typically been made based on their fatty acid composition, particularly is it relates to monounsaturated, polyunsaturated, and saturated fats [31–33]. Recent evidence, however, suggests that the relationship of vegetable oils to atherosclerosis may be based on other constituents such as flavonoids, which exhibit anti-inflammatory properties [59]. In the PREDIMED study, for example, the addition of added EVOO in the context of the Mediterranean diet showed decreased risk of stroke, myocardial infarction, or death when compared to the control. It is important to note that over half of EVOO has additional monounsaturated fats compared to regular olive oil.

  Tropical oils, such as palm or coconut oil, have considerable amounts of saturated fat. The literature in this area, however, is evolving concerning whether or not saturated fats in these oils increase the risk of atherosclerosis. Growing research suggests that increased consumption of vegetable oils in place of refined grains, starches, sugars, and meat may actually result in a reduction in risk of atherosclerosis. Another factor may be the processing of oils. For example, EVOO is produced with lower-temperature refining, which may help preserve phenolic compounds. Thus, the area of the effects of various tropical oils remains mixed and in need of further research.

- Alcohol
  Heavy alcohol consumption is responsible for a variety of cardiovascular problems and may play a role in increasing atherosclerosis. Some lowering of the risk of atherosclerosis appears to occur from moderate consumption of alcohol (no more than two alcoholic drinks per day for men and one alcoholic drink per day for women) [37,38]. As already noted, phenols are present in wine and beer as well, which may reduce atherosclerosis. The AHA and Centers for Disease Control and Prevention (CDC) recommend that individuals who consume alcohol do so in moderation, and those who do not drink alcohol should be advised not to begin [60].
- Coffee and tea
  Coffee not only contains caffeine but since it is the liquid extract of legumes (coffee beans), it contains many other active compounds, which may decrease the likelihood of atherosclerosis. With regard to CHD and atherosclerosis, the lowest risk is seen at three to four cups per day [61,62].

  Tea consumption is also associated with a lower risk of atherosclerotic heart disease [63–65]. Black tea and green tea can lower BP and may also lower LDL cholesterol, both of which could potentially lower the risk of atherosclerosis.

  In the final analysis, both tea and coffee consumed at moderate levels do not increase the risk of atherosclerosis and may actually reduce the risk of CVD.

11.5 NUTRIENTS

The consumption of various nutrients can lower the risk of atherosclerosis, including fiber and some micronutrients.

- Fiber
  A number of studies have shown that dietary fiber decreases cholesterol concentrations and BP and thereby lowers the risk of atherosclerosis [66–69]. In addition, several clinical trials have shown that dietary fiber decreases inflammation and downregulates the expression of oxidative stress related to cytokines and the inflammatory response, which can be mediated by gut microbiota. Good sources of fiber include fruits and vegetables and whole grains, which may contribute to their effects of lowering the risk of atherosclerotic disease.
- Micronutrients
  Good evidence exists from a variety of sources that some micronutrients may protect against atherosclerosis [70–72]. This may be a result of their effect on reducing endothelial cell damage, improving production of nitric oxide, and inhibiting the oxidation of LDL cholesterol. Dietary antioxidants such as zinc, selenium, and vitamin C and E may also contribute to

lowering inflammation. In addition, there is some evidence that magnesium supplementation can significantly reduce inflammation.

- Sodium

In the Western diet, most of the sodium (approximately 75%) comes from packaged goods and food consumption at restaurants, while a minority comes from home cooking or table salt. The amount of salt in the diet is associated with BP levels, with particularly strong effects in older individuals and people who already have hypertension and Black people [73–76]. For all of these reasons, sodium increases the risk of atherosclerosis. Lowering sodium in the diet is recommended by the AHA (less than 2,300 mg/day) [77].

Reducing the amount of salt in the diet results in significant lowering of BP and lowers the risk of atherosclerotic diseases. Some data have also suggested that salt reduction to less than 1,500 mg per day may further lower risk of atherosclerosis, although the research in this area is nonconclusive.

- Carbohydrates, added sugars, and fructose

Carbohydrates have been considered for many years as the foundation of a healthful diet. Modern nutrition research, however, indicates that total carbohydrate has little influence on cardiometabolic health [78–80]. It is the types and quality of carbohydrates that exert a major impact.

Whole grains as well as carbohydrate-containing foods such as fruits, vegetables, and legumes have been shown to lower the risk of atherosclerosis. In contrast, foods rich in refined grains such as white bread, white rice, crackers, cereals, and baked desserts, as well as starches such as white potatoes and added sugars exert adverse effects. Thus, the focus should be on eating healthful carbohydrates. While there has been an attempt to alert people to potential adverse effects of added sugar, the more realistic approach is to recommend overall carbohydrate quality, which includes lower added sugars but also measured complex carbohydrates.

Considerable attention has been focused on the potential harm of fructose and high fructose corn syrup [81,82]. There are, however, no data to suggest that fructose or high fructose corn syrup is more associated with atherosclerosis than is sucrose. Thus, once again, focus should be on overall carbohydrate quality.

- Dietary fats

The Dietary Guidelines for Americans (DGAs) 2020–2025 recommend limiting dietary fat to less than 35% of calories. As already indicated, however, low-fat diets have not been demonstrated to lower the risk of atherosclerosis. Given recent data that suggest that some types of saturated fat may not be associated with increased risk of atherosclerosis, whereas monounsaturated fat and polyunsaturated fat have both been demonstrated to lower the risk of atherosclerotic disease, it is important to take a more nuanced approach to the types of fat rather than a blanket reduction in fats [83,84]. For example, with the Mediterranean diet, which contains 35% fat, two-thirds of this fat is composed of monounsaturated fats, which are thought to contribute to lowering the risk of CVD as found in the PREDIMED study.

In contrast, trans fatty acids (TFAs), which are often used in industrial production with partially hydrogenated vegetable oil (which may contain 30–60% TFAs), have been shown to have unique adverse effects on blood lipids, including raising LDL cholesterol and lowering HDL cholesterol. For this reason, TFAs should be minimized in the diet.

11.6 BIOACTIVE COMPOUNDS

A variety of bioactive compounds including omega-3 fatty acids, lycopene, and polyphenols have been associated with a lower risk of atherosclerosis. All of these compounds reduce levels of LDL-C and improve inflammatory and oxidative stress biomarkers.

- Omega-3 fatty acids
  Omega-3 fatty acids and polyunsaturated fatty acids have been reported as an anti-atherogenic agent [83–90]. Potential mechanisms for reducing the risk of atherosclerosis by omega-3 fatty acids include improvements in lipoprotein profile, reduction in oxidative stress, and improvement in endothelial function and plaque stability. Omega-3 fatty acids also modulate the concentration or expression of pro-inflammatory markers such as adhesion molecules, cytokines, and immune cells. Fish, in particular oily fish, are excellent sources of omega-3 fatty acids.
- Lycopene
  Lycopene is a carotenoid and is the most prevalent of the carotenoids in the human diet [91–97]. It is present in red-colored fruits and vegetables such as tomatoes, papaya, and watermelon, along with others. Observational and interventional studies have suggested that lycopene may reduce atherosclerotic risk and prevent endothelial dysfunction as well as enhance LDL oxidation. Lycopene may also modulate the expression of pro-inflammatory markers and platelet aggregation. Lycopene is a potent antioxidant that further lowers the risk of atherosclerosis.
- Phytosterols
  A significant body of scientific evidence has demonstrated that a daily dose of two to three grams of plant sterols (phytosterols) is associated with LDL cholesterol reduction of 6–15% [98–101]. In addition, phytosterols lower pro-inflammatory markers. Phytosterols are found in all plant foods; the highest concentrations, however, are found in unrefined plant oils including vegetable, nut, and olive oil (particularly EVOO). Nuts, seeds, whole grains, and legumes are also good dietary sources of phytosterols.

11.7 POLYPHENOLS

Polyphenols are the most abundant dietary antioxidant present in most plant foods and beverages. They possess a wide range of healthy effects in the prevention of atherosclerosis. The most important food sources of polyphenols are fruits and vegetables, red wine, black and green tea, coffee, EVOO, and chocolate, as well as nuts, seeds, herbs, and spices [102–104]. Polyphenols appear to exert positive effects by delaying progression of atherosclerosis and inhibiting pro-inflammatory cytokines. They also appear to reduce BP due to the enhanced nitrous oxide production as well as improving lipometabolism, coagulation activity, and endothelial function.

11.8 MINERALS

- Zinc
  Zinc is an important trace mineral that is found in cells throughout the body. It is needed to support the function of the immune system and the breakdown of carbohydrates [105–107]. Zinc is obtained in the diet mainly from animal tissue sources such as meat, fish, and seafood. It also plays a major role in the immune response and is an important contributor to reducing atherosclerosis. It is an antioxidant. Zinc also reduces the risk of vascular calcification, which is present in severe stages of atherosclerosis.
- Potassium
  Potassium is necessary for normal cellular function. The human diet requires a constant source of potassium, since it is excreted in the urine. Vegetables and fruits are examples of potassium-rich foods [108,109]. The Atherosclerosis Risk in Communities (ARIC) study showed an inverse correlation between serum potassium and the risk of diabetes. A significant study from Korea showed that in the highest quartile of potassium intake, there was a 39% lower odds of metabolic syndrome. The DASH diet found that consumption of fruits and vegetables was important in lowering BP, and this was largely attributed to the high potassium content [109,110].
- Magnesium
  Magnesium is involved in multiple biochemical processes and is widely distributed in plant and animal foods [111]. Green, leafy vegetables such as spinach, legumes, nuts, seeds, and whole grains are rich sources of magnesium. Magnesium may reduce the risk of atherosclerosis by modulating smooth muscle tone and endothelial cell function.
- Methyl nutrients
  Epigenetics is defined as a field where changes in gene expression occur without changes in DNA sequence (see also Chapter 32). It is thought that methylation of DNA plays an important role in this [112–114]. Nutrients that contribute to this process are called methyl nutrients and include vitamins such as folate, riboflavin, vitamin B_{12}, vitamin B_6, and choline as well as amino acids such as methylamine, cystine, glycine, and serene.
- Folate
  Folate is a B vitamin found in a variety of foods such as liver, peas, mushrooms, green leafy vegetables [115], and fortified cereals. Human beings are unable to produce folate except through de novo synthesis by intestinal microbiota. Folate plays multiple roles in various aspects of DNA and lowers the risk of atherosclerosis. Other B vitamins, as already indicated, such as riboflavin, vitamin B_{12}, and B_6 may

contribute to enhancing epigenetic factors. B vitamins are also antioxidants, which may further contribute to their effects of lowering the risk of atherosclerosis.

11.9 MICROBIOME

There has been a dramatic increase in research in the area of the gut microbiota and its relationship to atherosclerosis in the past decade [116]. Adverse changes in the gut microbiota have been identified as playing a role in the pathogenesis of atherosclerosis. This connection may result from the influence of gut microbiota on host BP as well as alteration in the prevalence of bacteria genera affecting vascular tone and development of high BP. Emerging research suggests that microbiota may represent a therapeutic target for prevention of atherosclerosis. These issues are discussed in detail in Chapter 24.

11.10 OTHER LIFESTYLE PRACTICES AND HABITS

While nutrition plays a critical and diverse role in the initiation and progression of atherosclerosis, other lifestyle habits and practices also factor into the risk of developing atherosclerotic plaque. These include level of physical activity [117], maintenance of healthy body weight, and not smoking cigarettes. All of these are discussed in multiple chapters throughout this book.

11.11 CONCLUSIONS

Atherosclerosis is a systemic condition involving a complex series of steps resulting in plaque formation in various portions of the arterial tree. Atherosclerosis is the underlying condition in various chronic diseases including CHD, stroke, CKD, and ED. Nutrition plays a critical role in atherosclerosis. Multiple advances have occurred in our understanding of the atherosclerotic process and how nutrition interacts with it. In contrast to previous understandings which focused on a low-fat diet, modern nutrition emphasizes dietary patterns that interact with the vasculature in such areas as antioxidants and anti-inflammatory components. A wide variety of foods contained in the MedDiet and the DASH diet are thought to play critical roles in an overall approach to lowering atherosclerosis and thereby lowering the risk of various vascular diseases.

Clinical Applications

- Clinicians should understand modern research, which suggests that multiple plant attributes lower the risk of atherosclerosis, which is the underlying cause of multiple chronic diseases such as CHD, stroke, PAD, CKD, and ED.
- The process of atherosclerosis involves not only levels of fat in the bloodstream but also oxidation and inflammation.
- Various plant-based diets such as the MedDiet and the DASH diet have multiple plant-based components that contribute to their effectiveness in lowering the risk of atherosclerosis.

REFERENCES

1. Herrington W, Lacey B, Sherliker P, et al. Epidemiology of atherosclerosis and the potential to reduce the global burden of atherothrombotic disease. Circ Res. 2016;118(4):535–546.
2. Libby P, Bornfeldt KE, Tall AR. Atherosclerosis: Successes, surprises, and future challenges. Circ Res. 2016;118(4):531–534.
3. Shapiro MD, Fazio S. From lipids to inflammation: New approaches to reducing atherosclerotic risk. Circ Res. 2016;118(4):732–749.
4. Moran AE, Forouzanfar MH, Roth GA, Mensah GA, Ezzati M, Murray CJ, et al. Temporal trends in ischemic heart disease mortality in 21 world regions, 1980 to 2010: The Global Burden of Disease 2010 study. Circulation. 2014;129(14):1483–1492.
5. Bennett DA, Krishnamurthi RV, Barker-Collo S, et al. The global burden of ischemic stroke: Findings of the GBD 2010 study. Glob Heart. 2014;9(1):107–112.
6. Owen K, Sullivan V, Kris-Etherton P, et al. Nutrition and cardiovascular disease—an update. Curr Atheroscler Rep. 2018;30;20(2):8.
7. Casas R, Castro-Barquero S, Estruch R, et al. Nutrition and cardiovascular health. Int J Mol Sci. 2018;11;19(12):3988.
8. Getz GS, Reardon CA. Nutrition and cardiovascular disease. Arterioscler Thromb Vasc Biol. 2007;27(12):2499–2506.
9. Riccardi G, Giosuè A, Calabrese I, et al. Dietary recommendations for prevention of atherosclerosis. Cardiovasc Res. 2021;118(5):1188–1204.
10. Torres N, Guevara-Cruz M, Velazquez-Villegas L, et al. Nutrition and atherosclerosis. Arch Med Res. 2015;46(5):408–426.
11. Wei T, Liu J, Zhang D, Wang X, Li G, Ma R, Chen G, Lin X, Guo X. The relationship between nutrition and atherosclerosis. Front Bioeng Biotechnol. 2021;19;9:635504.
12. Jimenez-Torres J, Alcalá-Diaz J, Torres-Peña J, et al. Mediterranean diet reduces atherosclerosis progression in coronary heart disease: An analysis of the CORDIOPREV randomized controlled trial. Stroke. 2021;52(11):3440–3449.
13. Sacks FM, Svetkey LP, Vollmer WM, et al. Effects on blood pressure of reduced dietary sodium and the Dietary Approaches to Stop Hypertension (DASH) diet. DASH-Sodium Collaborative Research Group. N Engl J Med. 2001;344(1):3–10.
14. Healthy U.S.-Style Dietary Pattern for Adults Ages 19 through 59, with Daily or Weekly Amounts from Food Groups, Subgroups, and Components. *Dietary Guidelines for Americans, 2020–2025* | Chapter 4: Adults | Page 96. www.dietaryguidelines.gov/sites/default/files/2020-12/Dietary_Guidelines_for_Americans_2020-2025.pdf (Accessed January 2024).
15. Gimbrone MA, Jr, Garcia-Cardena G. Endothelial cell dysfunction and the pathobiology of atherosclerosis. Circ Res. 2016;118(4):620–636.
16. Bennett MR, Sinha S, Owens GK. Vascular smooth muscle cells in atherosclerosis. Circ Res. 2016;118(4):692–702.
17. Muller WA. How endothelial cells regulate transmigration of leukocytes in the inflammatory response. Am J Pathol. 2014;184(4):886–896.
18. Gerhardt T, Ley K. Monocyte trafficking across the vessel wall. Cardiovasc Res. 2015;107(3):321–330.
19. Li J, Ley K. Lymphocyte migration into atherosclerotic plaque. Arterioscler Thromb Vasc Biol. 2015;35(1):40–49.
20. Moore KJ, Sheedy FJ, Fisher EA. Macrophages in atherosclerosis: A dynamic balance. Nat Rev Immunol. 2013;13(10):709–721.
21. Robbins CS, Hilgendorf I, Weber GF, et al. Local proliferation dominates lesional macrophage accumulation in atherosclerosis. Nat Med. 2013;19(9):1166–1172.

22. Libby P, Lichtman AH, Hansson GK. Immune effector mechanisms implicated in atherosclerosis: From mice to humans. Immunity. 2013;38(6):1092–1104.
23. Bentzon JF, Otsuka F, Virmani R, et al. Mechanisms of plaque formation and rupture. Circ Res. 2014;114(12):1852–1866.
24. Lichtenstein A, Appel L, Vadiveloo M, et al. 2021 Dietary guidance to improve cardiovascular health: A scientific statement from the American Heart Association. Circulation. 2021;144(23):e472–e487.
25. Eckel R, Jakicic J, Ard J, et al. 2013 AHA/ACC Guideline on lifestyle management to reduce cardiovascular risk: A report of the American College of Cardiology/American Heart Association Task Force on Practice Guidelines. Circulation. 2014;129(25 Suppl 2):S76–S99.
26. Estruch R, Ros E, Salas-Salvado J, et al. Primary prevention of cardiovascular disease with a Mediterranean diet. N Engl J Med. 2013;368(14):1279–1290.
27. U.S. Department of Health and Human Services and U.S. Department of Agriculture. 2015–2020 Dietary Guidelines for Americans, 8th edition. 2015: 144.
28. Khosravi-Boroujeni H, Mohammadifard N, Sarrafzadegan N, et al. Potato consumption and cardiovascular disease risk factors among Iranian population. Int J Food Sci Nutr. 2012;63(8):913–920.
29. Khosravi-Boroujeni H, Saadatnia M, Shakeri F, et al. A case-control study on potato consumption and risk of stroke in central Iran. Arch Iran Med. 2013;16(3):172–176.
30. Lou-Bonafonte JM, Gabás-Rivera C, Navarro NA, Osada J. PON1 and Mediterranean diet. Nutrients. 2015;7(6):4068–4092.
31. Scotece M, Conde J, Abella V, et al. New drugs from ancient natural foods. Oleocanthal, the natural occurring spicy compound of olive oil: A brief history. Drug Discov Today. 2015;20:406–410.
32. Tresserra-Rimbau A, Rimm E, Medina-Remon A, et al. PREDIMED study investigators. Inverse association between habitual polyphenol intake and incidence of cardiovascular events in the PREDIMED study. Nutr Metable Cardiovasc Dis. 2014;24:639–647.
33. Beauchamp G, Keast R, Morel D, et al. Phytochemistry: Ibuprofen-like activity in extra-virgin olive oil. Nature. 2005;437:45–46.
34. Afshin A, Micha R, Khatibzadeh S, et al. Consumption of nuts and legumes and risk of incident ischemic heart disease, stroke, and diabetes: A systematic review and meta-analysis. Am J Clin Nutr. 2014;100:278–288.
35. Ronksley P, Brien S, Turner B, et al. Association of alcohol consumption with selected cardiovascular disease outcomes: A systematic review and meta-analysis. BMJ. 2011; 342:d671.
36. Willcox B, Willcox D, Todoriki H, et al. Caloric restriction, the traditional Okinawan diet, and healthy aging: The diet of the world's longest-lived people and its potential impact on morbidity and life span. Ann N Y Acad Sci. 2007;1114:434–455.
37. Brien S, Ronksley P, Turner B, et al. Effect of alcohol consumption on biological markers associated with risk of coronary heart disease: Systematic review and meta-analysis of interventional studies. BMJ. 2011;342:d636.
38. Arranz S, Chiva-Blanch G, Valderas-Martinez P, et al. Wine, beer, alcohol and polyphenols on cardiovascular disease and cancer. Nutrients. 2012;4:759–781.
39. Pan A, Sun Q, Bernstein A, et al. Red meat consumption and risk of type 2 diabetes: 3 cohorts of US adults and an updated meta-analysis. Am J Clin Nutr. 2011;94:1088–1096.
40. Chen G, Lv D, Pang Z, et al. Red and processed meat consumption and risk of stroke: A meta-analysis of prospective cohort studies. Eur J Clin Nutr. 2013;67:91–95.
41. Abete I, Romaguera D, Vieira A, et al. Association between total, processed, red and white meat consumption and all-cause, CVD and IHD mortality: A meta-analysis of cohort studies. Br J Nutr. 2014;112:762–775.

42. Al-Solaiman Y, Jesri A, Mountford W, et al. DASH lowers blood pressure in obese hypertensives beyond potassium, magnesium and fibre. J Hum Hypertens. 2010;24:237–246.
43. Nagao M, Iso H, Yamagishi K, et al. Meat consumption in relation to mortality from cardiovascular disease among Japanese men and women. Eur J Clin Nutr. 2012;66:687–693.
44. Takata Y, Shu X, Gao Y, et al. Red meat and poultry intakes and risk of total and cause-specific mortality: Results from cohort studies of Chinese adults in Shanghai. PLoS One. 2013;8:e56963.
45. Lee J, McLerran D, Rolland B, et al. Meat intake and cause specific mortality: A pooled analysis of Asian prospective cohort studies. Am J Clin Nutr. 2013;98:1032–1041.
46. Haring B, Gronroos N, Nettleton J, et al. Dietary protein intake and coronary heart disease in a large community based cohort: Results from the Atherosclerosis Risk in Communities (ARIC) study [corrected]. PLoS One. 2014 Oct;10;9(10):e109552.
47. Rong Y, Chen L, Zhu T, et al. Egg consumption and risk of coronary heart disease and stroke: Dose-response meta-analysis of prospective cohort studies. BMJ. 2013;346:e8539.
48. Shin J, Xun P, Nakamura Y, et al. Egg consumption in relation to risk of cardiovascular disease and diabetes: A systematic review and meta-analysis. Am J Clin Nutr. 2013;98:146–159.
49. Mozaffarian D, Rimm E. Fish intake, contaminants, and human health: Evaluating the risks and the benefits. JAMA. 2006;296:1885–1899.
50. Mozaffarian D, Wu J. Omega-3 fatty acids and cardiovascular disease: Effects on risk factors, molecular pathways, and clinical events. J Am Coll Cardiol. 2011;58:2047–2067.
51. Zheng J, Huang T, Yu Y, et al. Fish consumption and CHD mortality: An updated meta-analysis of seventeen cohort studies. Public Health Nutr. 2012;15:725–737.
52. Larsson S, Orsini N, Wolk A. Long-chain omega-3 polyunsaturated fatty acids and risk of stroke: A meta-analysis. Eur J Epidemiol. 2012;27:895–901.
53. Soedamah-Muthu S, Verberne L, Ding E, et al. Dairy consumption and incidence of hypertension: A dose response meta-analysis of prospective cohort studies. Hypertension. 2012;60:1131–1137.
54. Hu D, Huang J, Wang Y, et al. Dairy foods and risk of stroke: A meta-analysis of prospective cohort studies. Nutr Metable Cardiovasc Dis. 2014;(24):460–469.
55. Qin L, Xu J, Han S, et al. Dairy consumption and risk of cardiovascular disease: An updated meta-analysis of prospective cohort studies. Asia Pac J Clin Nutr. 2015;(24):90–100.
56. Gao D, Ning N, Wang C, et al. Dairy products consumption and risk of type 2 diabetes: Systematic review and dose-response meta-analysis. PLoS One. 2013;8:e73965.
57. Ericson U, Hellstrand S, Brunkwall L, et al. Food sources of fat may clarify the inconsistent role of dietary fat intake for incidence of type 2 diabetes. Am J Clin Nutr. 2015;101:1065–1080.
58. Smith JD, Hou T, Ludwig DS, et al. Changes in intake of protein foods, carbohydrate amount and quality, and long-term weight change: Results from 3 prospective cohorts. Am J Clin Nutr. 2015;101(6):1216–1224.
59. O'Sullivan TA, Hafekost K, Mitrou F, et al. Food sources of saturated fat and the association with mortality: A meta-analysis. Am J Public Health. 2013;103(9):e31–e42.
60. Baliunas DO, Taylor BJ, Irving H, Roerecke M, Patra J, Mohapatra S, Rehm J. Alcohol as a risk factor for type 2 diabetes: A systematic review and meta-analysis. Diabetes Care. 2009;32(11):2123–2132.
61. Ding M, Bhupathiraju S, Satija A, et al. Long term coffee consumption and risk of cardiovascular disease: A systematic review and a dose-response meta-analysis of prospective cohort studies. Circulation. 2014;129:643–659.

62. Steffen M, Kuhle C, Hensrud D, et al. The effect of coffee consumption on blood pressure and the development of hypertension: A systematic review and meta-analysis. J Hypertens. 2012;30:2245–2254.
63. Zhang C, Qin Y, Wei X, et al. Tea consumption and risk of cardiovascular outcomes and total mortality: A systematic review and meta-analysis of prospective observational studies. Eur J Epidemiol. 2015;30:103–113.
64. Liu G, Mi X, Zheng X, et al. Effects of tea intake on blood pressure: A meta-analysis of randomised controlled trials. Br J Nutr. 2014;(112):1043–1054.
65. Yarmolinsky J, Gon G, Edwards P. Effect of tea on blood pressure for secondary prevention of cardiovascular disease: A systematic review and meta-analysis of randomized controlled trials. Nutr Rev. 2015;73:236–246.
66. Sánchez-Muniz F. Dietary fibre and cardiovascular health. Nutr. Hosp. 2012;27:31–45.
67. Huang T, Xu M, Lee A, et al. Consumption of whole grains and cereal fiber and total and cause-specific mortality: Prospective analysis of 367,442 individuals. BMC Med. 2015;(24);13:59.
68. Yang Y, Zhao L, Wu Q, et al. Association between dietary fiber and lower risk of all-cause mortality: A meta-analysis of cohort studies. Am J Epidemiol. 2015;(181):83–91.
69. McRae M. Dietary fiber is beneficial for the prevention of cardiovascular disease: An umbrella review of meta-analyses. J Chiropr Med. 2017;(16):289–299.
70. Toole J, Malinow M, Chambless L, et al. Lowering homocysteine in patients with ischemic stroke to prevent recurrent stroke, myocardial infarction and death: The Vitamin Intervention for Stroke Prevention (VISP) randomized controlled-trial. JAMA. 2004;291:565–575.
71. Spence J, Bang H, Chambles L, et al. Vitamin intervention for stroke prevention trial: An efficacy analysis. Stroke. 2005;36:2404–2409.
72. Root M, McGinn M, Nieman D, et al. Combined fruit and vegetable intake is correlated with improved inflammatory and oxidant status from a cross-sectional study in a community setting. Nutrients. 2012;4:29–41.
73. Brown I, Tzoulaki I, Candeias V, et al. Salt intakes around the world: Implications for public health. Int J Epidemiol. 2009;38:791–813.
74. Aburto N, Ziolkovska A, Hooper L, et al. Effect of lower sodium intake on health: Systematic review and meta-analyses. BMJ. 2013;346:f1326.
75. Poggio R, Gutierrez L, Matta M, et al. Daily sodium consumption and CVD mortality in the general population: Systematic review and meta-analysis of prospective studies. Public Health Nutr. 2015;18:695–704.
76. Li X, Cai X, Bian P, et al. High salt intake and stroke: Meta-analysis of the epidemiologic evidence. CNS Neurosci Ther. 2012;18:691–701.
77. Muntner P, Shimbo D, Carey RM, et al. Measurement of blood pressure in humans: A scientific statement from the American Heart Association. Hypertension. 2019;73(5):e35–e66.
78. Tang G, Wang D, Long J, et al. Meta-analysis of the association between whole grain intake and coronary heart disease risk. Am J Cardiol. 2015;115:625–629.
79. Aune D, Norat T, Romundstad P, et al. Whole grain and refined grain consumption and the risk of type 2 diabetes: A systematic review and dose-response meta-analysis of cohort studies. Eur J Epidemiol. 2013;28:845–858.
80. Wu Y, Qian Y, Pan Y, et al. Association between dietary fiber intake and risk of coronary heart disease: A meta-analysis. Clin Nutr. 2015;34:603–611.
81. Stanhope KL. Sugar consumption, metabolic disease and obesity: The state of the controversy. Crit Rev Clin Lab Sci. 2016;53(1):52–67.

82. Malik V, Hu F. Fructose and cardiometabolic health: What the evidence from sugar-sweetened beverages tells us. J Am Coll Cardiol. 2015;66:1615–1624.
83. Hamer M, Steptoe A. Influence of specific nutrients on progression of atherosclerosis, vascular function, haemostasis and inflammation in coronary heart disease patients: A systematic review. Br J Nutr. 2006;95:849–859.
84. Burke MF, Burke FM, Soffer DE. Review of cardiometabolic effects of prescription Omega-3 fatty acids. Curr Atheroscler Rep. 2017;7;19(12):60.
85. Calder PC. The role of marine omega-3 (Ω-3) fatty acids in inflammatory processes, atherosclerosis and plaque stability. Mol Nutr Food Res. 2012;56:1073–1080.
86. Wang Q, Liang X, Wang L, et al. Effect of omega-3 fatty acids supplementation on endothelial function: A meta-analysis of randomized controlled trials. Atherosclerosis. 2012;(221):536–543.
87. Leslie MA, Cohen DJ, Liddle DM, et al. A review of the effect of omega-3 polyunsaturated fatty acids on blood triacylglycerol levels in normolipidemic and borderline hyperlipidemic individuals. Lipids Health Dis. 2015;6;14:53.
88. Yagi S, Aihara K, Fukuda D, et al. Effects of docosahexaenoic acid on the endothelial function in patients with coronary artery disease. J Atheroscler Thromb. 2015;22:447–454.
89. Thies F, Garry J, Yaqoob P, et al. Association of Ω-3 polyunsaturated fatty acids with stability of atherosclerotic plaques: A randomised controlled trial. Lancet. 2003;8; 361(9356):477–485.
90. Robinson JG, Stone NJ. Antiatherosclerotic and antithrombotic effects of omega-3 fatty acids. Am J Cardiol. 2006;98:39i–49i.
91. Kaliora AC, Dedoussis GV. Natural antioxidant compounds in risk factors for CVD. Pharmacol Res. 2007;56:99–109.
92. Valderas-Martinez P, Chiva-Blanch G, Casas R, et al. Tomato sauce enriched with olive oil exerts greater effects on cardiovascular disease risk factors than raw tomato and tomato sauce: A randomized trial. Nutrients. 2016;8(3):170.
93. Mozos I, Stoian D, Caraba A, et al. Lycopene and vascular health. Front Pharmacol. 2018;23;9:521.
94. Costa-Rodrigues J, Pinho O, Monteiro P. Can lycopene be considered an effective protection against cardiovascular disease? Food Chem. 2018;245:1148–1153.
95. Cheng H, Koutsidis G, Lodge J. Tomato and lycopene supplementation and cardiovascular risk factors: A systematic review and meta-analysis. Atherosclerosis. 2017;257:100–108.
96. Wang Y, Chung S, McCullough M. Dietary carotenoids are associated with cardiovascular disease risk biomarkers mediated by serum carotenoid concentrations. J Nutr. 2014;(144):1067–1074.
97. Xu XR, Zou ZY, Huang YM, et al. Serum carotenoids in relation to risk factors for development of atherosclerosis. Clin Biochem. 2012;(45):1357–1361.
98. Ras R, Geleijnse J, Trautwein E. LDL-cholesterol-lowering effect of plant sterols and stanols across different dose ranges: A meta-analysis of randomised controlled studies. Br J Nutr. 2014;112(2):214–219.
99. Cabra C, Klein MS-T. Phytosterols in the treatment of hypercholesterolemia and prevention of cardiovascular diseases. Arq Bras Cardiol. 2017;(109):475–482.
100. Rocha V, Ras R, Gagliardi A, et al. Effects of phytosterols on markers of inflammation: A systematic review and meta-analysis. Atherosclerosis. 2016;48:76–83.
101. Ras R, Fuchs D, Koppenol W, et al. Effect of a plant sterol-enriched spread on biomarkers of endothelial dysfunction and low grade low grade inflammation in hypercholesterolaemic subjects. J Nutr Sci. 2016;6;5:e44.
102. Tressera-Rimbau A, Arranz S, Eder M, et al. Dietary polyphenols in the prevention of stroke. Oxid Med Cell Longev. 2017;7467962.

103. González-Gallego J, García-Mediavilla M, Sánchez-Campos S, et al. Fruit polyphenols immunity and inflammation. Br J Nutr. 2010;104:S15–S27.
104. Bahramsoltani R, Ebrahimi F, Farzaei M, et al. Dietary polyphenols for atherosclerosis: A comprehensive review and future perspectives. Crit Rev Food Sci Nutr. 2019;59(1):114–132.
105. Wong CP, Ho E. Zinc and its role in age-related inflammation and immune dysfunction. Mol Nutr Food Res. 2012;56:77e87.
106. Wong CP, Rinaldi NA, Ho E. Zinc deficiency enhanced inflammatory response by increasing immune cell activation and inducing IL6 promoter demethylation. Mol Nutr Food Res. 2015;59:991e999.
107. Brand IA, Kleineke J. Intracellular zinc movement and its effect on the carbohydrate metabolism of isolated rat hepatocytes. J Biol Chem. 1996;271:1941e1949.
108. Binia A, Jaeger J, Hu Y, et al. Daily potassium intake and sodium-to-potassium ratio in the reduction of blood pressure: A meta-analysis of randomized controlled trials. J Hypertens. 2015;33(8):1509–1520.
109. D'Elia L, Barba G, Cappuccio FP, et al. Potassium intake, stroke, and cardiovascular disease a meta-analysis of prospective studies. J Am Coll Cardiol. 2011;57:1210–1219.
110. Sacks FM, Svetkey LP, Vollmer WM, et al. Effects on blood pressure of reduced dietary sodium and the Dietary Approaches to Stop Hypertension (DASH) diet. DASH-Sodium Collaborative Research Group. N Engl J Med. 2001;344:3–10.
111. Bolland MJ, Grey A, Avenell A, et al. Calcium supplements with or without vitamin D and risk of cardiovascular events: Reanalysis of the women's health initiative limited access dataset and meta-analysis. BMJ. 2011;342:d2040.
112. Glier MB, Green TJ, Devlin AM. Methyl nutrients, DNA methylation, and cardiovascular disease. Mol Nutr Food Res. 2014;58:172–182.
113. Waterland RA, Jirtle RL. Transposable elements: Targets for early nutritional effects on epigenetic gene regulation. Mol Cell Biol. 2023;23:5293–5300.
114. Law JA, Jacobsen SE. Establishing, maintaining and modifying DNA methylation patterns in plants and animals. Nat Rev Genet. 2010;11:204–220.
115. Lin S, Lee W, Su Y, et al. Folic acid inhibits endothelial cell proliferation through activating the cSrc/ERK 2/NF-kappaB/p53 pathway mediated by folic acid receptor. Angiogenesis. 2012;15:671–683.
116. Sanchez-Rodriguez E, Egea-Zorrilla A, Plaza-Díaz J, et al. The gut microbiota and its implication in the development of atherosclerosis and related cardiovascular diseases. Nutrients. 2020;26;12(3):605.
117. Huang WC, Tung CL, Yang YSH, et al. Endurance exercise ameliorates Western diet-induced atherosclerosis through modulation of microbiota and its metabolites. Sci Rep. 2022;7;12(1):3612.

12 Nutrition and Coronary Heart Disease

Key Points

- Cardiovascular disease (CVD) remains the leading killer of both men and women in the United States, resulting in over 37% of annual mortality.
- Nutritional practices play a pivotal role in the likelihood of developing CVD and, if already present, treating it.
- Dietary patterns, including increases in fruits and vegetables, whole grains, seafood (particularly oily fish), legumes and nuts, and lower nonfat dairy products, as well as decreases in red meats and processed meats, reduced sugar-sweetened beverages, and refined grains have all been shown to lower the risk of CVD and are central to the recommendations from the Dietary Guidelines for Americans (DGA) 2025 and the 2021 nutritional recommendations from the American Heart Association (AHA).
- Implementing heart-healthy diets should be a key mandate for clinicians to help their patients adopt healthier eating habits
- Clinicians should be aware of challenges in the environment such as misinformation, socioeconomic factors, and adverse targeted advertising, which may make it more difficult to convince many individuals to follow heart-healthy guidelines.

12.1 INTRODUCTION

CVD remains the largest source of morbidity and mortality in the United States and elsewhere in the developed world [1]. While CVD comprises coronary heart disease (CHD), stroke, hypertension, and heart failure, this chapter will focus specifically on CHD.

There has been a decades-long decline in CVD mortality; however, it still accounts for over 37% of all mortality in the United States. There are thousands of studies that support the concept that daily lifestyle habits and practices exert a profound likelihood of developing all aspects of CVD, and CHD in particular [2]. Lifestyle practices are associated with positive benefits, both in prevention and treatment of CVD and CHD, and nutrition clearly plays a pivotal role [3].

It has been estimated that over 700,000 Americans will experience their first myocardial infarction (MI) each year. That means that an American experiences a significant coronary event every 34 seconds. With the staggering impact of CHD on the lives of many individuals, both in the United States and around the world, important, ongoing work continues in an attempt to understand how to lower the risk of this often-fatal condition.

DOI: 10.1201/9781003452607-12

Multiple studies have demonstrated that nutritional practices including a diet containing more fruits and vegetables, fish (particularly oily fish), whole grains, and fiber, as well as maintaining a caloric balance to avoid weight gain, all lower the risk of CHD. Positive lifestyle decisions such as following a heart-healthy nutritional plan, maintaining a proper body weight, regular physical activity (engaging in at least 30 minutes per day of physical activity), and avoiding smoking or tobacco products all reduce the risk of CHD. The Nurses Health Trial and the Physicians' Health Study demonstrated that these practices can reduce the risk of CHD by over 80% and diabetes by over 90% in both men and women [4,5]. In addition, adoption of only one of these lifestyle habits or practices on a regular basis can reduce the risk of both CHD and diabetes by over 50%.

While mortality from CHD decreased by over 40% in the decades between 1980 and 2000, these still have a long way to go [6]. Reductions in the risk of CHD have resulted from improved lifestyle risk factors such as increased physical activity, smoking cessation, and better control of cholesterol and blood pressure. Unfortunately, obesity and diabetes have moved in the opposite direction and have the potential to reverse the gains made in other lifestyle-related practices.

Worldwide between 1990 and 2013, deaths from all aspects of CVD rose from 26% to 36% [7]. This has been attributed to epidemiologic transitions that have occurred during this period of time [8]. Nutritional factors play a significant role in many of the components of either positive or negative lifestyle decisions and practices.

While this chapter will focus on healthy nutrition, these dietary practices will be placed in the broader context of other lifestyle factors, including an emphasis on physical activity and energy balance.

This overall approach is consistent with the approach taken by the DGA 2020–2025 [9] as well as the 2021 Nutritional Guidelines from the AHA and guidance from multiple other sources including the Academy of Nutrition and Dietetics [10].

Multiple nutritional guidelines offered by the AHA, including not only the 2021 Dietary Guidelines to Improve Cardiovascular Health but also the 2013 AHA/American College of Cardiology (ACC) Guidelines on Lifestyle Management to Reduce Cardiovascular Risk [11] and the Guidelines for Lipid Management [12] and the Guidelines for Prevention and Treatment of High Blood Pressure, all focus on healthy nutritional practices and increasing physical activity [13]. All of these guidelines are similar and place an emphasis on not only heart-healthy nutrition but a broader approach toward positive lifestyle factors to improve cardiovascular health and lower the risk of CHD.

12.2 BACKGROUND

The recommendations from a variety of prestigious organizations regarding nutritional strategies for improving cardiovascular health are similar. These recommendations have typically drawn upon the same database, including large cohort studies and randomized controlled trials. These published consensus statements form the basis of the recommendations made in this chapter and include the following:

- AHA Diet and Lifestyle Recommendations Revision 2021: A Scientific Statement from the American Heart Association Nutrition Committee [3].

- Defining and Setting National Goals for Cardiovascular Health Promotion and Disease Reduction: American Heart Association Strategic Impact Goals Through 2020 and Beyond [14].
- 2013 AHA/ACC Guidelines for Lifestyle Management to Reduce Cardiovascular Risk: A Report of the American College of Cardiology/AHA Task Force on Practice Guidelines [11].
- DGA 2020–2025 Advisory Committee Report [9].
- AHA/ACC/AACVPR/AAPA/ABC/ACPM/ADA/AGS/APhA/ASPC/NLA/PCNA Guideline on the Management of Blood Cholesterol: Executive Summary: A Report of the American College of Cardiology/American Heart Association Task Force on Clinical Practice Guidelines [12].
- 2017 ACC/AHA/AAPA/ABC/ACPM/AGS/APhA/ASH/ASPC/NMA/PCNA Guideline for the Prevention, Detection, Evaluation, and Management of High Blood Pressure in Adults: A Report of the American College of Cardiology/American Heart Association Task Force on Clinical Practice Guidelines [13].

These consensus statements are uniformly based on dietary patterns rather than individual foods or nutrients and emphasize a dietary pattern that is higher in fruits and vegetables, whole grains (particularly high fiber), nonfat dairy, seafood, legumes, and nuts. The guidelines also recommend that individuals who consume alcohol (among adults) do so in moderation. They also uniformly recommend diets that are lower in red and processed meats, refined grains, sugar-sweetened beverages, and saturated and trans fats. The guidelines emphasize the importance of balancing calories and physical activity as strategies for maintaining healthy weight and, thereby, reducing risk of CHD.

To provide one example, the 2020 Strategic Plan from the AHA defines dietary goals in the context of a diet that is appropriate in energy balance pursuing an overall dietary plan consistent with the Dietary Approach to Stop Hypertension (DASH) diet [15] and the Mediterranean diet [16]. While the AHA recognizes that nutrition is complicated, the 2020 AHA Strategic Plan provides the following basic recommendations for components of the diet:

- Fruits and vegetables ≥4.5 cups/day.
- Fish two or more 2½-ounce servings/week (preferably oily fish).
- Fiber rich/whole grain ≥1.1 grams fiber/10 grams carbohydrate, three 1-ounce equivalent servings/day.
- Sodium ≤1500 milligrams/day.
- Sugar-sweetened beverages ≤460 calories (36 ounces)/week.

The AHA recognizes that nutrition is much more complex than these simple guidelines, but they provide a good starting point.

Nutrition guidelines have also shifted to the important aspect of how to actually implement available guidelines. It is recognized by the AHA and other organizations that only a distinct minority of Americans follow most of the guidelines. For example, only 12% of individuals consume their recommended number of servings of fruits, and only 7% follow the guidance for the recommended servings of vegetables

[2]. In the area of hypertension, less than 20% of individuals with high blood pressure currently follow the DASH diet. Thus, encouraging people to actually implement heart-healthy guidelines in their daily lives remains an important topic, which will be discussed toward the end of this chapter.

Modern nutritional practice has focused on dietary patterns as opposed to individual foods or components of food. This is the approach that has been taken by the AHA and their Dietary Guidelines 2021 as well as the DGA 2020–2025. Dietary patterns reflect more accurately how people actually eat and encompass balance, variety, and combinations of foods and beverages that people typically consume—foods prepared and consumed at home as well as outside of the home.

Research studies have shown that adherence to heart-healthy dietary patterns is associated with optimum cardiovascular health. The food based Healthy U.S.-Style Dietary Pattern outlined in the DGA 2020–2025 is designed to achieve nutrient adequacy and support heart health and general well-being as well as encompassing personal preferences, ethnic and religious practices, and life stages. As already indicated, heart-healthy dietary patterns that are associated with CHD risk reduction contain primarily fruits and vegetables, foods made with whole grains, healthy sources of protein (including plants, fish, and seafood), low-fat or fat-free dairy products, and if meat or poultry are desired, lean cuts in unprocessed forms, liquid plant oils, and minimally processed foods. Heart-healthy patterns also are low in beverages and foods containing added sugar and salt.

Heart-healthy dietary patterns are also those emphasized in the DASH diet, Mediterranean diet, DGA 2020–2025, Healthy U.S.-Style Dietary Pattern, and healthy vegetarian diets. The Dietary Patterns Methods Project showed 14–28% lower CVD risk for individuals adhering to this type of diet. It should be noted, however, that research on dietary patterns has typically been conducted in Western populations, and future research should also be conducted in non-Western countries. It should also be noted that there is no evidence supporting existing popular and fad diets with regard to lowering the risk of CVD.

The 2020–2025 DGA approached dietary patterns through food pattern modeling and the analysis of the current intake of the U.S. population, which allowed the development of the "Healthy U.S.-Style Dietary Pattern" [9]. This allowed flexibility in the amounts of foods from all food groups to establish healthy eating patterns that meet nutrient needs and accommodate temptations for saturated fats, sugars, and sodium. This approach also allowed analysis of current intakes to identify areas of potential public health concerns. Using this approach, the DGA stated the following [9]:

> Within the body of evidence, higher intakes of vegetables and fruits consistently have been identified as characteristic of healthy eating patterns; whole grains have been identified as well although slightly less consistently. The characteristics of healthy eating patterns have been identified with less consistency including fat free and low-fat dairy, seafood, legumes, and nuts, lowering intakes of meats including processed meats, poultry, sugar sweetened foods, particularly beverages and refined grains have also been identified as characteristics of healthy eating patterns.

The Healthy U.S.-Style Dietary Pattern for a 2,000-calorie level is found in Table 12.1. In addition, the DGA 2020–2025 emphasize that calories should be balanced to reduce the risk of weight gain and that calories from added sugars, saturated fats, and alcohol be limited to not exceed acceptable macronutrient distribution ranges of calories from protein, carbohydrates, and total fat. The following dietary patterns are all associated with lower risk of CVD.

TABLE 12.1
Composition of the Healthy U.S.-Style, Healthy Mediterranean Style, and Healthy Vegetarian Eating Patterns at the 2,000-Calorie Level, with Daily or Weekly Amounts from Food Groups, Subgroups, and Components

Food Group[a]	Healthy U.S.-Style Dietary Pattern	Healthy Mediterranean Style Eating Pattern	Healthy Vegetarian Eating Pattern
Vegetables	2½ c eq/day	2½ c eq/day	2½ c eq/day
--Dark green	1½ c eq/week	1½ c eq/week	1½ c eq/week
--Red and orange	5½ c eq/week	5½ c eq/week	5½ c eq/week
--Legumes (beans and peas)	1½ c eq/week	1½ c eq/week	3 c eq/week
--Starchy	5 c eq/week	5 c eq/week	5 c eq/week
--Other	4 c eq/week	4 c eq/week	4 c eq/week
Fruits	2 c eq/day	2½ c eq/day	2 c eq/day
Grains	6 oz eq/day	6 oz eq/day	6½ oz eq/day
--Whole grains	>3 oz eq/day	>3 oz eq/day	>3½ oz eq/day
--Refined grains	<3 oz eq/day	<3 oz eq/day	<3 oz eq/day
Dairy	3 c eq/day	2 c eq/day	3 c eq/day
Protein Foods	5½ oz eq/day	6½ oz eq/day	3½ oz eq/day
--Seafood	8 oz eq/week	15 oz eq/week	--
--Meat, poultry, eggs	26 oz eq/week	26 oz eq/week	3 oz eq/week (eggs)
--Nuts, seeds, soy products	5 oz eq/week	5 oz eq/week	14 oz eq/week
Oils	27 g/day	27 g/day	27 g/day
Limit on Calories for Other Uses (% of calories)[b]	270 kcal/day (14%)	260 kcal/day (13%)	290 kcal/day (15%)

[a] Food group amounts shown in cup (c) or ounce equivalents (oz eq). Oils are shown in grams (g). Amounts will vary for those who need <2,000 or >2,000 calories per day. Quantity equivalents for each food group are:

- Vegetables and fruits, 1 cup-equivalent is: 1 cup raw or cooked vegetable or fruit, 1 cup vegetable or fruit juice, 2 cups leafy salad greens, ½ cup dried fruit or vegetables.
- Grains, 1 ounce-equivalent is: ½ cup cooked rice, pasta, or cereal; 1 ounce dry pasta or rice; 1 medium (1 ounce) slice bread; 1 ounce of ready-to-eat cereal (about 1 cup of flaked cereal).

Source: Dietary Guidelines for Americans 2015–2020, pages 18 and 35.

- The Healthy U.S.-Style Dietary Pattern
  The Healthy U.S.-Style Dietary Pattern is also designed to meet recommended daily allowances (RDA) as well as acceptable macronutrient distribution ranges (AMDRs) set by the Food and Nutrition Board of the Institute for Medicine (IOM). Flexibility within this dietary pattern allows for minor modifications to allow use of the Mediterranean diet or DASH diet followed within these overall guidelines.
- Low-Fat Diets
  Clinical guidelines for CHD prevention have generally adopted the concept of low-fat diets. The pattern of low-fat eating forms the basis of numerous other diets that are discussed in this chapter.

  Low-fat diets are based on total fat consumption of between 25% and 35% of total calories with saturated fats (SFAs) no more than 7–10%; trans fats (TFAs) of less than 1%; increased unsaturated fat, monounsaturated fat, and omega-3 fats; and polyunsaturated fat (PUFA) consisting of the rest of the calories from fat [17,18]. These dietary plans also call for dietary cholesterol to be less than 300 milligrams/day, although this latter recommendation has become somewhat controversial since some research shows that dietary cholesterol does not significantly impact on blood cholesterol.

  Low-fat diets can be met by emphasizing the core recommendations from the 2021 AHA Dietary Guidelines as well as the DGA 2020–2025, which emphasize fruits and vegetables, whole grains, low-fat dairy products, and low-fat meats, if meat is desired. It is important to emphasize that saturated fats should be replaced by unsaturated or monounsaturated fats and not simple carbohydrates. It should also be noted that the food matrix of SFAs has been an area of recent research. This research has suggested that SFAs coming from dairy products may be less likely to cause adverse increases in risk factors for CVD compared to other sources of SFAs. The 2013 AHA/ACC Guidelines for Lifestyle Management recommend that consumption of SFAs not exceed 7% of calories.
- Low-Carbohydrate Diets
  Low-carbohydrate diets are typically defined as containing less than 45% of total calories from carbohydrates (30 grams of carbohydrates/day) [19,20]. Low-carbohydrate diets have been shown to reduce triglycerides (TG) and increase high-density lipoprotein (HDL) cholesterol (HDL-C). One study that compared low-carbohydrate to low-fat and Mediterranean diets showed greater weight loss in low-carbohydrate diets over the course of one year. One randomized control trial (DRIFT) showed that low-carbohydrate diets yielded more weight loss in modestly obese individuals after two years. At four years, however, there were no significant differences among the three arms.

  There are insufficient data from long-term trials to demonstrate that low-carbohydrate diets compared to low-fat or Mediterranean diets further reduce the risk of CHD.
- Mediterranean Diet
  The Mediterranean diet was originally described as the type of diet usually consumed in countries bordering the Mediterranean Sea. It is characterized

by relatively high fat intakes (40–50% of daily calories) of which SFA comprises less than or equal to 8% and monounsaturated fat (MUFA) 15–25% of calories [16,21,22]. The Mediterranean diet is also characterized by high omega-3 fatty acid intake from fish or plant sources and low omega-6/omega-3 ratios. This diet features seasonal, fresh, local vegetables; fruits; whole grain bread; legumes; nuts; and olive oil. Red meat is avoided. Moderate amounts of low-fat dairy products, as well as eggs, chicken, and fish are allowed. Small-to-moderate amounts of wine are encouraged with meals in non-Islamic countries.

A recent multicenter, randomized controlled trial in Spain in individuals with high cardiovascular risk but no overt evidence of CVD showed that the Mediterranean diet supplemented with extra virgin olive oil or with mixed nuts, compared to a control diet, resulted in a decrease of approximately 30% of the major cardiovascular events in the olive oil or nuts cohort compared to the control diet.

- DASH Diet

The DASH diet was originally formulated in the 1990s and has undergone several modifications and iterations since that time [15]. The initial goal of the DASH diet was to lower blood pressure and CHD incidence by nutritional means. Consistent with other low-fat diets, the DASH diet features vegetables and fruits, as well as low-fat dairy products, whole grains, chicken, fish, and nuts. It is low in fat, red meat, sweets, and soft drinks. The DASH diet provides more potassium, calcium, and magnesium and less fat and sodium than the typical Western diet. A typical composition of the DASH diet is found in Table 12.2.

Subsequent studies have substituted some of the carbohydrates with MUFAs and have further decreased the sodium in the diet. The modified DASH diets have reduced both systolic and diastolic blood pressure by 7–9 mm/Hg compared to a typical Western diet [23]. A study that combined the DASH Diet with a lifestyle program aiming to reduce overweight and increase physical activity while restricting sodium and alcohol intake (the ENCORE trial) showed additional decreases in both systolic and diastolic

TABLE 12.2
Typical Composition of the DASH Diet

- Fruits and vegetables ≥4.5 cups/day
- Fish two or more 2½-ounce servings/week (preferably oily fish)
- Fiber rich/whole grain ≥1.1 grams fiber/10 grams carbohydrate, three 1-ounce equivalent servings/day
- Sodium ≤1500 milligrams/day
- Sugar-sweetened beverages ≤460 calories (36 ounces)/week

Source: National Heart, Lung and Blood Institute. DASH Eating Plan. www.nhlbi.nih.gov/education/dash-eating-plan. These recommendations represent a reasonable starting point and have been expanded upon in other guidelines and recent reviews.

blood pressure, which were reduced by 14.2 mm/Hg and 17.4 mm/Hg, respectively [24]. This suggests that combining these lifestyle medicine components further decreases blood pressure. Unfortunately, even in individuals with high blood pressure, less than 20% currently follow the DASH diet.

- Vegetarian Diets
  A variety of vegetarian diets are available. These include vegan (consuming no animal products), lacto-ovo vegetarian (consuming milk and eggs), and pesco-vegetarian (consuming fish) along with vegetarian diet [25–28]. No data are available to suggest that one form of vegetarian diet is superior to others with regard to CHD risk. Few randomized controlled trials (RCTs) have been performed on vegetarian diets, and they have typically been small. These diets have typically resulted in lower risk of CHD and lower blood pressure compared to Western diets. It should be noted, however, that vegetarians are often more health conscious than other individuals, and these factors may compound the benefits of the nutritional pattern in a vegetarian diet.
- Japanese Diet
  There has been recent interest in Japanese diets, particularly those from Okinawa, which has the lowest CVD risk in the world [29]. Traditional Japanese diets emphasize seaweed, vegetables, fish, and soybean products, as well as fruits and green tea, and are low in meat. It should be noted that Japanese diets are often high in sodium from soy sauce and have been linked to a higher risk of strokes [30]. There have been relatively few studies of Japanese diets, so the link to reduced risk of CHD has not yet been determined.
- Prudent Diets
  In essence, all of the diets already discussed in this section could be considered to fall in the "prudent diet" category. A recent publication compared the prudent dietary pattern to a typical Western pattern and showed that the Western diet was associated with higher risk of mortality from CVD (22% higher), cancer (15% higher), and all-cause mortality (21% higher) [31].
- Plant-Based Diets
  There has been a recent surge in publications concerning plant-based diets. Essentially all the diets in this section may be considered plant based since they emphasize fruits and vegetables, legumes, and nuts and limit red meats, processed meats, sweets, and oils [32]. It should be noted, however, that it is possible to have a plant-based diet that does not lower the risk of heart disease [33], particularly if it has a lot of fat in it. A recent study compared a "healthy" plant-based diet to an "unhealthy" plant-based diet. Only the "healthy" plant-based diet resulted in decreased risk of CVD, while the "unhealthy" plant-based diet did not.

12.3 INDIVIDUAL FOOD ITEMS

As already indicated, most recent research in nutrition and CHD risk reduction involves dietary patterns. However, there have been studies of certain specific foods which also suggest that individual foods may either increase or decrease the risk of

CHD. The good news is that many of these food items are contained in heart-healthy dietary patterns.

12.4 AHA/ACC DIET AND LIFESTYLE RECOMMENDATIONS

In 2021, the AHA summarized diet and lifestyle recommendations in a scientific statement from the AHA Nutrition Committee [3]. These recommendations updated previous guidelines issued by the AHA in 2006 and also the 2013 AHA/ACC Guidelines for Lifestyle Management to Reduce Cardiovascular Risk. The 2021 Dietary Guidelines and its previous recommendations also include a broader approach not to just diet, but overall lifestyle combinations of diet and physical activity, in particular, were emphasized. The following goals were outlined in the 2021 Dietary Guidelines to improve cardiovascular health from the AHA:

- Balance Energy Intake and Expenditure to Maintain a Healthy Body Weight

  Maintaining a healthy body weight is an important component of CVD risk reduction. Over the past 40 years, the combination of increased energy intake and sedentary lifestyle has resulted in positive energy balance and accumulating excess body weight across the population in the United States. A combination of healthy dietary patterns and portion control to balance energy intake and expenditure is a key strategy for lowering the risk of heart disease. Numerous diet assessment tools are available for physicians to help patients achieve balance and healthy nutrition. Tracking diet through electronic medical records may also help facilitate this goal.
- Consume Increased Amounts and a Wide Variety of Fruits and Vegetables

  As already indicated in this chapter, dietary patterns rich in fruits and vegetables are associated with decreased risk of CVD. Deeply colored fruits and vegetables (tomatoes, leafy greens, peaches, etc.) tend to be more nutrient dense than lighter colored and white fruits and vegetables. Whole fruits and vegetables also supply dietary fiber and increase satiety due to their fiber. A variety of forms of fruits and vegetables (fresh, frozen, canned, and dried) can be incorporated in heart-healthy dietary patterns. Types of prepared fruits and vegetables with added salt and sugar should be limited.
- Emphasize Whole Grains

  Multiple studies have documented associations of the intake of the foods with whole grains and lower risk of CHD, stroke, metabolic syndrome, and cardiometabolic risk factors. Whole grains contain the endosperm, germ, and bran and are also a rich source of fiber. Products are allowed to be classified as whole grains if 51% of the grain in the product is a whole grain.
- Select Healthy Sources of Protein

  This recommendation involves selecting mostly protein from plants. These are typically plants that are either legumes or nuts, soybeans, lentils, chickpeas, and split peas. As already indicated, higher nut intake is also associated with lower risk of CVD. It should be noted that there has been an emergence of plant-based meat alternatives, although those should be used with caution because many are ultra-processed and contain saturated fat, added sugar, salt, stabilizers, and preservatives.

Regular fish and seafood intake is also recommended since these are good sources of protein. The preparation of fish matters since fried forms are not associated with benefits. The current recommendation, as already indicated, is to consume two fish meals per week. The greatest benefits are present when seafood replaces foods that are high in saturated fat.

Low-fat or fat-free dairy products are also recommended rather than full-fat products. The 2020–2025 DGA recommended low-fat dairy products citing a lower risk of all-cause mortality, CVD, overweight, and obesity. The DASH dietary pattern also includes low-fat and nonfat dairy products. It should be noted that the recommendation to consume low-fat and fat-free dairy products is still debated, as already indicated earlier in this chapter.

If meat or poultry is desired, chose lean cuts over processed forms. "Processed meats" include meat, poultry, or seafood products produced by smoking, curing or salting, in addition to chemical preservatives. Some common examples of processed meats include bacon, sausage, hot dogs, deli meat, pepperoni, and salami. Processed meats are typically high in salt and saturated fat, cholesterol, and polycyclic aromatic hydrocarbons.

- Chose liquid plant oils instead of tropical oils such as coconut, palm, or palm kernel oils or animal fats such as butter, lard, and margarine which contain partially hydrogenated fats.
- A strong body of scientific evidence supports the benefits of unsaturated fats (polyunsaturated and monounsaturated fats), particularly if they are chosen to replace trans fats. Unsaturated fat comes largely from plant oils. Major sources of polyunsaturated fat include plant oils such as soybean, corn, safflower, and sunflower oils; walnuts; and flax seed. Major sources of monounsaturated fat include canola and olive oils as well as nuts, including tree nuts and peanuts. Fish with a high fat content are a good source of omega-3 fatty acids. The goal is to use nontropical liquid plant oils as a substitute for saturated and trans fats (particularly animal and dairy fats).
- Chose Minimally or Unprocessed Foods Instead of Ultra-processed Foods.

  It should be noted that there is not a common definition of ultra-processed foods although these are typically products exposed with industrial food processing. There is a system that groups processed food according to the amount of processing. It is called the "NOVA" system. It should be noted that sales of processed foods have increased dramatically in the past two decades. These foods have been associated with overweight and obesity, CVD, and type 2 diabetes as well as all-cause mortality. A good general guideline is to emphasize unprocessed or minimally processed foods in a heart-healthy diet.
- Minimize or Decrease Foods and Beverages with Added Sugars

  Added sugars are those which are added to either food or beverages during preparation or processing. Many different types of added sugars exist including high fructose corn syrup, glucose, dextrose, honey, maple syrup, and concentrated fruit juices. Added sugars have been associated with a higher risk of CHD, diabetes, and overweight or obesity. The Dietary Guidelines 2020–2025 recommend that individuals minimize the intake of added sugars, and the Food and Drug Administration (FDA) has included added sugars on food labels with the recommendation to consume no more than 10% of calories from added sugars.

Low-calorie sweeteners have been suggested as an alternative for sugar-sweetened products. However, the research on potential health benefits from these products is mixed.

- Chose and Prepare Foods with Little or No Salt

  As indicated previously in this chapter, there is a positive relationship between salt (sodium chloride) and blood pressure. A number of studies have shown that reduced sodium intake is associated with decreased risk of age-related elevation of systolic blood pressure and diastolic blood pressure.

  In general, sodium restriction in Black individuals, middle-aged and older-aged people, and individuals with hypertension yields the most significant benefits. One suggestion that has been made includes the replacement of regular salt with potassium-rich salts, particularly during food preparation.

- Limit Alcohol Consumption

  Both the DGA 2020–2025 and the 2021 Dietary Guidelines from the AHA recommend limiting alcohol consumption and make the further recommendation that individuals who do not drink alcohol should not start. The 2020–2025 DGAs concluded that those who drink alcohol should consume no more than one alcoholic drink per day for women and no more than two drinks per day for men.

- Follow Heart-Healthy Guidelines When Eating Away from Home or Anyplace Where Food Is Prepared

  The recommendations listed earlier should also apply irrespective of where food is prepared or consumed.

12.5 ADDITIONAL BENEFITS OF HEART-HEALTHY DIETARY PATTERNS

There are multiple benefits from heart-healthy dietary patterns in addition to lowering the risk of CVD and CHD. A heart-healthy diet pattern is rich in fiber and will fulfill essential nutrient requirements for most individuals. Healthy diets are also low in saturated fat, trans fat, cholesterol, added sugar, and salt. These may yield benefits including decreased risk of both diabetes and overweight or obesity. There is also emerging evidence that healthy dietary patterns are linked to better cognitive abilities and slower decline with advancing years. The Mediterranean diet was associated with slower decline of cognitive status. The Mediterranean-DASH Intervention for Neurodegenerative Delay (MIND) study is also associated with slower rates of age-related cognitive decline [34].

In addition to the health benefits already discussed, the dietary heart-healthy patterns discussed in this chapter such as DASH, Mediterranean, or Healthy U.S.-Style and healthy vegetarian patterns are also associated with a similar impact compared to the average U.S. diet. In addition, current food systems that favor animal-based food production have been shown to substantially increase human-generated greenhouse gas emissions and water and land usage.

12.6 STRATEGIES FOR IMPLEMENTING AND ADHERING TO HEART-HEALTHY DIETARY PATTERNS

The AHA has indicated that implementing heart-healthy diets is a priority [35]. This reflects the concern that despite enormous information about the health benefits of heart-healthy diets, a distinct minority of consumers follow them. A number of challenges exist in the environment which make it more difficult to adhere to heart-healthy dietary patterns. For example, enormous misinformation exists in the nutrition arena and even among public and healthcare professionals. Furthermore, there is scant attention to nutrition within not only educational curricula for K–12, but even medical schools have not devoted substantial energy to nutrition education [36]. These factors need to be corrected.

In addition, there are, in the current environment, disparities in dietary quality by income, race, ethnicity, and education. One particularly difficult problem is that of food insecurity. It has been estimated that 37 million Americans have limited or uncertain access to safe and nutritious food [37]. A disproportionate number of these individuals are Black or Hispanic.

Inequities of healthcare in general, and nutrition in particular, have been an issue addressed in the 2030 AHA Strategic Goals [38]. It is important that physicians, in general, and cardiologists, in particular, recognize the importance of addressing inequities particularly in the area of nutrition. This problem is compounded by marketing that targets particularly Black and Hispanic children emphasizing processed foods and beverages. Even online shopping, which was initially thought to be an opportunity for reducing disparities, may have actually resulted in the opposite, particularly with shoppers from low-income or underrepresented groups.

12.7 COMBINATION WITH OTHER HEART-HEALTHY LIFESTYLE HABITS

All of the major recommendations from the AHA, DGA 2020–2025, and the Academy of Nutrition and Dietetics emphasize that sound nutrition should be advocated in the context of other heart-healthy habits such as regular physical activity, weight management, stress reduction, and proper sleep. These are all cornerstones of lifestyle medicine and should be emphasized by all practitioners, in addition to the heart-healthy guidance contained in this chapter.

12.8 FUTURE DIRECTIONS

Both the National Institutes of Health and the 2030 Strategic Plan from AHA emphasize that new tools have become available that may allow a more precise way of advocating nutrition for individuals throughout the life course and recognizing individual differences. This area has been deemed "precision" nutrition and has great potential for the future to harness big data, bioinformatics, and information of behavioral sciences [39].

12.9 CONCLUSIONS

The core tenets of heart-healthy nutrition have been shared by the DGA 2020–2025 and the 2021 Dietary Guidelines to Improve Cardiovascular Health from the AHA. These guidelines include adjusting energy intake and expenditure to achieve a healthy body weight, consuming plenty of fruits and vegetables, increasing the amount of whole grain in the diet, selecting healthy sources of proteins (mostly plants), increasing intake of fish and seafood and low-fat dairy products, choosing liquid plant oils rather than tropical oils, choosing minimally processed foods instead of ultra-processed foods, minimizing the intake of beverages and foods with added sugars and salt, either abstaining from alcohol or consuming moderate amounts, and following this heart-healthy guidance wherever food is consumed. All of these recommendations can contribute to following a heart-healthy diet. In addition, the environment should be taken into consideration to attempt to reduce currently existing challenges to following a heart-healthy diet.

Clinical Applications

- Clinicians should address nutritional factors in every patient encounter.
- Heart-healthy guidelines include the following:
    - Adjusting energy intake and expenditure to achieve a healthy body weight.
    - Consume plenty and a variety of fruits and vegetables.
    - Consume more whole grains.
    - Choose healthy sources of protein (mostly plants but also fish and seafood) and low-fat dairy products.
    - Choose liquid plant oils rather than tropical oils.
    - Chose minimally processed foods rather than ultra-processed foods.
    - Minimize the intake of beverages and foods with added sugars.
    - Choose and prepare foods with little or no salt.
    - If consuming alcohol, do so in moderation.
- Follow these guidelines wherever food is prepared and consumed.

REFERENCES

1. American Heart Association. Heart and Stroke Statistics. www.heart.org/en/about-us/heart-and-stroke-association-statistics (Accessed January 23, 2024).
2. Rippe J. Lifestyle strategies for risk reduction, prevention and treatment of cardiovascular disease. Am J Lifestyle Med. 2018;13(2).
3. Lichtenstein A, Appel L, Vadiveloo M, et al. 2021 dietary guidance to improve cardiovascular health: A scientific statement from the American Heart Association. Circulation. 2021;144(23):e472–e487.
4. Nurses' Health Study. https://nurseshealthstudy.org/ (Accessed January 23, 2024).
5. Steering Committee of the Physicians' Health Study Research Group. Final report on the aspirin component of the ongoing physicians' health study. N Engl J Med. 1989;20; 321(3):129–135.
6. Ford E, Ajani U, Croft J, et al. Explaining the decrease in U.S. deaths from coronary disease, 1980–2000. N Engl J Med. 2007;356(23):2388–2398.

7. The Global Burden of Disease; World Health Organization. The Global Burden of Disease: 2004 Update. Geneva. 2008.
8. Omran A. The epidemiologic transition: A theory of the epidemiology of population change. 1971. Milbank Q. 2005;83(4):731–757.
9. U.S. Department of Agriculture and U.S. Department of Health and Human Services. *Dietary Guidelines for Americans, 2020–2025*, 9th edition. December 2020. DietaryGuidelines.gov. 2020; www.dietaryguidelines.gov/resources/2020-2025-dietary-guidelines-online-materials
10. Becker P, Nieman Carney L, Corkins M, et al. Consensus statement of the academy of nutrition and dietetics/American society for parenteral and enteral nutrition: Indicators recommended for the identification and documentation of pediatric malnutrition (undernutrition). J Acad Nutr Diet. 2014;114(12):1988–2000.
11. Eckel RH, Jakicic JM, Ard JD, de Jesus JM, Houston Miller N, Hubbard VS, et al. 2013 AHA/ACC guideline on lifestyle management to reduce cardiovascular risk: A report of the American College of Cardiology/American Heart Association task force on practice guidelines. J Am Coll Cardiol. 2014;63(25 Pt B):2960–2984. Epub 2013/11/19.
12. Grundy SM, Stone NJ, Bailey AL, Beam C, Birtcher KK, Blumenthal RS, et al. 2018 AHA/ACC/AACVPR/AAPA/ABC/ACPM/ADA/AGS/APhA/ASPC/NLA/PCNA guideline on the management of blood cholesterol: A report of the American College of Cardiology/American Heart Association task force on clinical practice guidelines. Circulation. 2019;139(25):e1082–e1143.
13. Whelton PK, Carey RM, Aronow WS, Casey DE, Collins KJ, Dennison Himmelfarb C, et al. 2017 ACC/AHA/AAPA/ABC/ACPM/AGS/APhA/ASH/ASPC/NMA/PCNA guideline for the prevention, detection, evaluation, and management of high blood pressure in adults: Executive summary. Hypertension. 2018;71:e13–e115.
14. American Heart Association Strategic Plan. www.heart.org/ (Accessed January 23, 2024).
15. Tangney C, Li H, Wang Y, et al. Relation of DASH-and Mediterranean-like dietary patterns to cognitive decline in older persons. Neurology. 2014;83(16):1410–1416.
16. Estruch R, Ros E, Salas-Salvado J, et al. Primary prevention of cardiovascular disease with a Mediterranean diet. N Engl J Med. 2013;368(14):1279–1290.
17. Perk J, de Backer G, Gohlke H, et al. European guidelines on cardiovascular disease prevention in clinical practice (version 2012): The fifth joint task force of the European society of cardiology and other societies on cardiovascular disease prevention in clinical practice (constituted by representatives of nine societies and by invited experts). Eur Heart J. 2012;33:1635–1701.
18. Hooper L, Summerbell C, Thompson R, et al. Reduced or modified dietary fat for preventing cardiovascular disease. Cochrane Database Syst Rev. 2012;16;2012(5):CD00213.7.
19. Nordmann A, Nordmann A, Briel M, et al. Effects of low-carbohydrate vs. low-fat diets on weight loss and cardiovascular risk factors: A meta-analysis of randomized controlled trials. Arch Intern Med. 2006;166:285–293.
20. Santos F, Esteves S, da Costa Pereira A, et al. Systematic review and meta-analysis of clinical trials of the effects of low carbohydrate diets on cardiovascular risk factors. Obes Rev. 2012;13:1048–1066.
21. Vardavas C, Linardakis M, Hatzis C, et al. Cardiovascular disease risk factors and dietary habits of farmers from Crete 45 years after the first description of the Mediterranean diet. Eur J Cardiovasc Prev Rehabil. 2010;17:440–446.
22. Sofi F, Abbate R, Gensini G, et al. Accruing evidence about benefits of adherence to the Mediterranean diet on health: An updated systematic review and meta-analysis. Am J Clin Nutr. 2010;92:1189–1196.

23. Appel L, Champagne C, Harsha D, et al. Effects of comprehensive lifestyle modification on blood pressure control: Main results of the premier clinical trial. JAMA. 2003;289:2083–2093.
24. Blumenthal J, Babyak M, Hinderliter A, et al. Effects of the DASH diet alone and in combination with exercise and weight loss on blood pressure and cardiovascular biomarkers in men and women with high blood pressure: The ENCORE study. Arch Intern Med. 2010;25;170(2):126–135.
25. Hakala P, Karvetti R. Weight reduction on lactovegetarian and mixed diets: Changes in weight, nutrient intake, skinfold thicknesses and blood pressure. Eur J Clin Nutr. 1989;43:421–430.
26. Barnard N, Cohen J, Jenkins D, et al. A low-fat vegan diet and a conventional diabetes diet in the treatment of type 2 diabetes: A randomized, controlled, 74-wk clinical trial. Am J Clin Nutr. 2009;89:1588S–1596S.
27. Burke L, Styn M, Steenkiste A, et al. A randomized clinical trial testing treatment preference and two dietary options in behavioral weight management: Preliminary results of the impact of diet at 6 months: PREFER Study. Obesity (Silver Spring). 2006;14:2007–2017.
28. Burke L, Hudson A, Warziski M, et al. Effects of a vegetarian diet and treatment preference on biochemical and dietary variables in overweight and obese adults: A randomized clinical trial. Am J Clin Nutr. 2007;86:588–596.
29. Willcox D, Willcox B, Todoriki H, et al. The okinawan diet: Health implications of a low-calorie, nutrient-dense, antioxidant-rich dietary pattern low in glycemic load. J Am Coll Nutr. 2009;28(Suppl):500S–516S.
30. Shimazu T, Kuriyama S, Hozawa A, et al. Dietary patterns and cardiovascular disease mortality in Japan: A prospective cohort study. Int J Epidemiol. 2007;36:600–609.
31. Heidemann C, Schulze M, Franco O, et al. Dietary patterns and risk of mortality from cardiovascular disease, cancer, and all causes in a prospective cohort of women. Circulation. 2008;15;118(3):230–237.
32. Greger M. Plant-based diets for the prevention and treatment of disabling diseases. Am J Lifestyle Med. 2015;(9):336–342.
33. Satija A, Bhupathiraju S, Spiegelman D, et al. Healthful and unhealthful plant-based diets and the risk of coronary heart disease in U.S. adults. J Am Coll Cardiol. 2017;25;70(4):411–422.
34. Liu X, Morris M, Dhana K, et al. Mediterranean-DASH Intervention for Neurodegenerative Delay (MIND) study: Rationale, design and baseline characteristics of a randomized control trial of the MIND diet on cognitive decline. Contemp Clin Trials. 2021;102:106270.
35. Gidding S, Lichtenstein A, Faith M, et al. Implementing American Heart Association pediatric and adult nutrition guidelines: A scientific statement from the American Heart Association nutrition committee of the council on nutrition, physical activity and metabolism, council on cardiovascular disease in the young, council on arteriosclerosis, thrombosis and vascular biology, council on cardiovascular nursing, council on epidemiology and prevention, and council for high blood pressure research. Circulation. 2009;119(8):1161–1175.
36. Aggarwal M, Singh Ospina N, Kazory A, et al. The mismatch of nutrition and lifestyle beliefs and actions among physicians: A wake-up call. Am J Lifestyle Med. 2020;14(3):304–315.

37. Feeding American website. www.feedamerica.org (Accessed January 23, 2024).
38. Angell SY, McConnell MV, Anderson CAM, et al. The American Heart Association 2030 impact goal: A presidential advisory from the American Heart Association. Circulation. 2020;141(9):e120–e138.
39. Leopold J, Loscalzo J. Emerging role of precision medicine in cardiovascular disease. Circ Res. 2018;122(9):1302–1315.

13 Nutrition and Hypertension

Key Points

- Hypertension is extremely common in the United States, with between 47% and 49% of individuals having elevated blood pressure or actual hypertension according to recent guidelines.
- Multiple dietary factors play a significant role in lowering blood pressure including weight loss, reduced salt intake, increased potassium intake, and moderation of alcohol intake.
- Several healthy dietary patterns have been shown to lower the risk of high blood pressure. These include the Dietary Approach to Stop Hypertension (DASH) diet, vegetarian diets, and the Mediterranean diet.
- Other factors that impact positively on blood pressure include physical activity, not smoking cigarettes, and weight control. However, healthy dietary patterns remain the cornerstone for blood pressure control.

13.1 INTRODUCTION

Hypertension is extremely common in the United States [1–4]. While multiple different definitions of hypertension have been utilized over the years, recently, based on findings from the Systolic Blood Pressure Intervention Trial (SPRINT) [5], the American Heart Association (AHA) and the Centers for Disease Control and Prevention together have adopted criteria that normal blood pressure (BP) is less than 120 mm/Hg systolic and less than 80 mm/Hg diastolic. Specific numbers related to these most recent guidelines will be spelled out in the next section.

While multiple factors contribute to hypertension, nutrition is perhaps the most critical underlying risk factor. Healthy nutritional practices have been shown to significantly lower the risk of blood pressure and help in its control [6,7]. Conversely, unhealthy nutritional practices contribute significantly to elevated blood pressure. Other lifestyle habits and practices including level of physical activity, weight control, alcohol consumption, and avoidance of tobacco products all contribute to lowering the risk of developing hypertension or assisting in its control. While all of these factors play roles and will be discussed briefly in this chapter, the main focus will be on the relationship between nutrition and hypertension.

13.2 DEFINITION OF HYPERTENSION

The most recent guidelines from the AHA [1] and Centers for Disease Control and Prevention (CDC) [2] define a normal systolic blood pressure of less than 120 mm/Hg

DOI: 10.1201/9781003452607-13

BP classification	SBP	DBP	Lifestyle habits	Drug treatment
Normal BP	<120 mmHg	<80 mmHg	Promote	None
Elevated BP	120–129 mmHg	<80 mmHg	Yes	None
Stage 1 hypertension	130–139 mmHg	80–89 mmHg	Yes	May be Indicated*
Stage 2 hypertension	>=140 mmHg	>=90 mmHg	Yes	Indicated*

FIGURE 13.1 Categories of blood pressure in adults.

Source: Adapted from 2017ACC/AHA Categories of BP in Adults.

and a diastolic blood pressure of less than 80 mm/Hg. The complete guidelines for normal, elevated, and stage 1 and stage 2 hypertension are found in Figure 13.1.

There are several reasons for utilizing these criteria. First, the SPRINT trial showed that individuals who have a systolic pressure of >120 mg Hg significantly increase their risk of symptomatic heart disease. These criteria are also consistent with the widely accepted Joint National Committee on Prevention, Detection and Treatment of High Blood Pressure (JNC-7) [4]. JNC-7 reported that the risk of CVD increases beginning at 115/75 mm/Hg. The risk of CVD doubles with each increment of 20 mm/Hg systolic or 10 mm/Hg diastolic.

It should be noted that to achieve the levels of less than 120 mm/Hg and less than 80 mm/Hg, the SPRINT Trial required the use of three antihypertensive medications. This raises issues about whether or not individuals would be willing to adhere to regimens that require this level of medication outside of a research setting. This adds further impetus to the need for adopting positive lifestyle factors to lower the risk of developing hypertension or controlling it.

Indeed, JNC-7 recommended that individuals with systolic blood pressure of 120–139 mm/Hg or diastolic blood pressure of 80–89 mm/Hg be counseled to engage in health-promoting lifestyle modifications such as healthy nutrition and regular physical activity to lower their risk of CVD [4].

13.3 PREVALENCE OF HYPERTENSION IN THE UNITED STATES

Utilizing the criteria outlined in the previous section, the CDC estimates that between 47% and 49% of adults in the United States have hypertension, defined as systolic blood pressure >130 mm/Hg or diastolic blood pressure > 80 mm/Hg or taking medicine for hypertension [2].

In 2020, more than 670,000 deaths in the United States listed hypertension as a primary or contributing cause [8]. Only about one in four adults without hypertension have their condition under control [9]. About 34 million adults are recommended to take medication for hypertension [9]. Recent data have suggested that only 39% of these individuals have their blood pressure under control. Indeed, almost two out of three people in this group have a blood pressure of 140/90 mm/Hg or higher. About half of adults (about 45%) with uncontrolled hypertension have a blood pressure of 140/90 mm/Hg or higher [9]. A greater percentage of men (50%) have high blood pressure than women (44%). High blood pressure is more common in non-Hispanic Black males (56%) than in non-Hispanic white adults (48%), non-Hispanic Asian adults (46%), or Hispanic adults (39%) [9].

It has been estimated that adults who are normotensive at the age of 50 have a lifetime risk of developing hypertension of greater than 90% [10]. Blood pressure is a consistent and strong risk factor for both CVD and renal disease. It should also be noted, however, that almost one-third of blood pressure–related deaths from coronary heart disease (CHD) occur in individuals who have a blood pressure in the nonhypertensive range.

13.4 GUIDANCE FOR MANAGING HYPERTENSION

Multiple lifestyle factors play a significant role in managing high blood pressure. In fact, the JNC-7 Guidelines for managing high blood pressure include the following recommendations [4]:

- Consuming a diet high in fruits and vegetables, whole grains, and including low-fat dairy products, poultry, fish, legumes, and nontropical nuts while eliminating sweets, sugar-sweetened beverages, and red meat.
- Consuming no more than more than 2,300 milligrams of sodium per day.
- Engaging in regular aerobic activity three to four sessions per week lasting an average of 40 minutes per session of moderate- to vigorous-intensive physical activity. (Consistent with the Physical Activity Guidelines for Americans 2018 recommendations of 150 minutes of moderate intensity physical activity per week.)

Unfortunately, despite the fact that lifestyle factors play a very important role in lowering the risk of hypertension and its treatment, pharmaceutical therapy remains a mainstay for many individuals while lifestyle factors may be largely ignored. Even in nonhypertensive individuals, dietary changes that lower blood pressure have the potential to prevent hypertension and work broadly to reduce BP and thereby lower the risk of BP-related clinical complications.

Dietary changes can serve as initial treatment before the start of drug therapy. Even among hypertensive individuals who are already on drug therapy, dietary changes, particularly reducing salt intake, can further lower BP and facilitate a reduction in medication.

13.5 DIETARY FACTORS THAT LOWER BLOOD PRESSURE

- Weight Management
  The association between obesity and hypertension is well established through multiple trials. The reduction of body weight of 5–10 kg in overweight individuals is shown to be a highly effective way of reducing BP, with reductions of 6–12 mm/Hg systolic and 5–8 mm/Hg diastolic [11–14].

The combination of caloric reduction as well as increased physical activity are both important components of weight loss and weight management. The combination of these two components, namely exercise and caloric reduction when utilized together, results in greater blood pressure reduction than individual strategies alone.

For these reasons, the AHA recommends that overweight adults with hypertension be counseled to begin lifestyle changes in the areas of caloric reduction and physical activity to achieve a sustained weight loss of 2–5% to achieve clinically meaningful health benefits, including blood pressure reduction [1].

Intervention trials that include components of these lifestyle medicine modalities such as the PREMIER [15] and the ENCORE [16] (Exercise and Nutrition Interventions for Cardiovascular Health) study both recorded significant reductions in blood pressure of 11–16 mm/Hg and 6–10 mm/Hg systolic and diastolic pressure, respectively. Both physical activity and weight loss are independently important lifestyle measures for reduction in the overall risk of CVD.

Some trials have documented that modest weight loss, with or without sodium reduction, can prevent hypertension in about 20% of overweight, pre-hypertensive individuals and can also facilitate medication step-down or drug withdrawal [17]. While increased physical activity by itself is unlikely to achieve significant weight loss, long-term maintenance of physical activity has been clearly recognized as a critical factor in maintaining weight loss [18]. In addition, healthy nutrition and physical activity are also important for individuals who are normal body weight to prevent weight gain.

- Reduce Salt Intake

  Considerable evidence exists that when dietary salt (sodium chloride) intake rises, so does BP [19]. Three trials that tested three different sodium levels all showed statistically significant direct progressive dose-response relationships from reduction of salt [20–22]. The largest of the dose response trials, the DASH Diet, Sodium Intake and Blood Pressure Trial (DASH-Sodium), showed significant reduction in blood pressure, with the greatest reductions in the arm that reduced sodium consumption to 1,500 mg per day [23,24].

  Clinical trials have also shown reduced sodium intake can prevent hypertension and can also lower BP in the setting of antihypertensive medication, as well as facilitating hypertension control. Reduced salt intake is also associated with reduced incidence of CVD and congestive heart failure.

  The effects of sodium reduction on BP tend to be greater in African Americans, middle age and older persons, and individuals who already have hypertension, diabetes, or chronic kidney disease [25]. It should be noted that some salt intake is required to maintain blood pressure, although the National Academy of Science Committee set 1,500 mg per day of sodium as an adequate level to ensure nutrient adequacy [26].

  To reduce salt intake, consumers should choose foods lower in salt and lower the amount of salt added to food. Since greater than 75% of consumed salt comes from processed foods, any meaningful strategy to reduce salt intake must involve reduction in processed foods. Many manufacturers are trying to reduce the amount of salt in their products.

- Increased Potassium Intake
  High potassium intake is associated with reduced BP both in non-hypertensive and hypertensive individuals [27–29]. Potassium reduces BP to a greater extent in African Americans than in Caucasians. Increased potassium consumption is another reason to consume a diet high in fruits and vegetables, which represents another reason to consume fruits and vegetables rather than processed foods.

  Increased intake of potassium has a greater BP lowering in the context of higher salt intake and lesser reduction in the setting of lower salt intake. Most research suggests that a recommended potassium intake of 4.7 g/day is reasonable for modest lowering of blood pressure [28]. In an otherwise healthy population with normal kidney function, potassium intake of foods will achieve this level without any risk since excess potassium is readily excreted in the urine. If potassium excretion is impaired, intake should be lower than 4.7 grams per day to avoid adverse cardiac events such as arrhythmias, which may occur in the setting of hyperkalemia. Some drugs that may impair potassium excretion include angiotensin-converting enzyme (ACE) inhibitors, angiotensin receptor blockers, and nonsteroidal anti-inflammatory agents as well as potassium-sparing diuretics.
- Moderation of Alcohol Intake
  There is a direct dose-dependent relationship between alcohol intake and BP, particularly if the intake of alcohol increases above greater than two drinks per day [30,31]. Some studies have also suggested that the relationship between alcohol consumption and hypertension may even extend to the light drinking range (fewer than or equal to two drinks per day), although this is the range at which alcohol may reduce CHD risk. Available research supports that moderate alcohol intake among those who drink is an effective approach to lowering BP. As indicated in other chapters in this book, alcohol consumption should be limited to less than or equal to two alcoholic drinks per day for most men and less than or equal to one alcoholic drink per day for women. One drink is defined as 12 ounces of regular beer, 5 ounces of wine (12% alcohol), or 1 ounce of 80 proof distilled spirits.
- Whole Dietary Patterns
  As indicated in multiple chapters in this book, modern nutrition research focuses on whole dietary patterns that have been shown to result in lower blood pressure [32,33]. These dietary patterns include vegetarian diets, the DASH diet, and related healthy dietary patterns such as the Mediterranean diet or the Healthy U.S.-Style Dietary. In the OmniHeart Trial (Optimal Macronutrient Intake Trial) [34] for heart health, three healthy dietary patterns were studied, including a diet rich in carbohydrates (58% of total calories), a diet rich in protein (about half from plant sources), and a diet rich in unsaturated fat (predominantly monounsaturated fat). Just as in the DASH diet,

the OmniHeart Trial diet reduced saturated fat and cholesterol and contained abundant fruit, vegetables, fiber, potassium, and other minerals at recommended levels [35]. The results showed that either substituting some of the carbohydrates with protein (about half from plant sources) or unsaturated fat (mostly from monounsaturated fat) lowered blood pressure.

It should be noted that the DASH diet has also been shown to lower indices of inflammation, which represents another reason to consume a diet high in fruits and vegetables and whole grains (issues related to inflammation are discussed in detail in Chapter 9).

13.6 DIETARY FACTORS WITH LIMITED OR UNCERTAIN EFFECT ON BLOOD PRESSURE

A number of other dietary factors have either limited or uncertain effect on BP. They include the following:

- Fish Oil Supplementation
  Several small trials have documented high-dose omega-3 polyunsaturated fatty acid (typically found in fish oil) supplements can lower BP in hypertensive individuals [36–38]. In hypertensive individuals, average systolic and diastolic BP reductions were lowered 4.0 and 2.0 mm/Hg, respectively. There are some side effects, including belching and a fishy taste, that commonly occur. Fish oil supplements are not routinely recommended as a means to lower blood pressure.
- Fiber
  There are several clinical trials suggesting that increased fiber intake may reduce BP. Reductions in BP are very modest in the studies that have specifically looked at fiber, with reductions in both systolic and diastolic BP of 1.6 and 2.0 mm/Hg, respectively [39–41]. Thus, data are insufficient to recommend increased fiber alone as a means to lower BP. Increased fiber consumption, however, has been clearly shown to reduce the risk of CVD, which provides a reason to increase fiber in the diet.
- Calcium and Magnesium
  Several small studies suggest that calcium intake might possibly affect BP. However, the effect is very modest, with systolic and diastolic BP reductions of 0.9–1.4 mm/Hg and 0.2–0.8 mm/Hg, respectively [42–44]. There are, of course, other reasons to increase calcium intake for bone health (see Chapter 23 on osteoporosis).

  The use of magnesium as a determinant of BP is inconsistent, and data are insufficient to recommend supplementation for magnesium as a means to lower BP [45].
- Carbohydrate
  Some evidence suggests that the amount and type of carbohydrate intake may affect BP [46]. Speculation results from findings in countries where people eat largely plant-based, low-fat diets have lower BP compared to

Western countries. The OmniHeart Trial suggests that replacing some carbohydrate with protein or monounsaturated fat may result in further BP reduction.

Some studies have shown that sugar consumption may increase BP [47,48]. The current research status of carbohydrate and BP is insufficient to make specific a recommendation on the amount or type of carbohydrate to lower BP.

- Omega-3 Polyunsaturated Fatty Acids
  Fatty fish and oil are rich in long-chain omega-3 polyunsaturated fats and may play a role in blood pressure regulation via the production of eicosanoids and prostaglandins. There are small studies of supplements of polyunsaturated fats which are associated with relatively small reductions in BP (2.3–4.0 mm/Hg systolic and 2.2–2.5 mm/Hg diastolic pressure) [49–52]. This is the basis of recommending two or more fatty fish meals per week for cardio-protective effects as well as their potential effect of lowering the risk of arrhythmias.
- Saturated Fat
  The few available trials that focused only on reducing saturated fat had no significant effect on BP [53,54]. There are other reasons for lowering saturated fat, which is a recommendation of virtually all of the heart-healthy diets.
- Omega-6 Polyunsaturated Fat Intake
  Dietary intake of omega-6 polyunsaturated fat (mainly linoleic acid in Western diets) has little effect on BP.
- Monounsaturated Fat Intake
  There are few available studies of monounsaturated fat in isolation and its effect on BP. The OmniHeart Trial did suggest that partial substitute of carbohydrate with monounsaturated fat lowered BP; however, this was coupled with concomitant reduction of carbohydrate intake [53,54]. The Mediterranean diet also has a significant component of monounsaturated fat; however, the monounsaturated fat intake itself on BP is uncertain.
- Protein Intake
  A number of studies have suggested a significant inverse association between protein intake and BP [54,55]. The International Collaborative Study of Macronutrients, Micronutrients and Blood Pressure (INTERMAP) showed that protein from plant sources was associated with lower BP, while protein from animal sources had no effect [55,56]. Typical research designs in this area substitute soy protein for some carbohydrates. This may potentially confound the effects of protein due to the reduction of carbohydrates.
- Cholesterol
  The Multiple Risk Factor Intervention Trial (MRFIT) study shows that there was a significant direct relationship between cholesterol intake and both systolic and diastolic BP [57]. There still are not adequate studies to demonstrate the relationship between dietary cholesterol and BP.

- Vitamin C
  Some data suggest that vitamin C intake is associated with lower BP, although the data in this area are mixed, plus it is unclear whether or not intake of vitamin C reduces BP [58].

13.7 GENE-DIET INTERVENTIONS

There is some evidence that genetic factors affect BP levels as well as BP response to dietary changes. Most of this research focuses on BP response to salt intake [59].

13.8 EFFECTS OF MULTIPLE DIETARY CHANGES

A number of different types of interventions have been recommended to help in the reduction of blood pressure. In one study, the combination of a healthy DASH-based diet, increased physical activity, and weight loss—The Diet, Exercise, and Weight Loss Intervention Trial (The DEW-IT Trial)—both systolic and diastolic blood pressures were decreased by 12.1 and 6.6 mm/Hg, respectively. A subsequent trial named PREMIER explored weight loss, sodium reduction, and increased physical activity in the DASH diet. Hypertensive patients who were not on medication showed systolic and diastolic blood pressure reductions of 14.2 and 7.4 mm/Hg, respectively [59]. In nonhypertensive individuals, corresponding BP reductions were 9.2 and 5.8 mm/Hg, respectively.

13.9 NUTRITION AND OTHER VASCULAR CONDITIONS

Healthy nutrition plays a significant role in multiple other vascular conditions which are based on systemic atherosclerosis. These include chronic kidney disease, peripheral artery disease, stroke, and erectile dysfunction. These conditions are handled in separate chapters in this book.

13.10 OTHER LIFESTYLE HABITS AND ACTIONS AND BP

While this chapter has focused on healthy nutrition and its role in reducing the risk of high blood pressure and helping in its control, multiple other lifestyle habits and actions also play prominent roles in helping to control blood pressure. These include regular physical activity, not smoking, and weight control or weight loss in individuals who are overweight or obese. As already indicated, trials that have employed multiple lifestyle habits and actions in controlling blood pressure have shown significant reductions in both systolic and diastolic blood pressure, suggesting that lifestyle interventions may be synergistic for BP control [15].

13.11 BEHAVIORAL INTERVENTIONS TO ACCOMPLISH LIFESTYLE MODIFICATIONS TO CONTROL BLOOD PRESSURE

Multiple behavioral intervention trials have tested effects on dietary change on BP [59,60]. The application of various behavioral modification strategies is beyond the scope of this chapter; however, a detailed description of these various techniques may be found in numerous reviews. It should be noted that the effects of behavioral change have typically been rather modest, which suggests that changes in the environment, in addition to behavioral theories, play a very significant role. It should be noted, however, that behavioral components involving dietary change such as the DASH diet, DASH sodium trial, and Mediterranean diet have all been shown to substantially improve blood pressure control and reduce the likelihood of developing high blood pressure in the first place [61]. Certainly, changes in nutrition as well as other lifestyle behaviors play an important role in BP control and are recommended by all significant national guidelines.

13.12 COMPLEMENTARY THERAPIES

Various complementary therapies have been suggested to play a role in the management of high blood pressure and lifestyle modification. Such therapies as stress reduction, various types of music, deep breathing exercises, mind/body therapy, and yoga have had some significant but small effects on blood pressure management.

13.13 SPECIAL POPULATIONS

- Children

  Recent research has suggested that elevated blood pressure may begin in the first two decades of life and perhaps even in utero [62]. Elevated BP levels, particularly in the presence of obesity in children and adolescents aged 8–17 years old, have increased over the past 20 years. Approximately 3–4% of children are hypertensive. Elevated BP in childhood is an accepted risk factor for elevated BP in adulthood, which in turn, is a major risk factor for multiple aspects of CVD [63–65].

  In 2017, the American Academy of Pediatrics issued a "Clinical Practice Guideline for Screening and Management of High Blood Pressure in Children and Adolescents" [66]. Among the recommendations are that children and adolescents should have blood pressure measurement assessed at every health maintenance visit. Furthermore, children and adolescents are recommended to be treated first with increased physical activity and a DASH-type diet as well as reduction in dietary sodium.
- Older Persons

  The age-related rise in blood pressure has been well documented. As already indicated, even individuals who are normotensive at age 50 have a 90% chance of developing hypertension before they die. The basic nutritional recommendations for all adults including dietary changes (following a healthy diet with abundant fruits and vegetables and whole grains), as well as weight loss if necessary, and dietary sodium reduction are also appropriate for individuals over the age of 65 [67,68].

- African Americans
  On average, African Americans have higher BP and are at greater risk for BP complications than Caucasians or Hispanics [69,70]. The good news is that African Americans can achieve greater BP reduction from sodium reduction, increased potassium intake, and the DASH diet than Caucasians. These are particularly appropriate because some data suggest that African Americans consume high levels of sodium, and their potassium intake is less than non-Blacks. Thus, dietary change could make a major impact on reducing elevated BP in African Americans.

13.14 THE ROLE OF PHYSICIANS IN BP CONTROL

Numerous studies have shown that physician recommendation is the single most powerful tool for behavior change. This applies to many of the recommendations made in this chapter. Unfortunately, as already indicated in Chapter 1, a distinct minority of physicians are skilled in nutrition counseling; however, this is essential to lower the risk of elevated BP and assist in its treatment. Physicians should check BP at every clinical visit and make recommendations such as those contained in this chapter to follow healthy dietary practices, reduce sodium, and weight loss, if necessary, as well as increasing potassium and avoiding tobacco products.

13.15 CONCLUSIONS

This chapter has focused largely on healthy nutrition for blood pressure control. Multiple lifestyle interventions are highly effective in lowering the risk of developing high blood pressure and playing important roles in its therapy. Hypertension remains the most prevalent and easily recognizable risk factors for CVD and is particularly prominent as a risk factor for stroke. For all of these reasons, nutritional therapy and other lifestyle therapies are important components of counseling for blood pressure control. Figure 13.2 summarizes the appropriate lifestyle modifications for reduction in the risk management of hypertension with a particular focus on healthy nutrition.

Clinical Applications

- High blood pressure is a significant and common risk factor for CVD.
- Recent guidelines for blood pressure control have emphasized that even small increases in blood pressure above 115 mm/Hg systolic and 75 mm/Hg diastolic significantly increased the risk of CVD.
- Multiple lifestyle interventions such as healthy nutrition (particularly with salt reduction), regular physical activity, weight management (if needed), and smoking cessation can all profoundly affect the likelihood of developing high blood pressure and assist in its treatment (Figure 13.2).

Modification	Recommendation	Blood pressure reduction
Weight reduction	Maintain a BMI between 18.5 and 24.9	5–20 mm Hg per 10 kg weight loss
Healthy diet	Consume a diet rich in fruits, vegetables, and whole grains; moderate in fat-free or low-fat dairy products; reduced saturated fat and cholesterol such as the DASH dietary pattern	8–14 mm Hg
Exercise	Regular aerobic exercise 120–150 min/week; Or 60–90 min/daily for weight reduction and maintenance; Dynamic resistance exercise 90–150 min/week; Isometric resistance exercise 3 sessions/week	4–9 mm Hg
Reduced sodium/salt intake	Lower salt intake as much as possible (1.5 g/d of sodium or 3.8 g/d of sodium chloride) or at least 1000 mg reduction in current intake	2–8 mm Hg
Limit alcohol consumption	No more than two drinks/day for men; No more than one drink/day for women	2–4 mm Hg
Increase potassium	Increase intake to 3500–5000 mg/day (level of DASH diet); Content from fruits, vegetables, and low-fat dairy products	2–5 mm Hg

FIGURE 13.2 Clinical applications/lifestyle modifications for management of hypertension.

Sources: Adapted from Chobanian AV, Bakris GL, Black HR, et al. The seventh report of the joint national committee on prevention, detection, evaluation, and treatment of high blood pressure: The JNC 7 report. JAMA. 2003;289:2560–2572.

Whelton PK, Carey RM, Aronow WS, et al. 2017 ACC/AHA/AAPA/ABC/ACPM/AGS/APhA/ASH/ASPC/NMA/PCNA guideline for the prevention, detection, evaluation and management of high blood pressure in adults: Executive summary: A report of the American College of Cardiology/American Heart Association Task Force on Clinical Practice Guidelines. Hypertension 2017.

Appel LJ, Brands MW, Daniels SR, et al. Dietary approaches to prevent and treat hypertension: A scientific statement from the American Heart Association. Hypertension. 2006;47:296–308.

REFERENCES

1. Whelton P, Carey R, Aronow W, et al. 2017 ACC/AHA/AAPA/ABC/ACPM/AGS/APhA/ASH/ASPC/NMA/PCNA guideline for the prevention, detection, evaluation, and management of high blood pressure in adults: Executive summary. Hypertension. 2018;71:e13–e115.

2. Centers for Disease Control and Prevention. High Blood Pressure Facts about Hypertension. www.bing.com/search?q=CDC+high+blood+pressure+facts+about+hypertension&form=ANNH01&refig=3ed7d978563444299eab1e602781d6f3&pc=U531 (Accessed October 2, 2023).
3. Hannan M, Jeamjivibool T, Bronas U. Lifestyle management and prevention of hypertension. In Rippe J (ed). Lifestyle Medicine, 4th edition. Boca Raton: CRC Press, 2024.
4. Chobanian A, Bakris G, Black H, et al. The seventh report of the joint national committee on prevention, detection, evaluation, and treatment of high blood pressure: The JNC 7 report. JAMA. 2003;289(19):2560–2572.
5. SPRINT Research Group. Wright JT, Jr, Williamson JD, Whelton PK, et al. A randomized trial of intensive versus standard blood-pressure control. N Engl J Med. 2015;373:2103–2116.
6. Bazzano L, Green T, Harrison T, et al. Dietary approaches to prevent hypertension. Curr Hypertens Rep. 2013;15(6):694–702.
7. Appel L, Brands M, Daniels S, et al. American Heart Association: Dietary approaches to prevent and treat hypertension: A scientific statement from the American Heart Association. Hypertension. 2006;47(2):296–308.
8. Centers for Disease Control and Prevention, National Center for Health Statistics. About Multiple Cause of Death, 1999–2020. CDC Wonder Online Database Website. Atlanta, GA. www.cdc.gov/nchs/index.htm (Accessed October 2, 2023).
9. Centers for Disease Control and Prevention. Hypertension Cascade: Hypertension Prevalence, Treatment and Control of Estimates among US Adults Aged 18 Years and Older Applying the Criteria from the American College of Cardiology and American Heart Association's 2017 Hypertension Guideline-NHANES 2015–2018. Atlanta, GA: US Department of Health and Human Services. 2021. (Accessed October 2, 2023).
10. Kannel W, Wolf P. Framingham study insights on the hazards of elevated blood pressure. JAMA. 2008;3;300(21):2545–2547.
11. Neter J, Stam B, Kok F, et al. Influence of weight reduction on blood pressure: A meta-analysis of randomized controlled trials. Hypertension. 2003; 42:878–884.
12. Stevens V, Corrigan S, Obarzanek E, et al. Weight loss intervention in phase 1 of the trials of hypertension prevention: The TOHP collaborative research group. Arch Intern Med. 1993;153:849–858.
13. Stevens V, Obarzanek E, Cook N, et al. For the trials for the hypertension prevention research group: Long-term weight loss and changes in blood pressure: Results of the trials of hypertension prevention, phase II. Ann Intern Med. 2001;134:1–11.
14. Huang Z, Willett W, Manson J, et al. Body weight, weight change, and risk for hypertension in women. Ann Intern Med. 1998;128:81–88.
15. Appel L, Champagne C, Harsha D, et al. For the writing group of the PREMIER collaborative research group: Effects of comprehensive lifestyle modification on blood pressure control: Main results of the PREMIER clinical trial. JAMA. 2003;289:2083–2093.
16. Blumenthal J, Babyak M, Hinderliter A, et al. Effects of the DASH diet alone and in combination with exercise and weight loss on blood pressure and cardiovascular biomarkers in men and women with high blood pressure: The ENCORE study. Arch Intern Med. 2010;170:126–135.
17. Kaplan NM. Hypertension curriculum review: Lifestyle modifications for prevention and treatment of hypertension. J Clin Hyperten. 2004;6(12):716–719.
18. Physical Activity Guidelines Advisory Committee. 2018 physical activity guidelines advisory committee. 2018 Physical Activity Guidelines Advisory Committee Scientific Report. Washington, DC: U.S. Department of Health and Human Services; 2018.

19. He F, MacGregor G. Effect of modest salt reduction on blood pressure: A meta-analysis of randomized trials: Implications for public health. J Hum Hypertens. 2002;16:761–770.
20. Johnson A, Nguyen T, Davis D. Blood pressure is linked to salt intake and modulated by the angiotensinogen gene in normotensive and hypertensive elderly subjects. J Hypertens. 2001;19:1053–1060.
21. MacGregor G, Markandu N, Sagnella G, et al. Double-blind study of three sodium intakes and long-term effects of sodium restriction in essential hypertension. Lancet. 1989;2:1244–1247.
22. Sacks F, Svetkey L, Vollmer W, et al. For the DASH-sodium collaborative research group: Effects on blood pressure of reduced dietary sodium and the Dietary Approaches to Stop Hypertension (DASH) diet: DASH-sodium collaborative research group. N Engl J Med. 2001;344: 3–10.
23. Vollmer W, Sacks F, Ard J, et al. For the DASH-sodium trial collaborative research group: Effects of diet and sodium intake on blood pressure: Subgroup analysis of the DASH-sodium trial. Ann Intern Med. 2001;135:1019–1028.
24. Bray G, Vollmer W, Sacks F, et al. for the DASH collaborative research group: A further subgroup analysis of the effects of the DASH diet and three dietary sodium levels on blood pressure: Results of the DASH-sodium trial. Am J Cardiol. 2004;94:222–227.
25. He F, Markandu N, MacGregor G. Importance of the renin system for determining blood pressure fall with acute salt restriction in hypertensive and normotensive whites. Hypertension. 2001;38:321–325.
26. Institute of Medicine. Dietary Reference Intakes: Water, Potassium, Sodium Chloride, and Sulfate, 1st edition. Washington, DC: National Academy Press, 2004.
27. Cappuccio F, MacGregor G. Does potassium supplementation lower blood pressure? A meta-analysis of published trials. J Hypertens. 1991;9:465–473.
28. Whelton P, He J, Cutler J, et al. Effects of oral potassium on blood pressure: Meta-analysis of randomized controlled clinical trials. JAMA. 1997;277:1624–1632.
29. Geleijnse J, Kok F, Grobbee D. Blood pressure response to changes in sodium and potassium intake: A metaregression analysis of randomised trials. J Hum Hypertens. 2003;17:471–480.
30. Klatsky A, Friedman G, Siegelaub A, et al. Alcohol consumption and blood pressure kaiser-permanente multiphasic health examination data. N Engl J Med. 1977;296:1194–1200.
31. Xin X, He J, Frontini M, et al. Effects of alcohol reduction on blood pressure: A meta-analysis of randomized controlled trials. Hypertension. 2001;38:1112–1117.
32. Sacks F, Rosner B, Kass E. Blood pressure in vegetarians. Am J Epidemiol. 1974;100:390–398.
33. Armstrong B, van Merwyk AJ, Coates H. Blood pressure in seventh-day adventist vegetarians. Am J Epidemiol. 1977;105:444–449.
34. Appel L, Sacks F, Carey V, et al. for the OmniHeart collaborative research group: Effects of protein, monounsaturated fat, and carbohydrate intake on blood pressure and serum lipids: Results of the OmniHeart randomized trial. JAMA. 2005;294:2455–2464.
35. Ahiawodzi P, Furtado J, Mukamal K. Dietary macronutrients and circulating non-esterified fatty acids: A secondary analysis of the OMNI heart crossover trial. J Nutr. 2023;14;152(12):2802–2807.
36. Appel L, Miller ER 3rd, Seidler A, et al. Does supplementation of diet with "fish oil" reduce blood pressure? A meta-analysis of controlled clinical trials. Arch Intern Med. 1993;153:1429–1438.
37. Morris M, Sacks F, Rosner B. Does fish oil lower blood pressure? A meta-analysis of controlled trials. Circulation. 1993;88:523–533.

38. Geleijnse J, Giltay E, Grobbee D, et al. Blood pressure response to fish oil supplementation: Metaregression analysis of randomized trials. J Hypertens. 2002;20:1493–1499.
39. Whelton S, Hyre A, Pedersen B, et al. Effect of dietary fiber intake on blood pressure: A meta-analysis of randomized, controlled clinical trials. J Hypertens. 2005;23:475–481.
40. He J, Whelton P. Effect of dietary fiber and protein intake on blood pressure: A review of epidemiologic evidence. Clin Exp Hypertens. 1999;21:785–796.
41. He J, Streiffer R, Muntner P, et al. Effect of dietary fiber intake on blood pressure: A randomized, double-blind, placebo-controlled trial. J Hypertens. 2004;22:73–80.
42. Cappuccio F, Elliott P, Allender P, et al. Epidemiologic association between dietary calcium intake and blood pressure: A meta-analysis of published data. Am J Epidemiol. 1995;142:935–945.
43. Allender P, Cutler J, Follmann D, et al. Dietary calcium and blood pressure: A meta-analysis of randomized clinical trials. Ann Intern Med. 1996;124:825–831.
44. Bucher H, Cook R, Guyatt G, et al. Effects of dietary calcium supplementation on blood pressure: A meta-analysis of randomized controlled trials. JAMA. 1996;275:1016–1022.
45. Mizushima S, Cappuccio F, Nichols R, et al. Dietary magnesium intake and blood pressure: A qualitative overview of the observational studies. J Hum Hypertens. 1998; 12:447–453.
46. Hodges R, Rebello T. Carbohydrates and blood pressure. Ann Intern Med. 1983;98(Pt 2): 838–841.
47. Rebello T, Hodges R, Smith J. Short-term effects of various sugars on antinatriuresis and blood pressure changes in normotensive young men. Am J Clin Nutr. 1983;38:84–94.
48. Israel K, Michaelis O 4th, Reiser S, et al. Serum uric acid, inorganic phosphorus, and glutamic-oxalacetic transaminase and blood pressure in carbohydrate-sensitive adults consuming three different levels of sucrose. Ann Nutr Metable. 1983;27:425–435.
49. Geleijnse J, Giltay E, Grobbee D, et al. Blood pressure response to fish oil supplementation: Metaregression analysis of randomized trials. J Hypertens. 2002;20(8):1493–1439.
50. Appel L, Miller ER 3rd, Seidler A, et al. Does supplementation of diet with 'fish oil' reduce blood pressure? A meta-analysis of controlled clinical trials. Arch Intern Med. 1993;153(12):1429–1438.
51. Campbell F, Dickinson H, Critchley J, et al. A systematic review of fish-oil supplements for the prevention and treatment of hypertension. Eur J Prevent Cardiol. 2013;20(1):107–120.
52. Morris M, Sacks F, Rosner B. Does fish oil lower blood pressure? A meta-analysis of controlled trials. Circulation. 1993;88(2):523–533.
53. Ascherio A, Rimm E, Giovannucci E, et al. A prospective study of nutritional factors and hypertension among US men. Circulation. 1992;86:1475–1484.
54. Ascherio A, Hennekens C, Willett W, et al. Prospective study of nutritional factors, blood pressure, and hypertension among US women. Hypertension. 1996;27:1065–1072.
55. Obarzanek E, Velletri P, Cutler J. Dietary protein and blood pressure. JAMA. 1996;275:1598–1603.
56. Elliott P, Stamler J, Appel L, et al. for the INTERMAP cooperative research group: Relationship of dietary protein to blood pressure: The INTERMAP study. Arch Intern Med. 2006;9;166(1):79–87.
57. Stamler J, Caggiula A, Grandits G, et al. Relationship to blood pressure of combinations of dietary macronutrients: Findings of the Multiple Risk Factor Intervention Trial (MRFIT). Circulation. 1996;94:2417–2423.
58. Ness A, Chee D, Elliott P. Vitamin C and blood pressure: An Overview. J Hum Hypertens. 1997;11:343–350.
59. Lifton R, Wilson F, Choate K, et al. Salt and blood pressure: New insight from human genetic studies. Cold Spring Harb Symp Quant Biol. 2002;67:445–450.

60. Watson D, Tharp R. Self-Directed Behavior: Self-Modification for Personal Adjustment, 5th edition. Pacific Grove, Calif: Brooks/Cole, 1989.
61. Guasch-Ferré M, Salas-Salvadó J, Ros E, et al. PREDIMED investigators: The PREDIMED trial, Mediterranean diet and health outcomes: How strong is the evidence? Nutr Metable Cardiovasc Dis. 2017;27(7):624–632.
62. Barker D, Osmond C, Golding J, et al. Growth in utero, blood pressure in childhood and adult life, and mortality from cardiovascular disease. BMJ. 1989;298:564–567.
63. Gillman M, Cook N, Rosner B, et al. Identifying children at high risk for the development of essential hypertension. J Pediatr. 1993;122:837–846.
64. Bao W, Threefoot S, Srinivasan S, et al. Essential hypertension predicted by tracking of elevated blood pressure from childhood to adulthood: The Bogalusa heart study. Am J Hypertens. 1995;8:657–665.
65. Dekkers J, Snieder H, Van Den Oord E, et al. Moderators of blood pressure development from childhood to adulthood: A 10-year longitudinal study. J Pediatr. 2002;141:770–779.
66. Simons-Morton D, Obarzanek E. Diet and blood pressure in children and adolescents. Pediatr Nephrol. 1997;11:244–249.
67. Applegate W, Miller S, Elam J, et al. Nonpharmacologic intervention to reduce blood pressure in older patients with mild hypertension. Arch Intern Med. 1992;152:1162–1166.
68. Cappuccio F, Markandu N, Carney C, et al. Double-blind randomised trial of modest salt restriction in older people. Lancet. 1997;350:850–854.
69. Shustak R, Brothers J, Daniels S. Identification and management of children with dyslipidemia. In Rippe J (ed). Lifestyle Medicine, 4th edition. Boca Raton: CRC Press, 2024.
70. Erlinger T, Vollmer W, Svetkey L, et al. The potential impact of nonpharmacologic population-wide blood pressure reduction on coronary heart disease events: Pronounced benefits in African-Americans and hypertensives. Prev Med. 2003;37:327–333.

14 Nutrition and Stroke

Key Points

- Stroke is the third leading cause of mortality in the United States and around the world.
- The underlying pathophysiology for stroke is typically atherosclerotic disease, which is a systemic disease involving arteries in the heart (coronary heart disease), stroke, peripheral artery disease, chronic kidney disease, and erectile dysfunction.
- Healthy plant-based eating has been shown to lower multiple risk factors for atherosclerotic disease including risk factors for stroke.

14.1 INTRODUCTION

Stroke is the third leading cause of death in the United States and around the world. It is also one of the top causes of disability worldwide. Nutrition plays a critically important role in both the prevention and treatment of stroke [1–8]. The underlying pathophysiology for 90% of strokes is atherosclerosis [9,10]. Atherosclerosis leads to ischemic strokes. Hemorrhagic strokes also occur, but the etiology of those is different and is caused by abnormalities leading to hemorrhages from blood vessels in the brain.

Atherosclerosis is a systemic and dynamic process that progresses through the individual life. (See Chapter 11 for more detail about atherosclerosis.) Thus, atherosclerosis of the carotid arteries and small vessels of the brain is responsible for most ischemic strokes. Various lifestyle medicine modalities can play a significant role in lowering the role of arthrosclerosis, as already discussed in multiple other chapters in this book. Nutrition is a key consideration for the underlying processes of atherosclerosis.

Each year almost 800,000 Americans have strokes (also called cerebrovascular accidents [CVAs]) [11]. More than 150,000 individuals die of this cause each year. Approximately 6.6 million Americans over the age of 20 have had a stroke. Stroke also remains the leading cause of severe long-term disability in the United States [9].

While nutrition is the key risk factor for stroke, many of the other risk factors contribute and are identical to those for coronary heart disease (CHD). For this reason, the American Heart Association and American Stroke Association joined forces to list the Presidential Advisory on Optimal Brain Health [2]. This advisory focuses not only on issues specifically related to stroke but also issues related to cognition and lowering the risk of dementia. Prevention of stroke, however, represents the key component for optimizing brain health. Nutrition is the key lifestyle-related component of either reducing the risk of stroke or optimizing its treatment.

As already indicated in the chapter on atherosclerosis, the modern understanding of atherosclerosis involves multiple nutritional components. These are related to issues not only of dietary fats and cholesterol, but perhaps, even more importantly,

DOI: 10.1201/9781003452607-14

issues related to inflammation and oxidation [9,10]. Thus, the nutritional components of lowering the risk of stroke and optimizing these considerations have undergone transition to overall healthy dietary patterns which lower inflammation and oxidation as well as dietary fats and cholesterol.

14.2 RISK FACTORS FOR STROKE

Optimal brain health and function and lowering the risk of stroke are highly dependent on preserving adequate delivery of oxygen and glucose, both of which are delivered through cerebral blood flow [12,13]. Optimal brain function depends on both cardiovascular and cerebrovascular health. Strong parallels exist between cardiovascular and cerebrovascular health [14,15]. These involve inflammation, oxidative stress, and DNA damage that contribute to epigenetic changes. Most of these factors are related to nutrition. Thus, the issue of lowering vascular risk factors to lower the risk of stroke is similar to controlling the risk factors for CHD.

The most important risk factors for stroke are high blood pressure, smoking, and age in addition to nutritional factors. Diabetes and hyperlipidemia are also risk factors for stroke. Thus, nutritional approaches to CHD (see Chapter 12) are also highly relevant to lowering the risk of stroke. Atherosclerotic plaque in the carotid arteries is highly vascularized. The rupture of atherosclerotic plaque can result in plaque hemorrhage or ulceration and thrombosis formation. Alternatively, large plaques can cause carotid stenosis and lead to stroke by obstructing cerebral blood flow.

The significant impact of dietary patterns as well as single nutrients as contributors to the development of atherosclerosis is well established (see Chapter 11). Healthy dietary patterns as emphasized in the Dietary Guidelines for Americans may help reduce the risk of atherosclerosis by 30%. Following dietary patterns with consumption of adequate amounts of fruits, vegetables, legumes, and nonrefined grains, as well as lower intake of animal foods has been found to play a role in reducing the risk of factors for stroke (i.e. high blood pressure, elevated serum cholesterol, and hyperglycemia).

14.3 DIETARY PATTERNS

As emphasized in multiple chapters in this book, modern nutrition science focuses on dietary patterns rather than single foods or nutrients. In particular, healthy dietary patterns that have been explored and demonstrated to yield benefits in research trials are very similar to each other. These include the Mediterranean diet (MedDiet) [16], Dietary Approach to Stop Hypertension (DASH) [17], and the Healthy U.S.-Style Dietary outlined in the *Dietary Guidelines for Americans 2020–2025* [18] and multiple diets recommended by the American Heart Association [19]. All of these diets recommend consumption of adequate amounts of fruits and vegetables, legumes, whole grains, and fish and lower intake of animal foods.

- **<u>The Mediterranean Diet (MedDiet)</u>**—The MedDiet is characterized by a high consumption of fruits and vegetables, whole grains, nuts, legumes, fish, and olive oil as the main fat source; moderate wine consumption; and low intake of dairy products and meat [20]. Thus, this diet contains multiple components that are both anti-inflammatory and antioxidative as well as high levels of monounsaturated fats (largely from the olive oil) and large amounts of fiber (from fruit, vegetables, and whole grains).

Several research studies have shown an inverse association between the degree of adherence to MedDiet and risk of stroke. The risk of stroke reported in one meta-analysis of studies employing the MedDiet was reduced by 30%. This benefit resulted from the inverse relationship with ischemic stroke (50% reduction) [20]. No significant reduction, however, in hemorrhagic stroke occurred. The PREDIMED study also showed a 32% decrease in risk of stroke for individuals who followed the MedDiet [21]. In the U.S. population, the REGARDS study showed a 21% reduced risk of ischemic stroke for high versus low adherence to MedDiet [22]. Thus, abundant scientific evidence exists that adherence to the MedDiet lowers the risk of stroke in addition to significantly lowering the risk of CHD.

- **DASH Diet**—The DASH diet was specifically developed to target lowering blood pressure and CVD risk. It is included as an example of healthy eating patterns in the 2020–2025 Dietary Guidelines for Americans. The DASH diet emphasizes high intake of fruits and vegetables, nuts and legumes, whole grains, and low-fat dairy products and low intake of sodium, red and processed meat, and sweetened beverages [23]. Since high blood pressure represents a significant risk factor for stroke, the DASH diet is particularly appropriate for lowering risk of stroke. The DASH diet segment of the EPIC study, as well as studies from Sweden and the United States, have all shown that the DASH diet lowers the risk of ischemic stroke [6].
- **A Priori Diets**—The Healthy Eating Index (HEI) measures the degree to which an individual's diet is aligned with the *Dietary Guidelines for Americans 2020–2025*. Utilizing this measurement, the EPIC study showed that individuals with a high score on the HEI achieved by following heart-healthy dietary patterns were associated with a 46% reduction in the risk of ischemic stroke [6]. Other dietary patterns that use the a priori methodology have shown similar dramatic reductions in the risk of stroke from following the healthy dietary pattern.
- **Low-Fat Diets**—Low-fat diets initially were thought to lower the risk of both heart disease and stroke. Findings from studies using a low-fat diet, however, have been disappointing. A low-fat diet has not substantially outperformed the controlled condition with regard to atherosclerosis. These findings point to the fact that risk of atherosclerosis requires more than single-nutrient emphasis such as in a low-fat diet. This provides further evidence of the reduction in mortality from healthy eating patterns such as the MedDiet and DASH diet.
- **Western Diet**—As indicated in multiple chapters in this book, the Western diet increases the risk of stroke largely due to the fact that it is associated with an increased risk of lipid abnormalities and high blood pressure [24,25]. The Western diet has also been shown to be inflammatory (see Chapter 2).

14.4 MACRONUTRIENTS AND STROKE

- **Carbohydrates**—Postprandial glycemia is an independent risk factor for stroke. It is important to recognize that the quality of carbohydrates plays a significant role in this association. Specifically, refined grains are more associated with stroke than complex carbohydrates. One of the ways of measuring carbohydrate quality combines the glycemic index and glycemic load of various carbohydrates. Refined carbohydrates typically have a high glycemic index and glycemic load [26,27]. These findings suggest that the emphasis on complex carbohydrates rather than refined carbohydrates found in healthy dietary patterns represents another reason why they lower the risk of stroke [28,29].
- **Fatty Acids**—Historically, individuals have been counseled to reduce the amount of saturated fatty acids (SFAs) in their diet as a way of lowering the risk of atherosclerosis. Recent studies, however, have suggested that saturated fatty acids are complex. Specifically related to risk of stroke, some research studies have shown that SFA intake does not increase the risk of stroke. Further research is needed in this area.

  Monounsaturated fats (MUFAs) have been shown to be a component of healthy dietary patterns and to lower the risk of stroke. This reduction of risk is thought to result from the effect of MUFA lowering blood pressure as well as lowering low-density lipoprotein (LDL) cholesterol and triglycerides [30,31]. SFAs, the anti-inflammatory and antioxidative effects of phenolic compounds in olive oil and wine, which were demonstrated in the PREDIMED [21] study, may also contribute to risk reduction. Polyunsaturated fats (PUFAs) yield modest reductions in the risk factors for stroke [32–34].

  Thus, the current state of science in the area of various types of fats provides only slight evidence of decreased risk of stroke based on their consumption.
- **Proteins**—A recent meta-analysis has reported only minimal effects of protein consumption for decreasing the risk of stroke [35]. At the current time, there is not sufficient evidence to support the association between dietary protein intake and stroke.

14.5 MICRONUTRIENTS

- **Sodium**—Several meta-analyses of randomized control trials support the blood pressure–lowering effect of reducing salt intake since lowering blood pressure is significant for lowering stroke risk [36–38]. The available evidence suggests that elevated salt intake increases stroke risk.
- **Potassium**—There is an inverse relationship between dietary potassium intake and blood pressure from multiple studies [39–42]. Thus, a large body evidence studies supports the benefit of intake of dietary potassium on stroke risk because of its well-recognized beneficial effect on BP [43,44].

- **Calcium**—Multiple studies have explored the issue of calcium intake and stroke. Some evidence exists of a protective effect of calcium from dairy products on the risk of stroke [45]. These findings may be due both to the effects that dairy products have on lowering blood pressure and reducing systemic inflammation.
- **Magnesium**—A large meta-analysis of seven prospective studies showed that total dietary magnesium intake was inversely associated with the risk of stroke, particularly ischemic stroke [46]. Magnesium is found in a variety of plant foods such as legumes, dark green leafy vegetables, nuts, seeds, whole grains, and fortified cereals. It is also found in fish, poultry, and beef.
- **Vitamins and Antioxidants**—Most of the literature on stroke prevention has focused on B vitamins including folate, B_6, and B_{12}, all of which are involved in the metabolism of homocysteine [47]. Homocysteine is a potential risk factor for atherosclerosis. Vitamins counteracting oxidative stress and inflammation, including A, C, and E, have also been studied extensively. Studies on the impact of dietary vitamins B_6 and B_{12} on the risk of stroke are few and controversial. Regular consumption of high folate containing foods, however, appears to exert some protective effect. A diet rich in vitamin C appears to be beneficial for prevention of ischemic stroke [48]. There is no association with either vitamin A or vitamin E intake in stroke incidence [49]. In summary, there is no research evidence to support the use of antioxidant vitamin supplements in the prevention of stroke.
- **Vitamin D**—Some evidence exists that low circulating levels of vitamin D are associated with increased risk of stroke. No convincing evidence exists, however, of a significant effect of vitamin D supplementation on the risk of stroke [50].
- **Dietary Fiber**—Dietary fiber has been shown to reduce the risk of hypertension, which is the strongest risk factor for stroke. Dietary fiber also positively influences LDL cholesterol, oxidation, and inflammation. On the basis of available meta-analyses of prospective studies, dietary fiber has been found to be associated with a lower risk of stroke [51,52]. The beneficial effect of dietary fiber appears to be greater for ischemic than hemorrhagic stroke. It also appears to be more pronounced for grain and vegetable fiber intake. Healthy U.S.-Style Dietary Patterns have abundant fruits and vegetables and whole grains. The fiber in these components plays a significant role in reducing the risk of stroke.

14.6 FOOD GROUPS

- **Vegetable Sources**—Research has demonstrated a direct association between fruit and vegetable intake and the risk of stroke. This finding was confirmed by a meta-analysis of 20 cohort studies by Hu et al. that found that 200 grams or higher daily intake of fruit or vegetables was associated with 32% lower risk of stroke [53]. The protective effect of fruit and vegetables appears to be related to the fact that both are rich sources of potassium, magnesium, folate, fiber, and antioxidant compounds such as vitamin C, beta carotene, and flavonoids.

- **Legumes**—A recent meta-analysis showed no association between the consumption of legumes and the risk of stroke [54,55]. This was a surprising finding given that legumes have been previously found to be associated with lower risk of atherosclerosis.
- **Nuts**—Multiple meta-analyses for observational studies and one randomized controlled trial have been demonstrated that consumption of nuts lowers the risk of all-cause mortality from stroke in women but not in men [55]. Thus, the overall benefit of nuts for stroke risk reduction remains controversial.
- **Whole Grains**—Several recent meta-analyses of available prospective studies showed that whole grain consumption reduced the risk of stroke [56,57]. Nutrients that may be associated with this finding are fiber, vitamins and minerals, and other phytochemical compounds that are removed during the refining process. These compounds in whole grains have antioxidant properties and may reduce chronic inflammation and blood pressure levels.
- **Olive Oil**—Olive oil is a central component of the MedDiet. Its effect on the risk of stroke has been reviewed in two recent meta-analyses and one randomized controlled trial (RCT) that provided evidence of extra-virgin olive oil (EVOO) to lower the risk of stroke [58].
- **Chocolate**—A meta-analysis of five prospective studies has shown that chocolate consumption appears to be beneficial for reducing the risk of stroke [59]. The nutrients in chocolate that are hypothesized to be responsible for this finding are flavonoid antioxidants, which increase the level of high-density lipoprotein (HDL) and decrease the LDL cholesterol oxidation, thereby proving endothelial function and reducing blood pressure.

14.7 ANIMAL SOURCES

- **Fish**—Meta-analyses and prospective studies involving over 400,000 people have shown that fish consumption lowers the risk of stroke [32]. The potential benefit of fish consumption may result from the combined effect of long-chain omega-3 fatty acids and a wide array of nutrients abundant in fish (vitamins B and D) as well as essential amino acids and trace elements.
- **Meat and Processed Meat**—Meat consumption is a common source of protein, fat, and energy in humans [60,61]. Strong evidence exists that consumption of red and processed meats is associated with increased risk of ischemic stroke. The leading hypothesis for this association is based on the high content of saturated fatty acids and cholesterol and the high salt content found in processed meat.
- **Milk and Dairy Products**—Two meta-analyses have conducted data on milk and dairy products and stroke [62,63]. Both have shown modest decreases in the risk of stroke. The association is more consistent with low-fat milk. There is a hypothesis that the protective effects are due to milk's

content of calcium, magnesium, potassium, and bioactive compounds, all of which have been associated with reduction in hypertension and stroke.
- Eggs—No evidence exists that eggs are associated with decreased risk of ischemic stroke [64,65]. There may be slight protection against hemorrhagic stroke, however, based on two recent meta-analyses.

14.8 BEVERAGES

- Coffee—The association between coffee drinking and stroke was addressed in a meta-analysis of ten prospective observational studies. This meta-analysis showed a high reduction in risk of stroke of about 11% with 2–3 cups of coffee a day [66]. Higher intakes (mean of 5.5 cups per day) did not show any further reduction of risk of stroke.
- Tea—A meta-analysis of 14 prospective studies found that three or more cups per day of tea decrease the risk of total stroke and cerebral infarction. Thus, regular consumption of tea, particularly green tea, appears to be beneficial for reduction of risk of stroke [67,68].
- Sweetened Beverages—Several prospective studies have shown that sugar-sweetened beverages are somewhat associated with an increased risk of total stroke [69].
- Alcohol—An association of moderate alcohol consumption with reduced risk of cardiovascular disease has been shown in many epidemiologic studies [70–73]. Alcohol abuse, however, is unquestionably harmful. Moderate alcohol consumption or no consumption is associated with lower risk of stroke. Heavy alcohol consumption, however, increases both the risk of both ischemic and hemorrhagic stroke.

14.9 NUTRITION FOLLOWING STROKE

Less research is available for nutrition following stroke than in the area of nutrition to lower the risk of stroke. The few studies that have been done have focused on the potential of malnutrition following stroke [74,75]. Awareness of the possibility of malnutrition following stroke is essential to identifying malnourished patients. The studies that have been conducted on the frequency of malnutrition following stroke have found prevalence varied between 8% and 34% depending on criteria utilized. Poor nutrition is associated with reduced muscle strength, reduced resistance to infection, and impaired wound healing. All of these factors may result in increased risk of poor outcomes. The criteria for identifying malnutrition are discussed in considerable detail in Chapter 7. The potential for malnutrition following stroke is an issue that all clinicians should be aware of and look for.

14.10 MICROBIOME

The role of the intestinal microbiome in the risk of atherosclerosis has been a topic of multiple recent research trials (see Chapter 24). High levels of toxic metabolites produced by intestinal bacteria from meat (particularly red meat) have been demonstrated. In contrast, healthy plant diets have been demonstrated to support diverse and healthier bacteria in the microbiome. Fiber appears to be particularly important in this area. Metabolites emanating from the microbiome may either increase or decrease the risk of both stroke and cardiovascular disease.

14.11 OTHER LIFESTYLE FACTORS AND THE RISK OF STROKE

Hypertension, obesity, smoking, and diabetes all contribute to an increased risk of stroke and resultant cognitive impairment and dementia [76,77]. Considerable synergy exists between risk factors related to CHD and stroke. For that reason, the joint Presidential Advisory from the American Heart Association (AHA) and American Stroke Association (ASA) has recommended an intervention to lower risk factors for both CHD and stroke.

14.12 DEFINING OPTIMAL BRAIN HEALTH

The criteria for optimal brain health outlined by the AHA and ASA recommend utilizing the framework for CHD reduction developed by the AHA. Initially this framework was called "Life's Simple Seven" [78]. It has now been modified to include sleep and the name changed to "Life's Essential Eight" [79]. Components of this framework include multiple other lifestyle factors in addition to healthy nutrition to lower the risk of both heart disease and stroke. Included in the "Life's Essential Eight" framework are sound nutrition, increased physical activity, not utilizing tobacco, managing weight, controlling cholesterol, and managing blood sugar. Thus, multiple lifestyle factors impact on the risk of stroke. This framework is something that all clinicians should discuss with patients during regular clinical encounters.

Optimal brain health emphasizes the concept of the absence of vascular or neurogenic degenerative injury from stroke and Alzheimer's disease [76]. In the Presidential Advisory from the AHA and ASA, optimal brain health is defined as the "optimal capacity to function adaptably to the environment which could be assessed in terms of competencies across domains of thinking, moving and feeling." These domains are largely attributable to functions of the brain; thus lowering the risk of stroke is a key component in achieving optimal brain health.

14.13 CONCLUSIONS

Healthy nutrition plays a critically important role in reducing the risk of stroke. The underlying mechanism of 90% of strokes is atherosclerotic disease. Atherosclerosis is a systemic disease involving the vessels of the heart, cerebral vasculature (both large and small vessels), peripheral arteries, and issues related to chronic kidney disease and erectile dysfunction. Since atherosclerosis is a systemic disease, the nutritional components that are critically important to lowering the risk of atherosclerosis are common to risk reduction of all of these vascular diseases.

Numerous studies have now shown that healthy nutritional patterns such as the MedDiet, DASH diet, Healthy U.S.-Style Dietary, and various diets recommended by the AHA are all considered to be healthy plant-based diets. Numerous research studies have shown that these diets lower the risk of all forms of vascular disease, including risk factors for stroke. Thus, issues related to healthy plant-based eating should be discussed with every patient during clinical encounters.

Clinical Applications

- Modern understandings of nutritional science indicate that the underlying disease process of atherosclerosis is the underlying cause of 90% of strokes (ischemic strokes).
- Following healthy plant-based nutritional patterns such as the MedDiet or the DASH diet has been demonstrated to significantly lower the risk of stroke. Components of the healthy plant-based diet include abundant fruits and vegetables, whole grains, fish, seeds, nuts, and legumes. Following a lifelong healthy plant-based diet can significantly lower the risk of stroke and other atherosclerotic diseases including CHD, chronic kidney disease, peripheral artery disease, and erectile dysfunction.
- Following healthy plant-based diets should be discussed with all patients at clinical encounters as an important strategy for reducing the risk of stroke and other vascular diseases.

REFERENCES

1. Iacoviello L, Bonaccio M, Cairella G, et al. Diet and primary prevention of stroke: Systematic review and dietary recommendations by the ad hoc working group of the Italian society of human nutrition. Nutr Metab Cardiovasc Dis. 2018;28(4):309–334.
2. Gorelick P, Furie K, Iadecola C, et al. Defining optimal brain health in adults: A presidential advisory from the American Heart Association/American Stroke Association. Stroke. 2017;48(10):e284–e303.
3. Spence J. Nutrition and risk of stroke. Nutrients. 2019;11(3).
4. Foroughi M, Akhavanzanjani M, Maghsoudi Z, et al. Stroke and nutrition: A review of studies. Int J Prev Med. 2013;4(Suppl 2):S165–S179.
5. Huang C. Nutrition and stroke. Asia Pac J Clin Nutr. 2007;16(Suppl 1):266–274.
6. Tong T, Appleby P, Key T, et al. The associations of major foods and fibre with risks of ischaemic and haemorrhagic stroke: A prospective study of 418 329 participants in the EPIC cohort across nine European countries. Eur Heart J. 2020;41(28):2632–2640.
7. NHS. Stroke. Stroke—Prevention—NHS. (www.nhs.uk) (Accessed January 12, 2024).
8. Spence J. Diet for stroke prevention. Stroke Vasc Neurol. 2018;3(2):44–50.
9. Meschia J, Bushnell C, Boden-Albala B, et al. Guidelines for the primary prevention of stroke: A statement for healthcare professionals from the American Heart Association/American Stroke Association. Stroke. 2014;45(12):3754–3832.
10. Kernan W, Ovbiagele B, Black H, et al. Guidelines for the prevention of stroke in patients with stroke and transient ischemic attack: A guideline for healthcare professionals from the American Heart Association/American Stroke Association. Stroke. 2014;45(7):2160–2236.
11. Virani S, Alonso A, Aparicio H, et al. Heart disease and stroke statistics-2021 update: A report from the American Heart Association. Circulation. 2021;143(8):e254–e743.
12. Iadecola C. Neurovascular regulation in the normal brain and in Alzheimer's disease. Nat Rev Neurosci. 2004;5(5):347–360.

13. Cipolla M. The Cerebral Circulation. San Rafael, CA: Morgan & Claypool Life Sciences, 2009: 1–59.
14. Tahsili-Fahadan P, Geocadin R. Heart-brain axis: Effects of neurologic injury on cardiovascular function. Circ Res. 2017;120(3):559–572.
15. Young C, Davisson R. Angiotensin-II, the brain, and hypertension: An update. Hypertension. 2015;66(5):920–926.
16. Psaltopoulou T, Sergentanis TN, Panagiotakos DB, et al. IN: Kosti R, Scarmeas N. Mediterranean diet, stroke, cognitive impairment, and depression: A meta-analysis. Ann Neurol. 2013;74(4):580–591.
17. Struijk E, May A, Wezenbeek N, et al. Adherence to dietary guidelines and cardiovascular disease risk in the EPIC-NL cohort. Int J Cardiol. 2014;176(2):354–359.
18. U.S. Department of Agriculture and U.S. Department of Health and Human Services. *Dietary Guidelines for Americans, 2020–2025*, 9th edition. December 2020. DietaryGuidelines.gov. 2020; www.dietaryguidelines.gov/resources/2020-2025-dietary-guidelines-online-materials
19. Lichtenstein A, Appel L, Vadiveloo M, et al. 2021 dietary guidance to improve cardiovascular health: A scientific statement from the American Heart Association. Circulation. 2021;144(23): e472–e487.
20. Kontogianni M, Panagiotakos D. Dietary patterns and stroke: A systematic review and re-meta-analysis. Maturitas. 2014;79(1):41–47.
21. Estruch R, Ros E, Salas-Salvado J, et al. Primary prevention of cardiovascular disease with a Mediterranean diet. N Engl J Med. 2013;368(14):1279–1290.
22. Ronksley P, Brien S, Turner B, et al. Association of alcohol consumption with selected cardiovascular disease outcomes: A systematic review and meta-analysis. BMJ. 2011;342:d671.
23. Zhang C, Qin Y, Chen Q, et al. Alcohol intake and risk of stroke: A dose-response meta-analysis of prospective studies. Int J Cardiol. 2014;174:669e77.
24. Zhang X, Shu L, Si C, et al. Dietary patterns and risk of stroke in adults: A systematic review and meta-analysis of prospective cohort studies. J Stroke and Cerebrovasc Dis: The Off J Nat Stroke Ass. 2015;24(10):2173–2182.
25. Rodriguez-Monforte M, Flores-Mateo G, Sanchez E. Dietary patterns and CVD: A systematic review and meta-analysis of observational studies. Br J Nutr. 2015;114(9):1341–1359.
26. Jenkins DJ, Wolever TM, Taylor RH, et al. Glycemic index of foods: A physiologic basis for carbohydrate exchange. Am J Clin Nutr. 1981;34:362–366.
27. Salmerón J, Manson JE, Stampfer MJ, et al. Dietary fiber, glycemic load, and risk of non-insulin-dependent diabetes mellitus in women. JAMA. 1997;12;277(6):472–477.
28. Cai X, Wang C, Wang S, et al. Carbohydrate intake, glycemic index, glycemic load, and stroke: A meta-analysis of prospective cohort studies. Asia Pac J Public Health. 2015;27(5):486–496.
29. Mazzone T, Chait A, Plutzky J. Cardiovascular disease risk in type 2 diabetes mellitus: Insights from mechanistic studies. Lancet. 2008;371:1800e9.
30. Alonso A, Ruiz-Gutierrez V, Martínez-González M. Monounsaturated fatty acids, olive oil and blood pressure: Epidemiological, clinical and experimental evidence. Public Health Nutr. 2009;9:251e7.
31. Appel L, Sacks F, Carey V, et al. Effects of protein, monounsaturated fat, and carbohydrate intake on blood pressure and serum lipids: Results of the Omni heart randomized trial. JAMA. 2005;294:2455e64.
32. Chowdhury R, Stevens S, Gorman D, et al. Association between fish consumption, long chain omega 3 fatty acids, and risk of cerebrovascular disease: Systematic review and meta-analysis. BMJ. 2012;30;345:e6698.

33. Larsson S, Orsini N, Wolk A. Long-chain omega-3 polyunsaturated fatty acids and risk of stroke: A meta-analysis. Eur J Epidemiol. 2012;27:895e901.
34. Pan A, Chen M, Chowdhury R, et al. A-Linolenic acid and risk of cardiovascular disease: A systematic review and meta-analysis. Am J Clin Nutr. 2012;96:1262e73.
35. Zhang X, Yang Z, Li M, et al. Association between dietary protein intake and risk of stroke: A meta-analysis of prospective studies. Int J Cardiol. 2016;223:548e55.
36. Tobian L, Hanlon S. High sodium chloride diets injure arteries and raise mortality without changing blood pressure. Hypertension. 1990;15:900e3.
37. Oberleithner H, Riethmüller C, Schillers H, et al. Plasma sodium stiffens vascular endothelium and reduces nitric oxide release. Proc Natl Acad Sci USA. 2007;104:16281e6.
38. Dickinson K, Keogh J, Clifton P. Effects of a low-salt diet on flow-mediated dilatation in humans. Am J Clin Nutr. 2009;89:485e90
39. Whelton P, He J. Potassium supplementation. In Whelton PK, He J, and Louis GT (eds). Lifestyle Modification for the Prevention and Treatment of Hypertension. New York, NY: Marcel Dekker, Inc., 2003: 185e95.
40. Ascherio A, Rimm E, Giovannucci E, et al. A prospective study of nutritional factors and hypertension among US men. Circulation. 1992;86:1475e84.
41. Witteman J, Willett W, Stampfer MJ, et al. A prospective study of nutritional factors and hypertension among US women. Circulation. 1989;80:1320e7.
42. Aburto N, Hanson S, Gutierrez H, et al. Effect of increased potassium intake on cardiovascular risk factors and disease: Systematic review and meta-analyses. BMJ. 2013;346:f1378.
43. Larsson S, Orsini N, Wolk A. Dietary potassium intake and risk of stroke: A dose response meta-analysis of prospective studies. Stroke. 2011;42:2746e50.
44. D'Elia L, Iannotta C, Sabino P, et al. Potassium rich-diet and risk of stroke: Updated meta-analysis. Nutr Metable Cardiovasc Dis. 2014;24:585e7.
45. Larsson S, Orsini N, Wolk A. Dietary calcium intake and risk of stroke: A dose-response meta-analysis. Am J Clin Nutr. 2013;97:951e7.
46. Larsson S, Orsini N, Wolk A. Dietary magnesium intake and risk of stroke: A meta-analysis of prospective studies. Am J Clin Nutr. 2012;95:362e6.
47. McCully K. Homocysteine metabolism, atherosclerosis, and diseases of aging. Compr Physiol. 2015;6:471e505.
48. May J, Harrison F. Role of vitamin C in the function of the vascular endothelium. Antioxid Redox Signal. 2013;19:2068e83.
49. Juraschek S, Guallar E, Appel L, et al. Effects of vitamin C supplementation on blood pressure: A meta-analysis of randomized controlled trials. Am J Clin Nutr. 2012;95:10.
50. Sun Q, Shi L, Rimm EB, et al. Vitamin D intake and risk of cardiovascular disease in US men and women. Am J Clin Nutr. 2011;94:534e42.
51. Threapleton DE, Greenwood DC, Evans CE, et al. Dietary fiber intake and risk of cardiovascular disease: Systematic review and meta-analysis. BMJ. 2013;19;347:f6879.
52. Zhang Z, Xu G, Liu D, et al. Dietary fiber consumption and risk of stroke. Eur J Epidemiol. 2013;28(2):119–130.
53. Hu D, Huang J, Wang Y, et al. Fruits and vegetables consumption and risk of stroke a meta-analysis of prospective cohort studies. Stroke. 2014;45:1613e9.
54. Afshin A, Micha R, Khatibzadeh S, et al. Consumption of nuts and legumes and risk of incident ischemic heart disease, stroke, and diabetes: A systematic review and meta-analysis. Am J Clin Nutr. 2014;100(1):278–288.
55. Shi ZQ, Tang JJ, Wu H, et al. Consumption of nuts and legumes and risk of stroke: A meta-analysis of prospective cohort studies. Nutr Metable Cardiovasc Dis. 2014;24(12):1262–1271.

56. Mellen PB, Walsh TF, Herrington DM. Whole grain intake and cardiovascular disease: A meta-analysis. Nutr Metable Cardiovasc Dis. 2008;18(4):283–290.
57. Fang L, Li W, Zhang W, et al. Association between whole grain intake and stroke risk: Evidence from a meta-analysis. Int J Clin Exp Med. 2015;15;8(9):16978–16983.
58. Martínez-González MA, Dominguez LJ, Delgado-Rodríguez M. Olive oil consumption and risk of CHD and/or stroke: A meta-analysis of case-control, cohort and intervention studies. Br J Nutr. 2014;28;112(2):248–259.
59. Larsson SC, Virtamo J, Wolk A. Chocolate consumption and risk of stroke: A prospective cohort of men and meta-analysis. Neurology. 2012;18;79(12):1223–1229.
60. Yang C, Pan L, Sun C, et al. Red meat consumption and the risk of stroke: A dose-response meta-analysis of prospective cohort studies. J Stroke Cerebrovasc Dis. 2016;25:1177e86.
61. Haring B, Misialek J, Rebholz C, et al. Association of dietary protein consumption with incident silent cerebral infarcts and stroke: The Atherosclerosis Risk In Communities (ARIC) study. Stroke. 2015;46:3443e50.
62. Qin L, Xu J, Han S, et al. Dairy consumption and risk of cardiovascular disease: An updated meta-analysis of prospective cohort studies. Asia Pac J Clin Nutr. 2015;24:90e100.
63. de Goede J, Soedamah-Muthu S, et al. Dairy consumption and risk of stroke: A systematic review and updated dose-response meta-analysis of prospective cohort studies. J Am Heart Assoc. 2016;5(5).
64. Shin J, Xun P, Nakamura Y, et al. Egg consumption in relation to risk of cardiovascular disease and diabetes: A systematic review and meta-analysis. Am J Clin Nutr. 2013; 98:146e59.
65. Rong Y, Chen L, Zhu T, et al. Egg consumption and risk of coronary heart disease and stroke: Dose response meta-analysis of prospective cohort studies. BMJ. 2013;7; 346:e8539.
66. Malerba S, Turati F, Galeone C, et al. A meta-analysis of prospective studies of coffee consumption and mortality for all causes, cancers and cardiovascular diseases. Eur J Epidemiol. 2013;28:527e39.
67. Kokubo Y, Iso H, Saito I, et al. The impact of green tea and coffee consumption on the reduced risk of stroke incidence in Japanese population: The Japan public health center-based study cohort. Stroke. 2013;44:1369e74.
68. Shen L, Song L, Ma H, et al. Tea consumption and risk of stroke: A dose-response meta-analysis of prospective studies. J Zhejiang Univ—Sci B. 2012;13:652e62.
69. Xi B, Huang Y, Reilly K, et al. Sugar-sweetened beverages and risk of hypertension and CVD: A dose-response meta-analysis. Br J Nutr. 2015;113:709e17.
70. Costanzo S, Di Castelnuovo A, Donati M, et al. Wine, beer or spirit drinking in relation to fatal and non-fatal cardiovascular events: A meta-analysis. Eur J Epidemiol. 2011;26:833e50.
71. Di Castelnuovo A, Costanzo S, di Giuseppe R, et al. Alcohol consumption and cardiovascular risk: Mechanisms of action and epidemiologic perspectives. Future Cardiol. 2009;5:467e77.
72. Patra J, Taylor B, Irving H, et al. Alcohol consumption and the risk of morbidity and mortality for different stroke types—a systematic review and meta-analysis. BMC Pub Health. 2010;18;10:258.
73. Poli A, Marangoni F, Avogaro A, et al. Moderate alcohol use and health: A consensus document. Nutr Metable Cardiovasc Dis. 2013;23(6):487–504.
74. Sato Y, Yoshimura Y, Abe T. Nutrition in the first week after stroke is associated with discharge to home. Nutrients. 2021;15;13(3):943.
75. Dennis M. Nutrition after stroke. Br Med Bull. 2000;56(2):466–475.

76. World Health Organization and Alzheimer's Disease International. Dementia: A Public Health Priority. Paper presented at: World Health Organization; April 11, 2012. Geneva, Switzerland.
77. Centers for Disease Control and Prevention (CDC). Self-reported increased confusion or memory loss and associated functional difficulties among adults aged ≥ 60 years—21 States, 2011. MMWR Morb Mortal Wkly Rep. 2013;62:347–350.
78. Reis JP, Loria CM, Launer LJ, et al. Cardiovascular health through young adulthood and cognitive functioning in midlife. Ann Neurol. 2013;73(2):170–179.
79. American Heart Association. Life's Essential 8. Life's Essential 8 | American Heart Association. (Accessed January 12, 2024).

15 Nutrition and Cancer

Key Points

- Certain foods have been shown to decrease the risk of cancer including whole grains, vegetables, fruits, and legumes (such as beans).
- Key recommendations from a variety of sources, including the World Cancer Research Fund (WCRF) and the American Institute for Cancer Research (AICR), strongly recommended consumption of these foods to decrease the risk of cancer.
- Prestigious organizations in this area have also strongly recommended decreased consumption of foods that may increase cancer risk, including processed meats, red meat, alcoholic beverages, and salt-preserved foods.
- Patients should be advised to eat a variety and balanced diet from healthy food groups rather than consuming supplements.
- The WCRF/AICR report strongly discourages consumption of supplements as a means for reducing the risk of cancer.
- Nutrition should be placed in the context of other lifestyle habits and practices such as increased physical activity, weight management, and avoidance of tobacco products, all of which have been shown to decrease the risk of cancer.
- Caloric balance is also important. Fourteen percent of cancers in men and 20% of cancers in women are related to overweight or obesity.

15.1 INTRODUCTION

Cancer accounted for one in six deaths around the world in 2020, making it the second leading cause of worldwide deaths [1]. There are multiple underlying causes of cancer. Most are influenced by lifestyle factors, age, and environment, although some are found to be hereditary. The fact that 90% of lifetime risk of cancer comes from environmental and lifestyle factors suggests that risk factors for initiating cancer for most people are potentially modifiable [2].

"Cancer" is a generic term which encompasses more than 100 diseases and numerous different etiologies. Cancer is typically classified according to the organs or the tissues where the disease originates. In some classifications, cancers also may be described by the type of cell that forms them. The prevalence of cancer is very high. For example, in 2016, an estimated 1,685,210 new cancers were diagnosed in the United States, while 595,690 individuals died from the disease [3]. Worldwide the number of new cancers is predicted to rise by about 70% in the next two decades. It is particularly a problem in lower- and middle-income countries, although cancer is very prevalent in all countries [4].

The important role of lifestyle habits and actions in initiating cancer was strongly articulated in an important 1981 publication by Doll and Peto entitled "The Causes

DOI: 10.1201/9781003452607-15

of Cancer: Quantitative Estimates of Avoidable Risks of Cancer in the United States Today" [5]. This paper suggested that environmental and lifestyle intervention could profoundly impact on the likelihood of developing cancer. Within the Doll and Peto framework, 35% of the cancer burden at that time was thought to be initiated by dietary factors. This high prevalence of dietary causes of cancer includes both nutrition and alcohol.

While the linkage between nutrition and cancer has been hypothesized for several hundred years, only recently has the National Academy of Sciences (NAS) published an important institutional report on diet and nutrition in 1982. This report provided the first evidence-based dietary guidelines for the prevention of cancer. The report included recommendations to increase plant-based foods and decrease dietary fat intake and derive nutrients from whole foods rather than supplements. With this as background, the shift in nutrition research and cancer has moved toward whole dietary patterns, which will be largely the approach adopted in this chapter.

It is important to note that the influence of nutrition on prevention of cancer has been shown to vary by cancer type. Furthermore, it should also be noted that dietary intervention studies such as randomized, double-blind, control trials where all foods and liquids are provided for participants for the duration of the study can be very difficult and expensive to carry out.

Tools are now available that make recommendations for guidelines for cancer prevention as well as guidelines made in public health medicine. For example, the *Dietary Guidelines for Americans 2020–2025* now includes a section on cancer risk reduction [6]. The National Cancer Institute (NCI) has provided dietary assessment tools such as the Healthy Eating Index (HEI)-2015 to help evaluate dietary patterns [7]. In addition, the WCRF has provided a global Cancer Update Program (CUP) to analyze how diet, nutrition, and physical activity impact on cancer risk and survival. The most recent CUP was published in 2018 and included the WCRF and the AICR Cancer Prevention Recommendations [8]. These recommendations are summarized in Figure 15.1. This report concluded that an adherence to its guidelines substantially reduced total cancer risks.

Recent research has underscored that cancer is no longer recognized as an inevitable consequence of aging. The NCI has estimated that in the United States the overall cancer death rate fell by 13% between 2004 and 2013 [9]. This positive result is thought to reflect improvements in prevention, early detection, and treatment of different types and causes of cancer. Following nutritional guidelines represents a practical and cost-effective approach to cancer prevention in addition to promoting overall good health since many of the recommendations for cancer prevention are quite similar to those for the prevention of cardiovascular disease, diabetes, and many other chronic diseases.

15.2 DIETARY PATTERNS: AVAILABLE TOOLS

As already indicated, dietary patterns have largely replaced focus on individual foods or nutrients as the research basis for the association between nutrition and cancer prevention. Most prominently in this area are plant-based dietary patterns which emphasize consumption of a variety of fruits, vegetables, whole grains and

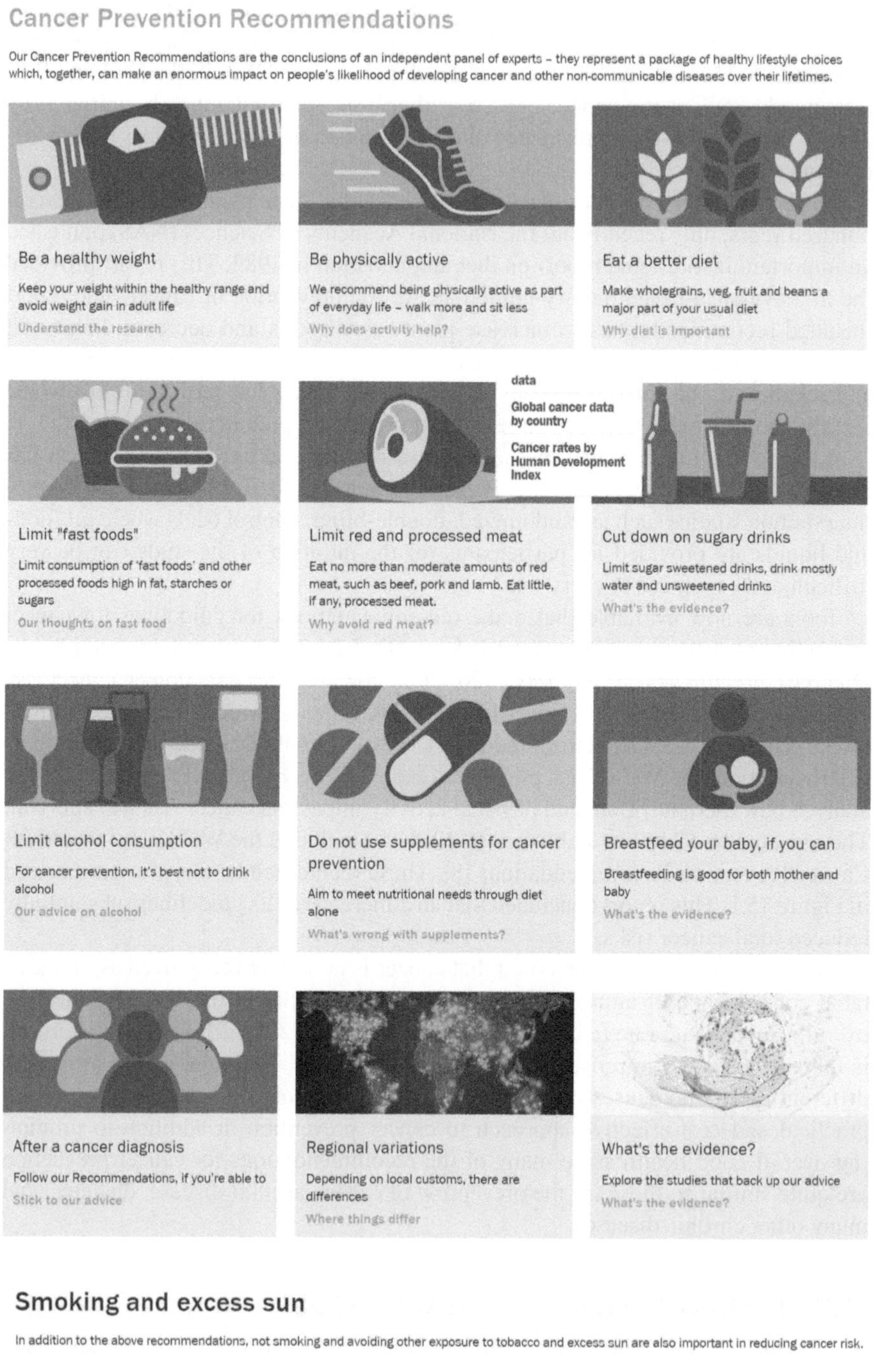

Cancer Prevention Recommendations
Our Cancer Prevention Recommendations are the conclusions of an independent panel of experts – they represent a package of healthy lifestyle choices which, together, can make an enormous impact on people's likelihood of developing cancer and other non-communicable diseases over their lifetimes.
Be a healthy weight
Keep your weight within the healthy range and avoid weight gain in adult life
Understand the research
Be physically active
We recommend being physically active as part of everyday life – walk more and sit less
Why does activity help?
Eat a better diet
Make wholegrains, veg, fruit and beans a major part of your usual diet
Why diet is important
data
Global cancer data by country
Cancer rates by Human Development Index
Limit "fast foods"
Limit consumption of 'fast foods' and other processed foods high in fat, starches or sugars
Our thoughts on fast food
Limit red and processed meat
Eat no more than moderate amounts of red meat, such as beef, pork and lamb. Eat little, if any, processed meat.
Why avoid red meat?
Cut down on sugary drinks
Limit sugar sweetened drinks, drink mostly water and unsweetened drinks
What's the evidence?
Limit alcohol consumption
For cancer prevention, it's best not to drink alcohol
Our advice on alcohol
Do not use supplements for cancer prevention
Aim to meet nutritional needs through diet alone
What's wrong with supplements?
Breastfeed your baby, if you can
Breastfeeding is good for both mother and baby
What's the evidence?
After a cancer diagnosis
Follow our Recommendations, if you're able to
Stick to our advice
Regional variations
Depending on local customs, there are differences
Where things differ
What's the evidence?
Explore the studies that back up our advice
What's the evidence?
Smoking and excess sun
In addition to the above recommendations, not smoking and avoiding other exposure to tobacco and excess sun are also important in reducing cancer risk.

FIGURE 15.1 Cancer prevention recommendations.

Source: World Cancer Research Fund, American Institute for Cancer Research. Diet, Nutrition, Physical Activity and Cancer: A Global Perspective. A Summary of the Third Expert Report. Diet, Nutrition, Physical Activity and Cancer: A Global Perspective (wcrf.org).

cereals, nuts, seeds, legumes, herbs, and spices. There is widespread consensus not only from the WCRF/AICR recommendations but also the European Prospective Investigation into Cancer and Nutrition (EPIC) study that plant-based diets lower the risk of cancer [10]. Of course, these diets are also prominent in lowering the risk of many other metabolic-based diseases. Plants contain numerous bioactive compounds (phytochemicals) including fiber, vitamins, minerals, and polyphenols. As already noted, these compounds are most beneficial when consumed in whole foods.

As indicated in previous chapters on nutrition and various other positive health factors, whole grains contain bran, endosperm, and germ layers, as well as soluble and insoluble fibers, protein, starch (carbohydrate), fats, and micronutrients such as B vitamins (e.g. thiamin, niacin and folate), which are important to the nutritional recommendations for lowering cancer risk. Whole grains and fiber intake has been consistently shown to reduce risk of gastrointestinal cancers including colorectal, colon, gastric, pancreatic, and esophageal cancers. Fruits and vegetables also are a good source of both soluble and insoluble fiber as well as other beneficial phytochemicals. Similar to whole grains, higher intake of nonstarchy vegetables and fruits is associated with decreased risk of gastrointestinal cancers and is also associated with decreased risk of lung cancer, breast cancer, and bladder cancer.

15.3 TOTAL FRUITS AND VEGETABLES

Numerous studies have shown that consumption of fruits and vegetables provides some protection against cancer [11]. Research supporting this concept is mostly from epidemiologic studies, but there are also animal and cell culture studies. Fruits and vegetables are high in fiber, vitamins, minerals, and other phytochemicals and also low in energy density. It should be noted that consumption of fruits and vegetables in these studies excludes starchy vegetables such as potato, yam, sweet potato, or cassava. There are multiple nonstarchy vegetables including spinach, cauliflower, kale, broccoli, carrots, lettuce, and tomatoes. These nonstarchy vegetables are associated with reduced risk of cancer of the esophagus, stomach, mouth, pharynx, and larynx. There is also some evidence that these vegetables may protect against cancer of the lung, colorectum, ovary, and endometrium.

Fruits may protect against cancer of the mouth, pharynx, larynx, esophagus, lung, and stomach. It is possible that fruits may protect also against cancers of the pancreas, nasal passages, and colorectum. Fruit and vegetable consumption as assessed by the CUP with reduced risk of lung cancer, but only in current smokers, not in former or never smokers. The relationship between fruit and vegetable intake and breast cancer survival is inconclusive.

It should be noted that most of the studies involving fruits and vegetables have been conducted in populations that have relatively homogenous diets and are not smokers. It should also be noted that the magnitude of fruit and vegetable consumption and cancer risk reduction may also be produced by other factors including many other environmental factors; other lifestyle factors; and the type, quantity, and duration of consumption of these foods. Recommendations from the WCRF conclude that individuals should eat at least five servings of a variety of nonstarchy vegetables and fruits every day particularly those of highly colored foods in a spectrum of red, green, yellow, white, purple, and orange. Allium vegetables such as garlic have also been recommended by the WCRF.

15.4 ENERGY BALANCE

One additional benefit of plant-based diets is that they are typically less calorie dense and more nutrient dense than other dietary patterns. Thus, plant-based diets, in addition to the nutrients they provide, may help reduce cancer risk by aiding and maintaining a healthy body weight. The 2018 WCRF/AICR Cancer Prevention Recommendation is to maintain a healthy body weight [8]. Six of the other recommendations (e.g. be physically active, eat a plant-based diet, limit fast foods, limit red and processed meats, cut down on sugary drinks, limit alcohol consumption) all are designed to influence energy balance and maintain the healthy weight recommendation. It is important to note that overweight and obesity are significant risk factors for both the initiation and propagation of cancer [11]. Indeed, 14% of all cancer mortality in men and 20% of all cancer mortality in women is associated with overweight and obesity [12–14].

Positive energy balance due to increased caloric consumption from foods and drinks contributes in a significant way to increased body fat, obesity, and other metabolic alterations. There are numerous mechanisms that link obesity to cancer, and the complete picture has not been completely elucidated. Obesity results in chronic inflammation and insulin resistance and increased incidence of cytokines and growth hormones, which promote both cancer initiation and progression.

Overweight and obesity and metabolic syndrome are associated with an increased risk of at least 13 cancers. According to the 2018 WCRF/AICR report, these include cancers of the esophagus, pancreas, liver, colorectal, postmenopausal breast, endometrial, and kidney cancers [8]. This report also reported a positive, powerful relationship between body fatness and risk of stomach, ovary, and prostate cancers.

The dietary pattern typically consumed by Americans is usually energy dense and can consist of a considerable amount of processed food, red and processed meat, and high-fat and high-sugar foods. It is also lower in whole grain, vegetables, and fruits. All of these contribute to the increased likelihood that American adults will become overweight or obese. These issues are dealt with in much greater detail in the chapter on obesity and cancer.

15.5 DIETARY FIBER

Dietary fiber includes a complex mix of mostly nondigestible plant substance compounds with variable effects on gut physiology. Fiber is roughly divided into two large categories: Either soluble, meaning that it dissolves in water, or insoluble meaning that it does not. Dietary fiber comes from a variety of sources and varies considerably in composition. It is likely that not all fiber will be equally protective against cancer. Soluble fiber is typically found in oats, barley, beans, and various fruits and vegetables. Insoluble fiber is found in whole grains, legumes, seeds, nuts, and dark green leafy vegetables. Fiber exerts numerous biological effects including slowing digestion, creating increased satiety, lowering blood sugar levels, and, perhaps, aiding insulin sensitivity, lowering blood cholesterol concentrations, and diluting harmful substances in the colon, while preventing constipation and protecting the lining of the colon which, in turn, prevents development of cancerous cells. Fermentation of fiber yields products such as short-chain fatty acids (SCFAs) produced by the gut microflora from a wide range of dietary fibers. These SCFAs have numerous benefits including induced apoptosis, cell cycle arrest, and differentiation of cancer cells.

Numerous organizations have recommend consuming at least 25 grams of fiber each day. This fiber should be divided throughout the day [15]. Whole grains and beans should be consumed at most meals. Fiber supplements are not recommended since they do not provide vitamins, minerals, antioxidants, and phytochemicals that work synergistically to prevent cancer [16]. The WCRF/AICR report cited 23 studies looking at foods containing dietary fiber and colon cancer. Overall evidence from these studies consistently showed a decreased risk of colon cancer with consumption of dietary fiber. These studies cited a 9% decreased risk of developing colorectal adenomas per 10 grams/day increase in dietary fiber [17]. Thus, the WCRF/AICR reported that it was probable that foods containing dietary fiber are protective against colorectal cancer. These findings are also consistent with a number of randomized intervention trials. It should be noted that a Cochran meta-analysis of five randomized controlled trials of increased dietary fiber did not reach the same conclusion [18]. It did not find that a difference between intervention and control groups with regard to development of adenomas. However, the consensus remains that increased fiber in the diet lowers the risk of colon cancer.

The effect of dietary fiber on mammary and prostate cancer has also been inconsistent. However, once again, the WCRF/AICR report identified three studies looking at food containing fiber before the diagnosis of primary breast cancer and found a significant 32% decreased risk per 10 grams increase/day. It should be noted, however, that the findings remain under investigation [19].

15.6 MICRONUTRIENTS AND PHYTOCHEMICALS

The micronutrients and phytochemicals that are found in fruits and vegetables may also complete the biological responses that play a role in preventing cancer. There are a wide variety of phytochemicals. Only a few will be mentioned here. Extensive reviews of the wide range of phytochemicals may be found elsewhere.

- **Garlic and allium vegetables**—The allium family contains approximately 500 species including garlic, onions, leeks, chives, and scallions. Allium vegetables are used worldwide to enhance taste, but also may potentially have apparent health benefits. Epidemiologic studies and some cell culture studies have suggested that garlic and other related sulfur constituents can reduce cancer risk by altering the biological behavior of tumors [20]. The WCRF/AICR report stated that garlic probably protects against colorectal cancer. Recent studies have suggested that garlic and other allium vegetables may exert protective effects against gastric, colorectal, and other digestive tract cancers. This evidence comes from randomized controlled trials as well as cohort studies. These have suggested between 18% and 29% reduction in cancer for consistent consumption of allium vegetables. There is also evidence of reduced risk of various cancers from animal studies. It has been hypothesized that these allium vegetables reduce the risk of cancer by inhibiting cancer cell metabolism in various ways.

- **Folate**—A folate is a water-soluble B vitamin. It is found in large quantities in green leafy vegetables. Folic acid, which is a synthetic form of folate, is also fortified in cereal products, flours, grains, and spreads. Folate is thought to influence cancer development by a specific action of assisting in the transfer of one carbon units. If folate is limited, normal DNA repair is inhibited. Some evidence also suggests that folate deficiency is associated with DNA strand break and impaired DNA repair. A recent study suggested that high dietary intake of folate protects against upper GI cancer including esophageal, gastric, and pancreatic cancer [21].
- **Carotenoids**—Carotenoids represent another example of a phytochemical where high-dose supplementation may actually create adverse effects related to cancer [11]. Typical green, yellow/red, and yellow/orange vegetables and fruits contain a wide variety of carotenoids including lutein, cryptoxanthin, lycopene, beta-carotene, and alpha-carotene. Studies have demonstrated that lessened concentrations of these nutrients significantly increases the risk of lung cancer. Studies have suggested that high-dose supplements of carotenoids may actually promote cancer. These findings were particularly prominent in heavy smokers. These studies suggest that caution must be observed when supplements are employed outside of normal food products. The highest source of carotenoids in the American diet is tomatoes.

15.7 SUPPLEMENTS

The 2018 WCRF/AICR Cancer Prevention Recommendations state that supplements should not be used for cancer prevention [11]. This conclusion is also consistent with that made by the NAS in 1982. In the United States, supplement use is common and has increased over the past decade in adult individuals [22]. According to the National Health and Nutrition Examination Survey (NHANES), over 57% of adults and 80% of women age 60 and over use dietary supplements. These are typically vitamin and mineral supplements, vitamin D, or omega-3 fatty acid supplements. There have been a variety of studies on dietary supplements, typically antioxidants, for prevention of certain cancers. These studies have typically provided no evidence of cancer prevention and, in some instances, even an increased risk of certain cancers. With regard to antioxidants, beta-carotene, vitamin E, vitamin C, vitamin A, and selenium are typically used in cancer prevention trials. Data on these studies have not demonstrated a reduction in the incidence of cancer. Several studies reported increased risk with supplementation. Studies using folic acid supplementation with the goal of reducing the risk of cancer have not demonstrated decreased risk. Randomized controlled trials (RCTs) using vitamin D and/or calcium supplementation have also demonstrated mixed results regarding cancer outcomes. For all these reasons, the 2018 WCRF/AICR report does not recommend use of supplements for cancer prevention.

15.8 PROCESSED FOODS

There are various definitions of what constitutes a processed food. Indeed, processed foods encompass a wide range of products. The U.S. Farm and Agriculture Service defines a processed food as one that has undergone any changes from its natural state. These include mechanical changes such as milling or cutting [23]. There are also other changes such as pasteurizing, cooking, canning, drying, fermenting, packaging, and addition of other ingredients. Based on this wide-ranging definition, most of the foods within our food supply have been processed to some degree. It is important to note that not all foods with some processing are unhealthy. Food processing can increase food safety and extend the shelf life of foods. However, food processing methods can also decrease nutritional properties and add less desirable nutritional ingredients such as added salt, sugars, and saturated or trans fats.

A variety of frameworks may be utilized to define processed foods that typically revolve around the level of processing. The multicenter EPIC study based food processing on the level of physical change made to the food and type of food and not the technique used [24]. Another widely used system, the NOVA System, classified foods based on the extent and purpose of industrial processing [25]. Within this system ultra-processed foods are defined as foods processed in such a way that nutrient density decreases and energy density increases through the addition of sugars and fats. Foods that are typically in this category are sugar-sweetened beverages, cookies, packaged goods, salty snacks, fast foods, and frozen dinners. Consumption of ultra-processed foods is strongly related to dietary quality. Unfortunately, the typical American diet contains over half of calories from ultra-processed foods. Chronic consumption of ultra-processed foods contributes to positive energy balance, weight gain, and increased body fat and is associated with higher overall cancer risk and breast cancer risk.

15.9 RED AND PROCESSED MEAT

In 2015, the AICR classified processed meat as a carcinogen [26]. There are abundant epidemiologic data supporting the association between red and processed meat intake and colorectal cancer. The WCRF/AICR report stated that processed meat is strongly associated with an increase in colorectal cancer and a possible risk of cancers of the nasal phalanxes, esophagus, lungs, stomach, and pancreas [8]. Red meat is listed as a probable cause of colorectal cancer. The hypothesis for this association is linked to the heme iron in red meat, which can lead to production of reactive oxygen species and lead to DNA damage in the GI tract. There is also some research suggesting an interaction between red and processed meat with gut microbiota which may also increase the risk of colorectal cancer [27]. It should be noted that there are some potential benefits from consumption of red meat, including that it is an excellent source of protein, vitamin B_{12}, niacin, vitamin B_6, zinc, and phosphorous [28]. Weighing both the risk and benefit of red meat, the WCRF/AICR recommended limiting the intake of red meat to a total of 12–18 ounces (three portions) per week in conjunction with a plant-based diet.

It is important to put into perspective that the lifetime risk for an individual to develop colon cancer is 5%, and the increased risk from regularly eating a pound of red or processed meat in the IARC report would raise the average lifetime risk to almost 6%. It should also be noted that the increased cancer risk may not be a function of the meat per se, but may reflect high fat intake as well as carcinogens generated through various meat cooking or processing methods. It should also be noted that the high energy density of meat increases the likelihood of obesity, in itself a major risk factor for cancer. Total meat consumption was possibly associated with weight gain in a large cohort of over 235,000 men. While research is ongoing on the potential linkages between meat consumption and cancer, it is important to remember that recommended amounts of red meat from the WCRF/AICR report may be mitigated by consumption of these products in the context of an overall plant-based diet.

15.10 ALCOHOL

Alcohol is a common term that encompasses ethanol or ethyl alcohol, which is a chemical substance found in beer, wine, and liquor. Ethanol has been classified by the IARC as a human carcinogen. In addition, the WCRF/AICR panel concluded that there was convincing evidence that alcoholic drinks may lead to mouth, pharynx, larynx, esophageal, colorectal (in men), and breast cancer. Alcoholic drinks are also a probable cause of liver cancer and colorectal cancer in women [8].

The amount of alcohol an individual consumes over time, and not the specific alcoholic beverage, appears to be the most important factor influencing cancer risk. Alcohol is thought to increase reactive oxygen species, often in cells. Ethanol is also metabolized into acetaldehyde. Both reactive oxygen species and acetaldehyde can damage DNA, increasing carcinogen potential. Alcohol also decreases the absorption and utilization of some micronutrients such as vitamin A; B complex; and vitamin C, D, and E. It also increases estrogen levels.

Current recommendations are for men to consume no more than two alcoholic drinks per day and women no more than one alcoholic drink per day. These recommendations are incorporated in the *Dietary Guidelines for Americans 2020–2025* [6].

15.11 THE WORLD CANCER RESEARCH FUND/AMERICAN INSTITUTE FOR CANCER RESEARCH THIRD EXPERT REPORT

The WCRF/AICR report represents the most comprehensive, detailed, and objective analysis of the issues related to nutrition, physical activity, and their impact on cancer. The WCRF/AICR report is updated approximately every five years and, most recently, in 2018 [8]. The report is designed to not only provide the guidance for healthcare practitioners whose patients may benefit from diet and lifestyle changes but also defines priorities for future research. A summary of the recommendations from the WCRF/AICR is found in Figure 15.2.

Additional information from this report provides issues related to public health and is found in Figure 15.3.

15.12 NUTRITION AND THE MOST COMMON CANCERS

The definitive evidence base related to nutrition and specific cancers comes from the EPIC study [10]. This is a cooperative study conducted in 23 centers in ten European countries. The systematic review forms the basis of the EPIC study. It represents the definitive, current database relating to nutritional practices and the risk of cancer. The findings are consistent with the WCRF/AICR recommendations but provide more granular detail about nutrition and specific cancers. This would be an important complementary study for individuals who are interested in this topic to have at their disposal.

The full Third Expert Report, *Diet, Nutrition, Physical Activity and Cancer: a Global Perspective*, is available online at dietandcancerreport.org It comprises the components listed below:	Abbreviated information from different parts of the Third Expert Report is available in this Summary as listed below:
A summary of the Third Expert Report Overview of the whole report, with a particular focus on the Cancer Prevention Recommendations and on public health and policy implications. See right column.	This publication is the Summary of the Third Expert Report. The Summary is available online at dietandcancerreport.org and can also be ordered in print.
Cancer trends Cancer statistics (available online only).	Not included in this Summary.
The cancer process Summarises the wealth of evidence on how diet, nutrition and physical activity can influence the biological processes that underpin the development and progression of cancer.	**Section 1:** Diet, nutrition, physical activity and the cancer process
Judging the evidence Outlines the rationale and methodology of the CUP, describing the rigorous scientific processes involved in gathering, presenting, assessing and judging evidence.	**Section 2:** Judging the evidence
Exposures sections ***Collating evidence and judgements by exposure*** Each of the 10 exposure sections covers definitions and background information, issues relating to interpretation of the evidence, the evidence itself (from epidemiological studies featured in CUP systematic literature reviews and from research into biological mechanisms) and judgements on the evidence. • **Wholegrains, vegetables and fruit and the risk of cancer** • **Meat, fish and dairy products and the risk of cancer** • **Preservation and processing of foods and the risk of cancer** • **Non-alcoholic drinks and the risk of cancer** • **Alcoholic drinks and the risk of cancer** • **Other dietary exposures and the risk of cancer** • **Physical activity and the risk of cancer** • **Body fatness and weight gain and the risk of cancer** • **Height and birthweight and the risk of cancer** • **Lactation and the risk of cancer**	**Section 3:** The evidence for cancer risk: a summary matrix

FIGURE 15.2 Contents of the Third Expert Report and a Summary

Source: World Cancer Research Fund, American Institute for Cancer Research. Diet, Nutrition, Physical Activity and Cancer: A Global Perspective. A Summary of the Third Expert Report. Diet, Nutrition, Physical Activity and Cancer: A Global Perspective (wcrf.org).

The full Third Expert Report, ***Diet, Nutrition, Physical Activity and Cancer: a Global Perspective***, is available online at dietandcancerreport.org It comprises the components listed below:	Abbreviated information from different parts of the Third Expert Report is available in this Summary as listed below:
CUP cancer reports and systematic literature reviews (SLRs) ***Collating evidence and judgements by cancer*** CUP cancer reports, which summarise the CUP systematic literature reviews, focus on a particular cancer site, covering trends in incidence and survival, pathogenesis, other established causes, methodology, issues relating to interpretation of the evidence, the evidence itself (from epidemiological studies featured in CUP systematic literature reviews and from research into biological mechanisms) and judgements on the evidence. Diet, nutrition, physical activity and: • cancers of the mouth, pharynx and larynx • nasopharyngeal cancer[1] • oesophageal cancer • lung cancer • stomach cancer • pancreatic cancer • gallbladder cancer • liver cancer • colorectal cancer • breast cancer • ovarian cancer • endometrial cancer • cervical cancer[2] • prostate cancer • kidney cancer • bladder cancer • skin cancer[1] • breast cancer survivors	**Section 3:** The evidence for cancer risk: a summary matrix
Diet, nutrition and physical activity: Energy balance and body fatness[1] Presents information, evidence and judgements on exposures that increase or decrease the risk of weight gain, overweight and obesity.	**Section 3:** The evidence for cancer risk: a summary matrix
Survivors of breast and other cancers Presents information on current knowledge of the importance of diet, nutrition and physical activity for cancer survivors, with a particular emphasis on breast cancer. Also includes current advice and research priorities.	**Section 4:** Survivors of breast and other cancers
Recommendations and public health and policy implications Presents the latest Cancer Prevention Recommendations, with information on the reasons behind each Recommendation. Also includes other findings of the CUP relating to regional and special circumstances, as well as public health and policy implications, along with a new policy framework.	**Section 5:** Recommendations and public health and policy implications
Changes since the 2007 Second Expert Report Important shifts in emphasis since the 2007 Second Expert Report (webpage only).	**Section 6:** Changes since the 2007 Second Expert Report
Future research directions Outlines areas where further research is needed.	**Section 7:** Future research directions

FIGURE 15.2 (*Continued*) Contents of the Third Expert Report and a Summary

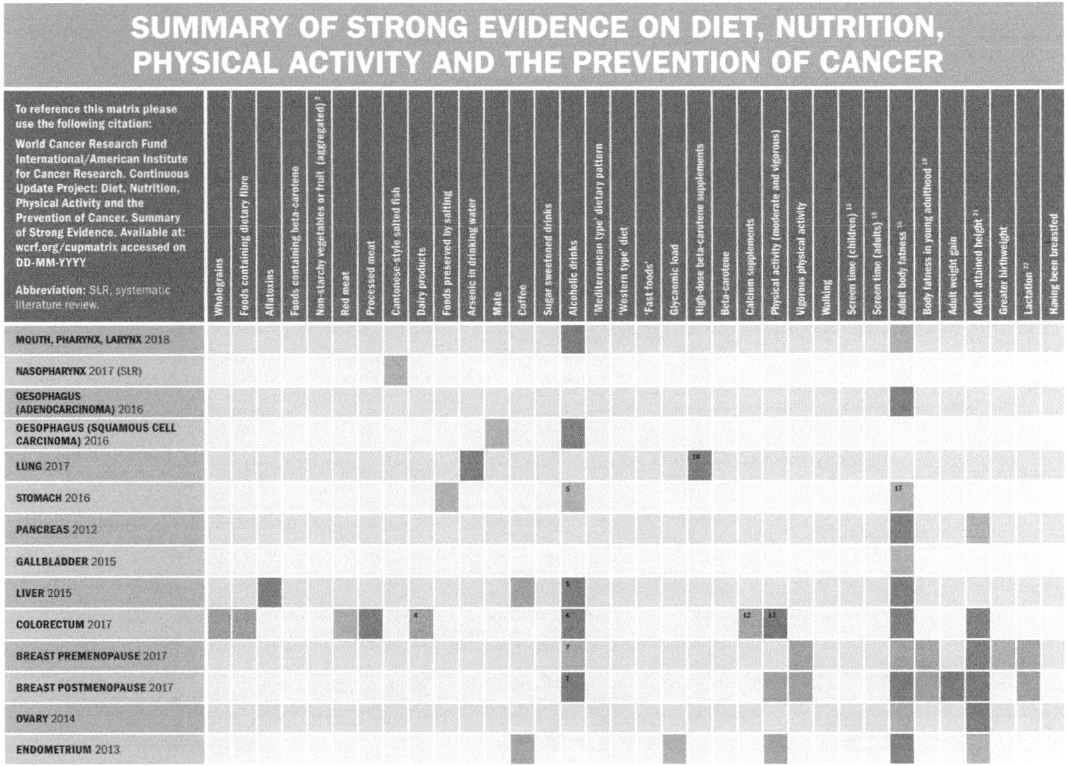

FIGURE 15.3 Summary of Strong Evidence on Diet, Nutrition, Physical Activity, and the Prevention of Cancer

Source: World Cancer Research Fund, American Institute for Cancer Research. Diet, Nutrition, Physical Activity and Cancer: A Global Perspective. A Summary of the Third Expert Report. Diet, Nutrition, Physical Activity and Cancer: A Global Perspective (wcrf.org). If lifestyle medicine practitioners are interested in only one definitive report related to nutrition and cancer, this would be the one to obtain.

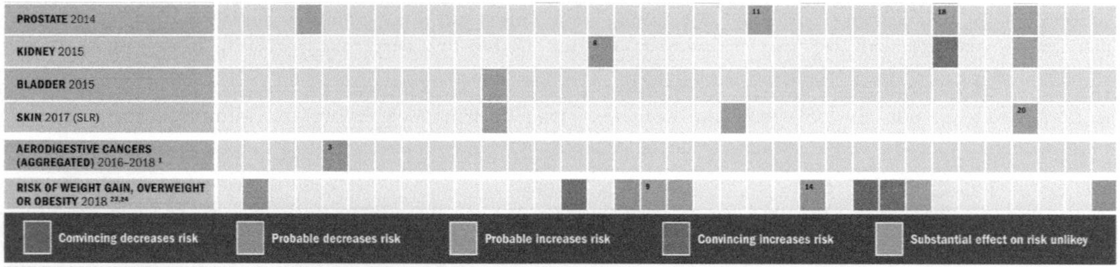

1 Includes mouth, pharynx and larynx, nasopharynx, oesophagus (squamous cell carcinoma and adenocarcinoma), lung, stomach and colorectal cancers.
2 Aggregated exposure which contains evidence for non-starchy vegetables, fruit and citrus fruit.
3 The Panel notes that while the evidence for links between individual cancers and non-starchy vegetables or fruits is limited, the pattern of association is consistent and in the same direction, and overall the evidence is more persuasive of a protective effect.
4 Includes evidence on total dairy, milk, cheese and dietary calcium intakes.
5 Stomach and liver: Based on intakes above approximately 45 grams of ethanol per day (about 3 drinks).
6 Based on intakes above approximately 30 grams of ethanol per day (about 2 drinks per day).
7 No threshold level of intake was identified.
8 Based on intakes up to 30 grams of ethanol per day (about 2 drinks per day). There is insufficient evidence for intake greater than 30 grams per day.
9 Such diets are characterised by high intakes of free sugars, meat and dietary fat; the overall conclusion includes all these factors.
10 Evidence is from studies of high-dose supplements in smokers.
11 Includes both foods naturally containing the constituent and foods which have the constituent added and includes studies using supplements.
12 Evidence derived from studies of supplements at dose >200 milligrams per day.
13 Colon cancer only.
14 Aerobic physical activity only.
15 Screen time is a marker of sedentary behaviour.
16 Body fatness is marked by body mass index (BMI) and where possible waist circumference and waist-hip ratio.
17 Stomach cardia cancer only.
18 Advanced prostate cancer only.
19 Young women aged about 18 to 30 years; body fatness is marked by BMI.
20 Malignant melanoma only.
21 Adult attained height is unlikely to directly influence the risk of cancer. It is a marker for genetic, environmental, hormonal and nutritional factors affecting growth during the period from preconception to completion of growth in length.
22 Evidence relates to effects on the mother who is breastfeeding and not to effects on the child who is being breastfed. Relates to overall breast cancer (unspecified).
23 The factors identified as increasing or decreasing risk of weight gain, overweight or obesity do so by promoting positive energy balance (increased risk) or appropriate energy balance (decreased risk), through a complex interplay of physiological, psychological and social influences.
24 Evidence comes mostly from studies of adults but, unless there is evidence to the contrary, also apply to children (aged 5 years and over).

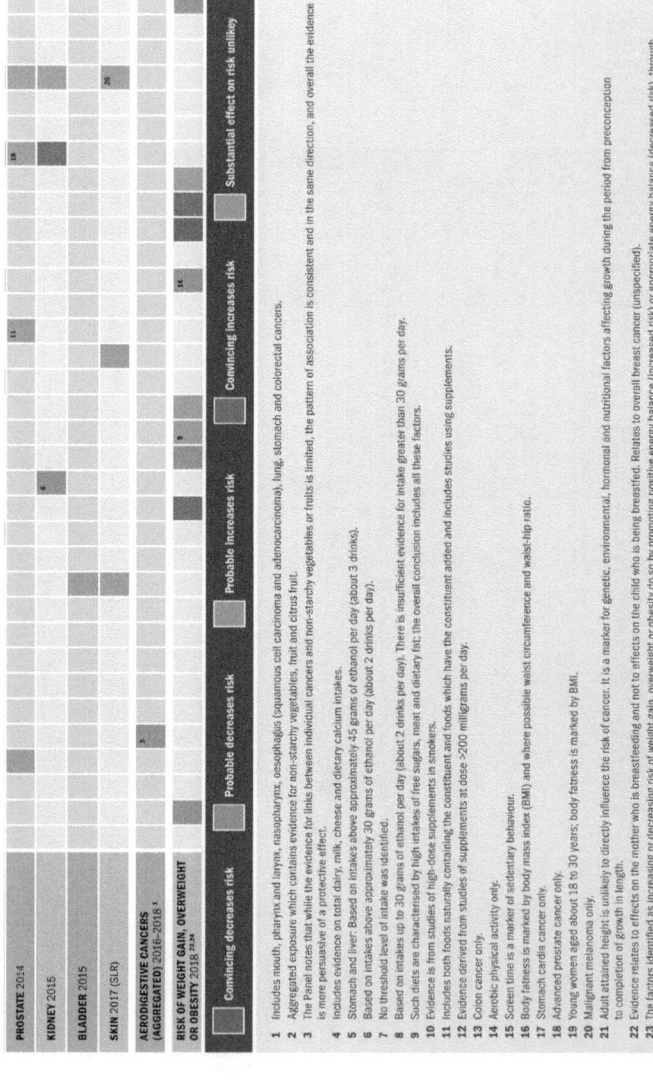

FIGURE 15.3 (*Continued*) Summary of Strong Evidence on Diet, Nutrition, Physical Activity, and the Prevention of Cancer

15.13 NUTRITION THERAPY FOR THE CANCER PATIENT

While this chapter has focused largely on nutrition in the prevention of cancer, it is also important that practitioners provide some advice concerning the importance of nutrition and lifestyle strategies in managing cancer treatment [29]. The metabolic response to cancer is varied, and certain tumors cause more nutritional alterations than others. In addition, cancer and cancer treatment often lead to symptoms that can impair dietary intake and digestion. These symptoms may result in a variety of side effects such as anorexia, nausea, vomiting, diarrhea, constipation, stomatitis, mucositis, dysphagia, and alterations in taste and smell. Since practitioners of lifestyle medicine may be in contact with individuals undergoing cancer treatment, it is worthwhile to have a sense for side effects that may occur during treatment. These are summarized in Figure 15.4.

15.14 CONCLUSIONS

There are strong links between nutrition and risk of cancer. On the positive side, numerous prestigious research organizations in this area including the WCRF and the AICR, have both recommended that individuals follow a plant-based diet including whole grains, more fruits and vegetables, and increased fiber, all of which have been shown to reduce the risk of various cancers. In addition, these organizations have recommended that red and processed meats, alcohol, and foods preserved by salting, as well as foods that are energy dense but nutrient poor should be limited as a means of further reducing the risk of cancer.

SYMPTOMS	SUGGESTIONS
Altered sense of taste or smell	○ Rinse mouth or brush teeth before eating. ○ Season foods with fruit marinades for meats, or use lemon, herbs and spices, pickles or hot sauce if tolerated. ○ Try sugar-free lemon drops, gum, or mints to improve mouth taste. ○ For foods that have an **off taste**, try fruity or salty flavors. ○ For **metallic tastes**, try spices or seasonings such as onion, garlic or onion powder, or add a little sweetener, agave nectar, or maple syrup or a nut butter (peanut butter, almond butter). ○ For **too salty, bitter, or acid tastes,** choose food naturally sweet rather than salty or acidic. Use low-sodium products. Also, try ¼ teaspoon of lemon juice to get rid of the salt taste. ○ For **too sweet**, add 6 drops of lemon or lime juice and add until the sweetness is muted. ○ For general **muted tastes**, add a spritz of lemon juice, but focus on adding more sea salt until the flavor becomes present. ○ For **bitter or strange-tasting meats,** add a sweetener like a fruit-based marinade or sweet and sour sauces to meats or choose meat alternative protein sources, i.e., eggs, tofu, dairy, or beans.

FIGURE 15.4 Managing Side Effects during Treatment

Source: World Cancer Research Fund, American Institute for Cancer Research. Diet, Nutrition, Physical Activity and Cancer: A Global Perspective. A Summary of the Third Expert Report. Diet, Nutrition, Physical Activity and Cancer: A Global Perspective (wcrf.org).

SYMPTOMS	SUGGESTIONS
Constipation	○ Focus on adequate hydration: aim for 64 ounces (8 cups) of fluid a day and a slow increase to 25–35 grams of fiber/day as tolerated. ○ Try a hot beverage, hot cereal, or high fiber food to stimulate bowel movements. ○ Incorporate probiotics such as yogurt, miso soup, and/or other supplements that help facilitate bowel movements. ○ Engage in light activity and/or stretching to improve bowel regularity. ○ Discuss medications that affect bowel function or stool softeners with a health professional as needed. ○ Schedule adequate bathroom time to facilitate bowel movements.
Diarrhea	○ Identify problem foods and decrease consumption. ○ Try a low-fat, low-fiber, and/or lactose-free diet, avoiding gas-producing foods, caffeine, and alcohol. ○ Try bulking agents, pectin, or soluble fiber foods (applesauce, banana, oatmeal, potatoes, rice). ○ Avoid sorbitol or other products containing sugar alcohol (e.g. sugarless gum and candy).
Fatigue	○ Encourage use of easy-to-prepare meals, snacks, prepared foods, and energy-dense foods. ○ Keep nonperishable snacks at the bedside (e.g. trail mix, nuts). ○ Eat small, frequent meals and snacks. ○ Eat well when appetite is best, i.e. breakfast. ○ Limit duties or chores as much as possible. ○ Try to apply energy-saving strategies to your activities. ○ Encourage light activity/movement. ○ Consider a physical therapy consult for strengthening. ○ Be evaluated for anemia as a cause of lack of energy and consider the use of a multivitamin and mineral supplement if medically appropriate.
Loss of appetite	○ Eat small, frequent meals of calorie-dense foods and fluids. ○ Eat in pleasant surroundings, avoiding stress or conflict at meal time. ○ Eat by the clock rather than waiting for appetite or hunger cues. ○ Consume smoothies or medical beverages when eating is too tiring. ○ Engage in light physical activity even for just ten minutes to stimulate appetite. ○ Use easy-to-prepare and easy-to-serve foods to preserve energy.
Nausea and vomiting	○ Eat five to six small meals/day that include lean protein choices like fish, chicken, beans, and tofu. ○ Limit exposure to smells by avoiding food preparation areas. ○ Consider eating cool, light foods with little odor. ○ Avoid greasy, high-fat foods. ○ Consume liquids between meals, rather than with meals. ○ Avoid/limit strong-smelling lotions, perfumes, soaps, and air fresheners. ○ Rest with head elevated for 30 minutes after eating. ○ Consider using complementary therapies such as ginger tea, ginger ale, and 0.5–1 gram ginger extract.

FIGURE 15.4 (*Continued*) Summary of Strong Evidence on Diet, Nutrition, Physical Activity, and the Prevention of Cancer

SYMPTOMS	SUGGESTIONS
Oral candidiasis, mucositis/ esophagitis, cold sores, inflammation in the mouth or esophagus	○ Choose foods lower in acidity and avoid tomato products, citrus juice, and pickled foods. ○ Choose foods that are less spicy; stay away from chili, chili powder, curry, cloves, black pepper, hot sauce, ginger, red pepper flakes, and other strong spices. ○ Choose foods softer in texture, with added moisture, sauce, or gravy. ○ Choose cream soups, mashed cauliflower and/or potatoes, yogurt, eggs, tofu, and pudding. ○ Serve foods cool or at room temperature. ○ Prepare smoothies with low-acid fruits like melons, bananas, or peaches and add yogurt, milk, or silken tofu. ○ For pain in the mouth—sip one tablespoon honey dissolved in one cup of warm water and avoid carbonated drinks. ○ Consume ice chips or frozen ice pop.
Early satiety	○ Choose calorie-dense foods or medical nutrition beverages. ○ Maximize intake when most hungry. ○ Eat small, frequent meals and snacks that include protein sources like eggs, cod, legumes, and seeds throughout the day. ○ Consume liquids between meals rather than with meals. ○ Engage in light physical activity to help move food through the GI tract.
Xerostomia, dry mouth, or reduced saliva	○ Alternate bites and sips at meals. ○ Add broth, gravies, and sauces to meals and dunk dry food in liquids. ○ Sip liquids throughout the day; aim for 8–10 cups/day. ○ Chew on carrots or celery. ○ Swish and spit using club soda or carbonated water. ○ Use a humidifier at home to moisten air. ○ Practice good oral hygiene. ○ Suck on hard candy, frozen grapes, or melon balls. ○ Avoid alcohol and alcohol-containing mouthwashes.

FIGURE 15.4 (*Continued*) Summary of Strong Evidence on Diet, Nutrition, Physical Activity, and the Prevention of Cancer

Clinical Applications

- All patients should be counseled on the importance of nutritional factors related to either the increased or decreased risk of cancer.
- The WCRF/AICR has recommended a plant-based diet including increased whole grains, fruits, and vegetables and increased fiber, all of which have been shown to decrease the risk of various cancers.
- Red meat, processed meat, alcohol, sugar-sweetened beverages, and foods preserved by salt should all be limited.
- Nutritional factors should be supplemented with other lifestyle habits and practices such as increased physical activity and maintenance of a healthy weight to further reduce the risk of cancer.

REFERENCES

1. American Cancer Society. Cancer facts and figures 2023. Cancer Facts & Figures 2023| American Cancer Society. (Accessed June 16, 2023).
2. Wu S, Powers S, Zhu W, et al. Substantial contribution of extrinsic risk factors to cancer development. Nature. 2016;529(7584):43–47.
3. Siegel R, Miller K, Jemal A. Cancer statistics, 2017. CA: A Cancer Journal for Clinicians. 2017;67(1):7–30.
4. World Health Organization: Cancer. Cancer (who.int) (Accessed June 16, 2023).
5. Doll R, Peto R. The causes of cancer: Quantitative estimates of avoidable risks of cancer in the United States today. J Nati Cancer Inst. 1981;66(6):1191–1308.
6. U.S. Department of Agriculture and U.S. Department of Health and Human Services. *Dietary Guidelines for Americans, 2020–2025*, 9th edition. December 2020. Dietary Guidelines.gov. 2020; www.dietaryguidelines.gov/resources/2020-2025-dietary-guidelines-online-materials
7. Krebs-Smith S, Pannucci T, Subar A, et al. Update of the healthy eating index: HEI-2015. J Acad Nutr Diet. 2018;118(9):1591–1602.
8. World Cancer Research Fund/American Institute for Cancer. Diet, Nutrition, Physical Activity and Cancer: A Global Perspective: A summary of the Third Expert Report. 2018, World Cancer Research Fund International: London, UK.
9. National Cancer Institute. Cancer Statistics. Cancer Statistics—NCI. (Accessed June 16, 2023).
10. Ubago-Guisado E, Rodriguez-Barranco M, Ching-Lopez A, et al. Evidence update on the relationship between diet and the most common cancers from the European Prospective Investigation into Cancer and Nutrition (EPIC) study: A systematic review. Nutrients. 2021;13(10).
11. World Cancer Research Fund/American Institute for Cancer Research. Food, Nutrition, Physical Activity, and the Prevention of Cancer: A Global Perspective, Washington, DC. 2007.
12. Calle E, Kaaks R. Overweight, obesity and cancer: Epidemiological evidence and proposed mechanisms. Nat Rev Cancer. 2004;4(8):579–591.
13. Calle E, Rodriguez C, Walker-Thurmond K, et al. Overweight, obesity, and mortality from cancer in a prospectively studied cohort of U.S. adults. N Engl J Med. 2003;348(17):1625–1638.
14. Calle E, Thun M, Petrelli J, et al. Body-mass index and mortality in a prospective cohort of U.S. adults. N Engl J Med. 1999;341(15):1097–1105.
15. American Institute for Cancer Research Fact Sheet on Fiber. Facts on Fiber and Whole Grains—American Institute for Cancer Research % (aicr.org) (Accessed June 28, 2023).
16. World Cancer Research Fund International/American Institute for Cancer Research. Continuous Update Project Report: Diet, Nutrition, Physical Activity and Colorectal Cancer. 2017. wcrf.org/colorectal-cancer-2017. All CUP reports are available at wcrf.org/cupreports (Accessed June 29, 2023).
17. Ben Q, Sun Y, Chai R, et al. Dietary fiber intake reduces risk for colorectal adenoma: A meta-analysis. Gastroenterology. 2014;146(3):689–699 e6.
18. Asano T, McLeod R. Dietary fibre for the prevention of colorectal adenomas and carcinomas. Cochrane Database Syst Rev. 2002(2):CD003430.
19. World Cancer Research Fund Continuous Update Project. Diet, Nutrition, Physical Activity and Breast Cancer Survivors. Breast-Cancer-Survivors-2014-Report.pdf (wcrf.org) (Accessed on June 28, 2023).

20. Nicastro H, Ross S, Milner J. Garlic and onions: Their cancer prevention properties. Cancer Prevention. 2015;8(3):181–189.
21. Liu W, Zhou H, Zhu Y, et al. Associations between dietary folate intake and risks of esophageal, gastric and pancreatic cancers: An overall and dose-response meta-analysis. Oncotarget. 2017;8(49):86828–86842.
22. Mishra S, Stierman B, Gahche J, et al. Dietary supplement use among adults: United States, 2017–2018. NCHS Data Brief. 2021(399):1–8.
23. Jones J. Food processing: Criteria for dietary guidance and public health? Proc Nutr Soc. 2019;78(1):4–18.
24. Slimani N, Deharveng G, Southgate D, et al. Contribution of highly industrially processed foods to the nutrient intakes and patterns of middle-aged populations in the European prospective investigation into cancer and nutrition study. Eur J Clin Nutr. 2009;63(Suppl 4):S206–S225.
25. Monteiro C, Levy R, Claro R, et al. A new classification of foods based on the extent and purpose of their processing. Cadernos de saude publica. 2010;26(11):2039–2049.
26. Grosso G, Bella F, Godos J, et al. Possible role of diet in cancer: Systematic review and multiple meta-analyses of dietary patterns, lifestyle factors, and cancer risk. Nutr Rev. 2017;75(6):405–419.
27. Abu-Ghazaleh N, Chua W, Gopalan V. Intestinal microbiota and its association with colon cancer and red/processed meat consumption. J Gastroenterol Hepatol. 2021;36(1):75–88.
28. U.S. Department of Agriculture, Agricultural Research Service. FoodData Central, 2019. fdc.nal.usda.gov (Accessed February 2, 2024).
29. Kaur S, Trujillo E. Nutrition therapy for the cancer patient. In Rippe JM (ed). Lifestyle Medicine, 3rd edition. Boca Raton: CRC Press, 2019.

16 Nutrition, Cognition, and Mental Health

Key Points

- Dietary patterns that are high in fruits and vegetables and whole grains and low in red meat, saturated fats, sugar, and salt have been shown to lower the risk of cognitive decline and Alzheimer's disease (AD).
- These diets are high in antioxidants and B vitamins.
- Nutritional strategies to lower the risk of cognitive decline should be combined with other lifestyle habits and actions to maximize their benefit.
- Most prominent in these dietary patterns which have yielded decreases in the likelihood of cognitive decline include the Mediterranean diet (MedDiet), DASH diet, and the Mediterranean-DASH Intervention for Neurodegenerative Delay (MIND) diet.

16.1 INTRODUCTION

Brain health and adequate brain function are critical to maintaining a satisfying and productive life [1–3]. As worldwide populations, but particularly in high-income countries, have continued to age, issues related to cognitive impairment have become a critically important health consideration across the world. To provide one example, AD, which is the most common form of dementia, has rapidly increased around the world. The United States and China have the largest number of individuals suffering from this debilitating, chronic form of dementia. In the United States, it is estimated that there are 4.9 million individuals suffering from AD, while in China there are over 5.4 million individuals suffering from this condition [1–3]. It has been hypothesized that AD cases around the world may be essentially amenable to modifiable risk factors. Indeed, it has been estimated that up to one-third of all AD cases could be mitigated or perhaps eliminated by modifiable environmental factors.

Nutrition represents a key modifiable environmental factor that has been clearly related to a variety of metabolic chronic diseases such as diabetes, cardiovascular disease, and even cancer. There is now increasing evidence that lifelong nutrition may have a direct effect on brain function [4–11]. For example, a number of longitudinal cohort studies have identified associations between a variety of nutrients and dietary patterns and a decrease in cognition, brain volume loss, or brain integrity [8]. Some randomized control trials (RCTs) have also confirmed these results [6,7,9,10]. Observational studies have also suggested a direct role for lifelong nutrition on clinical measures of cognitive status in older adults [12,13]. Thus, the relationship between nutrition and cognition is critically important in the study of lifestyle medicine. It

DOI: 10.1201/9781003452607-16

should be emphasized that healthful nutrition is only one component of potentially maintaining adequate cognition and lowering the risk of cognitive impairment. Other factors such as regular physical activity, avoidance of tobacco products, and weight management have also been demonstrated to play roles in maintaining cognition and lowering the risk of cognitive impairment [14–17]. The good news is that many of the habits and practices which are central to the study of lifestyle medicine and can lower the risk of cognitive impairment also have been shown to yield multiple other benefits for chronic diseases such as type 2 diabetes mellitus (T2DM), cardiovascular disease (CVD), and cancer.

Emerging data also show the most effective mechanisms for reducing the likelihood of cognitive impairment in general, and AD, in particular, relate to lifelong pursuit of healthy habits such as sound nutrition and regular physical activity. These studies have fundamentally changed the modern approach to AD [1–3]. In the past, a great deal of research focused on reversing tau bodies and neurologic tangles in the brain. Current thinking reflects the potential role of inflammation in contributing to AD. Thus, regular practices that lower the likelihood of inflammation such as consuming a plant-based diet and engaging in regular physical activity are playing increasing roles in lowering the risk of cognitive impairment [18–24].

As emphasized in multiple chapters in this book, modern nutrition research focuses more on dietary patterns rather than individual foods and nutrients. This approach is buttressed by numerous studies of chronic diseases including CVD, T2DM, cancer, and, increasingly, cognition. The approach to utilizing dietary patterns to yield multiple health benefits is advocated both in the *Dietary Guidelines for Americans 2020–2025* [25] and the 2021 Nutritional Recommendations from the American Heart Association [26].

The purpose of the current chapter is to summarize how nutritional habits and practices impact on both short- and long-term cognition and reduction in risk of cognitive impairment.

16.2 NUTRIENTS AND BIOLOGICALLY ACTIVE COMPOUNDS

- **Antioxidants**—Numerous nutrients found in fruits and vegetables including vitamin C, vitamin E, and carotenoids as well as polyphenolic phytochemicals (e.g. anthocyanins and polyphenols) have direct antioxidant properties. A number of other essential elements also act as co-factors for proteins and enzymes and possess antioxidant activity.

  Just like the cardiovascular system, the brain is highly susceptible to oxidative damage. It has been postulated that inadequate antioxidant defenses might stimulate the process and progression of dementia [27–29]. Therefore, dietary antioxidants can influence the development of cognitive impairment. Some of the major dietary sources of antioxidants include the B vitamins (B_6 and B_{12} and folate) as well as nutrients such as vitamin C [30,31], vitamin E [32,33], carotenoids [34], flavonoids, vitamin D, and various omega-3 fatty acids.

  Fruits such as berries, citrus fruits and kiwis, and some vegetables including brussels sprouts, cauliflower, and cabbage as well as tomatoes are good sources of vitamin C. Even some spices (parsley, sorel, and chives) are also good sources of vitamin C.

Vegetable oils, nuts, and seeds as well as some fatty fish (e.g. salmon, herring, and swordfish) as well as egg yolk and whole grain cereals are good sources of vitamin E. Carotenoids are largely found in yellow and orange vegetables (sweet potatoes, carrots, pumpkins, and tomatoes) as well as dark leafy vegetables (spinach, broccoli, and endive) and yellow or orange fruits (apricots, peaches, mangos, and melons).

Flavonoids are typically found in fruits, particularly citrus fruits, bananas, and berries as well as some vegetables (e.g. parsley and onions) and tea (both black and brewed) [35–39].

Vitamin D is found in fish (particularly oily fish) and either full-fat or fortified dairy products, egg yolk, meat, and meat products [40]. Omega-3 fatty acids are found in fish and some vegetable oils and nuts [41].

It should be noted that the effects of vitamin C on cognitive function are somewhat disputed. Evidence exists, however, that vitamin C consumption lowers the incidence of AD. However, beta carotene has not yielded consistent benefits on cognitive function. Those who had higher plasma carotenoid concentration in some studies experienced a lower incidence of dementia and AD. Thus, studies of vitamin E have been mixed.

The potential positive protective effect of vitamins D and E on risk of AD has been found to be more pronounced in current smokers, which suggests that dietary antioxidants are more clinically relevant under conditions of high oxidative stress.

The use of supplements containing antioxidants (as opposed to obtaining antioxidants from food sources) has been associated with decreased risk of cognitive impairment in one study and decreased risk for AD in another study. It should be noted, however, that these studies did not adjust for overall antioxidant status, so the potential benefit of antioxidant supplementation has not been definitely demonstrated in these studies. It also remains possible that those who take these supplements may be more health conscious, which could also mediate the observed association.

- **B vitamins**—Research on B vitamins related to cognitive function has largely focused on their role in homocysteine metabolism [42]. It has been established that there is an association between homocysteine concentration and cognitive decline. Homocysteine is produced by methylation of methionine. Homocysteine is eliminated from the body via two pathways, one of which requires folate and vitamin B_{12} while the other requires vitamin B_6. Dietary sources of vitamin B_6 and vitamin B_{12} have already been enumerated in this chapter.

  The relationship of folate to cognitive function was demonstrated in one study of elderly people who were in the highest quintile of folate intake. Most clinical trials of B vitamins, however, have found no association with cognitive function [43]. One study reported that supplementation with folate improved cognitive function in participants 50–70 years old. Combinations of folate, B_6, and B_{12} have also been demonstrated to improve cognitive function in a study of men 45–80 years old who took these supplements for four years [44]. Memory was also found to improve in these individuals. Taken together these observations suggest that individuals with high baseline level homocysteine concentrations (greater than 12.9 micromoles/ per liter) and low baseline vitamin B concentration or who have established CVD or cerebrovascular disease might benefit the most from vitamin B supplementation.

- **Vitamin D**—Vitamin D is associated with decreased neurodegeneration induced by inflammation. Vitamin D levels are also associated with decreases in amyloid B production and its appearance [40]. Sources of vitamin D have already been enumerated in this chapter. Several studies have found a protective association between concentration of vitamin D and reduced cognitive decline or dementia or AD in men or women aged 65 or older. It should be noted that there is little research on vitamin D supplementation. The single clinical trial exploring vitamin D supplementation reported no effect. In this study, however, vitamin D was examined only in conjunction with calcium and only in women.
- **Macronutrients**—Little scientific evidence exists on macronutrient intake and cognitive function. Within this category, most studies have focused on dietary lipids. Studies regarding dietary lipids have been focused on the significant role that they play in both cardiovascular and cerebral vascular health, both of which are potentially important contributors to dementia. Omega-3 fatty acids (particularly docosahexaenoic acid [DHA]) play critical roles in neuronal membrane and may also play a role as anti-inflammatory products. Dietary sources of omega-3 fatty acids have been listed in the previous section of this chapter. Higher intakes of omega-3 fatty acids have been associated with slower rates of cognitive decline in some, but not all, studies. Numerous clinical trials exploring supplementation with omega-3 fatty acids have suggested a protective effect. Some studies of omega-3 fatty acids have shown improved components of cognition including episodic memory in individuals of the age of 55.

  Observational studies on dietary lipids and cognitive function have shown mixed results. Studies related to polyunsaturated fats and monounsaturated fats have yielded mixed results in terms of cognitive function [45,46]. In one study, a higher intake of monounsaturated fats showed some protection against mild cognitive impairment in men aged 60–64 years old.

  Findings have also been mixed for saturated and trans fats. Several studies in individuals over the age of 50 have shown increased incidence of cognitive impairment and AD in subjects who consumed more saturated fat. Several observational studies have reported an association between trans fat and cognitive decline. It must be emphasized, however, that ample research has demonstrated that trans fats result in adverse effects on cardiovascular risk because of raising low-density lipoprotein (LDL) and lowering high-density lipoprotein (HDL).
- **Water/Hydration**—Numerous studies have shown that dehydration acutely leads to decreased cognitive function [47,48]. This supports the understanding

that individuals who exercise on a regular basis or who live in a very warm environment should be strongly advised to maintain adequate hydration. A recent study showed that 1,000 individuals who were followed for a decade who were adequately hydrated throughout that period of time increased their longevity by approximately 5 years. Levels of fluid consumption for adequate hydration averages 8–12 cups of water or other fluids a day for men and 6–9 cups of water or other fluids for women.

Even small amounts of dehydration (2% decline in body water) can lead to cognitive decline, particularly in young athletes. The exact pathophysiology for why this is true has yet to be totally elucidated. However, it is quite possible that decrease blood flow to the brain may result in diminished cognition.

In older individuals research has shown that even small amounts of dehydration (again on the order of about 2%) can lead to delirium and dementia. One important study followed 11,255 adults over a 30-year period. These investigators showed that individuals who were not adequately hydrated (as measured by serum sodium level ≥142 mEq/L had a 64% increased risk of building chronic disease including heart failure, stroke, atrial fibrillation, and peripheral artery disease, as well as chronic lung disease, diabetes, and dementia [49]. This study provided important information that chronic dehydration can also contribute to dementia.

It has been speculated that individuals who are dehydrated may increase inflammation in the body, and inflammation has been clearly shown to result in increased likelihood of dementia. For all of these reasons it is important to counsel individuals about maintenance of adequate hydration throughout all stages of life.

The National Academy of Medicine suggests that women consume around 6–9 cups (1.5–2.2 liters) of fluids daily and for men 8–12 cups (2–3 liters) each day. While water is recommended, other fluids such as coffee or tea or even alcoholic beverages such as beer can contribute to overall fluid consumption. Although in situations where alcohol or added sugar is consumed, the potential negative effects of beverages containing these substances must be considered before recommending them as part of an overall fluid intake. Water is certainly the safest and most reasonable recommendation for hydration.

16.3 FOOD GROUPS AND BEVERAGES

As already indicated, the vast majority of research in the area of nutrition and cognition now utilizes overall dietary patterns. Nonetheless, some literature exists that focuses on various food groups and beverages which also supports the role for nutrition in slowing cognitive decline.

- **Fruits and Vegetables**—Slower rates of cognitive decline and decreases of dementia have been reported in individuals who consume more vegetables and fruits. The highest level of benefits was found in individuals who consumed green leafy vegetables, which are a source of folate and flavonoids. Berries are also a good source of flavonoids.

- **Fish and Seafood**—Some support exists from observational studies for a potential beneficial association between fish and seafood consumption and improved cognitive outcomes [50,51]. These improved outcomes have been shown particularly in individuals who are carriers of APOE4, which suggests that the benefit of fish consumption for slowing the risk of dementia may pertain to those individuals with certain genetic backgrounds [52].
- **Meat, Legumes, and Dairy Products**—No association between meat or legume consumption and cognitive decline has been shown in the few studies that have examined these food groups. With regard to dairy products, few studies have been reported, and the results have been mixed. One study that followed individuals for 25–30 years showed the lower instance of vascular dementia in individuals over the age of 30 who consumed milk every day [52]. Another study found that the incidence of AD was reduced in participants over the age of 60 who reported daily consumption of milk.
- **Alcoholic Beverages**—The issue of alcoholic consumption, overall health, and cardiovascular health is complicated. Some studies support that consumption of moderate amounts of alcohol (two or fewer alcoholic drinks a day in men and one alcoholic drink in women) lowers the risk of cardiovascular disease, although this literature is mixed [53]. Regarding cognitive outcomes, similar benefits have been found in lower-risk cognitive decline with moderate consumption of alcoholic beverages. The same cautions about excessive alcohol drinking that applied to overall health and cardiovascular health also apply to cognitive health.
- **Nuts and Olive Oil**—Increased consumption of both nuts and olive oil in several clinical trials (components of PREDIMED) suggests there may be additional benefits in decreasing cognitive decline from nuts and olive oil; however, these occurred in the context of an overall Mediterranean diet (see next section) [54].
- **Coffee and Tea**—Coffee and tea are commonly consumed and the most common source of not only caffeine but also other biologically active compounds such as polyphenols [55–57]. It has been suggested that coffee ingredients include antioxidants and anti-inflammatory as well as neuro-protective effects. Once again, the studies are mixed with regard to coffee and tea consumption and reduction of risk of cognitive decline. Some studies have shown that moderate consumption of either tea or coffee (approximately three cups per day) may result in reduced likelihood of cognitive decline.

16.4 DIETARY PATTERNS

The most robust evidence supporting linkages between nutrition and cognition as well as lowering the risk of dementia comes from studies of dietary patterns rather than individual foods or nutrients. A number of different dietary patterns have been studied. The three most prominent ones, however, where evidence exists concerning the link between nutrition and reduced cognitive deterioration is the Mediterranean diet, the DASH Diet, and the MIND diet.

The Mediterranean diet is the most extensively studied healthy dietary pattern. The MedDiet features high intake of folate, vitamin E, carotenoids, and other antioxidants as well as monounsaturated fats and dietary fiber [54]. It also features a balanced intake of unsaturated fats and a moderately high intake of omega-3 fatty acids as well as low intake of saturated fatty acids. The MedDiet features high consumption of fruits, vegetables, whole grains, and olive oil, as well as nuts and seeds, It emphasis is on plant protein (legumes and seafood instead of red meat), wine in moderation (except in Muslim countries), and fermented berries. In some studies, the MedDiet has been supplemented with extra olive oil and extra nuts, which has further increased its benefits with regard to lowering the risk of cognitive decline. The MedDiet has been associated with reduced decline in performance on various cognitive test batteries as well as lowering the risk of dementia, mild cognitive impairment, and progression from mild cognitive impairment to dementia.

These findings have been supported by two large clinical trials that tested the Mediterranean Diet pattern in combination with nuts or olive oil versus advice for reduced dietary fat. These trials were included within a larger trial (PREDIMED) [54]. Another trial with fewer participants reported only six months follow-up [58]. The MedDiet improved performance on several neuropsychological test batteries compared to the habitual diet control group.

Meta-analyses of perspective cohort studies using the Mediterranean Diet have also been published and have reported a beneficial effect with adherence to the Mediterranean Diet to reduce risk of mild cognitive impairment, dementia, and AD.

The DASH diet has also been shown in a number of studies to lower the risk of cognitive decline [59–62]. This diet is high in potassium, magnesium, calcium, fiber, and protein and low in saturated fats, total lipids, cholesterol, and sodium. The DASH diet also features a high intake of folate, vitamin E, carotenoids, and other antioxidants. The DASH diet features a high consumption of fruits and vegetables, low-fat dairy products, and whole grains. It has a moderately high consumption of animal protein with low consumption of red meat and emphasizes foods that are low in saturated and trans lipids, sodium, and sugar.

The DASH diet was originally formulated for reducing systolic blood pressure. Subsequent versions of this diet, which include a more stringent reduction of sodium as well, have yielded further reductions in blood pressure. A study combining the DASH diet with increased physical activity resulted in even more substantial reductions in both systolic and diastolic blood pressure [63]. The MIND diet has been demonstrated to decrease the risk of AD and result in a slower decline in cognitive performance. This diet also emphasizes a high intake of folate, vitamin E, carotenoids, flavonoids, and other antioxidants as well as monounsaturated fats and decreased and trans fatty acids and maintaining a high intake of dietary fiber. The MIND diet increases the consumption of green leafy and other vegetables, nuts, berries, and beans and whole grains, fish, poultry, olive oil, and wine and a decrease in consumption of red meats, butter, margarine, cheese, pastries, sweets, and fried or fast foods [64].

Other diets that are currently being explored to examine the relationship between nutrition and lower the risk of cognitive decline include the Nordic diet [23], prudent diet, the anti-inflammatory Diet, the Healthy U.S.-Style Diet recommended by the Dietary Guidelines 2020–2025, and low GI diet.

A number of studies have also examined consumption of components of dietary patterns discussed earlier (MedDiet, DASH, and MIND diet) without formally utilizing these diets but emphasizing much of the components of these diets. These are called a priori studies and report numerous situations with components of the dietary patterns outlined here and appear to lower the risk of cognitive decline. Most of these studies involve data reduction methods rather than utilization of the specific dietary patterns employed in the MedDiet, DASH, and MIND diet.

16.4.1 DASH Diet

In one large study of 3,831 men age 65, individuals who were most adherent to either the DASH or MedDiet over a 11-year period of evaluation had consistently higher levels of cognitive function [6]. Whole grains, nuts, and legumes were also strongly associated with higher cognitive function. They represent protective foods common to various healthy plant-centered diets around the globe.

16.4.2 MIND Diet

It has been argued that the MIND diet is easier to follow than the Mediterranean diet, which calls for daily consumption of fish and three or four daily servings of each of the fruits and vegetables [64]. The MIND diet has 15 dietary components including 10 "brain healthy food groups" which are the following: Green leafy vegetables, other vegetables, nuts, berries, beans, whole grains, fish, poultry, and olive oil and also recommends decreased or minimal consumption of red meats, butter or stick margarine, cheese, pastries and sweets, and fried or fast food.

The recommendations for the MIND diet involve consuming at least three servings of whole grains, a salad, and one other vegetable every day along with a glass of wine. It also recommends snacking on most days on nuts or eating beans every other day or so. In addition, poultry and berries should be consumed at least once a week and fish at least once a week.

Individuals following this diet must limit eating the designated unhealthy foods (listed earlier) such as butter (less than one tablespoon a day), cheese, or fried or fast foods (less than a serving a week for any of the three). Berries are the only fruit that is specially included in the MIND diet, blueberries in particular with regard to brain health. Blueberries contain anthocyanins, which are potent antioxidants [65]. Research published by several investigators suggests that the MIND diet may reduce brain disease and decrease the risk of developing AD.

16.5 POTENTIAL MECHANISMS

One potential mechanism by which the MedDiet may protect against cognitive decline is through improving cardiovascular health and preventing cardiovascular disease due to better lipid composition featuring poly- and monounsaturated fats as opposed to saturated fats. In addition, the components of this diet may also yield antidiabetic effects, which can improve cognition by maintaining relatively stable blood glucose levels and reducing insulin. The brain is highly dependent on stable glucose levels, and insulin may exert inflammatory effects. In addition, the MedDiet, MIND, and DASH diets also feature increased consumption of antioxidants. Oxidative stress has been associated with declined cognitive performance. Some inflammation may damage the blood-brain barrier, contributing to a diminished cognitive performance. Additional potential mechanisms for linkages between nutrition and improved cognitive performance and decreased cognitive decline are currently topics of considerable research.

16.6 POTENTIAL CONFOUNDING FACTORS

It should be noted that when the MedDiet was studied, there were differences and outcomes between Mediterranean and non-Mediterranean countries. This finding suggests that possible effects of cognition may vary across geographic cultures and social demographic context. For example, cultural values and lifestyle in the Mediterranean area such as social connections and sense of community, meals cooked at home due to slower cooking methods, and times shared with family and friends rather than meals may partly contribute to discrepancies reported in these studies. It should be noted, however, that when the modified MedDiet has been utilized in Asian countries, similar results have been achieved, suggesting that the principles of the Mediterranean diet should be adapted to suit local food, cultures, and eating habits.

16.7 RELATIONSHIP WITH OTHER LIFESTYLE MEDICINE COMPONENTS

The nutritional strategies that have been employed in the Mediterranean, DASH, and MIND diets are consistent with the plant-based nutritional recommendations, which serve as a cornerstone for one of the pillars of lifestyle medicine [66]. It is also highly likely that other components for positive lifestyle habits and actions such as increased physical activity, weight management, avoiding tobacco products, positive connections to others, stress relief, and sleep are likely to also contribute to the reduced risk of cognitive decline.

It is clear from the initial studies that the dietary patterns found in the MedDiet, DASH, and MIND diet yield multiple benefits. Since these diets are loaded with antioxidants and other components that have favorable profiles, it is highly likely that it will be further evidence that proper nutrition can lower cognitive decline.

This provides another area where lifestyle medicine can play a significant role in helping individuals achieve healthy and fulfilling lives. Indeed, there are some studies that have now suggested that various lifestyle modalities, when used in combination with each other, can further lower the risk of cognitive decline. For example, the FINISH Geriatric Intervention Study to prevent cognitive impairment and disability (FINGER) was conducted in individuals aged 60–77 years with a high risk of dementia [15]. In this study, individual and group sessions with nutritionists who tailored participants' diets for increased consumption of fruits and vegetables, whole grain cereals, fish, low-fat milk, and low-fat meats and reduced consumption of sugar and butter as well as increased physical activity, cognitive training, and social activity slowed the onset of cognitive impairment and dementia. A smaller study in Korea has yielded similar benefits [4]. The area of multicomponent strategies including healthy nutrition to lower the risk of cognitive decline has emerged as a powerful and important added benefit of lifestyle habits and actions.

The area of other lifestyle factors that may improve cognition—physical activity—is perhaps the one that is most advanced. Various studies have shown that physical activity enhances brain cognition throughout the lifespan. Physical activity improves biomarkers of brain health and also decreases the likelihood of various dementias including AD.

The effects of physical activity on various biological markers of the brain underscore the ability of physical activity to enhance cognitive reserve [17]. The biological aspects of physical activity that impact on cognition include an increase in neurotransmitters and neurotrophic factors, which allow increased growth and survival of neurons. In addition, physical activity enhances connections between neurons classified as synaptogenesis, as well as growth of neurons (neurogenesis) and increased cerebral blood flow (angiogenesis) [67]. In addition, several research projects have shown that regular physical activity results in a reduction of age-related cognitive decline and, in some instances, a reversal of neuro-decline (i.e. neurogenesis and synaptogenesis).

Several studies have shown an increase in brain volume of both gray and white matter after six months of aerobic exercise intervention [68]. Physical activity may also delay symptoms associated with dementia in the normal aging process [69]. Emerging literature on individuals with advanced AD have shown mixed results in the area of physical activity; however, it is important to emphasize that individuals who have mild cognitive impairment (MCI) have demonstrated significant improvement in executive function with increased physical activity. This is important since MCI is thought to often lead to AD. The fact that exercise seems to be more important to MCI than AD suggests that physical activity is more likely to yield benefits as a long-term intervention. Thus, changes in physical activity earlier in life are very important to lowering the risk of AD. Increased physical activity should join proper nutrition as lifelong strategies to lower the risk of dementias in general and AD in particular.

16.8 CONCLUSIONS

Emerging data have now suggested that positive dietary patterns such as the MedDiet, DASH, and MIND diet can all lower the risk of cognitive decline. These diets, which are basically plant based, feature increases in fruits and vegetables, whole grains, legumes, and nuts. They are loaded with antioxidants and contain high levels of health-enhancing vitamins while lowering saturated fat and reducing sugar and salt. All of these measures are key components of an overall healthy diet and have been shown to reduce the risk of cardiovascular disease and diabetes and obesity. It is clear that this field is rapidly emerging and suggests that lifelong strategies reduce the risk of all forms of dementia, including AD, and can be impacted in significant ways by nutritional patterns as well as other lifestyle modalities.

Clinical Applications

- Lifestyle medicine practitioners should emphasize to all patients that strategies of sound nutrition that increase fruits and vegetables, whole grains, nuts, seeds, and legumes are all likely to not only yield benefits for reducing metabolic disease but also likely to decrease the likelihood of cognitive decline.
- Recommendations to follow such dietary patterns as the MedDiet, DASH diet, and the MIND diet to lower the risk of cognitive decline add another layer of benefit for daily habits and actions to improve overall health and quality of life.

REFERENCES

1. Gorelick P, Furie K, Iadecola C, et al. American Heart Association/American Stroke Association: Defining optimal brain health in adults: A presidential advisory from the American Heart Association/American Stroke Association. Stroke. 2017;48(10): e284–e303.
2. Winblad B, Amouyel P, Andrieu S, et al. Defeating Alzheimer's disease and other dementias: A priority for European science and society. Lancet Neurol. 2016;15(5):455–532.
3. Alzheimer's Association 2013. Alzheimer's Disease Facts and Figures. Alzheimer's Dement. 2013;9(2):208–245.
4. Scarmeas N, Anastasiou C, Yannakoulia M. Nutrition and prevention of cognitive impairment. Lancet Neurol. 2018;17(11):1006–1015.
5. Chen X, Maguire B, Brodaty H, et al. Dietary patterns and cognitive health in older adults: A systematic review. J Alzheimers Dis. 2019;67(2):583–619. https://doi.org/10.3233/JAD-180468. Erratum in: J Alzheimers Dis. 2019;69(2):595–596.
6. Wengreen H, Munger R, Cutler A, et al. Prospective study of dietary approaches to stop hypertension-and Mediterranean-style dietary patterns and age-related cognitive change: The cache county study on memory, health and aging. Am J Clin Nutr. 2013;98(5):1263–1271.
7. Valls-Pedret C, Sala-Vila A, Serra-Mir M, et al. Mediterranean diet and age-related cognitive decline: A randomized clinical trial. JAMA Intern Med. 2015 Jul;175(7):1094–1103. Erratum in: JAMA Intern Med. 2018;1;178(12):1731–1732.
8. Radd-Vagenas S, Duffy S, Naismith S, et al. Effect of the Mediterranean diet on cognition and brain morphology and function: A systematic review of randomized controlled trials. Am J Clin Nutr. 2018;1;107(3):389–404.
9. Shannon O, Stephan B, Granic A, et al. Mediterranean diet adherence and cognitive function in older UK adults: The European Prospective Investigation into Cancer and Nutrition-Norfolk (EPIC-Norfolk) study. Am J Clin Nutr. 2019;1;110(4):938–948.
10. Gehlich K, Beller J, Lange-Asschenfeldt B, et al. Consumption of fruits and vegetables: Improved physical health, mental health, physical functioning and cognitive health in older adults from 11 European countries. Aging Ment Health. 2020;24(4):634–641.
11. Bianchi V, Herrera P, Laura R. Effect of nutrition on neurodegenerative diseases: A systematic review. Nutr Neurosci. 2021;24(10):810–834.
12. Hooshmand B, Mangialasche F, Kalpouzos G, et al. Association of vitamin B12, folate, and sulfur amino acids with brain magnetic resonance imaging measures in older adults:

A longitudinal population-based study. JAMA Psychiatry. 2016 Jun 1;73(6):606–613. Erratum in: JAMA Psychiatry. 2016 Jun 1;73(6):640.
13. Luciano M, Corley J, Cox S, et al. Mediterranean-type diet and brain structural change from 73 to 76 years in a Scottish cohort. Neurology. 2017;31;88(5):449–455.
14. Lee K, Lee Y, Back J, et al. Effects of a multidomain lifestyle modification on cognitive function in older adults: An eighteen month community-based cluster randomized controlled trial. Psychother Psychosom. 2014;83:270–278.
15. Ngandu T, Lehtisalo J, Solomon A, et al. A 2 year multidomain intervention of diet, exercise, cognitive training, and vascular risk monitoring versus control to prevent cognitive decline in at-risk elderly people (FINGER): A randomised controlled trial. Lancet. 2015;385:2255–2263.
16. Moll van Charante E, Richard E, Eurelings L, et al. Effectiveness of a 6-year multidomain vascular care intervention to prevent dementia (preDIVA): A cluster-randomised controlled trial. Lancet. 2016;388:797–805.
17. Rippe J, Petruzzello S. Influence of physical activity on brain aging and cognition. In Rippe JM (ed). Lifestyle Medine, 4th edition. Boca Raton: CRC Press, 2024.
18. Valls-Pedret C, Sala-Vila A, Serra-Mir M, et al. Mediterranean diet and age-related cognitive decline: A randomized clinical trial. JAMA Intern Med. 2015;175:1094–1103.
19. Martinez-Lapiscina E, Clavero P, Toledo E, et al. Mediterranean diet improves cognition: The PREDIMED-NAVARRA randomised trial. J Neurol Neurosurg Psychiatry. 2013;84:1318–1325.
20. Knight A, Bryan J, Wilson C, et al. The Mediterranean diet and cognitive function among healthy older adults in a 6-month randomised controlled trial: The MedLey study. Nutrients. 2016;8:E579.
21. Singh B, Parsaik A, Mielke M, et al. Association of Mediterranean diet with mild cognitive impairment and Alzheimer's disease: A systematic review and meta-analysis. J Alzheimer's Dis. 2014;39:271–282.
22. Sofi F, Abbate R, Gensini G, et al. Accruing evidence on benefits of adherence to the Mediterranean diet on health: An updated systematic review and meta-analysis. Am J Clin Nutr. 2010;92(5):1189–1196.
23. Shakersain B, Rizzuto D, Larsson S, et al. The Nordic prudent diet reduces risk of cognitive decline in the Swedish older adults: A population-based cohort study. Nutrients. 2018;10:E229.
24. Gu Y, Nieves J, Stern Y, Luchsinger J, et al. Food combination and Alzheimer disease risk: A protective diet. Arch Neurol. 2010;67:699–706.
25. U.S. Department of Agriculture and U.S. Department of Health and Human Services. *Dietary GuidelinesforAmericans, 2020–2025*, 9thedition. December2020. DietaryGuidelines.gov (Accessed January 3, 2024).
26. Lichtenstein A, Appel L, Vadiveloo M, et al. 2021 dietary guidance to improve cardiovascular health: A scientific statement from the American Heart Association. Circulation. 2021;144(23):e472-e487.
27. Hayden K, Beavers D, Steck S, et al. The association between an inflammatory diet and global cognitive function and incident dementia in older women: The women's health initiative memory study. Alzheimer's Dement. 2017;13(11):1187–1196.
28. Ozawa M, Shipley M, Kivimaki M, et al. Dietary pattern, inflammation and cognitive decline: The whitehall II prospective cohort study. Clin Nutr. 2017;36(2):506–512.
29. Mecocci P, Boccardi V, Cecchetti R, et al. A long journey into aging, brain aging, and Alzheimer's disease following the oxidative stress tracks. J Alzheimer's Dis. 2018;62: 1319–1335.
30. Engelhart M, Geerlings M, Ruitenberg A, et al. Dietary intake of antioxidants and risk of Alzheimer disease. JAMA. 2002;287:3223–3229.

31. Zandi P, Anthony J, Khachaturian A, et al. Reduced risk of Alzheimer's disease in users of antioxidant vitamin supplements: The cache county study. Arch Neurol. 2004;61:82–88.
32. Morris M, Evans D, Tangney C, et al. Relation of the tocopherol forms to incident Alzheimer disease and to cognitive change. Am J Clin Nutr. 2005;81:508–514.
33. Devore E, Grodstein F, van Rooij F, et al. Dietary antioxidants and long-term risk of dementia. Arch Neurol. 2010;67:819–825.
34. Feart C, Letenneur L, Helmer C, et al. Plasma carotenoids are inversely associated with dementia risk in an elderly French cohort. J Gerontol A Biol Sci Med Sci. 2016; 71:683–688.
35. Commenges D, Scotet V, Renaud S, et al. Intake of flavonoids and risk of dementia. Eur J Epidemiol. 2000;16:357–363.
36. Letenneur L, Proust-Lima C, Le Gouge A, et al. Flavonoid intake and cognitive decline over a 10-year period. Am J Epidemiol. 2007;165:1364–1371.
37. Kesse-Guyot E, Fezeu L, Andreeva V, et al. Total and specific polyphenol intakes in midlife are associated with cognitive function measured 13 years later. J Nutr. 2012;142:76–83.
38. Root M, Ravine E, Harper A. Flavonol intake and cognitive decline in middle-aged adults. J Med Food. 2015;18:1327–1332.
39. Devore E, Kang J, Breteler M, et al. Dietary intakes of berries and flavonoids in relation to cognitive decline. Ann Neurol. 2012;72:135–43.
40. Jayedi A, Rashidy-Pour A, Shab-Bidar S. Vitamin D status and risk of dementia and Alzheimer's disease: A meta-analysis of dose-response. Nutr Neurosci. 2018;21:1–10.
41. Eskelinen M, Ngandu T, Helkala E, et al. Fat intake at midlife and cognitive impairment later in life: A population-based CAIDE study. Int J Geriatr Psychiatry. 2008;23(7):741–747.
42. Kumar A, Palfrey H, Pathak R, et al. The metabolism and significance of homocysteine in nutrition and health. Nutr Metable (Lond). 2017;22;14:78.
43. Durga J, van Boxtel M, Schouten E, et al. Effect of 3-year folic acid supplementation on cognitive function in older adults in the FACIT Trial: A randomised, double blind, controlled trial. Lancet. 2007;369:208–216.
44. Andreeva V, Kesse-Guyot E, Barberger-Gateau P, et al. Cognitive function after supplementation with B vitamins and long-chain omega-3 fatty acids: Ancillary findings from the SU.FOL.OM3 randomized trial. Am J Clin Nutr. 2011;94:278–286.
45. Yurko-Mauro K, McCarthy D, Rom D, et al. Beneficial effects of docosahexaenoic acid on cognition in age-related cognitive decline. Alzheimer's & Dementia: The Journal of the Alzheimer's Association. 2010;6(6):456–464.
46. Devore E, Stampfer M, Breteler M, et al. Dietary fat intake and cognitive decline in women with type 2 diabetes. Diabetes Care. 2009;32(4):635–640.
47. NIH/National Heart, Lung and Blood Institute. Good hydration linked to healthy aging. News Release. January 2, 2023. www.nhlbi.nih.gov/news/2023/good-hydration-linked-healthy-aging (Accessed January 3, 2024).
48. Popkin B, D'Anci K, Rosenberg I. Water, hydration, and health. Nutr Rev. 2010;68(8): 439–458.
49. Dmitrieva N, Gagarin A, Liu D, et al. Middle-age high normal serum sodium as a risk factor for accelerated biological aging, chronic diseases, and premature mortality. eBio-Medicine. 2023:104404.
50. Samieri C, Morris M, Bennette D, et al. Fish intake, genetic predisposition to Alzheimer disease, and decline in global cognition and memory in 5 cohorts of older persons. Am J Epidemiol. 2018;187:933–940.
51. Barberger-Gateau P, Raffaitin C, Letenneur L, et al. Dietary patterns and risk of dementia: The three-city cohort study. Neurology. 2007;69:1921–1930.

52. Ozawa M, Ohara T, Ninomiya T, et al. Milk and dairy consumption and risk of dementia in an elderly Japanese population: The Hisayama study. J Am Geriatr Soc. 2014;62: 1224–1230.
53. O'Keefe E, Di Nicolantonio J, O'Keefe J, et al. Alcohol and CV health: Jekyll and Hyde J-curves. Prog Cardiovasc Dis. 2018;61:68–75.
54. Estruch R, Ros E, Salas-Salvadó J, et al. Primary prevention of cardiovascular disease with a Mediterranean diet. N Engl J Med. 2013;368:1279–1290.
55. Wang Y, Ho C. Polyphenolic chemistry of tea and coffee: A century of progress. J Agric Food Chem. 2009;57(18):8109–8114.
56. Islam M, Tabrez S, Jabir N, et al. An insight on the therapeutic potential of major coffee components. Curr Drug Metable. 2018;19:544–556.
57. Mirza S, Tiemeier H, de Bruijn R, et al. Coffee consumption and incident dementia. Eur J Epidemiol. 2014;29:735–741.
58. Psaltopoulou T, Sergentanis T, Panagiotakos D, Kosti R, Scarmeas N. Mediterranean diet, stroke, cognitive impairment, and depression: A meta-analysis. Ann Neurol. 2013;74:580–591.
59. Berendsen A, Kang J, van de Rest O, et al. The dietary approaches to stop hypertension diet, cognitive function, and cognitive decline in American older women. J Am Med Dir Assoc. 2017;1;18(5):427–432.
60. Morris M, Tangney C, Wang Y, et al. MIND Diet associated with reduced incidence of Alzheimer's disease. Alzheimer's Dement. 2015;11(9):1007–1014.
61. Solfrizzi V, Custodero C, Lozupone M, et al. Relationships of dietary patterns, foods, and micro-and macronutrients with Alzheimer's disease and late-life cognitive disorders: A systematic review. J Alzheimer's Dis. 2017;59(3):815–849.
62. Folsom A, Parker E, Harnack L. Degree of concordance with DASH diet guidelines and incidence of hypertension and fatal cardiovascular disease. Am J Hypertens. 2007;20(3):225–232.
63. Ai M, Morris T, Ordway C, et al. The Daily Activity Study of Health (DASH): A pilot randomized controlled trial to enhance physical activity in sedentary older adults. Contemp Clin Trials. 2021;106:106405.
64. Marcason W. What are the components to the MIND diet? J Acad Nutr Diet. 2015; 115:1744.
65. Di Fiore N. Diet may help prevent Alzheimer's: MIND diet rich in vegetables, berries, whole grains, nuts. Rush University Medical Center website. www.rush.edu/news/diet-may-help-prevent-alzheimers (Accessed February 1, 2024).
66. ACLM Website. https://lifestylemedicine.org/ (Accessed January 3, 2024).
67. Physical Activity Guidelines Advisory Committee. 2018 physical activity guidelines advisory committee. 2018 Physical Activity Guidelines Advisory Committee Scientific Report. Washington, DC. Department of Health and Health and Human Services. 2018.
68. Tan Z, Spartano N, Beiser A, et al. Physical activity, brain volume, and dementia risk: The framingham study. J Gerontol A Biol Sci Med Sci. 2017;1;72(6):789–795.
69. Kayes M. Hatfield B. Influence of physical activity on brain aging and cognition: The role of cognitive reserve, thresholds for decline, genetic influence, and the investment hypothesis. In Rippe JM (ed). Lifestyle Medicine, 3rd edition. Boca Raton: CRC Press, 2019.

17 Nutrition and Peripheral Artery Disease

Key Points

- Peripheral artery disease (PAD) is a common and serious manifestation of systemic atherosclerosis.
- Nutritional components of the risk reduction for PAD are important and include following healthy plant-based diets, perhaps supplemented with additional anti-inflammatory and antioxidative vitamins and nontropical plant-based oils.
- A two- to four-fold increase in the prevalence of PAD exists among smokers compared to nonsmokers.
- Structured exercise programs can play a very important role not only in reducing the risk of PAD but also in treating symptoms such as claudication.

17.1 INTRODUCTION

PAD is a narrowing of the arteries or blockage in the arteries that carry blood from the heart to either the legs or the arms. PAD is primarily caused by a buildup of plaque in the arteries which is due to the process of atherosclerosis [1]. While PAD can happen in any blood vessel, it is more common in the legs than in the arms.

Multiple risk factors for PAD have been demonstrated, but nutrition is one of the most significant ones [2–10]. Other risk factors include smoking, high blood pressure, diabetes, high cholesterol, age above 60 years, and a sedentary lifestyle [1,11,12]. All of these contribute to atherosclerosis (see Chapter 11). People with PAD demonstrate an increased risk for developing coronary heart disease (CHD) and cerebrovascular disease (stroke). (See also Chapters 12 and 14.)

PAD is highly prevalent. Atherosclerotic plaques of the femoral artery have been reported to affect up to two-thirds of subjects aged 56–77 years old. The prevalence of PAD increases linearly with age.

PAD is significantly underdiagnosed since it is often asymptomatic for over ten years prior to manifesting any symptoms. Symptoms may include pain in the legs during physical activity such as walking which improves with rest. It should be noted that up to 40% of people with PAD have no leg pain. Symptoms of pain, aches, or cramps with walking are called "claudication" and can happen in the buttock, hip, thigh, or calf [13]. Other physical signs that may indicate PAD include muscle atrophy (weakness), hair loss in the extremities, smooth shiny skin, or skin that is cool to the touch, especially accompanied by pain while walking [13,14]. Decreased or absent pulses in the feet are often present and sometimes sores or ulcers in the leg or feet that do not heal [14].

DOI: 10.1201/9781003452607-17

Since multiple factors contribute to PAD, it may be difficult to determine exactly which ones are most prominent. Various risk factors, however, are related to nutrition such as low serum high-density (HDL) cholesterol and elevated total serum cholesterol.

PAD is thought to represent typically a more advanced form of systemic atherosclerosis than simply coronary heart disease (CHD). Moreover, multiple nutritional factors either contribute to or lower the risk of PAD. PAD seems to be particularly sensitive to influences of oxidation and inflammation. These are vulnerabilities which may explain the role of certain nutrients in reducing the risk of PAD.

Multiple other lifestyle-related factors may also contribute to increased risk of PAD. These include an inactive lifestyle and cigarette smoking. Structured walking programs are a key component in the therapy of PAD and are often combined with nutritional recommendations. The consumption of a healthy diet as well as regular physical activity and smoking cessation are recognized by multiple organizations as keys to either lowering the risk of PAD or treating it if it already exists. PAD is typically diagnosed with the combination of symptoms (e.g. claudication) or an ankle/brachial index (ABI) of less than 0.90 [15].

17.2 PAD AND CVD

PAD affects practically 8–12 million Americans. As already indicated, it is often underdiagnosed, so a high level of suspicion should be practiced by all physicians as well as familiarity with the various ways that PAD can present itself [16,17]. The prevalence of PAD increases with age. PAD is present in only 2–3% of people under the age of 50 years, but up to 29% of individuals over the age of 70 years [18]. Up to 60% of individuals with PAD will also have concomitant CHD and/or cerebrovascular disease [18]. Patients with PAD have a two to four times increased risk of cardiovascular and total mortality. While nutritional factors for reducing the risk of PAD are similar to those for reducing atherosclerosis in the coronary and cerebral arteries, some differences exist that have been reported. This impacts on how nutrition should be approached by individuals who either have or are at risk for PAD.

17.3 NUTRITION AND PAD

Numerous studies have demonstrated that fruits, vegetables, and antioxidants as well as fats and nontropical plant oils, and dietary fiber, as well as nuts and polyunsaturated fat, all lower the risk of PAD [1–10]. In contrast, saturated fat, dietary cholesterol, and processed meat are all associated with higher cardiovascular events in patients suffering from PAD.

In one longitudinal study, moderate alcohol intake significantly lowered the risk of PAD. Vitamin C has also been hypothesized to possess an antiatherogenic effect based on the association between PAD and subclinical vitamin C levels [19–22]. In addition, omega-3 fatty acids (mostly found in fish), which have been demonstrated to be effective in both the prevention and treatment of CHD, have also been hypothesized to lower the risk of PAD [23–27]. Several studies have shown that vitamin E intake also may reduce the risk of PAD [28,29]. Presumably, the effects of both vitamin C and vitamin E relate to their antioxidant effects. Good sources of vitamin

E include vegetable oils such as wheat germ, sunflower, and safflower oils; nuts (such as peanuts, walnuts, and especially almonds); and seeds (such as sunflower seeds).

17.4 DIETARY PATTERNS AND PAD

The Prevención con Dieta Mediterránea (PREDIMED) multicenter trial, with a Mediterranean diet (MedDiet) supplemented with extra-virgin olive oil or supplemented with nuts, showed a reduction of risk of PAD of 34% in the MedDiet plus extra-virgin olive oil group and 50% reduction in the MedDiet plus nuts group compared to the control group. These findings suggest that other healthy dietary patterns could also substantially lower the risk of PAD [30]. These finding are also consistent with multiple trials which have shown that the MedDiet lowers the risk of CHD. This is not surprising given that the underlying pathophysiology of both conditions is atherosclerosis.

In contrast in the MedDiet, there was an adverse impact for PAD for saturated fat, fatty acids, meat, and refined grains. A retrospective study of premenopausal Italian women showed that low adherence to the MedDiet increased the risk of atherosclerosis compared to the Italian population in general. In the United States in 2015, daily consumption of nuts (more than twice weekly) was associated with 21% lower odds of developing PAD [7]. Another study of 294 Swedish adults utilized an inflammatory diet index consisting of 12 foods with anti-inflammatory potential, including fruits and vegetables, whole grains, olive oil and canola oil, chocolate, legumes, red wine, and beer, and showed a 16% reduction in risk of PAD compared to individuals in the pro-inflammatory diet, which included processed red meat, organ meats, potato chips, and soft drink beverages. These findings were only exhibited in current and past smokers but not in never smokers. Thus, a variety of different dietary patterns have been demonstrated to lower the risk of PAD.

17.5 DIETARY QUALITY AND PAD

Data from the Women's Health Initiative, which is a large trial of over 138,000 postmenopausal women with no PAD at baseline, showed that dietary quality was associated with PAD risk. Dietary quality was assessed with the alternative Mediterranean Diet Index [7], Alternative Healthy Eating Index 2010, the Dietary Approaches to Stop Hypertension Diet Index, and the Healthy Eating Index 2015 and showed between 21% and 34% decreased risk of PAD in individuals who adhered to healthy diets. Among the contributing food groups and nutrients associated with lower risk of PAD were intakes of legumes, dietary fiber, and vegetable protein. In contrast, intakes of red meat, processed meat, and regular soft drinks was associated with higher risk. These findings further suggest that following healthy nutritional pattern lowers the risk of PAD.

17.6 NUTRITION AND THE ENDOTHELIUM

As outlined in the chapter on atherosclerosis, the endothelium, which represents the inner lining of arteries, is a critically important defense against atherosclerosis

[31–38]. Most studies have shown that dysfunction of the endothelium is particularly significant as a risk factor for PAD. Dysfunction of the endothelium represents an early inciting event for atherosclerosis. In addition, endothelial dysfunction reduces the generation of nitric oxide (NO), which is the key element for allowing arterial vasodilation. Modulation of endothelial function is a likely mechanism through which medical nutrition therapy targeting the diet response of risk factors to pro-inflammatory and pro-oxidative nutrients may be the underlying reason why healthy plant-based diets lower the risk of PAD. Multiple nutritional components have been shown to have positive effects on the endothelium. These include red wine, which is a good source of the polyphenol resveratrol, and other polyphenols which modulate systemic pro-inflammatory and pro-oxidative factors associated with endothelial dysfunction. In addition, nutrients such as omega-3 fatty acids, L-arginine, folic acid, cacao, and green leaf tea have all been shown to have a positive effect on endothelial health.

17.7 MALNUTRITION AND FOOD INSECURITY AND PAD

Various forms of malnutrition are common in vascular surgery patients who are undergoing procedures for PAD [34]. In one tertiary care vascular surgery unit utilizing a standard screening tool for malnutrition (Malnutrition Universal Screen Tool—MUST) between 12% and 15% of individuals admitted with PAD were malnourished. When micronutrients were examined, 79% showed low vitamin C, 56% showed low vitamin D, and over 40% low zinc, B_{12}, and folate. These findings are consistent with food insecurity, particularly in the elderly population. Food insecurity may adversely impact on diet. Food-insecure individuals often consume a diet high in energy-dense foods containing large amounts of sodium and sugar, which tend to be less expensive than foods contained in healthy plant-based diets [34]. These data were confirmed in a large study of over 2,000 adults with PAD over the age of 60 which showed that older individuals who were food insecure increased their risk of PAD by 50%. While the exact etiology of this significant increase is not completely understood, previous literature suggests that a connection exists between food insecurity, diets, and chronic diseases such as diabetes and hypertension, which are significant risk factors for PAD. Thus, food insecurity needs to be taken into consideration when treating adults with PAD to help decrease poor health outcomes associated with insufficient amounts of nutritious food.

17.8 BEYOND THE HEART-HEALTHY DIET FOR PAD

While there are multiple similarities in the underlying pathophysiology between CHD and PAD, there are some nuanced differences which may make nutritional patterns for PAD more specific and efficacious in addition to the general dietary pattern recommended for CHD.

The 2013 American Heart Association (AHA) and American College of Cardiology (ACC) Guidelines endorsed a "heart-healthy lifestyle" [35]. This guidance included a general framework for incorporating health and nutrition into lifestyle management to improve blood pressure and lipid control. Broad nutrient categories are associated with improved cardiovascular outcomes (e.g. fruits and vegetables, whole grains, legumes). These guidelines also recommend employing nutritional strategies to reduce low-density lipoprotein cholesterol (LDL-C) including a maximum of 5–6% of total calories from saturated fat and minimizing foods in trans fats.

PAD is often present at the severe end of the atherosclerotic syndromes. Individuals with PAD tend to have greater systemic inflammatory burden, higher blood pressure, higher triglyceride levels, and deficiency in various antioxidants and minerals. They also experience significantly higher mortality than individuals with CHD only. For this reason, some researchers have advised that patients with PAD should follow a diet that is specialized to address nutritional alterations associated with the disease. Such a nutritional pattern promotes intake of further anti-inflammatory- and antioxidant-rich foods [3]. Individuals with PAD who already have claudication often have diets high in saturated fat, sodium, and cholesterol and low in fiber, vitamin E, and folate intake. Studies have shown that nutritional patterns high in vitamins A, C, E, B_6, and B_{12} are associated with lower odds of having PAD. In addition, intake of fiber and omega-3 polyunsaturated fatty acids (PUFAs) are correlated with reduced prevalence of PAD.

It is therefore recommended by some researchers that diets that contain these demonstrated anti-inflammatory and antioxidant measures should be emphasized in addition to following the general guidance from the AHA and ACC [10]. Further research will be needed in this area to confirm that these slight modifications to the AHA/ACC recommendations are appropriate for specifically lowering the risk of PAD.

17.9 OTHER LIFESTYLE MEASURES AND PAD

In addition to following healthy nutritional patterns to lower the risk of PAD, multiple other lifestyle measures have been demonstrated to help reduce the likelihood of developing PAD or, if it is already present, to assist with its treatment. These lifestyle measures include increases in physical activity, smoking cessation, and weight management. In the area of physical activity, research data suggest that individuals with claudication should participate in structured physical activity. Structured physical activity has been demonstrated to improve the symptoms of claudication [36–42]. Simply advising increased walking has not been demonstrated to improve claudication. Smoking cessation is essential, since cigarette smoking is strongly associated with PAD. Smoking exerts potent oxidated and inflammatory effects [43–49]. Weight management is also very important since it can reduce both inflammation and oxidative stress.

An overall comprehensive approach to lifestyle measures including healthy plant-based nutrition and increased physical activity, smoking cessation, and weight management in combination are effective for lowering the risk of and assisting in the treatment of PAD [36,50,51]. In the area of weight management, abdominal obesity has been clearly associated with increased PAD in both prospective and cross sectional studies [52].

17.10 CONCLUSIONS

PAD is a common manifestation of systemic atherosclerosis associated with multiple core morbidities and can be the result of poor-quality diet and low levels of physical activity. Many of the nutritional recommendations for reducing the risk of PAD are similar to those of demonstrated efficacy in healthy plant-based diets. There are some additional considerations that merit potential recommendations, including increasing the amount of anti-inflammatory and antioxidative vitamins and other nutrients over and above the healthy plant-based diet recommended by the AHA and ACC. Since PAD is often asymptomatic for the first ten years of its development, physicians should maintain a high level of suspicion for PAD, since individuals with the condition are particularly prone to have other manifestations of systemic atherosclerosis including CHD and stroke.

Clinical Applications

- Since a common underlying etiology of atherosclerosis exists for PAD, CHD, and stroke, clinicians should be highly suspicious to check for peripheral pulses during clinical examination and also inquire about symptoms that individuals may have.
- Treatment of PAD involves not only following healthy plant-based diets but also employing other nutritional considerations such as additional nutrients to lower inflammation and oxidative stress.
- Nutritional strategies should be supplemented with other lifestyle habits and practices such as increased physical activity, smoking cessation, and weight management to lower the risk of PAD.
- Since PAD is often asymptomatic for at least ten years, physicians should have a high level of suspicion particularly in patients over the age of 60 years old to inquire about any signs or symptoms of PAD as well as monitoring peripheral pulses and obtaining other measurements such as ABI in individuals with suspected PAD.

REFERENCES

1. Gerhard-Herman M, Gornik H, Barrett C, et al. 2016 AHA/ACC guideline on the management of patients with lower extremity peripheral artery disease: Executive summary: A report of the American College of Cardiology/American Heart Association task force on clinical practice guidelines. Circulation. 2017;135(12):e686–e725.
2. Delaney C, Smale M, Miller M. Nutritional considerations for peripheral arterial disease: A narrative review. Nutrients. 2019;11(6):1219.
3. Nosova E, Conte M, Grenon S. Advancing beyond the “heart-healthy diet” for peripheral arterial disease. J Vasc Surg. 2015;61(1):265–274.
4. Yuan S, Bruzelius M, Damrauer S, et al. Anti-inflammatory diet and incident peripheral artery disease: Two prospective cohort studies. Clin Nutr. 2022;41(6):1191–1196.
5. Antonelli-Incalzi R, Pedone C, McDermott M, et al. Association between nutrient intake and peripheral artery disease: results from the In CHIANTI study. Atherosclerosis. 2006;186(1):200–206.
6. Wan D, Li V, Banfield L, et al. Diet and nutrition in peripheral artery disease: A systematic review. Can J Cardiol. 2022;38(5):672–680.
7. Chen G-C, Arthur R, Mossavar-Rahmani Y, et al. Adherence to recommended eating patterns is associated with lower risk of peripheral arterial disease: Results from the women’s health initiative. Hypertension. 2021;78(2):447–455.

8. Adegbola A, Behrendt C-A, Zyriax B-C, et al. The impact of nutrition on the development and progression of peripheral artery disease: A systematic review. Clin Nutr. 2022;41(1):49–70.
9. Centers for Disease Control and Prevention. Peripheral Arterial Disease (PAD). Peripheral Arterial Disease (PAD) | cdc.gov (Accessed January 8, 2024).
10. NIH U.S. National Library of Medicine. Effects of plant-based diet on peripheral arterial disease. Effects of Plant-Based Diet on Peripheral Arterial Disease—Full Text View—ClinicalTrials.gov (Accessed January 8, 2024).
11. Bonaca M, Creager M. Peripheral artery disease. In Zipes, Libby, Bonow, Mann, and Tomaselli (eds). Braunwald's Heart Disease, 11th edition. Amsterdam: Elsevier, 2019: 1328–1347.
12. Brevetti G, Giugliano G, Brevetti L, et al. Inflammation in peripheral artery disease. Circulation. 2010;122(18):1862–1875.
13. McDermott M. Lower extremity manifestations of peripheral artery disease: The pathophysiologic and functional implications of leg ischemia. Circ Res. 2015;116(9):1540–1550.
14. Hiatt W, Armstrong E, Larson C, et al. Pathogenesis of the limb manifestations and exercise limitations in peripheral artery disease. Circ Res. 2015;116(9):1527–1539.
15. Aboyans V, Criqui M, Abraham P, et al. Measurement and interpretation of the ankle-brachial index: A scientific statement from the American heart association. Circulation. 2012;126(24):2890–2909.
16. Fowkes F, Rudan D, Rudan I, et al. Comparison of global estimates of prevalence and risk factors for peripheral artery disease in 2000 and 2010: A systematic review and analysis. Lancet. 2013;382(9901):1329–1340.
17. Pande R, Perlstein T, Beckman J, et al. Secondary prevention and mortality in peripheral artery disease: National health and nutrition examination study, 1999 to 2004. Circulation. 2011;124(1):17–23.
18. Criqui M, Aboyans V. Epidemiology of peripheral artery disease. Circ Res. 2015;116(9): 1509–1526.
19. Lopes AOC. Vitamin C, B-complex vitamins and inflammation. In Garg M (eds). Nutrition and Physical Activity in Inflammation Diseases. Oxfordshire, UK: CABI International. 2013: 99–111.
20. Ford ES, Liu S, Mannino DM, et al. C-reactive protein concentration and concentrations of blood vitamins, carotenoids, and selenium among United States adults. Eur J Clin Nutr. 2003;57(9):1157–1163.
21. Wannamethee SG, Lowe GD, Rumley A, et al. Associations of vitamin C status, fruit and vegetable intakes, and markers of inflammation and hemostasis. Am J Clin Nutr. 2006; 83(3):567–574.
22. Langlois M, Duprez D, Delanghe J, et al. Serum vitamin C concentration is low in peripheral arterial disease and is associated with inflammation and severity of atherosclerosis. Circulation. 2001;10;103(14):1863–1868.
23. Holy E, Forestier M, Richter E, et al. Dietary alpha-linolenic acid inhibits arterial thrombus formation, tissue factor expression, and platelet activation. Arterioscler Thromb Vasc Biol. 2011;31(8):1772–1780.
24. Casula M, Soranna D, Catapano A, et al. Long-term effect of high dose omega-3 fatty acid supplementation for secondary prevention of cardiovascular outcomes: A meta-analysis of randomized, placebo controlled trials [corrected]. Atheroscler Suppl. 2013; 14(2):243–251.
25. Rizos E, Ntzani E, Bika E, et al. Association between omega-3 fatty acid supplementation and risk of major cardiovascular disease events: A systematic review and meta-analysis. JAMA. 2012;308(10):1024–1033.

26. Kotwal S, Jun M, Sullivan D, et al. Omega 3 fatty acids and cardiovascular outcomes: systematic review and meta-analysis. Circ Cardiovasc Qual Outcomes. 2012;5(6):808–818.
27. Roncaglioni M, Tombesi M, Avanzini F, et al. Ω-3 fatty acids in patients with multiple cardiovascular risk factors. N Engl J Med. 2013;368(19):1800–1808.
28. Gardner A, Bright B, Ort K, et al. Dietary intake of participants with peripheral artery disease and claudication. Angiology. 2011;62(3):270–275.
29. Carrero JJ, Grimble RF. Does nutrition have a role in peripheral vascular disease? Br J Nutr. 2006;95(2):217–229.
30. Ruiz-Canela M, Estruch R, Corella D, et al. Association of Mediterranean diet with peripheral artery disease: The PREDIMED randomized trial. JAMA. 2014;311(4):415–417.
31. Moss J, Ramji D. Nutraceutical therapies for atherosclerosis. Nat Rev Cardiol. 2016;13(9):513–532.
32. Torres N, Guevara-Cruz M, Velazquez-Villegas L, et al. Nutrition and atherosclerosis. Arch Med Res. 2015;46(5):408–426.
33. Thomas J, Delaney C, Suen J, et al. Nutritional status of patients admitted to a metropolitan tertiary care vascular surgery unit. Asia Pac J Clin Nutr. 2019;28(1):64–71.
34. Redmond ML, Dong F, Goetz J, et al. Food insecurity and peripheral arterial disease in older adult populations. J Nutr Health Aging. 2016;20(10):989–995.
35. Eckel R, Jakicic J, Ard J, et al. 2013 AHA/ACC guideline on lifestyle management to reduce cardiovascular risk. Circulation. 2014;129(25 Suppl 2):S76–S99.
36. Coca-Martinez M, Kinio A, Hales L, et al. Combined exercise and nutrition optimization for peripheral arterial disease: A systematic review. Ann Vasc Surg. 2021;71:496–506.
37. Fokkenrood H, Bendermacher B, Lauret G, et al. Supervised exercise therapy versus non-supervised exercise therapy for intermittent claudication. Cochrane Database Syst Rev. 2013(8):CD005263.
38. Murphy T, Cutlip D, Regensteiner J, et al. Supervised exercise, stent revascularization, or medical therapy for claudication due to aortoiliac peripheral artery disease: The CLEVER study. J Am Coll Cardiol. 2015;65(10):999–1009.
39. Lane R, Ellis B, Watson L, et al. Exercise for intermittent claudication. Cochrane Database Syst Rev. 2014;(7):CD000990.
40. Hageman D, Fokkenrood H, Gommans L, et al. Supervised exercise therapy versus home-based exercise therapy versus walking advice for intermittent claudication. Cochrane Database Syst Rev. 2018;4(4):CD005263.
41. Cheetham D, Burgess L, Ellis M, et al. Does supervised exercise offer adjuvant benefit over exercise advice alone for the treatment of intermittent claudication? A randomised trial. Eur J Vasc Endovasc Surg. 2004;27(1):17–23.
42. Kruidenier L, Viechtbauer W, Nicolai S, et al. Treatment for intermittent claudication and the effects on walking distance and quality of life. Vascular. 2012;20(1):20–35.
43. Hennrikus D, Joseph AM, Lando HA, et al. Effectiveness of a smoking cessation program for peripheral artery disease patients: a randomized controlled trial. J Am Coll Cardiol. 2010;56:2105–2112.
44. Stead LF, Buitrago D, Preciado N, et al. Physician advice for smoking cessation. Cochrane Database Syst Rev. 2013:CD000165.
45. Hoel AW, Nolan BW, Goodney PP, et al. Variation in smoking cessation after vascular operations. J Vasc Surg. 2013;57:1338–1344.
46. Rigotti NA, Pipe AL, Benowitz NL, et al. Efficacy and safety of varenicline for smoking cessation in patients with cardiovascular disease: A randomized trial. Circulation. 2010;121:221–229.
47. Rigotti NA, Regan S, Levy DE, et al. Sustained care intervention and postdischarge smoking cessation among hospitalized adults: A randomized clinical trial. JAMA. 2014;312:719–728.

48. Tonstad S, Farsang C, Klaene G, et al. Bupropion SR for smoking cessation in smokers with cardiovascular disease: A multicentre, randomised study. Eur Heart J. 2003;24: 946–955.
49. Tan CE, Glantz SA. Association between smoke-free legislation and hospitalizations for cardiac, cerebrovascular, and respiratory diseases: A meta-analysis. Circulation. 2012;126:2177–2183.
50. Parvar SL, Fitridge R, Dawson J, et al. Medical and lifestyle management of peripheral arterial disease. J Vasc Surg. 2018;68(5):1595–1606.
51. O'Neill BJ, Rana SN, Bowman V. An integrated approach for vascular health: A call to action. Can J Cardiol. 2015;31(1):99–102.
52. Brostow D, Hirsch A, Collins T, et al. The role of nutrition and body composition in peripheral arterial disease. Nat Rev Cardiol. 2012;9(11):634–643.

18 Nutrition and Chronic Kidney Disease

Key Points

- Chronic kidney disease (CKD) is common, with 11–13% of individuals in the United States having some level of CKD.
- Current research suggests that healthy plant-based diets lower the risk of CKD and can assist in its treatment.
- Risk factors for CKD, including obesity, type 2 diabetes mellitus (T2DM), hypertension, and cardiovascular disease (CVD), are also positively affected by healthy plant-based diets, which lower the risk of CKD.

18.1 INTRODUCTION

CKD is prevalent both in the United States and around the world. It is estimated that CKD affects between 11% and 13% of adults worldwide, and thus, it poses a major global health problem [1].

There is good evidence that lifestyle modifications, including consuming a healthier diet, may help reduce the risk of developing CKD and slow its progress or assist in its treatment [2–5]. As described in multiple chapters in this book, a healthy dietary pattern plays an important role in overall health and can be modified to delay or even prevent the onset of various chronic diseases such T2DM and CVD [5–12]. A healthy dietary pattern can also play an important role at various stages of CKD. Following a healthy dietary pattern such as the Dietary Approaches to Stop Hypertension (DASH) diet [13] and the Mediterranean diet [14,15] have been shown to lower the risk of multiple chronic conditions such as metabolic syndrome, T2DM, CVD, and cancer. Because CKD shares many risk factors with both T2DM and CVD, adherence to these healthy dietary patterns may also reduce the risk of CKD.

In addition, since the kidneys play a critical role in regulating fluid balance and moving waste products from the body, there are numerous nutritional changes which need to occur as CKD progresses [16]. Thus, nutritional factors are important not only to lower the risk factors for CKD but also play an important role in each stage of declining renal function as CKD progresses.

Individuals with CKD are at risk for a variety of nutritional disorders that may include undernutrition, protein energy wasting (PEW), and electrolyte disturbances. Furthermore, CKD may create unique challenges to maintain a high-quality diet in the constraints of a reduced glomerular filtration rate, which is a hallmark of CKD.

DOI: 10.1201/9781003452607-18

18.2 DEFINITION OF CHRONIC RENAL DISEASE

The basic role of the kidneys is to remove waste, toxins, and excess fluid [17]. They thus help to control blood pressure. The kidneys also stimulate the production of red blood cells, play a role in maintaining bone health, and regulate blood chemicals that are essential to life. Thus, kidneys are critical to maintaining good health.

Nutrition plays a fundamental and important role in maintaining the health of the kidneys. CKD is a condition where the kidneys are damaged and cannot filter blood as well as they should. Because of this, excess fluid and waste from the blood remain in the body and may cause other problems such as heart disease and stroke [18,19].

CKD has various levels of seriousness. It typically gets worse over time, although treatment, including various dietary patterns, may either lower the risk of developing CKD in the first place or slow its progression if it is present. To help prevent CKD and lower the risk of ultimate kidney failure, it is important to control risk factors for CVD (see next section). Making lifestyle changes, including nutritional changes, is important to lowering the risk and helping in the treatment of CKD [20]. As already indicated, it is estimated that 11–13% of adults in the United States have some level of CKD, and the majority remain undiagnosed [1,21]. For all these reasons, it is important to understand the risk factors for CKD and take appropriate measures.

18.3 RISK FACTORS FOR CKD

Multiple risk factors have been established for CKD. These include the following: age, obesity, T2DM, hypertension, smoking, and ethnicity. As will be discussed in subsequent sections of this chapter, initial diet and nutritional interventions to lower the risk of CKD include optimizing glycemic control with diet, weight loss if necessary, salt reduction, decrease in processed foods, following healthy nutritional patterns, and increase in physical activity.

18.4 NUTRITION AND CKD

Plant-based diets have been consistently shown to lower the risk of such conditions as obesity, T2DM, hypertension, and CVD [2,5,16,22–26]. Thus, plant-based diets are likely to decrease the risk of CKD. Indeed, higher adherence to the Mediterranean diet has been demonstrated to lower CKD incidence [23] as has the DASH diet [22]. These diets will be discussed in subsequent sections of this chapter. In contrast, recent data from the National Health and Nutrition Examination Survey (NHANES) showed that individuals who had CKD and consumed meat-based diets such as the typical Western diet, demonstrated elevated acid loads, which are known to increase the risk of progression of CKD [24]. A recent study of dietary sources of protein and CKD found that when one serving of red or processed meat was replaced by plant proteins, the risk of CKD was significantly lower. Protein obtained from plants was associated in preliminary studies with lower risk of CKD [25].

As nutritional needs change, while CKD progresses, it will typically be useful to engage a nutritionist who is specifically trained in CKD and diabetes to provide nutritional counseling for such a patient [16]. This type of consultation is called medical nutrition therapy (MNT) [27]. There are nutritionists who are specifically trained in both kidney disease and diabetes who can assist in this effort. They can be located through the Academy of Nutrition and Dietetics. Many hospitals will also have individuals who are specifically trained in this area. Be sure to inquire if the individual has specific background and training in kidney disease before hiring them as a consultant.

18.5 THE ROLE DIETARY CONSTITUENTS IN KIDNEY DISEASE

- Protein
  A long-standing debate exists about whether or not ingesting protein is a risk factor for CKD. There is some evidence that shows that long-term dietary protein intake, exceeding 1.5 gram/kg, may hinder glomerular filtration and exert pro-inflammatory effects—both of which are risk factors for kidney disease [27]. The weight reduction approach of high-protein diets has been shown to increase proteinuria in individuals with diabetes or hypertension, although its effect on kidney health is not clear. The effects of low-protein diets in human beings are inconsistent and controversial. Restricting dietary protein, however, results in reduction of urea generation. The recommendation of 0.6–0.8 grams of protein/kg is typically recommended for adults with moderate to advanced kidney disease (glomerular filtration rate [GFR] less than 45 mL/min) [27]. Within this recommendation, typically half the protein should be of "high biologic value" (e.g. dairy products) and the other half may be plant proteins.
- Sodium and Fluids
  Sodium consumption of less than 2,300 mg/day is recommended to help lower high blood pressure. In individuals with established CKD, sodium restriction is typically recommended to control fluid retention as well as hypertension and to improve the CVD risk profile [28]. Whether or not a low-sodium diet slows the progression of CKD remains in dispute. The recommendation of less than 2,300 grams of sodium for individuals with CVD has not yielded evidence for individuals with CKD. Thus, the recommended dietary sodium for individuals with CKD is less than 2,000 mg/day.
- Potassium
  Many fresh fruits and vegetables are considered healthy choices for most people given their high fiber and vitamin content and low production of acid in such foods [29]. Since potassium intake is associated with lower sodium intake, a relatively high daily potassium intake of 4.7 grams is recommended for healthy adults [29–32]. However, in patients with advanced chronic kidney disease, higher potassium intake is not recommended and may result in increased risk of CKD progression. In patients with hyperkalemia (greater than 5.5 mmol), dietary potassium less than 3 grams per day is recommended [33]. However, it is important that this intake not eliminate foods such as fresh fruits and vegetables with high fiber, which should not be compromised.

- Phosphorous
  In the general population, higher plasma phosphorous totals have been associated with increased risk of kidney disease [34]. In individuals with moderate-to-advanced CKD, dietary phosphorous intake of less than 800 mg per day is recommended, and processed foods with a high phosphorus to protein ratio should be minimized.
- Calcium and Vitamin D
  The suggested calcium intake for individuals without CKD is 1,000–1,300 mg per day; however, in individuals with moderate-to-advanced CKD, the recommendation is 800–1,000 mg of calcium per day from all sources [35–37].

  Vitamin D supplementation may be offered to individuals with CKD in whom low circulating vitamin D levels have been documented [38–39].

18.6 VEGETARIAN DIET, FIBER, AND THE MICROBIOME

Plant-based diets are recommended as part of any strategy for the prevention and management of CKD [40–42]. Foods in these diets contain small amounts of saturated fatty acids, protein, absorbable phosphorus, and meat and generate less acid while being rich in fiber [43,44], polyunsaturated and monounsaturated fats, magnesium, potassium, and iron. In patients with CKD, a diet with a higher portion of plant sources (greater than 50%), has been associated with better outcomes.

The protein in a vegetarian diet is coupled with high fiber content, which may yield better benefits for individuals with CKD. There are several mechanisms to which helpful plant-based diets may be associated with lowering the risk of CKD. Those individuals in the highest quintile of healthy plant-based diets have lower dietary acid loads and higher intake of fiber and micronutrients. In turn, higher dietary acid load (e.g. from meat products) has been associated with a higher risk of CKD and, therefore, modifying dietary acid load by increasing intake of fruits and vegetables is recommended. Improved markers of kidney injury and fiber intake, in particular, have a direct inverse association with incidence of CKD. Fiber has also been shown to improve glycemic control and insulin secretion, which is associated with a lower risk of microalbuminuria and proteinuria. Fiber can also reduce the risk of CKD by lowering risk factors for CKD such as hypertension and T2DM. Furthermore, as discussed in multiple chapters in this book, micronutrients found in fruits and vegetables and whole grains can reduce inflammation and oxidative stress as well as reducing endothelial dysfunction.

18.7 DIETARY MANAGEMENT OF ACIDOSIS

Considerable evidence suggests that elevated acid loads are detrimental to kidney health [42–47]. The bulk of acid production in the human body comes from diet, particularly Western diets, that favor animal-based, acid-inducing foods. Animal protein is acid-forming due to the presence of organic sulfur which is found in the amino acids in thiamine and cysteine, which are common in animal proteins and are oxidized to inorganic sulfate. In contrast, plant-based foods have natural dietary alkaline in the form of citrate and malate, which can be converted to bicarbonate. In the NHANES analysis of dietary and health records of nearly 1,500 adults, there was a significant association with increased risk of kidney failure in those at the highest third of daily acid load. Based on these findings, the National Kidney Foundation's Kidney Disease Outcomes Quality Initiative (KDOQI) nutrition guidelines suggest an increase in fruit and vegetable intake to decrease body weight, blood pressure, and acid production.

18.8 EATING PATTERNS AND CKD

As emphasized in multiple chapters in this book, modern nutrition science is based on overall eating patterns. While there is less known about the effects of various eating patterns on CKD, some emerging evidence exists that healthy plant-based eating patterns may lower the risk of progress of CKD.

- The Mediterranean Diet
  In the study from the Northern Manhattan Study Cohort, individuals who increasingly adhered to the Mediterranean diet showed reduced incidence of GFR of less than 60 mL/minute (GFR of less than 60 is considered mildly to moderately decreased kidney function) [23]. These findings are consistent with other research which has shown that eating patterns such as the DASH diet and outcomes from the Nurses' Health Study can lower the pace of progression of CKD [24].
- The DASH Diet
  The DASH diet in relationship to potential CKD was assessed in the Atherosclerosis Risk in Communities (ARIC) study, which evaluated 14,082 individuals over a mean follow-up of 23 years [2]. A total of 3,720 individuals developed kidney disease during this time period. Individuals who had a high DASH diet score were 16% less likely to develop CKD. The DASH diet is an eating pattern high in fruits, vegetables, and low-fat dairy products which has been demonstrated to substantially reduce blood pressure. Such a comprehensive healthy eating style incorporates many of the principles known to be effective for lowering the risk of CKD. Thus, the DASH approach appears to be a very viable approach to lowering the risk of CKD.

  Another study evaluating the DASH diet is called the CARDYA Study (Coronary Artery Risk Development in Young Adults) [20]. In this study of young adults (less than 40 years of age), poor diet quality associated with a low score from the DASH dietary inventory was associated with twice as much risk of developing microalbuminuria, which indicates the presence of chronic kidney disease compared to individuals who were more adherent to the DASH diet. These findings were consistent with another study conducted on a subgroup analysis of the Nurses Health Study involving older, White women which showed that individuals who followed a Western diet, compared to individuals who were adherent to the DASH diet, were at an increased risk of rapid GFR decline [24].

18.9 CONCLUSIONS

While there is less available literature on the relationship of nutrition to CKD taken as a whole, available research suggests that following healthy plant-based diets lowers the risk of developing CKD. This is, in a sense, not surprising given that healthy plant-based diets have been demonstrated to lower the risk of various chronic conditions such as obesity, T2DM, hypertension, and CVD, all of which are risk factors for CKD.

Since the kidneys play a critical role in maintaining proper fluid balance and ridding the body of waste products, paying close attention to nutritional parameters is vitally important in determining the risk of CKD and its treatment. As CKD progresses, changes will be required in areas such as protein, sodium, fluids, potassium, phosphorus, and calcium intake. Western diets generate a considerable amount of acid, which is also detrimental to kidney function. Thus, diets that maintain a high level of fruit and vegetable consumption, as well as fiber, are particularly valuable at all stages of risk factor reduction for CKD and in its treatment.

Clinical Applications

- Individuals should be counseled that plant-based diets not only are effective for lowering chronic diseases but the risk of chronic diseases such as obesity, T2DM, and CVD and also can play a role in lowering the risk of CKD.
- Once individuals have CKD, reduced salt intake and increased fruit and vegetable consumption are both important.
- Healthy eating patterns such as the Mediterranean diet and the DASH diet have been demonstrated to lower the risk of CKD and assist in its treatment.

REFERENCES

1. CDC. Centers for Disease Control and Prevention. Centers for Disease Control and Prevention (cdc.gov) (Accessed January 19, 2024).
2. Kim H, Caulfield L, Garcia-Larsen V, et al. Plant-based diets and incident CKD and kidney function. Clin J Am Soc Nephrol. 2019;14(5):682–691.
3. Rebholz C, Crews D, Grams M, et al. DASH (Dietary Approaches to Stop Hypertension) diet and risk of subsequent kidney disease. Am J Kidney Dis. 2016;68:853–861.
4. Chang A, Van Horn L, Jacobs D Jr., et al. Lifestyle-related factors, obesity, and incident microalbuminuria: The CARDIA (Coronary Artery Risk Development in Young Adults) Study. Am J Kidney Dis. 2013;62:267–275.
5. Hu E, Steffen L, Grams M, et al. Dietary patterns and risk of incident chronic kidney disease: the Atherosclerosis Risk in Communities study. Am J Clin Nutr. 2019;110(3):713–721.
6. Freeman A, Morris P, Barnard N, et al. Trending cardiovascular nutrition controversies. J Am Coll Cardiol. 2017;69:1172–1187.
7. McMacken M, Shah S. A plant-based diet for the prevention and treatment of type 2 diabetes. J Geriatr Cardiol. 2017;14:342–354.
8. Marsh K, Zeuschner C, Saunders A. Health implications of a vegetarian diet: A review. Am J Lifestyle Med. 2012;6:250–267.
9. Yokoyama Y, Nishimura K, Barnard N, et al. Vegetarian diets and blood pressure: A meta-analysis. JAMA Intern Med. 2014;174:577–587.
10. Orlich M, Singh P, Sabate J, et al. Vegetarian dietary patterns and mortality in Adventist Health Study 2. JAMA Intern Med. 2013;173:1230–1238.

11. Satija A, Bhupathiraju S, Rimm E, et al. Plant-based dietary patterns and incidence of type 2 diabetes in US men and women: Results from three prospective cohort studies. PLoS Med. 2016;13:e1002039.
12. Satija A, Bhupathiraju S, Spiegelman D, et al. Healthful and unhealthful plant-based diets and the risk of coronary heart disease in U.S Adults. J Am Coll Cardiol. 2017;70:411–422.
13. Sacks F, Svetkey L, Vollmer W, et al. Effects on blood pressure of reduced dietary sodium and the Dietary Approaches to Stop Hypertension (DASH) diet. DASH-Sodium Collaborative Research Group. N Eng J Med. 2001;344(1):3–10.
14. Gardener H, Wright CB, Gu Y, et al. Mediterranean-style diet and risk of ischemic stroke, myocardial infarction, and vascular death: the Northern Manhattan Study. Am J Clin Nutr. 2011;94(6):1458–1464.
15. Estruch R, Ros E, Salas-Salvado J, et al. Primary prevention of cardiovascular disease with a Mediterranean diet. N Eng J Med. 2013;368(14):1279–1290.
16. Kalantar-Zadeh K, Fouque D. Nutritional management of chronic kidney disease. N Eng J Med. 2017;377(18):1765–1776.
17. Levey A, de Jong P, Coresh J, et al. The definition, classification, and prognosis of chronic kidney disease: A KDIGO controversies conference report. Kidney Int. 2011;80(1):17–28.
18. Armstrong J, Laing D, Wilkes F, et al. Smell and taste function in children with chronic kidney disease. Pediatr Nephrol. 2010;25(8):1497–1504.
19. Vaziri N, Yuan J, Norris K. Role of urea in intestinal barrier dysfunction and disruption of epithelial tight junction in chronic kidney disease. Am J Nephrol. 2013;37(1):1–6.
20. Hsu CY, Iribarren C, McCulloch CE, Darbinian J, Go AS. Risk factors for end-stage renal disease: 25-year follow-up. Arch Intern Med. 2009;169(4):342–350.
21. Bello A, Levin A, Tonelli M, et al. Assessment of global kidney health care status. JAMA. 2017;9;317(18):1864–1881.
22. Lin J, Fung TT, Hu FB, Curhan GC. Association of dietary patterns with albuminuria and kidney function decline in older white women: A subgroup analysis from the Nurses' Health Study. Am J Kidney Dis. 2011;57(2):245–254.
23. Khatri M, Moon Y, Scarmeas N, et al. The association between a Mediterranean-style diet and kidney function in the Northern Manhattan Study cohort. Clin J Am Soc Nephrol. 2014;9(11):1868–1875.
24. Lin J, Fung T, Hu F, et al. Association of dietary patterns with albuminuria and kidney function decline in older white women: a subgroup analysis from the Nurses' Health Study. Am J Kidney Dis: The Off J Nat Kidney Found. 2011;57(2):245–254.
25. Joshi S, McMacken M, Kalantar-Zadeh K. Plant-based diets for kidney disease: A guide for clinicians. Am J Kidney Dis. 2021;77(2):287–296.
26. Clegg D, Hill Gallant K. Plant-based diets in CKD. Clin J Am Soc Nephrol. 2019;14(1):141–143.
27. MacLaughlin H, Friedman A, Ikizler T. Nutrition in kidney disease: Core curriculum 2022. Am J Kidney Dis. 2022;79(3):437–449.
28. Mente A, O'Donnell MJ, Rangarajan S, et al. Association of urinary sodium and potassium excretion with blood pressure. N Engl J Med. 2014;371:601–611.
29. Palmer B, Clegg D. Achieving the benefits of a high-potassium, paleolithic diet, without the toxicity. Mayo Clin Proc. 2016;91:496–508.
30. Araki S, Haneda M, Koya D, et al. Urinary potassium excretion and renal and cardiovascular complications in patients with type 2 diabetes and normal renal function. Clin J Am Soc Nephrol. 2015;10:2152–2158.
31. Institute of Medicine. Dietary Reference Intakes for Water, Potassium, Sodium, Chloride, and Sulfate. Washington, DC: The National Academies Press, 2005.

32. Chen Y, Sang Y, Ballew S, et al. Race, serum potassium, and associations with ESRD and mortality. Am J Kidney Dis. 2017;70:244–251.
33. St-Jules D, Goldfarb D, Sevick M. Nutrient non-equivalence: Does restricting high-potassium plant foods help to prevent hyperkalemia in hemodialysis patients? J Ren Nutr. 2016;26:282–287.
34. Sim J, Bhandari S, Smith N, et al. Phosphorus and risk of renal failure in subjects with normal renal function. Am J Med. 2013;126:311–318.
35. Spiegel D, Brady K. Calcium balance in normal individuals and in patients with chronic kidney disease on low- and high-calcium diets. Kidney Int. 2012;81:1116–1122.
36. Bushinsky D. Clinical application of calcium modeling in patients with chronic kidney disease. Nephrol Dial Transplant. 2012;27:10–13.
37. Hill K, Martin B, Wastney M, et al. Oral calcium carbonate affects calcium but not phosphorus balance in stage 3–4 chronic kidney disease. Kidney Int. 2013;83:959–966.
38. de Zeeuw D, Agarwal R, Amdahl M, et al. Selective vitamin D receptor activation with paricalcitol for reduction of albuminuria in patients with type 2 diabetes (VITAL study): A Randomised Controlled Trial. Lancet. 2010;376:1543–1551.
39. Powe C, Evans M, Wenger J, et al. Vitamin D—binding protein and vitamin D status of black Americans and white Americans. N Engl J Med. 2013;369:1991–2000.
40. Rebholz C, Coresh J, Grams ME, et al. Dietary acid load and incident chronic kidney disease: Results from the ARIC study. Am J Nephrol. 2015;42:427–435.
41. Mirmiran P, Yuzbashian E, Asghari G, et al. Dietary fibre intake in relation to the risk of incident chronic kidney disease. Br J Nutr. 2018;119:479–485.
42. Fogelman A. TMAO is both a biomarker and a renal toxin. Circ Res. 2015;116(3):396–397.
43. Wesson D, Buysse J, Bushinsky D. Mechanisms of metabolic acidosis—induced kidney injury in chronic kidney disease. J Am Soc Nephrol. 2020;31(3):469–482.
44. Raphael K, Carroll D, Murray J, et al. Urine ammonium predicts clinical outcomes in hypertensive kidney disease. J Am Soc Nephrol. 2017;28(8):2483–2490.
45. Scialla J, Anderson C. Dietary acid load: A novel nutritional target in chronic kidney disease? Adv Chronic Kidney Dis. 2013;20(2):141–149.
46. Goraya N, Simoni J, Jo C, et al. A comparison of treating metabolic acidosis in CKD stage 4 hypertensive kidney disease with fruits and vegetables or sodium bicarbonate. Clin J Am Soc Nephrol. 2013;8(3):371–381.
47. Goraya N, Simoni J, Jo C, et al. Dietary acid reduction with fruits and vegetables or bicarbonate attenuates kidney injury in patients with a moderately reduced glomerular filtration rate due to hypertensive nephropathy. Kidney Int. 2012;81(1):86–93.

19 Nutrition and Erectile Dysfunction

Key Points

- Erectile dysfunction (ED) is very common, with as many as 52% of males between the ages of 40 and 70 reporting ED.
- Nutritional factors can play a significant role in lowering inflammation and oxidative stress and improving levels of nitric oxide, which are critically important in terms of erectile function.

19.1 INTRODUCTION

ED is common in the United States and around the world. It is clinically defined as the inability to attain or maintain a penile erection "sufficient for satisfactory sexual performance" [1]. While there are many different potential causes and risk factors for ED, nutrition plays a central role in many of the etiologies. Furthermore, ED often precedes other vascular chronic illnesses such as coronary heart disease (CHD) and stroke [2]. This is not surprising given that atherosclerosis is the etiology for the most common form of ED. ED shares risk factors and pathophysiology with many other chronic vascular diseases. The underlying etiology of all these diseases is based on atherosclerosis. (See also Chapter 11.) Multiple studies have now shown that issues related to nutrition can either predispose to ED or lower the likelihood of it [3–6]. Thus, nutrition plays a very important role in virtually all aspects of ED.

The Massachusetts Male Aging Study (MMAS) in 1,290 men ages 40–70 years old reported a prevalence of 52% of ED [7]. In this age group of 40- to 70-year-olds, there was also an age-related prevalence of ED with increases in each decade and a tripling comparing men in the ages of 60–69 compared to 42–49. Estimates of ED prevalence vary widely based on different definitions and survey methods. However self-reported ED occurs in 15% of men ages 40–59 and 45% of those in their 60s and 70% in those 70 or older [8].

19.2 CAUSES OF ERECTILE DYSFUNCTION

There are three broad classifications for ED. They are organic, psychogenic, or mixed. Within the organic etiology, approximately 80% of cases include vascular, neurogenic, hormonal, or drug induced [9,10]. Vasculogenic ED now accounts for most of organic ED and is thought to be due to abnormalities in penile arterial inflow or venous outflow [10]. Symptomatic ED frequently precedes other manifestations of atherosclerotic cardiovascular disease, often developing two to three years before the onset of angina and three to five years before the development of other cardiovascular

DOI: 10.1201/9781003452607-19

events [9,11,12]. This appears to be due, in part, to the fact that penile arteries are smaller in diameter than coronary arteries, typically 1–2 or 3–4 mm in diameter [13]. Because ED typically precedes other manifestations of atherosclerotic disease, it has been called the "canary in the coal mine" for CHD [14]. Thus, it has been recommended that ED serves as an independent risk factor for CVD, and the consensus recommendation is that individuals with vasculogenic ED be screened for risk of CVD [15].

19.3 PATHOPHYSIOLOGY OF ERECTILE DYSFUNCTION

A great deal of knowledge has been gained in the past two decades concerning the underlying events related particularly to vasculogenic ED [16]. This research has demonstrated a central role for nitric oxide (NO) in the etiology of ED [17–20]. NO is now regarded as the principal mediator influencing ED and also has a very significant influence on cardiovascular health. Nutritional choices as well as other lifestyle factors play a significant role in the production of NO.

NO is generated both by cells in the endothelium and also by the parasympathetic nerve endings in the penis. NO-dependent relaxation of the cavernosal smooth muscle leads to enhanced dilatation of the penile arteries and also leads to compression of the small veins in blood flow, which creates an erection [21,22]. NO, in addition to its vasodilatory effect, also has antioxidant and anti-inflammatory effects on the vessel walls [23,24]. Plant-based foods contain bioactive polyphenolic compounds and have been linked to increased NO [25]. This, in turn, provides the hypothetical mechanism for why improved ED occurs in plant-based diets such as the Mediterranean diet [26,27]. In contrast, reactive oxygen species reduce the bioavailability of NO and promote endothelial cell dysfunction. These species are prominent in response to the Western diet. In contrast, plant-based foods contain compounds, particularly phenolic compounds, which are protective against reactive oxygen species and may enhance erectile function [27]. The pathophysiologic mechanism of NO provides a compelling picture for why plant-based diets such as the Mediterranean diet are associated with decreased likelihood of ED [4], while Western diets are associated with increased likelihood of ED. As will be discussed later in this chapter, regular exercise, weight loss, and cessation of tobacco products also enhance the availability of NO and may contribute to the demonstrated decrease in risk associated with these other lifestyle modalities [23,24].

19.4 MEASURES OF ERECTILE DYSFUNCTION

A variety of different measures have been used to quantify ED. The most commonly used one in clinical studies is the validated five-item International Index of Erectile Function (IIEF) Score [26]. This new empirical score is derived from five questions on the ability to achieve and maintain an erection and classifies ED into five categories: Severe [5–7], moderate [8–11], mild to moderate [12–16], mild [17–21], and no erectile dysfunction [22–25]. The IIEF questionnaire asks a variety of questions related to how well an erection was able to be maintained and how satisfactory the sexual intercourse was for the individual.

19.5 RELATIONSHIP OF ED TO CHD AND STROKE

Given the similarities of risk factors related between ED, CHD, and stroke, it is not surprising that vasculogenic ED is associated with atherosclerotic cardiovascular disease events including myocardial infarction, ischemic stroke, and cardiovascular death. In a meta-analysis of prospective cohort studies, ED was associated with between 40% and 50% increase in the likelihood of all forms of CVD and a 35% increase in the likelihood of coronary artery disease as well as a 19% increase in the risk of stroke [28]. In a prospective cohort study of 1,913 men living in Europe age 40–79, ED was associated with a 1.4 times higher risk of mortality.

19.6 RELATIONSHIP OF NUTRITION TO ED

As discussed in multiple other chapters in this book, the Mediterranean diet has been shown to lower the risk of CVD and diabetes. This diet is high in fruits and vegetables, olive oil, whole grains, tree nuts, and lean proteins, including beans, legumes, fish, and moderate in poultry and red wine. It discourages processed foods and red meat and refined grains.

Several trials have demonstrated that the Mediterranean diet pattern lowers the risk of ED. A study by Esposito et al. in 180 patients with metabolic syndrome showed that the Mediterranean diet lowered markers of endothelial dysfunction and vascular inflammation [29]. In another study of 65 men with ED, the same group showed after two years that three men in the intervention group and other two in the control group reported normal erectile dysfunction based on the IIEF Score [24]. In addition, measures in endothelial function and inflammatory markers (C-reactive protein) were improved in the intervention group but were unchanged in the control group. Research reported at the European Society of Cardiology also showed substantial improvements in ED in males with hypertension who had high levels of adherence to the Mediterranean diet. These data suggest that it is reasonable to counsel patients with ED to adhere to a Mediterranean-style dietary pattern that is rich in fruits, vegetables, and whole grains including nuts, olive oil, and fish for the purpose of slowing progression or improving ED.

19.7 OBSERVATIONAL DIET STUDIES

Observational studies have also supported a link between dietary components and ED. In the 25,096 men in the Health Professionals Follow-Up Study, those in the highest quintile of fruit intake had a 14% lower risk of incident ED over a ten-year period [30]. In a cross-sectional study of 1,500 Canadian men with diabetes, 26% of whom reported symptoms of ED, a daily serving of fruit or vegetables measured by a Food Frequency Questionnaire was associated with a 10% decrease of self-reported ED [31]. A study of 100 men in Italy with ED compared to 100 matched controls showed that higher intakes of fruits and vegetables and higher monounsaturated to saturated fat ratio were associated with reduced incidence of ED [32].

As described in detail in Chapter 2, the Western diet is rich in red and processed meats, dairy, and refined grains, processed foods, and artificial sweeteners and salt and has minimal intake of fruits, vegetables, fish, and whole grains. The Western diet has been shown to increase the risk of multiple chronic diseases, particularly vascular diseases. Between 50% and 70% of men with CHD also have ED. Thus, it seems reasonable to assume that the Western diet also increases the risk of ED. Increased prevalence of ED has been shown in individuals who have the metabolic syndrome and also individuals with obesity. (See the next section.)

19.8 OBESITY AND ERECTILE DYSFUNCTION

Several studies have shown increased risk of ED in males who are obese. In one study, males who had a waist circumference of 32 inches were compared to males who had a waist circumference of 42 inches. Individuals with the 32-inch waist were 50% less likely to have ED than individuals with the 42-inch waist [33]. Given the association between obesity and inflammation, the findings that there is an increased risk of ED in obese males are not surprising.

Several trials of weight loss in individuals with obesity and ED have shown a 30–40% decrease in ED following a weight loss of greater than 5%. In a study by Esposito et al., 209 subjects who had or were at risk for ED followed a weight loss program and increased exercise of at least 2.5 hours per week [34]. After two years, significantly more individuals in the lifestyle change arm achieved normal erectile function (increased from 34% to 56% in the intervention arm compared to 36–38% in the control arm). Other studies have shown improvements in the IIEF Score for individuals who followed a self-help exercise and diet program [33].

Although these studies are relatively small, they suggest that weight loss through calorie reduction and increased physical activity is appropriate to recommend to individuals with obesity as a means of improving ED.

19.9 DIETARY EFFECTS ON THE MICROBIOME

As discussed in detail in Chapter 24, the microbiome has been the subject of considerable recent research exploring how nutrition interacts with microbial cells and plays a role in multiple chronic diseases. An example of how the microbiome responds to the Western diet is the production of trimethylamine N-oxide (TMAO), which promotes atherosclerosis, vascular inflammation, and endothelial dysfunction, thereby increasing the risk of cardiovascular disease (CVD) [35]. The likely mechanism is through reduction in healthy endothelial cells. In addition, plant-based foods supply fiber, which has been shown in multiple studies to enable the production of short-chain fatty acids such as butyrate, which may reduce cholesterol synthesis, inflammation, and the burden of atherosclerosis [36]. Thus, nutritional practices are likely to impact on the microbiome in ways that further either increase or decrease the risk of ED.

19.10 EFFECT OF PHYSICAL ACTIVITY ON ERECTILE DYSFUNCTION

Numerous studies have shown that physical activity improves ED and lowers the risk of ED, as well as all forms of atherosclerotic vascular disease [37]. In the area of ED, physical activity may augment NO release from endothelial cells, thereby directly improving blood flow to the penile bed as it does to other vascular beds [38]. In addition, exercise has been associated with vascular protective effects including decreased markers of inflammation. Studies have now shown that the combination of exercise and plant-based nutrition lowers the risk of ED, presumably through synergistic effects through the NO pathway.

19.11 THE EFFECTS OF TOBACCO CESSATION ON ERECTILE DYSFUNCTION OUTCOMES

Smoking has been identified by the American Urologic Association as an independent risk factor for ED [39]. The likely mechanism for this is both reducing NO levels and promoting reactive oxygen species and inflammation [40]. There are, of course, multiple health benefits from smoking cessation, including reducing the risk of ED, as well as multiple other health benefits.

19.12 CONCLUSIONS

ED is common in males between 40 and 70 years of age. While there are multiple causes of ED, by far the largest percentage is vasculogenic ED, which functions largely through the vascular effects of NO. Various nutritional strategies, including consumption of a healthy plant-based diet rather than the Western diet, have been shown to lower the risk factors and prevalence of ED. Thus, ED is another vascular-related condition where healthy plant-based nutrition can play a significant role. Other lifestyle factors such as regular physical activity, weight loss, and tobacco cessation are also important and act synergistically with a healthy plant-based diet to lower the risk of ED. Since 50–70% of individuals with CHD also have ED, clinicians should address this topic and counsel patients in this area who have CHD. ED is also considered to be a sentinel event or, as some people have called it, the "canary in the coal mine," since ED often precedes symptomatic CHD by three to five years.

Clinical Applications

- ED is common in males between the ages of 40 and 70.
- Following a healthy plant-based diet and getting increased physical activity as well as smoking cessation and, if overweight or obese, weight loss have all been shown to lower the risk of ED.
- Individuals with ED should be counseled about the importance of healthy lifestyle practices such as plant-based nutrition, increased physical activity, and smoking cessation, as a means of helping to ameliorate symptoms of ED.
- Since ED often occurs three to five years prior to symptomatic CHD, individuals with ED should also be assessed for risk factors for CHD.

REFERENCES

1. NIH Consensus Conference. Impotence. NIH Consensus Development Panel on Impotence. JAMA. 1993;270–83–90.

2. Uddin S, Mirbolouk M, Dardari Z, et al. Erectile dysfunction as an independent predictor of future cardiovascular events. Circulation. 2018;138(5):540–542.
3. La J, Roberts N, Yafi F. Diet and men's sexual health. Sex Med Rev. 2018;6(1):54–68.
4. Aladesuru O, Stoddard M, Chughtai B. Western diet and erectile dysfunction. In Chughtai B (ed). Molecular Mechanisms of Nutritional Interventions and Supplements for the Management of Sexual Dysfunction and Benign Prostatic Hyperplasia. London, UK: Elsevier, 2021: 167–176.
5. Mediterranean diet shows promise in men with erectile dysfunction. Aug 25, 2021. European Society of Cardiology Press Release. Sophia Antipolis, France—25 Aug 2021. (Accessed June 28, 2023).
6. Esposito K, Marfella R, Ciotola M. et al. Effect of a Mediterranean-style diet on endothelial dysfunction and markers of vascular inflammation in the metabolic syndrome: A randomized trial. JAMA. 2004; 292(12):1440–1446.
7. Feldman H, Goldstein I, Hatzichristu D, et al. Impotence and its medical and psychosocial correlates: Results of the Massachusetts male aging study. J Urol. 1994;151:54–61.
8. Nehra A, Jackson G, Miner M, et al. The Princeton III consensus recommendations for the management of erectile dysfunction and cardiovascular disease. Mayo Clin Proc. 2012;87:766–778.
9. Shamloul R, Ghanem H. Erectile dysfunction. Lancet. 2013;381:153–165.
10. Yafi FA, Jenkins L, Albersen M, et al. Erectile dysfunction. Nat Rev Dis Primers. 2016;2:16003.
11. Feldman D, Cainzos-Achirica M, Billups K. Subclinical vascular disease and subsequent erectile dysfunction: The Multiethnic Study of Atherosclerosis (MESA). Clin Cardiol. 2016;39(5):291–298.
12. Gandaglia G, Briganti A, Jackson G, et al. A systematic review of the association between erectile dysfunction and cardiovascular disease. Eur Urol. 2014;65(5):968–978.
13. Jackson G. Erectile dysfunction and cardiovascular disease. Arab J Urol. 2013;11:212–216.
14. Meldrum D, Gambone J, Morris M, et al. The link between erectile and cardiovascular health: The canary in the coal mine. Am J Cardiol. 2011;108:599–606.
15. Nehra A, Jackson G, Miner M., et al. The Princeton III consensus recommendations for the management of erectile dysfunction and cardiovascular disease. Mayo Clin Proc. 2012;87(8):776–778.
16. Lue T. Erectile dysfunction. N Eng J Med. 2000;342(24):1802–1813.
17. NIH Consensus Conference. Impotence. NIH Consensus Development Panel on Impotence. JAMA. 1993:270–83–90.
18. Anderson K, Wagner G. Physiology of penile erection. Physiol Rev. 1998:75–191–236.
19. de Tejada I, Goldstein I, Azadzoi K, et al. Impaired neurogenic and endothelium-mediated relaxation of penile smooth muscle from diabetic men with impotence. N Engl J Med. 1989;320(16):1025–1030.
20. Ignarro, L, Bush P, Buga G. et al. Nitric oxide and cyclic GMP formation upon electrical field stimulation cause relaxation of corpus cavernosum smooth muscle. Biochem Biophys Res Commun. 1990;31;170(2):843–850.
21. Italiano G, Calabrò A, Spini S. et al. Functional response of cavernosal tissue to distension. Urol Res. 1998;26(1):39–44.
22. Gondré M, Christ G. Endothelin-1-induced alterations in phenylephrine-induced contractile responses are largely additive in physiologically diverse rabbit vasculature. J Pharmacol Exp Ther. 1998;286(2):635–642.
23. Sullivan M, Thompson C, Dashwood M. Nitric oxide and penile erection: Is erectile dysfunction another manifestation of vascular disease? Cardiovasc Res. 1999;43(3):658–665.

24. Esposito K, Ciotola M, Giugliano F, et al. Mediterranean diet improves erectile function in subjects with the metabolic syndrome. Int J Impot Res. 2006;18:405–410.
25. Cassidy A, Franz M, Rimm EB. Dietary flavonoid intake and incidence of erectile dysfunction. Am J Clin Nutr. 2016;103:534–541.
26. Sharma J, Al-Omran A, Parvathy S. Role of nitric oxide in inflammatory diseases. Inflammopharmacology. 2007;15:252–259.
27. Shannon O, Stephan B, Minihane A, et al. Nitric oxide boosting effects of the Mediterranean Diet: A potential Mechanism of Action. J Gerontol a Biol Sci Med Sci. 2018;73:902–904.
28. Mano R, Ishida A, Ohya Y, et al. Dietary intervention with Okinawan vegetables increased circulating endothelial progenitor cells in healthy young women. Atherosclerosis. 2009;204:544–548.
29. Robertson R, Smaha L. Can a Mediterranean-style diet reduce heart disease? Circ. 2001;103:1821–1822.
30. Shiri R, Ansari M, Falah Hassani, K. Association between comorbidity and erectile dysfunction in patients with diabetes. Int J Impot Res. 2006;18(4):348–353.
31. Wang F, Dai S, Wang M, et al. Erectile dysfunction and fruit/vegetable consumption among diabetic Canadian Men. Urology. 2013;82(6):1330–1335.
32. Esposito K, Ciotola M, Giuglian F, et al. Dietary factors in erectile dysfunction. Int J Impot Res. 2006;18:370–374.
33. Kolotkin R, Zunker C, Østbye T. Sexual functioning and Obesity: A Review. Obesity. 2012;20(12):2325–2333.
34. Esposito K, Giugiano F, DiPalo C, et al. Effect of lifestyle changes on erectile dysfunction in obese men: A randomized controlled trial. JAMA. 2004;291: 2978–2984.
35. Tang W, Hazen S. The gut microbiome and its role in cardiovascular diseases. Circ. 2017;135(11):1008–1010.
36. Dhingra D, Michael M., Rajput H, et al. Dietary fibre in foods: A review. J Food Sci Techno. 2012;49:255–266.
37. Duca Y, Calogero A, Cannarella R, et al. Erectile dysfunction, physical activity and physical exercise: Recommendations for clinical practice. Andrologia. 2019;51(5):e13264.
38. Meldrum D, Gambone J, Morris M, et al. Lifestyle and metabolic approaches to maximizing erectile and vascular health. Int J Impot Res. 2012;24(2):61–68.
39. Burnett A, Nehra A, Breau R, et al. Erectile dysfunction, AUA guideline. J Urol. 2018;200:633–641.
40. Tost R, Caneiro F, Lee A, et al. Cigarette smoking and erectile dysfunction: Focus on NO bioavailability and ROS generation. J Sex Med. 2008;5:1284–1295.

20 Nutrition for the Prevention and Treatment of Prediabetes

Key Points

- Prediabetes is very common in the United States.
- Prediabetes is caused by insulin resistance and often beta cell defects and is clearly an increased risk for type 2 diabetes as well as diabetes-related health complications.
- Prediabetes is diagnosed with fasting blood glucose 100–125 mg/dL or two-hour post-challenge plasma glucose of 140–199 mg/dL and a hemoglobin A1C of 5.7–6.4%.
- There is a high prevalence of prediabetes in all age groups, but particularly in individuals over the age of 65.
- It is incumbent upon physicians to counsel people about various lifestyle strategies, including healthy nutrition, increased physical activity, and weight management to lower the risk of prediabetes progressing to T2DM.

20.1 INTRODUCTION

Prediabetes (sometimes called glucose intolerance) is an extremely common condition. Both its prevention and its treatment comprise multiple lifestyle habits and actions, one of which is nutrition. In the United States, 34% of adults age 18 or older had prediabetes in 2015, while over 48% of adults age 55 or older had this condition [1]. Prediabetes is somewhat higher in men (36.6%) than in women (29.3%). Prediabetes may be diagnosed either with impaired fasting glucose (IGF) or impaired glucose tolerance (IGT) (more on this in the next section). IFG appears to be more common than IGT, with the prevalence of 26% compared to 14% [2]. IGT appears to be more common in women, and IFG appears to be more common in men [3]. There are no significant differences in prevalence among race or ethnic groups. Roughly similar susceptibility exists amongst African Americans, Whites, and Asians, although African Americans seem to have a somewhat higher prevalence of prediabetes [4] and Asian Indians seem to be particularly susceptible to prediabetes [5].

Numerous studies have shown the positive effects of lifestyle measures such as proper nutrition and increased physical activity to reduce the risk of prediabetes turning into type 2 diabetes mellitus (T2DM). For this reason, it is important to explore how nutritional recommendations can lower the risk of either developing prediabetes in the first place or lowering the risk of prediabetes turning into T2DM.

DOI: 10.1201/9781003452607-20

20.2 WHAT IS PREDIABETES?

Prediabetes reflects hyperglycemia, where blood glucose levels are higher than normal but lower than diabetes levels. There is strong evidence that lifestyle interventions which focus on achieving and maintaining a healthy weight, improving dietary patterns, and increasing physical activity can prevent or reverse prediabetes. Unfortunately, many physicians who focus in the area of diabetes ignore potentially significant therapies to lower the risk of prediabetes. Indeed, many clinicians simply do not make the diagnosis of prediabetes.

Prediabetes is diagnosed by a fasting plasma glucose of 100–125 mg/dL or a two-hour post-challenge plasma glucose of 140–199 mg/dL or hemoglobin A1C between 5.7% and 6.4% [6]. Each of these conditions reflect insulin resistance. IFG reflects primarily hepatic insulin resistance, while IGT reflects muscle insulin resistance. It should be noted that individuals may present with either or both of these conditions.

Glycated hemoglobin (A1C) measures the amount of red blood cells covalently bounded to a glucose molecule and elevates A1C chronic hyperglycemic over a two-month period in the lifespan of hemoglobin. A1C values between 5.7% and 6.4% are also recommended by the American Diabetes Association (ADA) to define prediabetes [6]. Some controversy exists about whether or not prediabetes diagnoses should be utilized. Some experts oppose the use of the prediabetes diagnosis because it may lead to unnecessary use of glucose management drugs and may further stigmatize patients and harm insurance or employment or economic benefits in healthcare systems [7]. However, most experts agree that the diagnosis of prediabetes should be detected and managed as early as possible to minimize morbidity of T2DM [8–11]. Lifestyle medicine interventions are highly effective in the prevention and treatment of prediabetes. These interventions involve behavioral changes featuring healthy eating patterns, achieving and maintaining healthy weights and body composition, and regular physical activity. These modalities have been clearly demonstrated to be efficacious, particularly in the area of reducing the risk of prediabetes turning into T2DM.

Individuals who have prediabetes have either moderate or severe insulin resistance in muscle and/or liver with impaired beta-cell function. Insulin resistance is most commonly linked to obesity and unhealthy lifestyles, while impaired beta-cell function involves both genetic and environmental contributions [12]. These abnormalities in glucose regulation increase the risk of T2DM as well as cardiovascular disease (CVD).

People with prediabetes have a 4–12 times possible higher risk of developing T2DM and almost twofold higher risk of CVD disease and mortality [8,9]. Higher degrees of hyperglycemia predict a higher risk of not only CVD but also cancer, infectious diseases, and mental health problems in people with prediabetes [13,14].

20.3 THE ROLE OF LIFESTYLE FACTORS IN THE DEVELOPMENT OF PREDIABETES

There are multiple potential causes of prediabetes. The common unifying pathway typically involves some or all of the following: Impaired insulin secretion, insulin resistance, subclinical inflammation, increased body fat, and body fat distribution.

All of these factors may also impact differently, depending on genetic background. For example, normal-weight South Asians have been shown to progress from prediabetes to T2DM more rapidly than individuals of European descent [15]. Concerning lifestyle behaviors, excessive caloric intake and decreased physical activity can contribute to overweight and obesity, which, in turn, can increase insulin resistance, which, in turn, increases the risk of developing prediabetes [16].

It is known that insulin resistance typically precedes T2DM by approximately 20 years in many individuals. Insulin resistance also increases with age, although major contributions in insulin resistance may be age-related increase in body fat and decreases in physical activity. Poor nutrition during various times in development can also be associated with adverse glucose metabolism later in life [17]. Exercise also impacts on glucose regulation both by glucose transport to skeletal muscle and insulin-deviated glucose regulation [18]. The role of inflammation in the process of hyperglycemia also contributes to other factors such as insulin resistance, increased blood pressure, abnormal lipid profile, and lower fitness level.

Interestingly, poor sleep quality is also associated with a two- to threefold increased risk in prediabetes among U.S. adults [19]. Smoking has also been associated with a significant increase in prediabetes and results in a 78% increase risk of IGT [20]. Alcohol consumption has also been associated with prediabetes risk in men with up to 42% increased risk and a 1.4-fold increase in risk for women [21]. Of course, all of these factors are central to the practice of lifestyle medicine.

There is an ongoing exploration of how to employ lifestyle medicine measures to combat these various adverse lifestyle factors. It is particularly important to focus on insulin resistance. Recent data have suggested that the largest component of insulin resistance comes from position of fat in a variety of areas [22], particularly unexercised muscle, which results in reduced glucose uptake. Free fatty acids, which are more readily produced in visceral abdominal fat, also decrease insulin sensitivity and impair vascular reactivity [23]. Intracellular diacylglycerol has recently been identified as a contributor to insulin resistance in the liver.

Reducing body weight and increasing physical activity are key lifestyle factors in the prevention or lowering of the risk of hyperglycemia found in prediabetes. Exercise decreases hyperglycemia through a variety of mechanisms including decreasing concentrations of fatty acid metabolites [24,25]. Exercise can also increase glucose uptake through the working muscle 7–20 times above the basal rate, which yields improvement in insulin sensitivity [26]. In addition, exercise seems to improve serum levels of adiponectin, a hormone that promotes insulin sensitivity.

The development of hyperglycemia results in impaired pancreatic B-cell function and also B-cell mass, which is largely due to apoptosis. Research has shown that B-cell mass is about 60% of normal in individuals with prediabetes [27]. Either of these mild B-cell defects can result in impaired fasting hyperglycemia. The B-cell defect that is mild is typically found in patients with prediabetes [28]. Lifestyle changes to reduce insulin resistance can often restore normal glycemia. In instances where B-cell defect is more severe, pharmacological therapy may be needed in addition to lifestyle changes.

It should be noted that not everyone who develops insulin resistance will develop prediabetes. However, due to the fact that prediabetes rates increase with age, obesity, and physical inactivity, it is essential to adopt a proactive approach emphasizing healthy lifestyle to reduce insulin resistance and develop glucose intolerance in individuals who are at risk. This is particularly important in individuals who have prediabetes, where these changes early in the course can often restore normal glycemia. For this reason, it is particularly important to utilize lifestyle changes early in the course of prediabetes.

20.4 LIFESTYLE INTERVENTION FOR PREDIABETES PREVENTION AND TREATMENT

Individuals with prediabetes are an important target population for lifestyle modification interventions not only for the high-risk diabetes that they have but also the likely presence of other cardiovascular risk factors.

Lifestyle interventions including both nutritional changes and physical activity modification have been clearly demonstrated to improve glucose regulation and cardiovascular risk factors. One meta-analysis that compared nutritional interventions alone to those combining physical activity and dietary strategies showed larger effects in the combined intervention. Of note, studies that employed only physical activity intervention had the weakest effect [29]. Lifestyle interventions can restore normal glucose handling in people with prediabetes. The evidence-based summary provided by the U.S. Community Preventive Services Task Force found that diet and physical activity intervention led to restoration of normal glycemia in as early as one year from the intervention start and ranged from 20% at two years to 52% at six years [30]. Individuals who received lifestyle interventions were 53% more likely to achieve normal glycemia than those who did not receive this intervention.

The most prominent study to demonstrate how powerful lifestyle intervention can be for individuals with prediabetes was the Diabetes Prevention Program (DPP) [31]. This study enrolled overweight individuals who had both IGT and IFT. They were randomized to a placebo arm, metformin (850 mg) twice per day, or intensive lifestyle intervention. The lifestyle modification arm included 16 weekly educational sessions followed by eight monthly sessions and focused on reducing body weight by 7% and increasing physical activity to greater than 150 minutes per week. In addition, healthy nutrition was emphasized with increased emphasis on fruits and vegetables and whole grains. Multiple other studies including the Tuebingen Lifestyle Intervention Program (TULIP) [32] study and the Lifestyle Medicine Modification Program in Japan showed similar decreases in the likelihood of progressing to T2DM [33]. The Intensive Lifestyle Modification Program in the DPP reduced the likelihood of progressing to T2DM by 58%.

20.5 COMPONENTS OF EFFECTIVE LIFESTYLE INTERVENTION PROGRAMS

A variety of lifestyle intervention programs have been developed to effectively reduce the risk of developing prediabetes or lower the risk of prediabetes converting to T2DM. Of the interventions attempted, dietary interventions have resulted in the largest reductions of fasting blood sugar, followed by interventions combining nutrition and physical activity strategies. Interventions employing physical activity strategies alone achieved smaller results. Studies exploring weight loss and changing body composition to glucose regulation, typically utilizing a combination of healthy nutrition and physical activity, have shown that when weight loss of 5–7% is achieved, this reduced the likelihood of developing T2DM by 58%, largely as a result of the weight loss [31].

As already indicated, the most successful lifestyle modification programs used interventions such as the DPP not only aimed at promoting weight loss but also improving diet and increasing physical activity. In the DPP, the goal was weight reduction of greater than 5%, reduced total fat intake to less than 30%, and reduced saturated fat intake to less than 10%, while increasing fiber intake to greater than 15 grams per 1,000 calories and engaging in moderate-intensity physical activity for at least 30 minutes per day. The success of the DPP program suggests that a combination of proper nutrition and regular physical activity are keys to lowering the risk of prediabetes converting to T2DM. These interventions are also very important as a strategy for risk factor reduction for multiple other metabolic diseases [32–34]. The guidelines for individuals in DPP of engaging in 150 minutes of moderate intensity or 75 minutes of vigorous intensity aerobic activity per week are consistent with many other recommendations from prestigious national bodies, including the Physical Activity Guidelines for Americans 2018 [35]. In the area of nutrition, decreasing calorie intake and improving dietary quality are both important as components of prediabetes prevention and management.

Diets low in saturated fat and high in unsaturated fat, fruit, vegetables, and fiber intake, such as the Mediterranean diet, have been shown to be beneficial for glucose control both for individuals with prediabetes and T2DM. In addition, the PREDIMED-REUS Nutrition Intervention, which utilized the Mediterranean-style diet supplemented with extra olive oil and mixed nuts, was associated with a 51–52% lower T2DM risk than simply a low-fat diet alone [36]. Behavioral change both in the areas of nutrition and physical activity should be gradual and supervised. Start with small changes such as decreasing fried foods and switching to more whole grain breads as well as consumption of more fruits and vegetables. Successful programs such as the DPP employed proven behavioral change techniques such as goal setting, action planning, and problem solving, which were essential to participants to developing the self-regulating skills needed to adopt the health behaviors. In addition, social support, such as that provided by group-based weight loss programs or walking groups, also represent an effective and important tool to help people in changing their behavior. Lifestyle messages should also be culturally appropriate, which would improve acceptability and adherence [37,38].

Finally, technology can also be used to promote behavior change. For example, a recent meta-analysis of smart phone applications as well as remote monitoring and coaching have been demonstrated to assist people in moderate improvements in A1C levels [39,40]. It is important to emphasize that lifestyle modification alone may not be completely successful in individuals who have severe insulin resistance and particularly for people who have body mass index (BMI) ≥ 35 kg/m^2. In those whose A1C is very high, lifestyle intervention in combination with pharmacologic treatment with metformin may be additionally helpful.

20.6 DIETARY PATTERNS TO REDUCE THE RISK OF DIABETES

As already discussed in multiple chapters in this book, modern nutritional research focuses on dietary patterns, rather than individual foods or nutrients. The same is true for strategies to lower the risk of prediabetes turning into diabetes. The most compelling research available for healthy eating patterns for prediabetes to prevent type 2 diabetes are the Mediterranean diet and the low-fat or low-carbohydrate eating plans. The PREDIMED trial, which was a large, randomized controlled trial (RCT), compared a Mediterranean-style diet to low-fat eating patterns for prevention of type 2 diabetes onset [36]. The Mediterranean-style diet resulted in a 30% lower risk. Other studies that include vegetarian and Dietary Approaches to Stop Hypertension (DASH) diets also demonstrated a lower risk of developing type 2 diabetes [41].

The diets that have been shown effective to lower the risk of developing prediabetes or lowering the risk of prediabetes advancing to type 2 diabetes are all very consistent with each other and are all consistent with the *Dietary Guidelines for Americans 2020–2025* [42]. The Healthy U.S.-Style Dietary Pattern contained in the *Dietary Guidelines for Americans 2020–2025* emphasizes a variety of vegetables from all the subgroups, fruits (especially whole fruits), grains (at least half of which are whole grains), and low-fat dairy and a variety of protein foods and nontropical oils. This healthy eating pattern limits saturated fats and trans fats as well as added sugars and sodium [42].

The Mediterranean-style diet also emphasizes plant-based foods including nuts and seeds, vegetables, beans, and whole grains, fish and other seafood, olive oil as a principal source of dietary fat, dairy products such as yogurt and cheese in low or moderate amounts and typically fewer than four eggs per week, red meat in low frequency, wine in low to moderate amounts (except in Islamic countries where it is forbidden), and reduced concentrated sugars or honey. This is typically the diet that is found in countries that border the Mediterranean Sea. It has been demonstrated to reduce the risk of diabetes, lower A1C and triglycerides, and reduce the risk of major CVD events.

Vegetarian or vegan plans emphasize plant-based eating and do not include flesh foods, but do include egg (ovo) and/or dairy (lacto) products. These patterns have been demonstrated to reduce the risk of diabetes, reduce A1C, and yield weight loss, while lowering low-density lipoprotein cholesterol (LDL-C) and non–high-density lipoprotein cholesterol (HDL-C).

Low-fat diets emphasize vegetables, fruits, and starches, particularly those made with whole grain, as well as lean protein sources including beans and low-fat dairy products. These diets are typically defined as containing ≤30% of calories from fat and ≤10% of saturated fat. These diets have been shown to reduce the risk of diabetes, and with appropriate caloric restrictions, yield weight loss.

The DASH diet [41] also emphasizes fruits and vegetables, low-fat dairy products, whole grains, poultry, fish, and nuts, while reducing saturated fat, red meat, and sugar-containing beverages, while reducing sodium. The DASH diet has been demonstrated to reduce the risk of diabetes and lower blood pressure as well as achieving weight loss, particularly if caloric restriction is present.

20.7 THE ROLE OF FAT IN THE PREVENTION OF T2DM

Consumption of polyunsaturated fat has been shown to lower the risk of T2DM when compared to diets that have more saturated fat [36,41]. In addition, supplementation with omega-3 fatty acids in prediabetes has been demonstrated to reduce serum triglycerides and in several instances has been demonstrated to improve glucose metabolism. The PREDIMED trial, when supplemented with either extra-virgin olive oil or nuts versus a control diet, reduced the incidence of T2DM in individuals who entered the study without diabetes who were at high risk for CVD at baseline. A number of other observational studies, however, have failed to demonstrate the adverse relationship with full-fat dairy intake and diabetes risk. These inconsistent results may be due to differences in food matrix variations found in food sources of fat.

20.8 WEIGHT LOSS IN INDIVIDUALS WITH PREDIABETES

There is robust evidence indicating that weight loss is highly effective in preventing the progression from prediabetes to type 2 diabetes as well as managing cardiometabolic health in both individuals with prediabetes and in T2DM [43]. Both medical nutrition therapy (MNT) and diabetes self-management education and support (DSMES) should be utilized with overall eating plans that result in an energy deficit in individuals who are overweight or obese, in turn resulting in a collaborative effort to achieve weight loss. Structured weight loss programs with regular visits and potential use of meal replacements have also been shown to enhance weight loss in people with diabetes. Nutritional therapy in the form of MNT is the cornerstone in weight loss programs. It is most effective when combined with regular physical activity.

In the DPP follow-up of over four years, individuals with prediabetes were observed to achieve 7–10% of weight loss. Similar results were obtained in the Look AHEAD trial. If pharmaceutical therapy or metabolic surgery are utilized in individuals with prediabetes, nutritional therapy remains a key component of an overall lifestyle medicine program. Evidence does not identify one specific eating plan that is superior to others for generating recommended weight loss in people with prediabetes or diabetes. As always, any weight loss plan recommended should take into account an individual's dietary preferences, culinary ability, and meal preparation skills. Physical activity should also be recommended. As always, both the intensity of the intervention and the degree of individuals' adherence to the program are critically important for successful weight loss.

20.9 SWEETENERS IN PREDIABETES AND PREVENTION OF DIABETES

Sugar-sweetened beverage (SSB) consumption in the general population as well as individuals with prediabetes and diabetes significantly increases the risk of type 2 diabetes, weight gain, heart disease, kidney disease, nonalcoholic fatty liver disease, and tooth decay. In one study, a single serving of SSBs per day increased the risk of type 2 diabetes in adults with prediabetes by 26% [44]. Conversely, the replacement of SSBs with an equal amount of water reduced the risk of type 2 diabetes by 7–8% [45]. A number of Food and Drug Administration (FDA)–approved sugar substitutes have been considered safe and approved for consumption by the general public. However, neither the American Heart Association (AHA) nor the ADA recommend sugar substitute usage as an evidence-based strategy for reducing body weight to reduce cardiometabolic risk factors.

20.10 ALCOHOL CONSUMPTION

The ADA recommends that adults who have prediabetes and drink alcohol should do so in moderation, which means one drink per day or less for adult women and two drinks per day or less for adult men [21]. It is also important to educate people who have diabetes about the potential of delayed hypoglycemia after drinking alcohol. Moderate alcohol consumption appears to have no long-term detrimental effects on glucose in people with type 2 diabetes, although there are some data showing improved glycemia and insulin sensitivity with moderate intake. Neither the AHA nor the ADA recommends people with prediabetes who do not currently drink alcohol begin to do so.

20.11 PERSONALIZED NUTRITION/PRECISION MEDICINE IN PREDIABETES

Given the high prevalence of prediabetes, it is important to find ways of helping individuals with this condition lower their risk of progressing to T2DM. There has been recent interest in the area of personalized nutrition as a component of precision medicine to optimize care for individuals with both prediabetes and diabetes [45]. This field includes nutrigenomics where genetic variants influence the metabolism of specific nutrients to predict an individual's responses to them, as well as metabolics, which are based on the metabolic fingerprints of food. These factors may also impact on changing the abundance and composition of gut microbiota, which are relevant to food metabolism and glycemic control. The field of precision nutrition also utilizes many of the aspects of "big" data [46]. All of these can contribute to lowering the risk of an individual's prediabetes developing to T2DM. For example, metabolomics can undercover novel biomarkers in dietary components at risk of type 2 diabetes. While these studies are in their infancy, they carry enormous potential for eventually helping the large number of individuals who have prediabetes lower their risk of converting to T2DM.

20.12 CONCLUSIONS

An enormous number of people in the United States and around the world have the condition of prediabetes. In the United States, it has been estimated that between 34% and 38% of individuals have prediabetes, which is a condition which often leads to T2DM. The fundamental underlying issue in individuals who have prediabetes is glucose intolerance, which is typically based on insulin resistance. A number of factors impact on insulin resistance. One of which is age, since over 48% of adults age 65 or older have prediabetes. An array of lifestyle medicine habits and practices can significantly impact on the likelihood of prediabetes leading to T2DM. Perhaps the largest body of data comes from the DPP, which demonstrated that a combination of healthy nutrition, physical activity, and weight loss can reduce the likelihood of prediabetes developing into T2DM by 58%.

Nutritional recommendations in individuals with prediabetes include dietary patterns that are also effective for lowering the risk of CVD and other metabolic conditions. These dietary patterns typically involve increased consumption of fruits and vegetables, whole grains, fiber, and oily fish and reducing the intake of red meat, SSBs, and sodium. Weight loss is also a highly effective strategy for lowering the risk of converting prediabetes to diabetes. This was demonstrated in both the DPP and the Look AHEAD Trial [47].

Given the high prevalence of prediabetes, it is important that all practitioners of lifestyle medicine counsel individuals who have elevated fasting blood sugar about the various nutritional and other strategies to lower their risk of developing T2DM.

Clinical Applications

- All patients should be screened for fasting blood sugars.
- Prediabetes is diagnosed with a fasting blood glucose of 100–125 mg/dL or two-hour post-challenge plasma glucose of 140–199 mg/dL or hemoglobin A1C of 5.7–6.4%.
- Lifestyle measures can significantly lower the risk of prediabetes progressing to T2DM. These measures include healthy nutrition, regular physical activity, and, if necessary, weight loss.
- While prediabetes is very common, physicians typically do not recognize how important and powerful lifestyle measures can be used to reduce the risk of prediabetes converting to diabetes.
- It is essential that physicians be on the lookout for prediabetes and make effective counseling decisions to help individuals who have prediabetes lower their risk of progressing to diabetes.

REFERENCES

1. Centers for Disease Control and Prevention. National Diabetes Statistics Report, 2017. Atlanta, GA: Centers for Disease Control and Prevention, U.S. Dept of Health and Human Services, 2017.
2. Cowie C, Rust K, Ford E, et al. Full accounting of diabetes and pre-diabetes in the U.S. population in 1988–1994 and 2005–2006. Diabetes Care. 2009;32(2):287–294.
3. DECODE Study Group. Age- and sex-specific prevalences of diabetes and impaired glucose regulation in 13 European cohorts. Diabetes Care. 2003;26(1):61–69.
4. Lee L, Alexandrov A, Howard V, et al. Race, regionality and pre-diabetes in the Reasons for Geographic and Racial Differences in Stroke (REGARDS) study. Prev Med. 2014;63:43–47.
5. Gujral U, Narayan K, Kahn S, et al. The relative associations of β-cell function and insulin sensitivity with glycemic status and incident glycemic progression in migrant Asian Indians in the United States: The MASALA study. J Diabetes Complicat. 2014;28(1):45–50.
6. American Diabetes Association. Standards of Medical Care in Diabetes-2017. Diabetes Care. 2017;40(Supplement 1):S4–S132.

7. Yudkin J, Montori V. The epidemic of pre-diabetes: The Medicine and the Politics. BMJ. 2014;349.g4485.
8. Levitan E, Song Y, Ford E, et al. Is nondiabetic hyperglycemia a risk factor for cardiovascular disease? A meta-analysis of prospective studies. Arch Intern Med. 2004;164(19):2147–2155.
9. Brunner E, Shipley M, Witte D, et al. Relation between blood glucose and coronary mortality over 33 years in the Whitehall study. Diabetes Care. 2006;29(1):26–31.
10. Gerstein H, Santaguida P, Raina P, et al. Annual incidence and relative risk of diabetes in people with various categories of dysglycemia: A systematic overview and meta-analysis of prospective studies. Diabetes Res Clin Pract. 2007;78(3):305–312. PMID: 17601626.
11. Tabák A, Herder C, Rathmann W, et al. Prediabetes: A high-risk state for developing diabetes. The Lancet. 2012;379(9833):2279–2290.
12. Shepherd P, Kahn B. Glucose transporters and insulin action—implications for insulin resistance and diabetes mellitus. N Eng J Med. 1999;341(4):248–257.
13. The Emerging Risk Factors Collaboration. Glycated hemoglobin measurement and prediction of cardiovascular disease. JAMA. 2014;311(12):1225–1233.
14. The Emerging Risk Factors Collaboration. Diabetes mellitus, fasting glucose, and risk of cause-specific death. N Eng J Med. 2011;364(9):829–841.
15. Ikehara S, Tabák A, Akbaraly T, et al. Age trajectories of glycaemic traits in non-diabetic South Asian and white individuals: The Whitehall II cohort study. Diabetologia. 2015;58:534–542.
16. Ferrannini E, Gastaldelli A, Iozzo P. Pathophysiology of prediabetes. Med Clin North Am. 2011;95(2):327–339.
17. Barres R, Zierath J. The role of diet and exercise in the transgenerational epigenetic landscape of T2DM. Nat Rev Endocrinol. 2016;12(8):441–451.
18. Fiuza-Luces C, Garatachea N, Berger N, et al. Exercise is the real polypill. Physiology. 2013;28(5):330–358.
19. Engeda J, Mezuk B, Ratliff S, et al. Association between duration and quality of sleep and the risk of pre-diabetes: Evidence from NHANES. Diabet Med. 2013;30(6):676–680.
20. Piatti P, Setola E, Galluccio E, et al. Smoking is associated with impaired glucose regulation and a decrease in insulin sensitivity and the disposition index in first-degree relatives of type 2 diabetes subjects independently of the presence of metabolic syndrome. Acta Diabetol. 2014;51(5):793–799.
21. Cullmann M, Hilding A, Ostenson C. Alcohol consumption and risk of pre-diabetes and type 2 diabetes development in a Swedish population. Diabet Med. 2012;29(4):441–452.
22. Furukawa S, Fujita T, Shimabukuro M, et al. Increased oxidative stress in obesity and its impact on metabolic syndrome. J Clin Invest. 2004;114(12):1752–1761.
23. Erion D, Shulman G. Diacylglycerol-mediated insulin resistance. Nat Med. 2010;16(4):400–402.
24. Samuel V, Petersen K, Shulman G. Lipid-induced insulin resistance: Unravelling the mechanism. Lancet. 2010;375(9733):2267–2277.
25. Schenk S, Horowitz J. Acute exercise increases triglyceride synthesis in skeletal muscle and prevents fatty acid-induced insulin resistance. J Clin Invest. 2007;117(6):1690–1698.
26. Sato Y, Nagasaki M, Nakai N, et al. Physical exercise improves glucose metabolism in lifestyle-related diseases. Exp Biol Med. 2003;228(10):1208–1212.
27. Butler A, Janson J, Bonner-Weir S, et al. Beta-cell deficit and increased beta-cell apoptosis in humans with type 2 diabetes. Diabetes. 2003;52(1):102–110.
28. Beaudry J, Riddell M. Effects of glucocorticoids and exercise on pancreatic beta-cell function and diabetes development. Diabetes Metab Res Rev. 2012;28(7):560–573.

29. Zhang X, Devlin H, Smith B, et al. Effect of lifestyle interventions on cardiovascular risk factors among adults without impaired glucose tolerance or diabetes: A systematic review and meta-analysis. PLoS One. 2017;12(5):e0176436.
30. Balk E, Earley A, Raman G, et al. Combined diet and physical activity promotion programs to prevent type 2 diabetes among persons at increased risk: A systematic review for the community preventive services task force. Ann Intern Med. 2015;163(6):437–451.
31. Diabetes Prevention Program Research Group. Reduction in the incidence of type 2 diabetes with lifestyle intervention or metformin. N Eng J Med. 2002;346(6):393–403.
32. Stefan N, Staiger H, Wagner R, et al. A high-risk phenotype associates with reduced improvement in glycaemia during a lifestyle intervention in prediabetes. Diabetologia. 2015;58(12):2877–2884.
33. Kosaka K, Noda M, Kuzuya T. Prevention of type 2 diabetes by lifestyle intervention: A Japanese trial in IGT males. Diabetes Res Clin Pract. 2005;67(2):152–162.
34. Zhang X, Imperatore G, Thomas W, et al. Effect of lifestyle interventions on glucose regulation among adults without impaired glucose tolerance or diabetes: A systematic review and meta-analysis. Diabetes Res Clin Pract. 2017;123:149–164.
35. Physical Activity Guidelines Advisory Committee. 2018 Physical Activity Guidelines Advisory Committee. 2018 Physical Activity Guidelines Advisory Committee Scientific Report. Washington, DC: U.S. Department of Health and Human Services, 2018.
36. Konstantinidou V, Ruiz L, Ordovás J. Personalized nutrition and cardiovascular disease prevention: From Framingham to PREDIMED. Adv Nutr: An Int Rev J. 2014;5(3):368S–71S.
37. Bhopal R. The inter-relationship of folk, traditional and Western medicine within an Asian community in Britain. Soc Sci Med. 1986;22(1):99–105.
38. Pardhan S, Mahomed I. Knowledge, self-help and socioeconomic factors in South Asian and Caucasian diabetic patients. Eye. 2004;18(5):509–513.
39. Cui M, Wu X, Mao J, et al. T2DM Self-Management via Smartphone Applications: A Systematic Review and Meta-Analysis. PLoS One. 2016;11(11):e0166718.
40. Bian R, Piatt G, Sen A, et al. The effect of technology-mediated diabetes prevention interventions on weight: A meta-analysis. J Med Internet Res. 2017;19(3):e76.
41. Sacks F, Svetkey L, Vollmer W, et al. Effects on blood pressure of reduced dietary sodium and the Dietary Approaches to Stop Hypertension (DASH) diet. DASH-Sodium Collaborative Research Group. N Eng J Med. 2001;344(1):3–10.
42. U.S. Department of Agriculture and U.S. Department of Health and Human Services. *Dietary Guidelines for Americans, 2020–2025*, 9th edition. December 2020. DietaryGuidelines.gov; www.dietaryguidelines.gov/resources/2020-2025-dietary-guidelines-online-materials.
43. Franz M, Boucher J, Green-Pastors J, et al. Evidence-based nutrition practice guidelines for diabetes and scope and standards of practice. J Am Diet Assoc. 2008 Apr;108 (4 Suppl 1):S52–S58.
44. Ziemer D, Berkowitz K, Panayioto R, et al. A simple meal plan emphasizing healthy food choices is as effective as an exchange-based meal plan for urban African Americans with type 2 diabetes. Diabetes Care. 2003;26(6):1719–1724.
45. Michie S, Ashford S, Sniehotta F, et al. A refined taxonomy of behaviour change techniques to help people change their physical activity and healthy eating behaviours: The CALO-RE taxonomy. Psychology & Health. 2011;26(11):1479–1498.
46. Collins F, Varmus H. A new initiative on precision medicine. N Engl J Med. 2015;372(9): 793–795.
47. Berger S, Huggins G, McCaffery J, et al. Comparison among criteria to define successful weight-loss maintainers and regainers in the Action for Health in Diabetes (Look AHEAD) and Diabetes Prevention Program trials. Am JClin Nutr. 2017;106(6):1337–1346.

21 Nutrition for Overweight and Obesity

Key Points

- Overweight and obesity result from an imbalance of energy intake versus energy output.
- To utilize nutrition to assist in weight management, it is essential to create a caloric deficit, typically between 500 and 700 kcals/day.
- It is important to maintain healthy nutritional habits during weight loss. This can be accomplished by following evidence-based diets such as the DASH diet, the Mediterranean diet, and Healthy U.S.-Style Dietary Pattern in conjunction with caloric restriction.
- Behavioral intervention is the cornerstone for treatment plans with overweight or obesity. The American Heart Association (AHA), the American College of Cardiology (ACC), and The Obesity Society (TOS) all recommend comprehensive programs of weight management to combat overweight and obesity including not only physicians but also registered dietary nutritionists (RDNs).
- Obesity is a chronic relapsing disease and requires long-term strategies and commitments and shared decision making between the patient and the healthcare team.

21.1 INTRODUCTION

Overweight and obesity are endemic in the United States and around the world [1–3]. Increasing data suggest that over 72% of the adult population in the United States is either overweight or obese. Obesity in particular, increases the risk of multiple chronic diseases including morbidity from hypertension, dyslipidemias, type 2 diabetes mellitus (T2DM), coronary heart disease (CHD), stroke, gallbladder disease, osteoarthritis, sleep apnea, and respiratory problems as well as some cancers [4–6]. The psychosocial economic consequences of obesity have enormous implications for the health and well-being of the U.S. population.

Numerous prestigious academic organizations have offered guidance on nutritional and other lifestyle-related factors for reducing the likelihood of overweight and obesity. Both the Nutritional Guidelines 2021 from the AHA [7] and the *Dietary Guidelines for Americans 2020–2025* [8] emphasize that nutritional plans that create an energy balance are important to maintaining a healthy weight. In addition, the Joint Guidelines from the AHA/ACC/TOS also emphasize the importance of balanced energy intake and expenditure to maintain a healthy weight [4]. In order to lose weight, an energy deficit is required, which involves the following considerations:

DOI: 10.1201/9781003452607-21

- Target and energy intake less than is required for energy balance, specifically, 1,000–1,500 kcals/day for women and 1500–1800 kcals/day for men. It should be noted that kilocalorie levels need to be adjusted for the individual's body weight and physical activity levels [4].
- Individual energy requirements need to be developed according to a variety of expert guidelines, with the goal of an energy deficit of 500 kcals/day or 700 kcals/day or a 30% energy deficit [9–11].
- *Ad libitum* approaches may also be employed that do not establish a formal energy deficit but are achieved by reduction or elimination of particular food groups, particularly those that are high in energy density.
- The AHA/ACC/TOS guidelines rate the level of evidence for this approach as high.
- Nutrition is a key consideration in all of these approaches. In addition, all of these approaches emphasize the consumption of healthy foods such as increased fruit and vegetables, whole grains, and other plant-based components. These are typically high in nutrient density and low in energy density.

A wide variety of dietary approaches can produce weight loss in overweight individuals [4]. A few of them are listed here, and all are associated with weight loss, provided that reduction in energy intake is achieved. These include the following:

- The diet from the European Association for the Study of Obesity Guidelines.
- High-protein diet (25% of full calories from protein, 30% from fat, and 45% of total calories for carbohydrates).
- Higher-protein-zone-type diet (40% of calories from carbohydrates, 30% of total calories from protein, and 30% of total calories from fat).
- Lacto-ovo vegetarian-style diet with energy restriction.
- Low-calorie diet with prescribed energy restriction.
- Low-carbohydrate diet (initially less than 20 grams of carbohydrate per day).
- Low-fat vegan-style diet (10–25% of total calories from fat).
- Low-fat diet (20% of total calories from fat).
- Low-glycemic-load diet.
- Lower fat (less than or equal to 30% fat), high dairy (four servings of low-fat dairy products/day).
- Mediterranean-style diet.
- The AHA-style Step 1 Diet with a prescribed energy restriction of 1500–1800 kcals/day and less than 30% of total calories from fat and less than 10% of total calories from saturated fat.

21.2 DIETARY INTERVENTION AND COMPOSITION OF WEIGHT LOSS OVER TIME WITH DIETARY INTERVENTIONS

Regardless of dietary intervention, energy restriction is appropriate in overweight and obese adults. The average weight loss is maximal at six months and smaller weight loss for up to two years during treatment follow-up tapers. These approaches include the following:

- Low-fat approach.
- Higher-protein approaches.
- Low-carbohydrate dietary patterns including Mediterranean style, vegetarian, and other dietary pattern approaches.

21.3 MEDICAL ASSESSMENT

Nutritional assessment for weight loss in overweight and obese individuals starts with a medical assessment [12]. The AHA/ACC/TOS guidelines recommend a comprehensive lifestyle intervention composed of diet, physical activity, and behavior therapy [4]. The principal components of an on-site comprehensive lifestyle intervention include the following:

- Reduced-Calorie Diet—Overweight or obese individuals are typically prescribed a diet designed to induce an energy deficit of greater than or equal to 500 kcals/day. This typically involves prescribing 1,200–1,500 kcals per day for women and 1,500–1,800 kcals/day for men [6].
- Increased Physical Activity—Comprehensive intervention programs typically prescribe increased aerobic activity such as brisk walking for greater than 150 minutes per week. This is consistent with both the *Dietary Guidelines for Americans 2020–2025* and the Physical Activity Guidelines for Americans 2018 [13].
- Behavior Therapy—Comprehensive lifestyle interventions include a structured behavioral change program that includes self-monitoring of food intake, physical activity, and weight. Recommendations from the AHA/ACC/TOS guidelines [4] include the following:
  1. Advise overweight and obese individuals who would benefit from weight loss to participate for longer than or equal to six months in a comprehensive lifestyle program.
  2. Advise overweight and obese individuals who have lost weight to participate in a long-term (longer than or equal to one year) comprehensive weight loss maintenance program.
  3. For weight loss maintenance, prescribe face-to-face or phone delivery of a weight loss maintenance program to provide monthly or more frequent contact with trained interventionists.
  4. For individuals with body mass index (BMI) greater than or equal to 40 kg/m^2 or BMI greater than or equal to 35 kg/m^2 with obesity or comorbid conditions who have not responded to behavioral treatment, bariatric surgery may be an appropriate option for improving health. These individuals should be referred to an experienced bariatric surgeon for consultation. As part of the initial medical evaluation, biometrics should be measured including height, weight, and calculation of BMI. This allows

classification of overweight and obesity according to current classification methods.

5. Measuring Waist Circumference—In individuals with BMI <35 kg/m^2, it is recommended to provide additional information about medical conditions associated with obesity such as cardiovascular risk (greater than 88 cm or greater than 35 inches for women; greater than 102 cm or greater than 40 inches for men). In addition, a medical history should be undertaken with questions related to cardiovascular risk factors such as high blood pressure, hyperlipidemia, and hyperglycemia. Blood pressure lipids and glucose should be measured to assess cardiovascular risk and allow treatment to be matched to risk profile. During the initial medical examination and history, syndromes such as endocrine disorders and hypothyroidism, Cushing's disease, polycystic ovary syndrome, and other metabolic conditions should be ruled out since they may contribute to a patient's weight status. Medication history is also essential in order to identify any drugs associated with weight gain that can be discontinued or modified. For female patients it is also important to inquire about the possibility of pregnancy before making weight loss recommendations. Recommendations for weight gain during pregnancy should be individualized based on pre-pregnancy BMI to improve pregnancy outcome, avoid excessive maternal postpartum weight retention, and reduce the risk of the child acquiring chronic disease later in life.

21.4 NUTRITION ASSESSMENT

A comprehensive nutrition assessment involves obtaining a variety of aspects of nutrition-related status as well as nutrition-related problems [4,6]. This involves generating a food- and nutrition-related history, anthropometric measurements, biochemical data, medical tests and procedures, nutrition-focused physical findings, and history of the individual to generate a comprehensive weight management program. The nutrition-related history relates to beliefs and attitudes including food preferences and motivation, access to fruits and vegetables, the food environment, and many other aspects including past diet history [14,15].

The patient's weight history should be obtained as well as social history, living situation, and socioeconomic status. Weight history involves questions about the highest and lowest adult body weight as well as usual body weight within the last six months and the stated individual's preference of preferred or desired body weight. Assessment of body composition can help further individualize the dietary intervention for weight loss; available technology for such body composition assessment may include dual energy x-ray absorptiometry (DEXA) or bioelectrical impedance analysis (BIA).

21.5 DIETARY ASSESSMENT

A patient's energy needs represent an initial step to create the personalized dietary plan which is essential for decreased energy deficit needed for weight loss [4,6].

Energy expenditure consists of three components, basal energy expenditure, thermal effect of food, and adjustment for the physical activity level. The most accurate and typically used equation for basal energy expenditure involving these three components is called the Miflin-St. Jeor equation [16,17]. These are the following: For females REE = 10 × body weight (kg) + 6.25 × height (cm) – 5 × age (years) – 161. For males REE = 10 × body weight (kg) + 6.25 × height (cm) – 5 × age (years) + 5.

Physical activity level must also be estimated applying the appropriate activity level to the Mifflin–St. Jeor equation results, which is REE × 1.2 (sedentary), or × 1.4 (low active or moderate active), or × 1.6 (active) [16,17]. These activity evaluations emphasize that the key modifiable components of energy balance include both physical activity and diet since they complement each other to create an energy deficit [18]. It should be noted that increased physical activity alone is not a highly effective way of losing weight in the short term; however, it is critically important in terms of long-term maintenance of weight loss. In addition, both physical activity and inactivity play roles in overall health considerations in addition to determining energy expenditure.

- Determining Energy Intake
  The next step is to determine an individual's total energy intake and dietary consumption. There are multiple ways to assess total dietary intake. These are listed in Table 21.1. Mobile applications are now available for assessing and monitoring intake.
- Determining Eating Environment and Readiness for Intervention
  The eating environment includes access to food, food budget, location of meals, cultural food practices, and with whom meals are eaten. The assessment of readiness to change is typically based on various behavior change frameworks, which include cognitive behavior therapy, post-transtheoretical model, social cognitive theory, and social learning theory. Patient motivation is a key component for success in weight loss. Motivational interviewing (MI) can also play an important role, as is the case for any change in behavior. The MI technique places the individual who desires to lose weight at the center of counseling and puts them in charge of their weight loss program.

21.6 DIETARY INTERVENTION

When starting an intervention, it is important to discuss expectations and have clear and realistic weight loss goals together with the individual's input. As little as 5–10% of weight loss improves cardiovascular risk factors. This amount of weight loss may differ from a patient's expectations. In fact, when individuals with obesity were specifically asked about their weight loss goals, they stated that a 5–10% weight loss would be extremely disappointing.

As already indicated, there are numerous dietary approaches that facilitate reduction in energy consumption. For individuals who have a BMI >30, very low-calorie diets (<800 kcals daily) may be appropriate as a starter approach. They are no more effective, however, than the 1,200–1,500 kcals per day with regard to long-term

TABLE 21.1
Dietary Intake Assessment Methods

Method	Strengths	Limitations
Food Record/Food Diary *Patients are asked to prospectively record intake for a specified period of time*	• Doesn't rely on patient memory • Can be completed in advance of dietetic visit • Portion sizes can be measured at time of consumption • Data can be entered into dietary analysis program • Records of multiple days provide valid measure of usual intake for most nutrients	• Patient intake may change as a result of keeping a food record • Requires patient to be literate, numerate, and have portion size knowledge • High patient burden, time consuming • Relies on self-reported information
24-hr Recall *Patients are retrospectively asked about intake from the past 24 hours*	• Unlikely to modify behavior • Inexpensive • Low patient burden • No patient literacy requirement • Can be conducted in person or by telephone • Data can be entered into dietary analysis program	• Dependent on patient memory • Relies on self-reported information • Requires skilled interviewer • High inter-interviewer variability • Time consuming • Not representative of usual intake
Food Frequency Questionnaire *Patients complete a survey that retrospectively queries how often certain foods/beverages were consumed in a specified period of time*	• Low patient burden • Quick, inexpensive • Easily standardized • Useful screening tool	• Requires patient to be literate and numerate • Dependent on patient memory • Can be cognitively difficult for patient because food lists are not meal-based • Doesn't provide valid estimate of total intake or meal patterns
Diet History *Patients are interviewed about their usual eating habits*	• No patient literacy requirement • Low patient burden • Enables assessment of meal patterning, usual nutrient, and food group intake in one interview	• Dependent on patient memory • Requires skilled interviewer • Time consuming

Source: From Crowley N, Arlinghaus, K. Dietary Management of Overweight and Obesity. In Rippe JM (ed): Lifestyle Medicine, 4th ed. CRC Press (Boca Raton), 2024. Used with permission.

weight loss. Meal replacements may have value because they provide a regulated amount of calories per serving and so constitute a departure from normal eating patterns. For most obese patients, however, caloric restriction using real foods is ultimately the best way to approach healthy, long-term weight loss.

Numerous studies have compared low-fat to low-carbohydrate diets. In some studies, low-carbohydrate diets have resulted in more initial weight loss; however, when studies have compared them for weight loss at two years, they are the equivalent.

Perhaps the most effective way of inducing weight loss involves utilizing diets which will also result in an overall healthy eating pattern with energy restriction and can also yield other cardiometabolic benefits. For example, the Dietary Approaches to Stop Hypertension (DASH) diet [19] may produce further reductions in blood pressure and the Mediterranean diet with energy restriction [20] may also yield further cardiovascular risk reduction improvements when compared to low-fat diets. As discussed in numerous chapters on metabolic disease in this book, dietary patterns that involve healthy nutrition such as those recommended in the *Dietary Guidelines for Americans 2020–2025*, coupled with energy restriction, can represent a very good starting point.

Eating foods with low energy density substitutes with higher energy density and allows a greater sense of fullness and a greater amount of food to be eaten [21,22]. It is also important to reduce sugar-sweetened beverage consumption since individuals typically compensate less for energy consumed in beverages when compared to energy from foods [22,23]. The Academy of Nutrition and Dietetics recommends non-nutritive sweeteners for this reason [24]. It should be noted, however, that not all studies with nutritive sweeteners have been successful for inducing long-term weight loss. It is also important to emphasize that while restricting calories, it remains important that essential nutrients be consumed. This can be accomplished by utilizing a basic plant-based healthy diet.

In the final analysis, it is essential that robust discussions take place with the individual who is attempting to lose weight to create a plan that is both realistic and likely to improve adherence. This can be most easily achieved by evaluating the strengths of the patient's current diet and making necessary modifications to achieve weight loss and manage any of the other conditions. It is also important to emphasize that energy balance may be very complicated and may vary considerably among individuals. Some of this variation may result from changes in the microbiome in the gut [25]. Variability from individual to individual emphasizes the importance of careful discussions with each patient.

One approach that has great promise in this area has been called "precision nutrition" for weight loss (see Chapter 32 for more detail). This concept is only beginning to be explored. It involves recognition that different individuals will lose weight at different speeds. A component of precision prevention may also involve the role of epigenetics.

21.7 SETTING REALISTIC GOALS

Setting goals that the overweight or obese individual will find to be realistic is critically important [25]. One way to approach this issue is to use MI. This is the type of interviewing that puts the individual patient in the center of the encounter. MI explores both barriers and strengths which the individual can recognize either to help facilitate or hinder success in any lifestyle change, but in particular, in weight loss [26]. The AHA/ACC/TOS guidelines recommend comprehensive lifestyle management for all individuals who are trying to lose weight including those for whom pharmaceutical or surgical intervention is also recommended. This, of course, is central to the central tenets of lifestyle medicine.

Frequency of contact is an important characteristic demonstrated to enhance the likelihood of weight loss success. Lifestyle medicine practitioners may want to engage along with either a weight management, comprehensive group, or at least an RDN to accomplish this frequency of contact. There is good evidence that at least 14 sessions of medical nutrition therapy (MNT) over a period of six months is most efficacious. This will increase the likelihood of achieving 5–10% of loss of initial weight.

It is also important to recognize that energy needs will change as weight is lost. This is why continued monitoring and evaluation of energy requirements are important since these allow adjustments of energy intake based on reduced body weight. This will help the individual work their way through, or perhaps even prevent, a weight loss plateau, which may occur at about six months for many patients. Of course, continuing to engage in regular physical activity is also very important.

For weight maintenance after weight loss, good evidence exists from both from the Diabetes Prevention Program [27] and the Look AHEAD trial [28,29] that at least monthly ongoing visits and continued MNT occur for at least one year. Increasing use of technology as a mode of delivery may also be helpful to meet weight loss goals.

An increasing number of weight loss medications are now available on the market which may also assist in short- and long-term weight loss. Perhaps the most thoroughly studied is the class of semaglutides. If weight loss medication is indicated, it may be worth consulting with a weight loss specialist to consider the options that are currently available.

If either pharmaceutical therapy or bariatric surgery is contemplated, it will be important for the lifestyle medicine practitioner to continue to play a central role, particularly when it comes to the area of nutrition and weight loss. There are a number of current Food and Drug Administration (FDA)–approved medications which may help facilitate weight loss use through appetite suppression or absorption of fat. A detailed description of these medications is beyond the scope of this chapter. However, the newer GLP-1 agonists such as semaglutide [30] and tirzepatide [31] have shown very promising results for weight loss.

For individuals who have a BMI >35 kg/m^2 or with obesity with comorbid conditions or BMI >40 kg/m^2 who are motivated to lose weight but for whom behavioral therapy has not resulted in sufficient weight loss, a referral may be appropriate for an experienced bariatric surgeon who has an interdisciplinary team of medical nutritional and psychological professionals for evaluation [32]. In this setting it will be essential to continue the appropriate nutritional therapy in collaboration with the bariatric surgical team [33].

In virtually every aspect of behavioral change including weight loss, physician recommendation remains a very powerful motivator. Studies have shown that physician recommendation stands as more powerful than any other factor for encouraging individuals who are overweight or obese to lose weight. It is essential that medical practitioners discuss weight with their patients and underscore that weight is a health concern and there are effective treatments for weight loss. Unfortunately, less than 40% of physicians routinely discuss weight with overweight or obese patients, which represents lost opportunity, since over 70% of individuals see their primary care physician on an at least an annual basis.

21.8 FOOD CHOICE

To help an overweight or obese individual adopt the most efficacious weight loss plan for them, it is central to understand that a variety of factors impact on how individuals chose foods. This involves addressing issues of what, when, and how much individuals eat. This can be impacted on by both environmental factors such as choosing healthy, nutrient-dense but lower energy-dense foods as well as discussions with whomever prepares food. Environmental cues such as food palatability and the neurobiologically rewarding effects of food should also be considered. Furthermore, neighborhood availability of healthy foods has been shown to be strongly associated with healthy weight status in a neighborhood. Such factors as cost and convenience must also be taken into consideration. Portion size of packaged foods and foods served away from home can also influence food choice. In addition, the social and media environment can impact on food choice since people typically eat in accordance with beliefs about what constitutes normal eating behavior. Food advertising can also strongly impact on food choices.

21.9 EVIDENCE-BASED DIETS

While a number of commercially based diet programs are available, it is important to consider how energy restriction can occur without compromising micronutrient intake. Dietary patterns that contain strong evidence of weight loss with appropriate healthy food choices will increase the likelihood of adequate micronutrient intake. Those include the DASH diet, the Mediterranean diet and the Healthy U.S.-Style Dietary Pattern contained in the Dietary Guidelines for Americans (DGAs) 2020–2025.

The DASH diet focuses on increasing vegetables, fruits, lean proteins, and whole grains with limited saturated fats, sweets, sugar-sweetened beverages, and sodium [19]. The DASH diet, combined with caloric restriction and exercise, has been demonstrated to reduce both weight and blood pressure.

The Mediterranean diet also emphasis vegetables and fruits but also contains olive oil, nuts, beans, legumes, seeds, and whole grains and contains limited meats and dairy and moderate wine consumption [20]. This diet is particularly rich in antioxidants. The Mediterranean diet has been shown to be an effective strategy for reducing weight and lowering cardiovascular risk factors. Overweight and obese individuals who followed the Mediterranean diet plan achieved weight loss of between 8.36 and 22.22 pounds in one study at 12 months.

The Healthy U.S.-Style Eating Pattern (HUSEP) also includes healthy intake of vegetables, fruits, whole grains, fat-free and low-fat dairy products, proteins, and mono- and polyunsaturated fats with limits on added sugars, saturated fats, trans fats, cholesterol, sodium, and alcohol [8]. The HUSEP can be used as a general eating pattern for adults as well as for weight loss when it is combined with modest caloric restriction.

21.10 MEAL REPLACEMENTS AND STRUCTURED MEAL PLANS

Meal replacements and structured meal plans may also represent a possible way to help achieve weight loss by helping overweight and obese individuals decrease caloric intake [33,34]. Structured meal plans in combination with behavioral weight loss interventions generally use low-caloric diets (1,200–1,500 kcals/day) with three meals and two snacks each day [35]. Meal replacements may be utilized to decrease consumption by replacing one to two primary meals a day with a lower-calorie alternative such as a bar, shake, soup, or hot chocolate.

21.11 BEHAVIORAL CONSIDERATIONS FOR TREATMENT

Both TOD [4,6] and the Academy of Nutrition and Dietetics recommend basic MNT for adult weight management but also include the use of behavioral change strategies to help individuals sustain a reduced-calorie diet and increase physical activity. Behavioral techniques are utilized to provide the individual with the skills they can use to improve their overall lifestyle [36]. This, of course, is a central concept for all of lifestyle medicine. Behavioral strategies that have been demonstrated to assist in weight loss include self-monitoring, problem solving, and various cognitive behavioral strategies [37].

21.12 COMMERCIAL WEIGHT LOSS PROGRAMS

Commercial weight loss programs, both "in person" and via the internet, represent a multibillion-dollar industry. Many obese individuals will have experienced one or more commercial weight loss programs. These programs are monitored by the Federal Trade Commission (FTC). When a diet or program is not keeping promises that they make, the FTC may intervene to take the program off the market or insist upon modifications. An evaluation of commercial weight loss programs is beyond the scope of this chapter; however, it is available through the Academy of Nutrition and Dietetics and also TOS.

21.13 GLUCAGON-LIKE PEPTIDE 1 (GLP-1) AGONISTS: ARE THEY SUCCESSFUL IN THE LONG TERM?

New research has suggested that GLP-1 agonists may produce a weight loss of 12–18%, which far exceeds any prior pharmacologic therapy. These results have generated enormous attention and utilization.

It should be noted that in the trials that establish efficacy for GLP-1 agonists, weight loss typically plateaus at 12–18 months, and when the medication is stopped, patients generally regain the lost weight within a year. This has led to a recommendation of chronic use. The big problem with the need for long-term use is the enormous expense of these medications. The U.S. list prices for these medicines are $12,000–$16,000 per year. Despite the health benefits of achieving substantial amounts of weight loss, the incremental costs of long-term use of GLP-2 agonists may reach between $270,000 and $483,000 per quality-adjusted life year [38].

Many obesity experts are now saying that to combat the problem of weight regain following use of GLP-1 agonists alone, they should be combined with careful nutrition counseling. Long-term trials such as the Diabetes Prevention Program and the Look AHEAD study have clearly demonstrated that sound long-term nutritional counseling with a structured approach is highly efficacious. Thus, it would appear that a reasonable approach to the use of GLP-1 agonists might combine them with ongoing structured nutrition counseling programs to ameliorate the problem of significant weight regain following cessation of these medications. Without such a strategy, the chronic use of these medications may be cost-prohibitive both for the individual and also for the overall health care budget of the United States [39].

21.14 NUTRITION WEIGHT LOSS MYTHS

Unfortunately, many individuals continue to look for a "secret" for weight loss [37]. This may also be buttressed by claims from various commercial programs to have discovered the secret for weight loss. Thus, it is important to understand there are many myths that further perpetuate unrealistic views of finding one "magical" secret for weight loss. Some of the most prevalent weight loss myths are the following:

- Drinking more water can aid in weight loss—While water is certainly preferable to sugar-sweetened beverages, there is no reason to exceed the recommended daily allowance (RDA) of water, which is 1 ml of water for every calorie consumed.
- Skipping breakfast causes weight gain—This has been demonstrated to be a myth through a variety of research studies.
- Small meals consumed more frequently—Numerous studies have examined the relationship between food timing and frequency. When this has been evaluated, the strategy of eating small meals frequently has not consistently resulted in improved outcomes.
- Eating after dinner will cause weight gain—Once again, the studies in this area are quite mixed. Ultimately, positive energy balance is what causes weight gain. It is possible that late evening meals may increase overall calorie intake, in which case this strategy is not unreasonable to decrease eating late at night.
- Obesity is caused by insulin resistance—Obesity certainly can lead to insulin resistance, but treating insulin resistance as a strategy for weight loss is putting the cart before the horse. Caloric restriction remains the strategy for weight loss, and when weight is lost, insulin resistance will naturally decrease.

21.15 CONCLUSIONS

Overweight and obesity are caused by imbalance between caloric consumption and caloric expenditure. Healthy weight loss involves both improving nutrition and, in many instances, increasing physical activity [37]. Multiple diets are available including the DASH diet, the Mediterranean diet and the HUSEP, which, when combined with modest caloric restriction, can play a critical role in safe and healthy weight loss while reducing the risk of other chronic conditions that are associated with overweight and obesity such as cardiovascular disease, diabetes, and even cancer while still maintaining proper nutritional balance.

Clinical Applications

- Healthy nutrition with caloric restriction is essential for weight loss as a strategy for overcoming overweight and obesity.
- A nutrition assessment utilizes tools to estimate energy expenditure and energy intake.
- During energy restriction, it is important to utilize evidence-based diets that are healthy including such diets as DASH, Mediterranean diet, and the HUSEP.
- Obesity is a chronic relapsing disease and requires long-term strategies and commitments shared between the overweight or obese individual and healthcare team.

REFERENCES

1. Centers for Disease Control and Prevention. DC US Obesity Stats Overweight and Obesity Data Statistics. www.cdc.gov/obesity/data/index.html (Accessed January 8, 2024).
2. Chong B, Jayabaskaran J, Kong G, et al. Trends and predictions of malnutrition and obesity in 204 countries and territories: An analysis of the blobal burden of disease Study 2019. eClinicalMedicine. 2023;57:101850.
3. Rippe J, Foreyt J. Obesity Prevention and Treatment: A Practical Guide. Boca Raton: CRC Press, 2021.
4. Flegal K, Graubard B, Williamson D, et al. Excess deaths associated with underweight, overweight, and obesity. JAMA. 2005;20;293(15):1861–1867.
5. Bray G. Obesity: The disease. J Med Chem. 2006;13;49(14):4001–4007.
6. Raynor H, Champagne C. Position of the academy of nutrition and dietetics: Interventions for the treatment of overweight and obesity in adults. J Acad Nutr Diet. 2016;116(1):129–147.
7. Lichtenstein A, Appel L, Vadiveloo M, et al. 2021 Dietary guidance to improve cardiovascular health: A scientific statement from the American Heart Association. Circulation. 2021;144(23):e472–e487.
8. U.S. Department of Agriculture and U.S. Department of Health and Human Services. *Dietary Guidelines for Americans, 2020–2025*, 9th edition. December 2020. Dietary Guidelines.gov (Accessed January 8, 2024).
9. The Joint FAO/WHO/UNU Expert Consultation on Energy and Protein Requirements. Energy and Protein Requirements: Report of Joint FAO/WHO/UNU Expert Organization Technical Report Series No. 724 Geneva: World Health Organization, 1985: 1–206.
10. Subak L, Wing R, West D, et al. PRIDE Investigators. Weight loss to treat urinary incontinence in overweight and obese women. N Engl J Med. 2009;29;360(5):481–490.
11. Svetkey L, Stevens V, Brantley P, et al. Weight Loss Maintenance Collaborative Research Group. Comparison of strategies for sustaining weight loss: The weight loss maintenance randomized controlled trial. JAMA: J Am Med Assoc. 2008;299(10):1139–1148.

12. Crowley N, Arlinghaus K. Dietary management of overweight and obesity. In Rippe JM (ed). Lifestyle Medicine, 4th edition. Boca Raton: CRC Press, 2024.
13. Physical Activity Guidelines Advisory Committee. 2018 Physical Activity Guidelines Advisory Committee Scientific Report. Washington, DC: U.S. Department of Health and Human Services, 2018.
14. Academy of Nutrition and Dietetics. Nutrition Terminology Reference Manual (eNCPT): Dietetics Language for Nutrition Care. http://ncpt.webauthor.com (Accessed January 8, 2024).
15. Academy of Nutrition and Dietetics Evidence Analysis Library. "Adult Weight Management: Executive summary of recommendations 2014" Academy of Nutrition and Dietetics. www.andeal.org/topic.cfm?menu=5276&cat=4690 (Accessed January 8, 2024).
16. Frankenfield D, Roth-Yousey L, Compher C. Comparison of predictive equations for resting metabolic rate in healthy nonobese and obese adults: A systematic review. J Am Diet Assoc. 2005;105(5):775–789.
17. Mifflin M, St Jeor S, Hill L, et al. A new predictive equation for resting energy expenditure in healthy individuals. Am J Clin Nutr. 1990;51(2):241–247.
18. Donnelly J, Blair S, Jakicic J, et al. American College of Sports Medicine Position Stand. Appropriate physical activity intervention strategies for weight loss and prevention of weight regain for adults. Med Sci Sports Exerc. 2009;41(2):459–471.
19. Sacks F, Svetkey L, Vollmer W, et al. Effects on blood pressure of reduced dietary sodium and the Dietary Approaches to Stop Hypertension (DASH) diet. DASH-Sodium Collaborative Research Group. N Engl J Med. 2001;344(1):3–10.
20. Estruch R, Ros E, Salas-Salvado J, et al. Primary prevention of cardiovascular disease with a Mediterranean diet. N Engl J Med. 2013;368(14):1279–1290.
21. Rolls B, Roe L, Meengs J. Portion size can be used strategically to increase vegetable consumption in adults. Am J Clin Nutr. 2010;91(4):913–922.
22. Perez-Escamilla R, Obbagy J, Altman J, et al. Dietary energy density and body weight in adults and children: A systematic review. J Acad Nutr Diet. 2012;112(5):671–684.
23. Tate D, Turner-McGrievy G, Lyons E, et al. Replacing caloric beverages with water or diet beverages for weight loss in adults: Main results of the Choose Healthy Options Consciously Everyday (CHOICE) randomized clinical trial. Am J Clin Nutr. 2012;95(3):555–563.
24. Fitch C, Keim K. Position of the Academy of Nutrition and Dietetics: Use of nutritive and nonnutritive sweeteners. J Acad Nutr Diet. 2012;112(5):739–758.
25. Krajmalnik-Brown R, Ilhan Z, Kang D, et al. Effects of gut microbes on nutrient absorption and energy regulation. Nutr Clin Pract. 2012;27(2):201–214.
26. Fifield P, Suzuki J, Minski S. Motivational interviewing and lifestyle change. In Rippe JM (ed). Lifestyle Medicine, 4th edition. Boca Raton: CRC Press, 2024.
27. Knowler W, Barrett-Connor E, Fowler S, et al. Reduction in the incidence of type 2 diabetes with lifestyle intervention or metformin. N Engl J Med. 2002;346(6):393–403.
28. Wing R, Bolin P, Brancati F, et al. The Look AHEAD Research Group. Cardiovascular effects of intensive lifestyle intervention in type 2 diabetes. N Engl J Med. 2013;369(2):145–154.
29. Wing R, Hamman R, Bray G, et al. Achieving weight and activity goals among diabetes prevention program lifestyle participants. Obes Res. 2004;12(9):1426–1434.
30. Weghuber D, Barrett T, Barrientos-Pérez M, et al. Once-weekly semaglutide in adolescents with obesity. N Engl J Med. 2022;387(24):2245–2257.
31. Jastreboff A, Aronne L, Ahmad N, et al. Tirzepatide once weekly for the treatment of obesity. N Engl J Med. 2022;387(3):205–216.
32. Kushner R. Surgery for severe obesity. In Rippe J (ed). Lifestyle Medicine, 4th edition. Boca Raton: CRC Press, 2024.

33. Ashley J, St Jeor S, Schrage J, et al. Weight control in the physician's office. Arch Intern Med. 2001;161(13):1599–1604.
34. Ditschuneit H, Flechtner-Mors M, Johnson T, et al. Metabolic and weight-loss effects of a long-term dietary intervention in obese patients. Am J Clin Nutr. 1999;69(2):198–204.
35. Ditschuneit H, Flechtner-Mors M. Value of structured meals for weight management: Risk factors and long-term weight maintenance. Obes Res. 2001;9(Suppl 4):284S–289S.
36. D'Zurilla T, Goldfried M. Problem solving and behavior modification. J Abnorm Psychol. 1971;78(1):107–126.
37. Ledoux T, Lopez T, Johnston C, et al. Nutrition in weight management and obesity. In Rippe J (ed). Nutrition in Lifestyle Medicine. Nutrition and Health. Humana Press, 2017.
38. Atlas SJ, Kim K, Nhan E, et al. Medications for obesity management: Effectiveness and value. J Manag Care Spec Pharm. 2023;29(5):569–657.
39. Mozaffarian D, Aspry K, Garfield K, et al. "Food is medicine" strategies for nutrition ecurity and cardiometabolic health equity. J Am Coll Cardiol. 2024;83(8):843–864.

22 Nutrition in the Prevention and Treatment of Diabetes

Key Points

- The prevalence of diabetes has grown substantially in the United States and around the world in the last 30 years.
- Over 10% of the population in the United States currently has diabetes
- Lifestyle interventions including proper nutrition, optimally delivered with medical nutrition therapy (MNT), weight loss if necessary, and increased physical activity, have all been shown to assist in the treatment of diabetes. These same modalities also have been shown to assist in the prevention of diabetes and lowering the risk of prediabetes being converted to diabetes.

22.1 INTRODUCTION

Diabetes is a chronic metabolic health condition that is extremely common in the United States and around the world. The prevalence of diabetes has grown considerably in the last two decades and mirrors, to some degree, the increase in overweight and obesity during that period of time.

According to the Centers for Disease Control and Prevention (CDC), in 2019 there were 37.3 million Americans (approximately 10%) who had diabetes [1]. Unfortunately, approximately 20% of people with diabetes do not know that they have it. Of equal importance, 96 million adults, more than 33% of the population, have prediabetes, and unfortunately a shocking 80% of these individuals do not know that they have this condition [2]. Diabetes is associated with a variety of other chronic conditions. For example, 69% of individuals with diabetes have high blood pressure, 44% have high cholesterol, and 39% have chronic kidney disease [3]. Diabetes is highest among Black and Hispanic/Latino adults in both men and women.

Multiple lifestyle modalities can play significant roles in both decreasing the likelihood that prediabetes will progress to diabetes and also in both the prevention and therapy of diabetes itself. Lifestyle therapies including MNT [4], increased physical activity, weight management, and educational counseling and support, all play critical roles in both the prevention and management of diabetes [5–9]. Indeed, lifestyle interventions in individuals with prediabetes can effectively prevent or delay type 2 diabetes mellitus (T2DM) in some instances for up to 15–20 years [10]. These same lifestyle interventions are effective throughout the disease process and have the greatest impact early in the course of the disease. Nutritional intervention, particularly in the form of MNT, plays a critical role in all phases of diabetes prevention and management.

DOI: 10.1201/9781003452607-22

22.2 THE DEFINITION OF NUTRITIONAL THERAPY FOR DIABETES

According to the National Academy of Medicine, nutrition therapy is the treatment of a disease or condition through modification of nutrient or whole food intake. This is particularly important in the area of diabetes [11].

The Dietary Guidelines for Americans (DGA) 2020–2025 provide an overall framework for healthy eating for all Americans [12]. The core of the DGA 2020–2025 contains the recommendation that people follow a healthy eating pattern with abundant fruits and vegetables while maintaining an appropriate calorie level.

Individuals with diabetes should follow the same basic pattern as the Healthy U.S.-Style Dietary; however, there are some recommendations that differ from the DGA. Typical nutrition therapy for diabetes is provided through a framework called MNT, which is typically provided by a registered dietitian nutritionist (RDN) [13]. Multiple components comprise MNT, including assessment, nutritional diagnosis, intervention (e.g. education and counseling), and monitoring with ongoing follow-up to support long-term lifestyle changes, evaluation outcomes, and modification of interventions as needed. The overall goal of MNT is to provide support for healthy eating patterns that emphasize nutrient-dense foods (particularly fruits and vegetables and whole grains) in appropriate portion sizes with the goal of improving hemoglobin A1C, blood pressure, and cholesterol levels.

Detailed recommendations for goals for MNT have been provided by the American Dietetic Association (ADA) and include the following emphasis: Achieve and maintain body weight goals and delay or prevent complications of diabetes. In addition, the goal of MNT is to make sure that nutritional needs are based on personal and cultural preferences, access to healthy food choices, and the willingness and ability to make behavioral changes [13]. Throughout MNT, positive messages about food choices are provided, and limiting food choices is only advised when there is strong scientific evidence.

The overarching goal for MNT is to provide the individual with diabetes the practical tools to meet day-to-day meal planning objectives and challenges. The Academy of Nutrition and Dietetics recommends that RDNs implement three to six MNT encounters within six months of the diagnosis of diabetes. Additional MNT encounters may be necessary based on the individual assessment.

The RDN is the ideal person to administer MNT, particularly if the RDN has met the standards for expert knowledge aligned by the Academy of Nutrition and Dietetics.

The overall framework for healthcare professionals in providing nutritional guidance can also be found in the Academy of Nutrition and Dietetics Scope of Practice [14]. In addition to providing MNT, individuals with diabetes should be counseled in the area of diabetes self-management education and support (DSMES), which has been demonstrated to improve real metabolic outcomes [15]. DSMES is essential to facilitate knowledge, skills, and abilities for the individual with diabetes to manage self-care throughout the lifespan [16].

Nutrition remains a core topic in these type of comprehensive programs. MNT has been demonstrated to be effective in improving hemoglobin A1C similar to or greater than expected with treatment available with medication for T2DM. MNT interventions are often shown to improve hemoglobin A1C with absolute decreases of up to 2% in T2DM in three to six months [13–15]. Ongoing MNT is also helpful in maintaining glycemic control. MNT has also been demonstrated in multiple studies to be a cost-effective type of lifestyle intervention [14].

22.3 RECOMMENDATIONS FOR NUTRITION THERAPY FOR PREVENTION OF DIABETES

The evidence for nutrition therapy in prediabetes comes from several large, randomized controlled trials. Prediabetes is the state where hyperglycemia is present but blood glucose levels are lower than the diabetes threshold. Compelling evidence exists that lifestyle interventions, particularly in nutrition intervention, focusing on achieving and maintaining healthy body weight, improving dietary patterns, and increasing physical activity can prevent or reverse prediabetes. Individuals with prediabetes may particularly benefit by modifying a variety of activities. Most prominently, these include diet, although physical activity also can improve glucose regulation and reduce cardiovascular risk factors.

- Diabetes Prevention Program

  In the Diabetes Prevention Program (DPP), overweight participants who had impaired glucose tolerance (IGT) and impaired fasting glucose (IFG) were randomized to a placebo, metformin (850 mg twice a day), or intensive lifestyle intervention that included 16 weekly educational sessions followed by 8 monthly session—all of which focused on proper nutrition and reducing body weight. At the end of the 2.8-year follow-up period, the lifestyle intervention program proved superior to either metformin or the placebo group by lowering the risk of advancing to T2DM by 58% [17].

  Other studies have shown similar results. For example, the Finnish Diabetes Prevention Study (FDPS) showed that weight loss of 7% improved insulin sensitivity and basal cell function while significantly reducing the incidence of T2DM. These studies showed that individuals with prediabetes should be referred to intensive behavioral lifestyle intervention programs, such as the one that was delivered in the DPP, and should receive MNT, which is typically provided by an RDN. The goal of MNT is to improve eating habits as well as increasing moderate-intensity physical activity to at least 150 minutes per week and achieving or maintaining a 7–10% loss of initial body weight.

  Of note, DPP-model intensive lifestyle interventions, including individualized MNT for prediabetes, has been demonstrated to achieve cost-effectiveness and should be covered by third-party payors and various other payment models. Individual health tools are now becoming available to make diabetes prevention programs more accessible to the public. These programs have thus far shown that they can yield weight loss, improve glycemia, and reduce risk of diabetes and cardiovascular disease (CVD) [17,18]. More studies are still needed in this area.

- Macronutrients
  The ADA has recommended that nutrient distribution be based on the individual assessment of current eating patterns, preferences, and metabolic goals [13]. There is not an ideal percentage of calories from carbohydrate, protein, or fat for all people who either have or are at risk for diabetes. In addition, the ADA recommends counseling individuals to optimize meal timing and food choices, which also guides medication and physical activity recommendations.
- Fiber
  The ADA recommends that individuals with diabetes be encouraged to consume recommended amounts of dietary fiber, preferably through food [13,19–23]. Fiber may help lower hemoglobin A1C. The ADA further recommends that people with diabetes should, on average, eat about the same portions of macronutrients as the general public. This comprises 45% calories from carbohydrate, 36–40% calories from fat, and the remainder (16–18%) from protein. The macronutrient mix should also be appropriate to either obtain weight management goals or lose weight. The quality of carbohydrate foods should be chosen for complex carbohydrates that are rich in dietary fiber, vitamins, and minerals. Regular intake of dietary fiber is associated with lower all-cause mortality in people with diabetes. At least half of grain consumption should be whole, intact grains. Dietary fiber should be consumed in whole foods rather than supplements.
- Dietary Fat
  Epidemiologic studies have found that the consumption of polyunsaturated fat is associated with lower risk of type 2 diabetes [24]. In addition, supplementation with omega-3 fatty acids in individuals with prediabetes has shown some benefit for serum triglycerides. The PREDIMED study, which compared the Mediterranean-style eating pattern supplemented with either extra-virgin olive oil or nuts versus a control diet, reduced the incidence of type 2 diabetes among people without diabetes at high risk for CVD at baseline [25]. Several studies have suggested and reported that increased saturated fat intake is associated with higher risk of diabetes [26].

22.4 EATING PATTERNS

The ADA has stated that a variety of different eating patterns are acceptable for the management of diabetes [27]. Eating patterns should focus on the following: Emphasize nonstarchy vegetables, minimize added sugars and refined grains, and chose whole foods over highly processed foods to the greatest extent possible.

It has also been recommended to reduce overall carbohydrate intake in individuals with diabetes. This recommendation can be applied to a variety of eating patterns.

Compelling research exists for managing prediabetes and lowering the risk of type 2 diabetes such as found in Mediterranean, low-fat, or low-carbohydrate eating patterns. This was demonstrated in the PREDIMED trial and also the DASH diet [28–32]. Several type 2 diabetes prevention randomized controlled trials (RCTs) utilized low-fat eating patterns to achieve weight loss and improve glucose control.

Within these options, it is not clear which eating pattern is optimal from the low-fat eating patterns. When the Mediterranean eating pattern was compared to low-fat eating, the need for glucose-lowering medications was lower in the Mediterranean-style eating group. In addition, when additional olive oil and nuts were added to the Mediterranean-style diet, CVD incidence was reduced both in people with and without diabetes [33].

Vegetarian and vegan eating patterns have shown good results related to glycemia and CVD risk factors; however, these patterns have also resulted in weight loss. For example, in the Look AHEAD (Action for Health and Diabetes) trial, individuals who followed a calorie-restriction, low-fat eating pattern in the context of a structured weight loss program achieved moderate success but did not consistently improve glycemia or CVD risk factors in individuals who have T2DM [34].

Given the complexity of research findings for eating patterns, there are some general guidelines for physicians to recommend. These should include:

1. Emphasis on nonstarchy vegetables.
2. Minimizing added sugars and refined grains.
3. Choosing whole foods over highly processed foods to the greatest extent possible.

It is important to emphasize that while there are some disparities among research results for various eating patterns, all recommend more healthy versus less healthy options—eating more fruits and vegetables and fish and decreased consumption of red meat.

A variety of plant-based diets are available, and some have demonstrated high levels of success in lowering hemoglobin A1C [35]. As always, recommendations should include patterns that fit into individuals' preferences to improve adherence.

22.5 ENERGY BALANCE AND WEIGHT MANAGEMENT

Individuals who are overweight or obese should be encouraged to lose weight to improve A1C, CVD risk factors, and quality of life [36–41]. This is true for individuals both with prediabetes and diabetes. MNT and DSMES will both be helpful in this area and should include individualized eating plans that result in an energy deficit. Enhanced physical activity should also be recommended. It is particularly important in individuals who are older or prone to hypoglycemia to be counseled about appropriate portion sizes for healthy eating [42]. In individuals with T2DM a 5% weight loss is recommended to achieve clinical benefits. Some individuals may additionally benefit from up to 15% weight loss.

Medication may also be utilized in individuals with T2DM to achieve and sustain a 7–10% weight loss [43]. Healthy eating plans such as the Mediterranean-style eating plan with energy restriction should be utilized. It is important that as DSMES and MNT modalities are applied, individuals be assessed for any disordered eating pattern. In the DPP, maximum prevention of diabetes over four years was observed in individuals who lost 7–10% of weight [17]. The DPP approach included both healthy eating and increased physical activity. Regular physical activity should be considered as an important part of a comprehensive lifestyle plan as demonstrated in the DPP. The Look AHEAD trial [37] and the Diabetes Remission Clinical Trial (DiRECT) [38] both showed partial diabetes remission. Diabetes remission is defined as maintenance of euglycemia (complete remission) or prediabetes level of glycemia (partial remission; no diabetic medication for at least one year) [44,45].

22.6 SWEETENERS

The ADA recommends sugar-sweetened beverages (SSBs) be replaced with water as often as possible [13]. Individuals should also be counseled to avoid increasing intake of calories from other sources if SSBs are reduced. These recommendations are based on the fact that SSB consumption in the general population is a significant contributor to T2DM, weight gain, heart disease, kidney disease, nonalcoholic fatty liver disease, and tooth decay.

A wide variety of noncaloric sugar substitutes are also available; however, the American Heart Association (AHA) and ADA have both concluded that enough evidence does not exist to determine whether or not noncaloric sugar substitutes eventually lead to long-term reduction in body weight or reduced metabolic risk factors including glycemia [46].

22.7 ALCOHOL

Similar to the AHA, the ADA has recommended that people with diabetes or prediabetes who drink alcohol should do so in moderation [47–51]. It should also be noted that delayed hypoglycemia can occur after drinking alcohol, which emphasizes why it is important to monitor glucose after drinking alcoholic beverages to reduce the risk of hypoglycemia. Generally, moderate alcohol consumption has minimal acute or long-term detrimental effects on glycemia in people with T2DM [52]. Moderate alcohol consumption is defined as one 12-oz beer, a 5-oz glass of wine, or 1.5 oz of distilled spirit.

The issue of delayed hypoglycemia when consuming alcohol may be the result of reduced hypoglycemia awareness because of the cerebral effects of alcohol. This is particularly an issue for those who use insulin [52]. Consuming alcohol with food can minimize the risk of nocturnal hypoglycemia and should be discussed with individuals with T2DM. With individuals with prediabetes, there may be a slight protective effect of moderate alcohol intake on CVD risk when compared to either alcohol abstainers or heavy consumers. None of these effects should lead healthcare providers to recommend starting to consume alcohol for an individual who does not currently consume alcohol. However, moderation for those who drink alcohol seems to be a reasonable recommendation.

22.8 MICRONUTRIENTS AND DIABETES

The American Dietetic Association states that scientific evidence does not support the use of dietary supplements in the form of vitamins or minerals to meet glycemia targets or improve CVD risk factors for people with diabetes or prediabetes [53–55]. It is essential that individuals maintain a balanced intake of food sources to provide the recommended daily allowance of nutrients and micronutrients. Multivitamin supplements may be justified for people who are following an eating plan that restricts calories or who are pregnant. Other chronic conditions such as celiac disease warrant further discussion with the RDN or physician involved in the team taking care of the individual with diabetes. It is also important to note that herbal products and nutritional supplements are not regulated or standardized by the Food and Drug Administration (FDA). Healthcare providers should ask about the supplements or herbal products, since over 70% of the adult population in the United States takes at least one form of them, and these may interfere with other medical therapies.

22.9 MNT AND ANTIHYPERGLYCEMIC MEDICATIONS

It is important that individuals providing MNT in diabetes care should assess and monitor medication change in relation to nutrition care plans [56–60]. It is essential that individuals with fixed daily insulin doses have a consistent carbohydrate intake with respect to time and amount, keeping in mind the insulin action time. This can result in improved glycemia and reduce the risk of hypoglycemia. When consuming a mixed meal, dosing should not be based solely on carbohydrate counting. Continuous glucose monitoring and self-monitoring of blood glucose should guide decision making for administration of insulin, particularly when nutritional changes have occurred.

22.10 THE ROLE OF NUTRITION THERAPY IN THE PREVENTION AND MANAGEMENT OF DIABETES COMPLICATIONS

Since CVD and elevated blood pressure are very common in individuals with diabetes, it is important to modify nutrition therapy to help prevent complications [61–65]. For example, lowering saturated fat and replacing it with unsaturated fat or monounsaturated fats will reduce total cholesterol and low-density lipoprotein cholesterol (LDL-C), which lowers the risk of CVD. It is also important to emphasize complex carbohydrates and, in some instances, replace high-carbohydrate foods (particularly, simple carbohydrates) with increased monounsaturated or polyunsaturated fat, which may improve glycemia and triglycerides. The recommendation for consuming more whole grains and fiber that is made to the general public is also appropriate for people with diabetes, as is the recommendation to eat one or two servings of fish (particularly oily fish) per week.

It is also important for individuals with diabetes to limit the amount of salt in their diet [66–70]. This is because high blood pressure is very common in individuals with diabetes. The AHA recommends the consumption of less than 2,300 mg/day for the general public, and this recommendation is also appropriate for individuals who have diabetes.

The question often comes up in individuals with diabetes who also have some evidence of kidney disease concerning whether or not to reduce dietary protein [71,72].

Research has shown that consuming dietary protein below the recommended daily allowance of 0.8 grams/kg of body weight/day does not alter the course of diabetic kidney disease.

22.11 PERSONALIZED NUTRITION/PRECISION MEDICINE

Considerable recent interest has been developed in the general area of precision medicine, particularly as it relates to individuals with diabetes or other metabolic conditions. This field is called "personalized nutrition" [73]. To date, an approach to personalized nutrition has not been demonstrated to improve outcome in individuals with T2DM or prediabetes.

There is some evidence that considerable differences in metabolism and genetic backgrounds exist among individuals, so the area of precision medicine and personalized nutrition may yield important data that will help guide more precise diabetes counseling in the area of nutrition in the future [74].

The goal of precision nutrition is to tailor dietary interventions and recommendations related to an individual's genetic background, metabolic profile, and environmental exposure to develop a more personalized way of preventing and managing this chronic disease. Precision nutrition is based on a variety of emerging technologies and information such as data that come from nutrigenomic studies. These studies may identify genetic variants that could influence intake and metabolism of specific nutrients, which may help predict an individual's response to dietary intervention. In addition, metabolomics studies have demonstrated metabolic fingerprints of food and nutrient consumption can uncover pathways that may be modified by diet. The area of gut microbiota has seen dramatic increases in research that are relevant to food metabolism and glycemic control.

These scientific advances, coupled with mobile apps and wearable devices, may help improve glycemic control and diabetes management. The field is in its infancy, although it holds great promise for the future of making diabetes care and management even more precise and individualized for people who have T2DM.

22.12 DIABETES SELF-MANAGEMENT EDUCATION AND SUPPORT

Individuals with diabetes are asked to make multiple daily self-management decisions and perform complex daily activities. For this reason, DSMES is important to the effective management of diabetes. DSMES has been strongly supported by a joint statement from the ADA, American Association of Diabetes Educators, and the Academy of Nutrition and Dietetics (AND) [15]. DSMES has been consistently shown to improve health outcomes. This is a process of helping individuals with diabetes with enhanced knowledge, skill, and ability for diabetes self-care. The specific particulars of DSMES are beyond the scope of this chapter. However, the reader is referred to the Joint Statement of the ADA, AND, and the Association of Diabetes Care and Education Specialists, which is found in the references.

22.13 THE ROLE OF OTHER LIFESTYLE HABITS AND PRACTICES IN THE PREVENTION AND MANAGEMENT OF PREDIABETES AND T2DM

Diabetes is a chronic disease that is amenable to many of the central tenets and practices of lifestyle medicine. Nutrition plays a particularly important role in management of diabetes and is best administered as MNT. Optimally, this should be done by diabetes educators such as RDNs who are specifically trained to deliver MNT. There is also a significant role for physical activity across the spectrum of diabetes. In addition to its role in reducing the risk of ever developing diabetes, regular physical activity can play an important role in the management of diabetes in individuals who already have this condition.

The role of physical activity in the prevention and management of diabetes is recognized both in the position statement from the ADA on Physical Activity/Exercise in Diabetes and the Physical Activity Guidelines for Americans 2018 Scientific Report [75]. Of course, increased physical activity not only is valuable for preventing or delaying T2DM but also confers multiple other health benefits for individuals with T2DM or prediabetes. Aerobic activity such as walking, cycling, jogging, or swimming is typically recommended, although there is some evidence that resistance training may also help individuals lower the risk of diabetes and/or treating it if already present. Other lifestyle medicine factors such as education, counseling, support, and psychosocial care are also very important for people who have diabetes. Physicians should counsel patients on all of the pillars of lifestyle medicine to optimize treatment of individuals who have diabetes or prediabetes.

22.14 CONCLUSIONS

Proper nutrition is critically important for an individual who either has diabetes or to prevent diabetes. Recommendations should be delivered by an RDN who is skillful in MNT. Also, participation in diabetes self-management education is critically important, since individuals will be making numerous decisions throughout the course of the day related to the treatment of their diabetes. Physicians should also counsel individuals in other areas of daily lifestyle habits and actions such as regular physical activity, weight management, and sleep. It is important that nutrition therapy recommendations are regularly updated based on changes in the individual's disease course, preferences, and life circumstances. It should also be noted that the type of nutritional recommendations made in this chapter, including nutrition therapy and formal diabetes education, are, unfortunately, not given to most people with diabetes. Therefore, physicians should play a role in strategies to improve access to these services for people who have diabetes.

Clinical Applications

- Proper nutrition therapy is a key component of the overall management of diabetes.

- MNT, optimally delivered by a skilled RDN, has been shown to significantly improve outcomes in people who have T2DM.
- Since diabetes is a chronic disease, where individuals will make multiple important decisions on a daily basis, DSMES is also critically important as recommended by the ADA, the American Association of Diabetes Educators, and the AND.
- Other lifestyle modalities such as increased physical activity, proper weight management, and lowering other risks for CVD should be emphasized in individuals who have diabetes to optimize its care.

REFERENCES

1. Centers for Disease Control and Prevention. National Diabetes Statistic Report. 2017. Atlanta, GA. US Centers for Disease Control and Prevention. US Department of Health and Human Services. (Accessed January 17, 2024).
2. Via M, Mechanic J. Integrating Lifestyle Medicine for Prediabetes, Type 2 Diabetes, and Cardiometabolic Disease. Boca Raton: CRC Press, 2023.
3. NCD Risk Factor Collaboration (NCD-RisC). Worldwide trends in diabetes since 1980: A pooled analysis of 751 population-based studies with 4.4 million participants. Lancet. 2016;387:1513–1530.
4. Knowler W, Fowler S, Hamman R, et al. Diabetes Prevention Program Group. 10-year follow-up of diabetes incidence and weight loss in the Diabetes Prevention Program Outcomes Study. Lancet. 2009;374:1677–1686.
5. Franz M, MacLeod J, Evert A, et al. Academy of nutrition and dietetics nutrition practice guideline for type 1 and type 2 diabetes in adults: Systematic review of evidence for medical nutrition therapy effectiveness and recommendations for integration into the nutrition care process. J Acad Nutr Diet. 2017;117:1659–1679.
6. Colberg S, Sigal R, Yardley J, et al. Physical activity/exercise and diabetes: A position statement of the American Diabetes Association. Diabetes Care. 2016;39:2065–2079.
7. Garber A, Abrahamson M, Barzilary J, et al. Consensus statement by the American Association of Clinical Endocrinologists and American College of Endocrinology on the comprehensive type 2 diabetes management algorithm—2016 executive summary. Endocr Pract. 2016;22:84–113.
8. Handelsman Y, Bloomgarden Z, et al. American Association of Clinical Endocrinologists and American College of Endocrinology: Clinical practice guidelines for developing a diabetes mellitus comprehensive care plan—2015. Endocr Pract. 2015;21 (Suppl 1):1–87.
9. Powers M, Bardsley J, Cypress M, et al. Diabetes self-management education and support in type 2 diabetes: A joint position statement of the American Diabetes Association, the American Association of Diabetes Educators, and the Academy of Nutrition and Dietetics. J Acad Nutr Diet. 2015;115:1323–1334.
10. Holman R, Paul S, Bethel M, et al. 10-Year follow-up of intensive glucose control in type 2 diabetes. N Engl J Med. 2008;359:1577–1589.
11. Inzucchi S, Bergenstal R, Buse J, et al. American Diabetes Association (ADA); European Association for the Study of Diabetes (EASD). Management of hyperglycemia in type 2 diabetes: A patient-centered approach: Position statement of the American Diabetes Association (ADA) and the European Association for the Study of Diabetes (EASD). Diabetes Care. 2012;35(6):1364–1379.

12. U.S. Department of Agriculture and U.S. Department of Health and Human Services. *Dietary Guidelines for Americans, 2020–2025*, 9th edition. December 2020. DietaryGuidelines.gov. 2020.
13. Evert A, Dennison M, Gardner C, et al. Nutrition therapy for adults with diabetes or prediabetes: A consensus report. diabetes care. 2019;42(5):731–754.
14. Briggs Early K, Stanley K. Position of the academy of nutrition and dietetics: The role of medical nutrition therapy and registered dietitian nutritionists in the prevention and treatment of prediabetes and type 2 diabetes. J Acad Nutr Diet. 2018;118(2):343–353.
15. Powers M, Bardsley J, Cypress M, et al. Diabetes self-management education and support in type 2 diabetes: A joint position statement of the American Diabetes Association, the American Association of Diabetes Educators, and the Academy of Nutrition and Dietetics. Diabetes Care. 2015;38(7):1372–1382.
16. Brunisholz K, Briot P, Hamilton S, et al. Diabetes self-management education improves quality of care and clinical outcomes determined by a diabetes bundle measure. J Multidiscip Healthc. 2014;21(7):533–542.
17. The Diabetes Prevention Program (DPP) Research Group. The Diabetes Prevention Program (DPP): Description of lifestyle intervention. Diabetes Care. 2002;25(12): 2165–2171.
18. Lindstrom J, Louheranta A, Mannelin M, et al. The Finnish Diabetes Prevention Study (DPS): Lifestyle intervention and 3-year results on diet and physical activity. Diabetes Care. 2003;26(12):3230–3236.
19. Vega-López S, Venn B, Slavin J. Relevance of the glycemic index and glycemic load for body weight, diabetes, and cardiovascular disease. Nutrients. 2018;10:E1361.
20. He M, van Dam R, Rimm E, et al. Whole-grain, cereal fiber, bran, and germ intake and the risks of all-cause and cardiovascular disease-specific mortality among women with type 2 diabetes mellitus. Circulation. 2010;121:2162–2168.
21. Burger K, Beulens J, van der Schouw Y, et al. Dietary fiber, carbohydrate quality and quantity, and mortality risk of individuals with diabetes mellitus. PLoS One. 2012;7:e4312.
22. Post R, Mainous A, King D, et al. Dietary fiber for the treatment of type 2 diabetes mellitus: A meta-analysis. J Am Board Fam Med. 2012;25:16–23.
23. Dahl W, Stewart M. Position of the Academy of Nutrition and Dietetics: Health implications of dietary fiber. J Acad Nutr Diet. 2015;115:1861–1870.
24. Wu J, Marklund M, Imamura F, et al. Cohorts for Heart and Aging Research in Genomic Epidemiology (CHARGE) Fatty Acids and Outcomes Research Consortium (FORCE). Omega-6 fatty acid biomarkers and incident type 2 diabetes: Pooled analysis of individual-level data for 39 740 adults from 20 prospective cohort studies. Lancet Diabetes Endocrinol 2017;5:965–974.
25. Salas-Salvadó J, Bulló M, Estruch R, et al. Prevention of diabetes with Mediterranean diets: A subgroup analysis of a randomized trial. Ann Intern Med. 2014;7;160(1):1–10.
26. Guasch-Ferré M, Becerra-Tomás N, Ruiz-Canela M, et al. Total and subtypes of dietary fat intake and risk of type 2 diabetes mellitus in the Prevención con Dieta Mediterránea (PREDIMED) study. Am J Clin Nutr. 2017;105(3):723–735.
27. US Department of Health and Human Services. US Department of Agriculture. 2015–2020 Dietary Guidelines for Americans, 8th ed. https://health.gov/our-work/nutrition-physical-activity/dietary-guidelines/previous-dietary-guidelines/2015 (Accessed January 17, 2024).
28. Chiu T, Pan W, Lin M, et al. Vegetarian diet, change in dietary patterns, and diabetes risk: A prospective study. Nutr Diabetes. 2018;8:12.

29. Becerra-Tomás N, Díaz-López A, Rosique-Esteban N, et al. PREDIMED Study Investigators. Legume consumption is inversely associated with type 2 diabetes incidence in adults: A prospective assessment from the PREDIMED study. Clin Nutr. 2018;37:906–913.
30. Lee Y, Park K. Adherence to a vegetarian diet and diabetes risk: A systematic review and meta-analysis of observational studies. Nutrients 2017;9:603.
31. Malik V, Li Y, Tobias D, et al. Dietary protein intake and risk of type 2 diabetes in US men and women. Am J Epidemiol. 2016;183:715–728.
32. Schwingshackl L, Bogensberger B, Hoffmann G. Diet quality as assessed by the healthy eating index, alternate healthy eating index, dietary approaches to stop hypertension score, and health outcomes: An updated systematic review and meta-analysis of cohort studies. J Acad Nutr Diet. 2018;118:74–100.
33. Estruch R, Ros E, Salas-Salvadó J, et al.; PREDIMED Study Investigators. Primary prevention of cardiovascular disease with a Mediterranean diet supplemented with extra-virgin olive oil or nuts. N Engl J Med. 2018;378:e34.
34. Pi-Sunyer X, Blackburn G, Brancati FL, et al. Look AHEAD Research Group. Reduction in weight and cardiovascular disease risk factors in individuals with type 2 diabetes: One-year results of the Look AHEAD trial. Diabetes Care. 2007;30:1374–1383.
35. Satija A, Bhupathiraju S, Rimm E, et al. Plant-based dietary patterns and incidence of type 2 diabetes in US men and women: Results from three prospective cohort studies. PLoS Med. 2016;13(6):e1002039.
36. Prinz N, Schwandt A, Becker M, et al. Trajectories of body mass index from childhood to young adulthood among patients with type 1 diabetes—a longitudinal group-based modeling approach based on the DPV Registry. J Pediatr. 2018;201:78–85.e4.
37. Wadden T, Neiberg R, Wing R, et al. Look AHEAD Research Group. Four-year weight losses in the Look AHEAD study: Factors associated with long-term success. Obesity (Silver Spring). 2011;19:1987–1998.
38. Lean M, Leslie W, Barnes A, et al. Primary care-led weight management for remission of type 2 diabetes (DiRECT): An open-label, cluster-randomised trial. Lancet. 2018;391:541–551.
39. Wing R; Look AHEAD Research Group. Long-term effects of a lifestyle intervention on weight and cardiovascular risk factors in individuals with type 2 diabetes mellitus: Four-year results of the Look AHEAD trial. Arch Intern Med. 2010;170:1566–1575.
40. Hamdy O, Mottalib A, Morsi A, et al. Long-term effect of intensive lifestyle intervention on cardiovascular risk factors in patients with diabetes in real-world clinical practice: A 5-year longitudinal study. BMJ Open Diabetes Res Care. 2017;5:e000259.
41. Wing R, Lang W, Wadden T, et al.; Look AHEAD Research Group. Benefits of modest weight loss in improving cardiovascular risk factors in overweight and obese individuals with type 2 diabetes. Diabetes Care. 2011;34:1481–1486.
42. Boulé N, Haddad E, Kenny G, et al. Effects of exercise on glycemic control and body mass in type 2 diabetes mellitus: A meta-analysis of controlled clinical trials. JAMA. 2001 Sep 12;286(10):1218–1227.
43. Norris S, Zhang X, Avenell A, et al. Pharmacotherapy for weight loss in adults with type 2 diabetes mellitus. Cochrane Database Syst Rev. 2005;1:CD004096.
44. Gregg E, Chen H, Wagenknecht L, et al.; Look AHEAD Research Group. Association of an intensive lifestyle intervention with remission of type 2 diabetes. JAMA. 2012;308:2489–2496.
45. Buse J, Caprio S, Cefalu W, et al. How do we define cure of diabetes? Diabetes Care 2009;32:2133–2135.

46. Johnson R, Appel L, Brands M, et al. American Heart Association Nutrition Committee of the Council on Nutrition, Physical Activity, and Metabolism and the Council on Epidemiology and Prevention. Dietary sugars intake and cardiovascular health: A scientific statement from the American Heart Association. Circulation. 2009;120:1011–1020.
47. Shai I, Wainstein J, Harman-Boehm I, et al. Glycemic effects of moderate alcohol intake among patients with type 2 diabetes: A multicenter, randomized, clinical intervention trial. Diabetes Care. 2007;30:3011–3016.
48. Ahmed A, Karter A, Warton E, et al. The relationship between alcohol consumption and glycemic control among patients with diabetes: The Kaiser Permanente Northern California Diabetes Registry. J Gen Intern Med. 2008;23:275–282.
49. Bantle A, Thomas W, Bantle J. Metabolic effects of alcohol in the form of wine in persons with type 2 diabetes mellitus. Metabolism. 2008;57:241–245.
50. Schrieks I, Heil A, Hendriks H, et al. The effect of alcohol consumption on insulin sensitivity and glycemic status: A systematic review and meta-analysis of intervention studies. Diabetes Care 2015;38:723–732.
51. Howard A, Arnsten J, Gourevitch M. Effect of alcohol consumption on diabetes mellitus: A systematic review. Ann Intern Med. 2004;140:211–219.
52. Timko C, Kong C, Vittorio L, et al. Screening and brief intervention for unhealthy substance use in patients with chronic medical conditions: A systematic review. J Clin Nurs. 2016;25:3131–3143.
53. Bantle J, Wylie-Rosett J, Albright A, et al. American Diabetes Association. Nutrition recommendations and interventions for diabetes: A position statement of the American Diabetes Association. Diabetes Care 2008;31(Suppl 1):S61–S78.
54. Sesso H, Christen W, Bubes V, et al. Multivitamins in the prevention of cardiovascular disease in men: The Physicians' Health Study II randomized controlled trial. JAMA. 2012;308:1751–1760.
55. Macpherson H, Pipingas A, Pase M. Multivitamin-multimineral supplementation and mortality: A meta-analysis of randomized controlled trials. Am J Clin Nutr. 2013;97:437–444.
56. Battista M, Labonté M, Ménard J, et al. Dietitian-coached management in combination with annual endocrinologist follow up improves global metabolic and cardiovascular health in diabetic participants after 24 months. Appl Physiol Nutr Metable. 2012;37:610–620.
57. Briggs Early K, Stanley K. Position of the academy of nutrition and dietetics: The role of medical nutrition therapy and registered dietitian nutritionists in the prevention and treatment of prediabetes and type 2 diabetes. J Acad Nutr Diet. 2018;118:343–353.
58. Møller G, Andersen H, Snorgaard O. A systematic review and meta-analysis of nutrition therapy compared with dietary advice in patients with type 2 diabetes. Am J Clin Nutr. 2017;106:1394–1400.
59. Kim J, Lee J, Chung H, et al. Impact of visit-to-visit fasting plasma glucose variability on the development of type 2 diabetes: A nationwide population-based cohort study. Diabetes Care. 2018;41:2610–2616.
60. Garber A, Abrahamson M, Barzilay J, et al. Consensus statement by the American Association of Clinical Endocrinologists and American College of Endocrinology on the comprehensive type 2 diabetes management algorithm. 2017 executive summary. Endocr Pract. 2017;23:207–238.
61. Wennehorst K, Mildenstein K, Saliger B, et al. A comprehensive lifestyle intervention to prevent type 2 diabetes and cardiovascular diseases: The German CHIP Trial. Prev Sci. 2016;17:386–397.

62. Sun Y, You W, Almeida F, et al. The effectiveness and cost of lifestyle interventions including nutrition education for diabetes prevention: A systematic review and meta-analysis. J Acad Nutr Diet. 2017;117:404–421.e36.
63. Delahanty L, Dalton K, Porneala B, et al. Improving diabetes outcomes through lifestyle change—a randomized controlled trial. Obesity (Silver Spring). 2015;23:1792–1799.
64. Liu H, Zhang M, Wu X, et al. Effectiveness of a public dietitian-led diabetes nutrition intervention on glycemic control in a community setting in China. Asia Pac J Clin Nutr. 2015;24:525–532.
65. Marincic P, Hardin A, Salazar M, et al. Diabetes self-management education and medical nutrition therapy improve patient outcomes: A pilot study documenting the efficacy of registered dietitian nutritionist interventions through retrospective chart review. J Acad Nutr Diet. 2017;117:1254–1264.
66. Zhang Z, Cogswell M, Gillespie C, et al. Association between usual sodium and potassium intake and blood pressure and hypertension among U.S. adults: NHANES 2005–2010. PLoS One. 2013;8:e75289.
67. Centers for Disease Control and Prevention (CDC) CDC grand rounds: Dietary sodium reduction—time for choice. MMWR Morb Mortal Wkly Rep. 2012;61:89–91.
68. Appel L, Frohlich E, Hall J, et al. The importance of population-wide sodium reduction as a means to prevent cardiovascular disease and stroke: A call to action from the American Heart Association. Circulation. 2011;123:1138–1143.
69. World Health Organization. Guideline: Sodium Intake for Adults and Children, 2012. www.who.int/publications/i/item/9789241504836 (Accessed January 17, 2024).
70. Institute of Medicine (US) Committee on Strategies to Reduce Sodium Intake. Strategies to Reduce Sodium Intake in the United States. Henney JE, Taylor CL, Boon CS (eds). Washington, DC: National Academies Press (US), 2010.
71. Wheeler M, Dunbar S, Jaacks L, et al. Macronutrients, food groups, and eating patterns in the management of diabetes: A systematic review of the literature, 2010. Diabetes Care. 2012 Feb;35(2):434–445.
72. American Diabetes Association; 4. Lifestyle management: Standards of medical care in diabetes—2018. Diabetes Care. 2018;41(Suppl 1):S38–S50.
73. Wang D, Hu F. Precision nutrition for prevention and management of type 2 diabetes. Lancet Diabetes Endocrinol. 2018;6(5):416–426.
74. Tanaka T, Ngwa J, van Rooij F, et al. Genome-wide meta-analysis of observational studies shows common genetic variants associated with macronutrient intake. Am J Clin Nutr. 2013 Jun;97(6):1395–1402.
75. Physical Activity Guidelines for Americans 2018. US Department of Health and Human Services. Office of Disease Prevention and Health Promotion. https://health.gov/our-work/nutrition-physical-activity/physical-activity-guidelines (Accessed January 17, 2024).

23 Nutrition and Osteoporosis

Key Points

- Osteoporosis is a potentially disabling disease resulting in increased fragility and bone fractures. Osteoporosis may result in high morbidity and mortality.
- Healthy habits are important for lowering the risk of osteoporosis.
- Chief among these habits and practices are nutritional factors to lower the risk of osteoporosis and improve bone mineral density through adequate intake of calcium and vitamin D. Protein also plays a role.
- Recent evidence suggests that other components of a healthy diet including fruits and vegetables, whole grains, monounsaturated fats, and polyunsaturated fats may all further contribute to lowering the risk of osteoporosis.
- A diet that has been demonstrated to lower the risk of osteoporosis is the Mediterranean diet (MedDiet), although other healthy diets, in all likelihood, also will lower the risk of osteoporosis.
- Like many other metabolic diseases, osteoporosis also appears to have a significant component of inflammation, which causes a decrease in bone mineral density and increases its risk.
- Bone and muscle exhibit a vigorous communication. Thus, in aging patients, clinicians should assess both osteoporosis risk and risk of muscle loss (sarcopenia).

23.1 INTRODUCTION

Osteoporosis is a common skeletal disorder based on a systemic reduction in bone mass, strength, and skeletal architecture. Osteoporosis significantly increases the risk of fractures and the subsequent loss of mobility, which can cause a major reduction in health-related quality of life (HRQoL) [1]. According to the World Health Organization (WHO), osteoporosis is a major cause of serious health problems and particularly increases mortality in elderly patients [1]. Approximately 8 million women and 1–2 million men had osteoporosis in the United States in 2012 [2]. In addition, it is estimated that approximately 22 million women and about 5.5 million men in the European Union also have osteoporosis [3]. In the developing world, 2–8% of men and 9–38% of women have osteoporosis [4].

Nutrition plays a significant role in osteoporosis [5–8]. The role of nutritional elements of calcium and vitamin D in osteoporosis development is well described and will be discussed in this chapter [5–8]. However, there is also compelling evidence that healthy diets that are high in fruits and vegetables and whole grains as well as

DOI: 10.1201/9781003452607-23

polyunsaturated fatty acids (PUFAs) also play a very significant role in the development of osteoporosis [9]. Furthermore, the Western diet (WD), which contains abundant red meat, processed meats, refined carbohydrates, and sugar and is low in fiber, has been shown to increase the likelihood of osteoporosis [10]. The leading theory for why the WD increases the risk of osteoporosis relates to the inflammatory nature of this diet.

Osteoporosis is also frequently combined with muscle wasting, which is called sarcopenia [11]. In addition, there is an association between osteoporosis and osteoarthritis [12]. An association also exists between osteoporosis and obesity. Dietary patterns such as the Mediterranean diet (MedDiet) have been shown to lower the risk of osteoporosis in contrast to WD. Other components of osteoporosis prevention include lifestyle measures such as weight-bearing exercise, avoiding tobacco products, and weight management. These lifestyle measures will also be discussed in this chapter.

23.2 DIAGNOSIS OF OSTEOPOROSIS

The diagnosis of osteoporosis is typically made during a routine screening for the disease. The U.S. Preventative Services Task Force recommends screening for women over the age of 65 or women of any age who have factors yielding increased chance for developing osteoporosis. There is no specific recommendation for osteoporosis screening in men.

The typical screening test for osteoporosis is performed with a dual energy x-ray absorptiometry (DEXA) scan, which assesses bone mineral density (BMD) in a specific area of bone, typically either the spine or hip [13]. BMD test results are compared with average bone density of healthy, young individuals and also the average bone density of other people of an individual's age, sex, and race. As defined by the World Health Organization (WHO), osteoporosis is present when a BMD is 2.5 standard deviations or more below the average value for healthy young women [13]. If the BMD is between 1 and 2.5 BMD in a deviation, it is below the average for healthy young women; this is considered to be osteopenia.

23.3 BONE METABOLISM

Many individuals suffer from the misperception that bone is an inert substance. In fact, bone is highly metabolically active. Cells that increase BMD are osteoblasts, whereas osteoclasts are largely related to bone reabsorption. Nutrients such as vitamin D are thought to act on both osteoblasts and osteoclasts [14]. Normally these cell types are in balance with each other. It is also important to recognize that other lifestyle measures such as regular weight-bearing exercise impact on bone BMD. A typical individual reaches their maximum BMD in their early twenties [15]. Thus, prevention of osteoporosis should begin at an early age [16].

23.4 NUTRITION AND OSTEOPOROSIS

Proper nutrition exerts a significant impact on osteoporosis because it is one of the few safely modifiable risk factors. Healthy, well-balanced nutrition can play an important role in the prevention and pathophysiology of osteoporosis and, in addition, support pharmacologic therapy, if necessary. In postmenopausal women it is also important to understand that low-grade inflammation, poor dietary habits, and sedentary and unhealthful lifestyles such as smoking and alcohol consumption can all contribute to increasing the risk and severity of osteoporosis.

Calcium is the main nutrient for bone health. Over 99% of calcium is found in the bone matrix. In addition, optimal dietary calcium intake is necessary for bone health at all stages of life. The dietary requirements for calcium are determined by the age-related need for bone development and maintenance. Thus, the recommended dietary allowance (RDA) for calcium varies throughout life. (See subsequent section.) Nutritional intake of calcium is the preferred method for calcium acquisition since it allows consumption of small quantities of the mineral throughout the day, thus optimizing this absorption and avoiding spikes. In addition, vitamin D plays a very important role in bone remodeling. (See subsequent section.)

Over the past two decades, numerous epidemiologic and experimental studies in nutrition have further clarified other nutrients and dietary patterns that can lower the risk of osteoporosis and/or assist in its treatment [5–8]. One of the most well studied is the Mediterranean diet (MedDiet). This diet has well-known health benefits protecting against a number of chronic Western diseases (both cardiovascular disease [CVD] and other metabolic diseases) [17,18]. In addition, the MedDiet diet has been shown to lower the risk of osteoporosis and assist in its treatment.

23.5 OSTEOPOROSIS, CALCIUM, AND VITAMIN D

Calcium is the single most important nutrient for bone health. Ninety-nine percent of calcium in the body is stored in the bones. In general, about two-thirds of the bone is made up of this mineral, specifically in the form of hydroxyapatite [19]. The remaining 32% is made up of various organic substances, such as collagen. The recommended amount of calcium in the diet depends on age (1,000 milligrams/day for adult men and women and 1,200 milligrams/day for people over the age of 50) [19]. If calcium intake in the diet is insufficient, serum calcium levels start decreasing, which results in a series of consequences.

- **Calcium**—If calcium intake is insufficient, there is an increased secretion of parathyroid hormone (PTH), which results in the absorption of bone to release calcium into the blood [20–23]. As this phenomenon continues, it results in a decrease in BMD and increases the risk of osteoporosis. There are also data that calcium intake increases BMD during growth periods and decreases BMD in the elderly, thereby reducing the risk of bone fracture [20–23].

  Calcium deficiency is associated with a number of other consequences. Dietary calcium deficiency is a major source of childhood rickets in developing countries.

  Calcium intake alone is not adequate for bone health, since vitamin D deficiency is also an important factor in increasing calcium uptake by the intestines [23]. In addition, glucose, fructose, and lactose increase the uptake of calcium in the intestines, thereby decreasing the risk for osteoporosis.

Before menopause, BMD remains relatively constant in women but starts decreasing immediately after menopause. Thus, even though intake of calcium and vitamin D is highly effective in increasing peak BMD, the dietary or pharmacologic intake of these substances can prevent excessive BMD loss after menopause [24].

The main dietary source of calcium is dairy products. However, if individuals do not receive adequate dairy dietary calcium, commercial calcium supplements may be appropriate. Calcium carbonate among the commercial supplements has the highest absorbability. If dairy products are chosen, they should be low fat [5]. Other good sources of calcium include dark green leafy vegetables such as bok choy, collards, and turnip greens and also broccoli, sardines, and salmon. Calcium-fortified foods such as soy milk, tofu, orange juice, cereals, and breads are also available.

- **Vitamin D**—Almost 90% of vitamin D requirement for the body is made in the skin in the exposure to sunlight [25]. A small amount of vitamin D is supplied from foods. Vitamin D deficiency is a widespread problem among the elderly in all countries, except for the United States, where foods are fortified with vitamin D [26].

  There is no scientific consensus about the vitamin D requirement for the body. Some researchers, however, consider a serum level of less than 20 mcg/mL the ideal level to define vitamin D deficiency [27,28]. The current recommendation for vitamin D intake is 10 micrograms/day in people age 50–70 years and 15 micrograms/day in older people [29].

  Vitamin D is hydroxylated in the liver to form 25-hydroxy-vitamin D. This substance is then converted into hydroxylated 1-25 (OH) D3 [30]. This hydroxylation in the liver is activated by PTH and inhibited by phosphate. Binding of this form of hydroxylated vitamin D to receptors in the intestines results in synthesis of proteins that are involved in transportation of calcium from the intestinal tract to the blood. This form of vitamin D, hydroxylated vitamin D_3, simulates osteoblasts, thereby increasing production of osteocalcin and alkaline phosphatase.

  Some foods actually contain significant amounts of vitamin D including fatty fish, fish oil, egg yolks, and liver [7,31]. Other foods that are fortified with vitamin D are major sources of the mineral including milk and cereals. The chart in Table 23.1 shows how much calcium and vitamin D is necessary per life stage.

- **Other aspects of nutrition**—In addition to vitamin D and calcium, the National Institutes of Health (NIH) recommends a healthy balanced diet that includes plenty of fruits and vegetables as well as the appropriate amount of calories for a person's age, height, and weight, as well as adequate amounts of protein [8]. All of these are important nutrients to help protect and maintain bone health.

TABLE 23.1
Recommended Dietary Allowances (RDAs) for Calcium

Age	Male	Female	Pregnant	Lactating
0–6 months*	200 mg	200 mg		
7–12 months*	260 mg	260 mg		
1–3 years	700 mg	700 mg		
4–8 years	1,000 mg	1,000 mg		
9–13 years	1,300 mg	1,300 mg		
14–18 years	1,300 mg	1,300 mg	1,300 mg	1,300 mg
19–50 years	1,000 mg	1,000 mg	1,000 mg	1,000 mg
51–70 years	1,000 mg	1,200 mg		
>70+ years	1,200 mg	1,200 mg		

Source: National Institutes of Health. Office of Dietary Supplements. Calcium Fact Sheet for Health Professionals. Updated January 3, 2024. https://ods.od.nih.gov/factsheets/Calcium-HealthProfessional/.

23.6 MACRONUTRIENTS AND OSTEOPOROSIS

The way the main macronutrients in the diet, namely proteins, lipids, and carbohydrates, influence bone health reflects on their ability to relate calcium metabolism to skeletal homeostasis.

- **Proteins**—Proteins support a variety of functions in the body. They can be either beneficial or harmful to bone health depending on the amount of protein ingested and the source of protein (plant versus animal). Dietary protein influences bone in several ways [32–35]:
  - It forms large components of organic bone matrix.
  - It regulates serum levels of insulin-like growth factor-1 (IGF1).
  - It may affect calcium metabolism.

  In addition, proteins account for approximately 30% of bone mass and 50% of bone volume.

  The current RDA of protein is 0.8 gm/kg body weight a day for adults and 1.5 gm/kg body weight a day for children and 1.0 gm/kg body weight a day for adolescents and older people [36]. A number of observational studies demonstrate that higher protein is associated with higher BMD in middle-aged and older adults and may exert a protective effect against spinal and femoral bone loss.

  A variety of sources of proteins are available. Proteins of animal origin are present in meat, fish, poultry, eggs, and dairy products. These have traditionally been called "complete proteins" since they contain a sufficient amount of essential amounts of vitamins and amino acids [32]. Vegetable proteins can be obtained from plant sources such as legumes, tofu, soy, tempeh, nuts, and seeds. They may have a lower nutritional quality due to variable amino acid profiles [32], although some plant proteins are considered "complete."

Various in vitro studies suggest that amino acids can affect bone health by a variety of mechanisms including osteoblast growth and differentiation. It should be noted that controversy exists about the difference between animal and plant proteins. Some investigators, however, have found that plant proteins convey an equal benefit of reducing the likelihood of fractures [37–39].

Insufficient dietary protein can also lead to muscle wasting resulting in unintentional body weight loss. (See subsequent section on osteoporosis and sarcopenia.) Lean muscle mass affects overall BMD and also cross-sectional bone parameters related to bone strength. Therefore, bone loss in elderly individuals is often preceded by loss of muscle mass and strength. Proteins are also the source of bioactive peptides, which can stimulate bone formation and may also have antioxidant and antimicrobial properties.

- **Lipids**—Lipids play a variety of roles in the body. For example, they are part of structural units of cell membranes, play a role in energy storage, and serve as a precursor of metabolic compounds involved in inflammatory and immune responses. Lipids are also important for absorption of fat-soluble vitamins (A, D, E, and K). For this reason, the WHO recommends that fats account for 20–35% of total energy intake.

  A variety of different classifications for lipids relate to chemical double bonds including saturated fatty acids (SFAs), monounsaturated fatty acids (MUFAs), and polyunsaturated fats (PUFAs) [40–42]. SFAs have generally been considered harmful to health, particularly in the area of cardiovascular disorders. The most common MUFA is oleic acid, which is present mainly in olive oil and meat. A MUFA-rich diet may provide beneficial health effects, particularly in the presence of coronary heart disease and type 2 diabetes mellitus (T2DM). Among the PUFAs, omega-3 acids and omega-6 fatty acids are the most significant [41]. The human body cannot synthesize them, so they must be obtained from food. The main sources of these acids are vegetable oils such as sunflower oil and soybean oil.

  Dietary lipids can also influence bone health. Increased lipid uptake may result in decreased BMD and elevated risk of fracture. In the Mediterranean diet, MUFAs were associated with increased BMD [18,43]. The beneficial effects of olive oil on BMD have been attributed to high contents of vitamin D and phenolic compounds. There are few data to indicate that consumption of PUFAs positively impacts on BMD.
- **Carbohydrates**—Dietary carbohydrates have a range of physiologic properties and health benefits. Carbohydrates are typically found in fruits, grains, vegetables, and milk products. Dietary fiber found in many of these dietary components also has significant effects on health [44,45]. In contrast, diets high in refined sugar adversely affect osteoblast proliferation and may result in decreased BMD.

  Carbonated and sugar-sweetened beverages have been associated with decreased BMD [46]. This may be partially a result of concomitant reduction in the consumption of milk and other nutrient-rich foods [47,48]. In addition, some research has suggested that consumption of carbonated beverages are negatively related to calcium intake. It should be noted that complex carbohydrates and fiber prevent a decrease in BMD.

Carbohydrates have a great impact on postprandial blood glucose levels (see also Chapter 20) and may play an important role in the management of diabetes. Patients with diabetes are often diagnosed with increased risk of bone fragility and fractures similar to osteoporosis. Diabetic bone disease is considered a significant secondary complication of diabetes.

23.7 MICRONUTRIENTS AND POLYPHENOLS AND OSTEOPOROSIS

Micronutrients include minerals and vitamins important for healthy development of the skeletal system as well as disease prevention and well-being. With the exception of vitamin D, they are not produced in the body and must therefore be consumed in food. The most important micronutrients for the prevention and treatment of osteoporosis are calcium and vitamin D. However, a variety of other minerals and vitamins are also involved in bone formation.

Minerals

- **Calcium**—The role of calcium has been discussed in detail in the previous section.
- **Phosphorous**—Phosphorous is an essential micronutrient with various physiologic roles. It is an important component of nucleic acids and high energy compounds (e.g. ATP, ADP, GTP, and GDP) and also plays an important role in biological membranes and phospholipids [49,50]. Biological membranes play an important role in energy metabolism, intercellular signaling, and acid-base balance. Phosphorous is the second basic component (after calcium) in bone tissue. The human body contains 550–770 grams of potassium [51]. Almost 85% of this phosphorus is stored in teeth and bones in the form of phosphorous proteins and hydroxy appetite crystals.

  Phosphorous deficiency results in rickets in children and osteomalacia in adults. Lack of phosphorous in the diet is very rare in humans due to its natural occurrence in large amounts of foods and the body's high ability to absorb it. In healthy adults, the current RDAs for phosphorous are 700 milligrams/day and 1,250 milligrams/day during adolescent growth. The impact of adequate phosphorous consumption in bone health is strongly supported by scientific evidence.

  Phosphorous can be found in foods in naturally occurring forms such as meat, dairy products and cereals, seeds, nuts, and legumes [49]. Phosphorous is also found in cola products, which are one of the most frequently consumed beverages. In cola products, it is found as phosphoric acid, which is easily absorbed [50,51]. Based on current evidence, most scientists agree that it is desirable to limit the intake of phosphorous additives [52,53].

- **Magnesium**—Magnesium is an essential micronutrient with a wide range of metabolic, regulatory, and structural functions [50,54]. Magnesium provides a basis for ATP and regulates the activity of about 300 enzymes involved in the synthesis of proteins, carbohydrates, and nucleic acids. Magnesium deficiency can be detrimental to bone health by interfering with vitamin D and PTH and supporting inflammation and consequent bone loss [54,55].

  The main sources of magnesium are green vegetables (such as spinach), legumes, nuts, seeds, whole grains, and almonds [45]. The current RDA for magnesium is 320 mg/day for women and 420 mg/day for men [56]. Insufficient physical activity can cause decreased magnesium [57] levels, as can smoking cigarettes [58]. Excessive intake of alcohol and coffee may also inversely influence the amount of magnesium in the body.
- **Vitamins**
  - *Vitamin D*—Vitamin D has already been discussed in the previous section in this chapter.
  - *Vitamin C*—Vitamin C is an essential vitamin required for many physiologic processes including the biosynthesis of collagen, various hormones, and a variety of other physiologic parameters [59–61]. Vitamin C is also an essential antioxidant and plays an important role in immune responses [62]. With regard to bone, vitamin C is an essential cofactor of collagen production as well as osteoblast synthesis and also has the ability to suppress osteoclast differentiation [63].

    Vitamin C deficiency can lead to scurvy, which is manifest by osteolysis, osteonecrosis, and decreased BMD, ultimately resulting in pathological fractures [64,65].

    The main sources of vitamin C are citrus fruits and juices, broccoli, tomato products, peppers, green leafy vegetables, potatoes, papaya, strawberries, and fortified breakfast cereals [59,60]. The recommended RDA for vitamin C is 75 milligrams/day for adult women and 90 milligrams/day for adult men [66]. The RDA for smokers increases by 35 milligrams/day because of increased oxidative stress and metabolic turnover of vitamin C.
  - *Vitamin K*—Vitamin K is a fat-soluble vitamin that occurs in two forms, vitamin K-1 and vitamin K-2. Vitamin K-1 is the more common form and can be achieved by consuming green vegetables such as spinach, kale, broccoli, cauliflower, cabbage, or supplements [59,62]. The current RDA for vitamin K is 90 micrograms/day for women and 120 micrograms/day for men [59,62]. Low vitamin K intake is associated with skeletal fragility [67]. Both vitamin K-1 and vitamin K-2 have been used to treat age-related bone loss and osteoporosis. The possible relationship for vitamin K-2 to decreased fracture risk needs to be further elucidated by a larger study.
- **Flavonoid polyphenols**—Polyphenols are secondary metabolites of plants which are abundant in vegetables and fruits. Flavonoid polyphenols have a wide variety of biological activities such as antioxidant, anti-inflammatory, anticarcinogenic, and antibacterial impact [68]. Polyphenols help delay

the aging process and reduce the risk of some chronic diseases [68–71]. Flavonoids are a group of polyphenols that are also common in the daily diet [72]. Both flavonoids and other polyphenols play a crucial role in skeletal health and prevention of osteoporosis [73–75]. The high level of polyphenols found in the Mediterranean diet has been credited as one possible reason for the decreased risk of osteoporosis in individuals who follow the Mediterranean diet. (See subsequent section.)

23.8 OSTEOPOROSIS AND INFLAMMATION

As discussed in multiple other chapters in this book, inflammation is a common underlying threat behind many chronic diseases including CVD, T2DM, obesity, metabolic syndrome, and some cancers. Excessive inflammation also has significant adverse effects on bone turnover. Excessive inflammatory cytokine production increases osteoclast activation in bone resorption. This may, in turn, contribute to bone loss in various clinical inflammatory conditions. In addition, inflammation decreases intestinal absorption of calcium, phosphate, and nutrients as well as vitamin D deficiency, which increases bone resorption [10].

A dietary inflammatory index has been developed that looks at either food components that increase inflammation or decrease inflammation [10]. Demonstration that multiple components in the Western diet increase inflammation has been confirmed in a variety of studies. In addition, the effects of the Mediterranean diet on reducing osteoporosis may partially be attributed to various anti-inflammatory components in the diet including fruits and vegetables that contain high levels of flavonoids.

23.9 OSTEOPOROSIS AND SARCOPENIA

As indicated earlier in this chapter, bone and muscle have an ongoing vigorous interaction [11]. In addition to the medical burden of osteoporosis related to fractures and diminished quality of life, sarcopenia is an additional syndrome that impacts on osteoporosis. Sarcopenia has a multifactorial origin, and the diagnosis requires a presence of both low muscle mass and low muscle function [76].

Many investigators define sarcopenia as an age-related syndrome characterized by a progressive and generalized loss of muscle mass and strength with adverse effects on human health. Sarcopenia increases the likelihood of falls and also leads directly to osteoporosis, obesity, and impaired metabolic health. Major treatment factors for sarcopenia include physical activity and proper nutrition, which also impact on osteoporosis [77–80]. There may be an additional benefit from increasing the amount of protein in the diet to reduce the risk of sarcopenia, although this remains controversial [81,82]. Adequate protein in the diet, as already mentioned, is also important for maintaining BMD.

23.10 OSTEOPOROSIS, OSTEOARTHRITIS, AND OBESITY

As discussed in multiple chapters in this book, obesity is associated with adipose tissue expansion and chronic low-grade inflammation. The inflammatory mediators released by adipocytes influence not only the comorbidities of obesity and metabolic diseases but also osteoporosis and osteoarthritis. Nutritional intervention is not only important for obesity but also may play an important role in reducing the secretion of inflammatory markers, which may adversely impact both osteoarthritis and osteoporosis [12]. The dietary intervention for obesity that may positively impact on osteoarthritis and osteoporosis is an area of intense current research. The same type of diet composition shown to be effective for weight loss in individuals with obesity also may play a significant role in lowering the level of inflammation that contributes to both osteoarthritis and osteoporosis.

23.11 OSTEOPOROSIS AND THE WESTERN DIET

The WD contains considerable processed protein foods, sweets and desserts, soft drinks, fried foods, meat and refined grains. (This diet is described in detail in Chapter 2.) The WD has been associated with lower BMD and a higher risk of fractures [83,84]. Moreover, high fat intake, such as found in this diet, as well as refined carbohydrates, may directly interfere with intestinal calcium absorption and increased fat accumulation, resulting in obesity, which can lead to decrease in osteoblast differentiation and bone formation. In addition, the higher sodium intake in WD can result in urinary loss of calcium, which may increase bone loss in new bones through remodeling [85].

An excessive intake in phosphorous, which is found in many processed food additives, may also disrupt the calcium-phosphorous ratio, affecting endocrine ratio and homeostasis, which may also be deleterious to bone health. Furthermore, the WD pattern results in endogenous acid production, which further negatively impacts bone, which serves as a provider of alkaline to maintain acid-base balance [86]. This leads to progressive bone loss.

23.12 OSTEOPOROSIS AND HEALTHY NUTRITION

As discussed in multiple chapters in this book, modern nutrition research focuses on overall dietary patterns rather than individual foods or nutrients. Healthy dietary patterns are associated with abundant intake of fruits, vegetables, low-fat dairy products, whole grains, poultry, fish, nuts, and legumes. These diets have been associated with decreased risk of multiple chronic diseases and have also been associated with positive effects on bone health, better BMD, and lower risk of fracture. Moreover, this type of diet is inversely associated with bone disruption markers.

- **Mediterranean diet**—Several recent studies have shown that adherence to the Mediterranean diet (MedDiet) is protective against osteoporosis [43,87,88]. It has been hypothesized that the antioxidant effects of fruits in the MedDiet play a significant role in this effect. Moreover, higher consumption of the MedDiet shows an increase in 25(OH)D, suggesting that higher vitamin D levels also play a role in reducing the risk of osteoporosis. In postmenopausal women, higher MedDiet scores not only were associated with higher BMD but also lower risk of hip fractures. This has been repeated in several other studies.

In addition, olive oil, which is featured in the MedDiet, has been reported as beneficial for bone status [89]. This may be due to a high proportion of polyphenols in olive oil, which appear to be beneficial for preventing loss of bone mass. These phenolic compounds also appear to modulate growth capacity and maturation of osteoblasts by increasing alkaline phosphate activity.

The dietary intake of olive oil was significantly associated with higher BMD in the cohort of Spanish women across a wide range of ages. A cohort of subjects analyzed as part of the PREDIMED study showed that participants with the highest intake of extra-virgin olive oil had the lowest incidence of osteoporosis-related fractures [17].

- **Asian diet**—Most Asian populations have dietary patterns in which soy and fish are elevated compared to that of Western populations. They also have a significantly lower incidence of osteoporotic fractures [90]. Several meta-analyses have demonstrated that supplements with soy osteo-flavonoids and omega-3 fatty acids (typically found in oily fish) improve bone health status in women [91]. These findings are supported by other epidemiologic studies. In one study of a Korean population, increased consumption of fruits and dairy products as part of the traditional Korean diet, which consists mainly of rice and vegetables, might decrease the risk of osteoporosis in postmenopausal women in Korea [92]. It should be noted that in many Asian societies, particularly those where there is increased affluence, more components of the WD are now being consumed, which may increase the risk of osteoporosis.
- **Vegetarian diets**—Vegetarian diets typically contain lower amounts of calcium, vitamin D, vitamin B_{12}, and protein, as well as omega-3 fatty acids, all of which play important roles in maintaining bone health [93]. Healthy vegetarian diets, however, typically contain higher quantities of various protective bone-related nutrients such as magnesium, potassium, and vitamin K, as well as antioxidant and anti-inflammatory phytonutrients. Limited available knowledge, however, suggests that, on balance, vegetarian diets, particularly vegan diets, may result in higher risk for lower BMD and fractures [94]. The vegan population should obtain calcium from other sources such as tofu, fortified soy products, or fortified orange juice.

23.13 NUTRITION AND OTHER LIFESTYLE MODALITIES TO REDUCE THE RISK OF OSTEOPOROSIS

While nutrition plays the primary role in reduction of risk for osteoporosis, numerous other lifestyle modalities can reduce the risk of osteoporosis. These include regular weight-bearing exercise, weight management, not smoking cigarettes, and minimizing or avoiding excessive alcohol [11]. All of these factors significantly reduce the risk of osteoporosis and should be discussed with every patient, particularly females and patients over the age of 65 (both men and women).

23.14 CONCLUSIONS

Osteoporosis is a common disease that can have disabling consequences, including fragility fractures and reduced quality of life. Promotion of healthy habits is particularly important for reducing the risk of osteoporosis. Chief among these patterns is healthy nutrition. Adequate intake of calcium, vitamin D, and protein is typical in most studies as a component of the healthy diet. Emerging evidence, however, has also been published that suggests that fruits and vegetables as well as whole grains and oily fish may all contribute to lowering the risk of osteoporosis. Prominent among the types of diets studied is the MedDiet, which features all of these factors. Conversely, the WD, which is high in red meats, processed meats, refined grains, and sugars as well as processed foods that are high in saturated fat may significantly increase the risk of osteoporosis, both through increased inflammation and potential weight gain. Thus, osteoporosis joins other metabolic conditions as an area where healthy nutrition can play a very significant role.

Clinical Applications

- Osteoporosis is often a disabling disease that may result in fragility fractures.
- Osteoporosis is particularly common in women over the age of 65, although it can occur in men as well.
- For younger individuals (particularly women) discussion should occur concerning peak years of building of BMD and strength. The peak of bone strength and BMD typically occurs in the twenties.
- While calcium and vitamin D are key nutrients, protein and various phytochemicals such as those found in fruits and vegetables also are important for bone health.
- A healthy diet following either a Mediterranean style or the Healthy U.S.-Style Dietary Pattern diet will also lower the risk of osteoporosis.
- Other lifestyle measures such as regular weight-bearing activity, not smoking, and reducing alcohol, as well as weight management, all contribute to lowering the risk of osteoporosis.

REFERENCES

1. Weng S, Hsu H, Weng Y, et al. Health-related quality of life and medical resource use in patients with osteoporosis and depression: A cross-sectional analysis from the National Health and Nutrition Examination Survey. Int J Envir Res Public Health. 2020; 17(3):1124.
2. Willson T, Nelson S, Newbold J, et al. The clinical epidemiology of male osteoporosis: A review of the recent literature. Clin Epidemiol. 2015;7:65–76.
3. Svedbom A, Hernlund E, Ivergard M, et al. The EU review panel of the IOF. Osteoporosis in the European Union: A compendium of country-specific reports. Arch Osteoporos. 2013;(8):137.
4. Wade S. Estimating prevalence of osteoporosis: Examples from industrialized countries. Arch Osteoporosis. 2014;(9):182.
5. Hejazi J, Davoodi A, Khosravi M, et al. Nutrition and osteoporosis prevention and treatment. Biom Res and Ther. 2020;7(4):3709–3720.

6. Martiniakova M, Babikova M, Mondockova V, et al. The role of macronutrients, micronutrients and flavonoid polyphenols in the prevention and treatment of osteoporosis. Nutrients. 2022;14(3):523.
7. Chen L, Hou P, Chen K. Nutritional support and physical modalities for people with osteoporosis: Current opinion. Nutrients. 2019;11(12):2848.
8. Muñoz-Garach A, García-Fontana B, Muñoz-Torres M. Nutrients and dietary patterns related to osteoporosis. Nutrients. 2020;12(7):1986.
9. Nieves J. Skeletal effects of nutrients and nutraceuticals, beyond calcium and vitamin D. Osteoporos Int. 2013;24(3):771–786.
10. Zhao S, Gao W, Li J, et al. Dietary inflammatory index and osteoporosis: The National Health and Nutrition Examination Survey, 2017–2018. Endocrine. 2022;78(3):587–596.
11. Papadopoulou S, Papadimitriou K, Voulgaridou G, et al. Exercise and nutrition Impact on osteoporosis and sarcopenia—the incidence of osteosarcopenia: A narrative review. Nutrients. 2021;13(12):4499.
12. Oliveira M, Vullings J, van de Loo F. Osteoporosis and osteoarthritis are two sides of the same coin paid for obesity. Nutrition. 2020;70:110486.
13. Kanis J, Melton L, Christiansen C, et al. The diagnosis of osteoporosis. J Bone Miner. Res. 1994;9:1137–1141.
14. Seeman E, Delmas P. Bone quality—the material and structural basis of bone strength and fragility. N Engl J Med. 2006;354:2250–2261.
15. Kanis J, Melton L, Christiansen C, et al. The diagnosis of osteoporosis. J Bone Miner Res. 1994;9(8):1137–1141.
16. Chen L, Wen Y, Kuo C, et al. Calcium and vitamin D supplementation on bone health: Current evidence and recommendations. Int J Gerontol. 2014;8:183–188.
17. Estruch R, Ros E, Salas-Salvado J, et al. Primary prevention of cardiovascular disease with a Mediterranean diet. N Engl J Med. 2013;368(14):1279–1290.
18. Quattrini S, Pampaloni B, Gronchi G, et al. The Mediterranean diet in osteoporosis prevention: An insight in a peri- and post-menopausal population. Nutrients. 2021;13(2):531.
19. Corwin R, Hartman T, Maczuga S, et al. Dietary saturated fat intake is inversely associated with bone density in humans: Analysis of NHANES III. J Nutr. 2006;136(1):159–165.
20. Stránský M, Rysava L. Nutrition as prevention and treatment of osteoporosis. Physiol. Res. 2009;58:S7.
21. Heaney R. Calcium, dairy products and osteoporosis. J Am Coll Nutr. 2000;19(Suppl 2):83S–99S.
22. Sanders K, Nowson C, Kotowicz M, et al. Calcium and bone health: Position statement for the Australian and New Zealand Bone and Mineral Society, Osteoporosis Australia and the Endocrine Society of Australia. Med J Aust. 2009;190(6):316–320.
23. Garriguet D. Bone health: Osteoporosis, calcium and vitamin D. Health Rep. 2011;22(3):7.
24. Rodrıguez-Martınez M, Garcıa-Cohen E. Role of Ca 2+ and vitamin D in the prevention and treatment of osteoporosis. Pharmacol Ther. 2002;93(1):37–49.
25. Holick M, Chen T. Vitamin D deficiency: A worldwide problem with health consequences. Am J Clin Nutr. 2008;87(4):1080S–1086S.
26. Mosekilde L. Vitamin D and the elderly. Clin Endocrinol. 2005;62(3):265–281.
27. Holick M, Binkley N, Bischoff-Ferrari H, et al. Evaluation, treatment, and prevention of vitamin D deficiency: An endocrine society clinical practice guideline. J Clin Endocrinol Metab. 2011;96(7):1911–1930.
28. Prentice A. Vitamin D deficiency: A global perspective. Nutr Rev. 2008;66(Suppl 2): S153–S164.
29. Malabanan A, Holick M. Vitamin D and bone health in postmenopausal women. J Womens Health. 2003;12(2):151–156.

30. Andersson U, Litton M, Fehniger T, et al. Detection and quantification of cytokine-producing cells by immunostaining. Techniques in Quantification and Localization of Gene Expression. Springer, 2000:55–79.
31. Reid I, Bolland M. Controversies in medicine: The role of calcium and vitamin D supplements in adults. Med J Aust. 2019;211:468–473.
32. Darling A, Millward D, Torgerson D, et al. Dietary protein and bone health: A systematic review and meta-analysis. Am J Clin Nutr. 2009;ajcn:27799.
33. Orwoll E. The effects of dietary protein insufficiency and excess on skeletal health. Bone. 1992;13(4):343–350.
34. Kerstetter J, Kenny A, Insogna K. Dietary protein and skeletal health: A review of recent human research. Curr opin Lipido. 2011;22(1):16–20.
35. Hunt J, Johnson L, Roughead Z. Dietary protein and calcium interact to influence calcium retention: A controlled feeding study. Am J Clin Nutr. 2009;89(5):1357–1365.
36. Rapuri P, Gallagher J, Haynatzka V. Protein intake: Effects on bone mineral density and the rate of bone loss in elderly women. Am J Clin Nutr. 2003;77(6):1517–1525.
37. Welch A, Mulligan A, Bingham S, et al. Urine pH is an indicator of dietary acid-base load, fruit and vegetables and meat intakes: Results from the European Prospective Investigation into Cancer and Nutrition (EPIC)-Norfolk population study. Br J Nutr. 2008;99(06):1335–1343.
38. Munger R, Cerhan J, Chiu B. Prospective study of dietary protein intake and risk of hip fracture in postmenopausal women. Am J Clin Nutr. 1999;69(1):147–152.
39. Dargent-Molina P, Sabia S, Touvier M, et al. Proteins, dietary acid load, and calcium and risk of postmenopausal fractures in the E3N French women prospective study. J Bone Miner Res. 2008;23(12):1915–1922.
40. Weiss L, Barrett-Connor E, von Mühlen D. Ratio of Ω-6 to Ω-3 fatty acids and bone mineral density in older adults: The Rancho Bernardo Study. Am J Clin Nutr. 2005;81(4):934–938.
41. Watkins B, Li Y, Lippman H, et al. Omega-3 polyunsaturated fatty acids and skeletal health. Exp Biol Med. 2001;226(6):485–497.
42. Go J, Song Y, Park J, et al. Association between serum cholesterol level and bone mineral density at lumbar spine and femur neck in postmenopausal Korean women. Korean J Fam Med. 2012;33(3):166–173.
43. Zupo R, Lampignano L, Lattanzio A, et al. Association between adherence to the Mediterranean diet and circulating vitamin D levels. Int J Food Sci Nutr. 2020;71(7):884–890.
44. Soliman G. Dietary fiber, atherosclerosis, and cardiovascular disease. Nutrients. 2019;23; 11(5):1155.
45. Ratajczak A, Rychter A, Zawada A, et al. Nutrients in the Prevention of Osteoporosis in Patients with Inflammatory Bowel Diseases. Nutrients. 2020;6;12(6):1702.
46. Ogur R, Uysal B, Ogur T, et al. Evaluation of the effect of cola drinks on bone mineral density and associated factors. Basic Clin Pharmacol Toxicol. 2007;100(5):334–338.
47. Ericsson Y, Angmar-Månsson B, Flores M. Urinary mineral ion loss after sugar ingestion. Bone Miner. 1990;9(3):233–237.
48. Vartanian L, Schwartz M, Brownell K. Effects of soft drink consumption on nutrition and health: A systematic review and meta-analysis. Am J Public Health. 2007;97:667–675.
49. Vorland C, Stremke E, Moorthi R, et al. Effects of excessive dietary phosphorus intake on bone health. Curr Osteoporos Rep. 2017;15:473–482.
50. Ciosek Z, Kot K, Kosik-Bogacka D, et al. The effects of calcium, magnesium, phosphorus, fluoride, and lead on bone tissue. Biomolecule. 2021;28;11(4):506.
51. Butusov M, Jernelov A. Phosphorus: An Element That Could Have Been Called Lucifer. New York, NY, USA: Springer, 2013; Vol. 9, ISBN 978-1-4614-6802-8.

52. Tucker K, Morita K, Qiao N, et al. Colas, but not other carbonated beverages, are associated with low bone mineral density in older women: The framingham osteoporosis study. Am J Clin Nutr. 2006;84:936–942.
53. Wyshak G. Teenaged girls, carbonated beverage consumption, and bone fractures. Arch Pediatr Adolesc Med. 2000;154:610–613.
54. Castiglioni S, Cazzaniga A, Albisetti W, et al. Magnesium and osteoporosis: Current state of knowledge and future research directions. Nutrients. 2013;31;5(8):3022–3033.
55. Capozzi A, Scambia G, Lello S. Calcium, Vitamin D, vitamin K2, and magnesium supplementation and skeletal health. Maturitas. 2020;140:55–63.
56. Rude R, Singer F, Gruber H. Skeletal and hormonal effects of magnesium deficiency. J Am Coll Nutr. 2009;28(2):131–141.
57. Jurkiewicz A, Wiechuła D, Loska K. Original article/artykuł oryginalny. J Orthop Trauma Surg Rel Res. 2008;2:17–24.
58. Zioła-Frankowska A, Kubaszewski Ł, Dabrowski M, et al. The content of the 14 metals in cancellous and cortical bone of the hip joint affected by osteoarthritis. Biomed Res Int. 2015;2015:815648.
59. Nieves J. Osteoporosis: The role of micronutrients. Am J Clin Nutr. 2005;81(5):1232S–1239S.
60. Devaki S, Raveendran R. Vitamin C: Sources, Functions, Sensing and Analysis; London, UK: Intech Open, 2017; ISBN 978-953-51-3422-0.
61. Dosedel M, Jirkovský E, Macáková K, et al. Vitamin C-sources, physiological role, kinetics, deficiency, use, toxicity, and determination. Nutrients. 2021;13;13(2):615.
62. Dennehy C, Tsourounis C. A review of select vitamins and minerals used by postmenopausal women. Maturitas. 2010;66:370–380.
63. Finck H, Hart A, Jennings A, et al. Is there a role for vitamin C in preventing osteoporosis and fractures? A review of the potential underlying mechanisms and current epidemiological evidence. Nutr Res Rev. 2014;27(2):268–283.
64. Brzezinska O, Łukasik Z, Makowska J, et al. Role of vitamin C in osteoporosis development and treatment—a literature review. Nutrients. 2020;12:2394.
65. Fain O. Musculoskeletal manifestations of scurvy. Joint Bone Spine. 2005;72(2):124–128.
66. Institute of Medicine (US). Panel on dietary antioxidants and related compounds. In Dietary Reference Intakes for Vitamin C, Vitamin E, Selenium, and Carotenoids, Washington, DC, USA: National Academies Press (US), 2000; ISBN 978-0-309-06949-6.
67. Feskanich D, Weber P, Willett W, et al. Vitamin K intake and hip fractures in women: A prospective study. Am J Clin Nutr. 1999;69(1):74–79.
68. Šikuten I, Štambuk P, Andabaka Ž, et al. Grapevine as a rich source of polyphenolic compounds. Molecules. 2020;28;25(23):5604.
69. Arts I, Hollman P. Polyphenols and disease risk in epidemiologic studies. Am J Clin Nutr. 2005;81(Suppl 1):317S–325S.
70. Pojer E, Mattivi F, Johnson D, et al. The case for anthocyanin consumption to promote human health: A review. Compr Rev Food Sci Food Saf. 2013;12:483–508.
71. Minatel I, Borges C, Ferreira M, et al. Phenolic Compounds: Functional Properties, Impact of Processing and Bioavailability. London, UK: Intech Open, 2017; ISBN 978-953-51-2960-8.
72. Taleb-Contini S, Salvador M, Balanco J, et al. Antiprotozoal effect of crude extracts and flavonoids isolated from chromolaena hirsuta (asteraceae). Phytother Res. 2004;18 (3):250–254.
73. Wong S, Chin K, Ima-Nirwana S. The osteoprotective effects of kaempferol: The evidence from in vivo and in vitro studies. Drug Des Dev Ther. 2019;13:3497–3514.
74. Kim T, Jung J, Ha B, et al. Effects of luteolin on osteoclast differentiation, function in vitro and ovariectomy-induced bone loss. J Nutr Biochem. 2011;22(1):8–15.

75. Niu Y, Yang Y, Xiao X, et al. Quercetin prevents bone loss in hindlimb suspension mice via stanniocalcin 1-mediated inhibition of osteoclastogenesis. Acta Pharmacol Sin. 2020;41(11):1476–1486.
76. Edwards M, Dennison E, Sayer A, et al. Osteoporosis and sarcopenia in older age. Bone. 2015;80:126–130.
77. Papadopoulou S, Tsintavis P, Potsaki G, et al. Differences in the prevalence of sarcopenia in community-dwelling, nursing home and hospitalized individuals: A systematic review and meta-analysis. J Nutr Health Aging. 2020;24(1):83–90.
78. Benedetti M, Furlini G, Zati A, et al. The effectiveness of physical exercise on bone density in osteoporotic patients. BioMed Res Int. 2018;23;2018:4840531.
79. Centers for Disease Control and Prevention. Healthy aging for older adults. Older Adults and Healthy Aging. (cdc.gov) (Accessed February 5, 2024).
80. McMillan L, Zengin A, Ebeling P, et al. Prescribing physical activity for the prevention and treatment of osteoporosis in older adults. Healthcare. 2017;6;5(4):85.
81. Ganapathy A, Nieves J. Nutrition and sarcopenia—what do we know? Nutrients. 2020; 11;12(6):1755.
82. Devries M, McGlory C, Bolster D, et al. Leucine, not total protein, content of a supplement is the primary determinant of muscle protein anabolic responses in healthy older women. J Nutr. 201;148:1088–1095.
83. Sahni S, Mangano K, McLean R, et al. Dietary approaches for bone health: Lessons from the framingham osteoporosis study. Curr Osteoporos Rep. 2015;13:245–255.
84. Movassagh E, Vatanparast H. Current evidence on the association of dietary patterns and bone health: A scoping review. Adv Nutr. 2017;8:1–16.
85. Cao J. Effects of obesity on bone metabolism. J Orthop Surg Res. 2011;15;6:30.
86. Nicoll R, McLaren Howard J. The acid-ash hypothesis revisited: A reassessment of the impact of dietary acidity on bone. J Bone Miner Metab. 2014;32(5):469–475.
87. Rivas A, Romero A, Mariscal-Arcas M, et al. Mediterranean diet and bone mineral density in two age groups of women. Int J Food Sci Nutr. 2013;64(2):155–161.
88. Palomeras-Vilches A, Viñals-Mayolas E, Bou-Mias C, et al. Adherence to the Mediterranean diet and bone fracture risk in middle-aged women: A case control study. Nutrients. 2019;18;11(10):2508.
89. García-Martínez O, Rivas A, Ramos-Torrecillas J, et al. The effect of olive oil on osteoporosis prevention. Int J Food Sci Nutr. 2014;65:834–840.
90. Messina M. Soy foods, isoflavones, and the health of postmenopausal women. Am J Clin Nutr. 2014;100:423S–430S.
91. Zheng X, Lee S, Chun O. Soy isoflavones and osteoporotic bone loss: A review with an emphasis on modulation of bone remodeling. J Med Food. 2016;19(1):1–14.
92. Shin S, Joung H. A dairy and fruit dietary pattern is associated with a reduced likelihood of osteoporosis in Korean postmenopausal women. Br J Nutr. 2013;110:1926–1933.
93. Tucker K. Vegetarian diets and bone status. Am J Clin Nutr. 2014;100(Suppl 1):329S–335S.
94. Ho-Pham L, Nguyen N, Nguyen T. Effect of vegetarian diets on bone mineral density: A bayesian meta-analysis. Am J Clin Nutr. 2009;90(4):943–950.

24 Nutrition and the Microbiome

Key Points

- The microbiome consists of over 100 trillion microorganisms (most of which are bacteria but also viruses, fungi, and protozoa) which exist in the human gastrointestinal tract.
- Researchers have suggested that the microbiome is best thought of as a virtual organ.
- There are multiple interactions between the microbiome and other organs in the body, including the lungs and the brain. This is an area of intense research.
- Eating a healthy diet such as the Mediterranean diet has been shown to enhance the balance of gut microbiota, which creates another reason for plant-based diets which are high in fruits and vegetables, whole grains, fiber, and healthy fats.

24.1 INTRODUCTION

There multiple important health-related considerations related to the human microbiome and how nutrition interacts with it [1–4]. The *microbiome* is the collective genomes of the microorganisms in a particular environment—in this case, it would be the human gut. In contrast, the *microbreiota* is the community of microorganisms themselves.

An extensive number of microbiota live in the human gut. Approximately 100 trillion microorganisms (most of them bacteria but also viruses, fungi, and protozoa), exist in the human gastrointestinal (GI) tract [1–4]. Some investigators feel that the microbiome should best be considered a virtual organ of the body [5,6]. It is indeed a very complex organ. The human genome consists of about 23,000 genes, whereas the microbiome contains approximately 4 million genes and produces thousands of metabolites [7]. It plays an important role in replacing many of the functions of the host, and thus, significantly influences the host phenotype and health.

What we eat dramatically affects the human microbiome with significant and diverse impacts ranging from immune, metabolic, and neurobehavioral traits [8–13]. Of all the environmental factors that impact on the human microbiome, diet is perhaps the most important, although physical activity, drugs, and anthropometric measures also have an impact on the microbiota composition.

The purpose of this chapter is to examine various roles of nutrition on the microbiota and, in turn, explore how the microbiome interacts with human health.

DOI: 10.1201/9781003452607-24

24.2 FUNCTION OF THE MICROBIOTA

The gut microbiota function to metabolize nondigestible substrates such as dietary fibers [14]. This metabolism is conducted through a process of fermentation, and this supports the growth of specialized microbiomes that produce short-chain fatty acids (SCFAs) and gases [15]. The major SCFAs produced are acetate, propionate, and butyrate [16].

Butyrate is the main energy source for human colonocytes (cells that line the colon). It can also activate intestinal gluconeogenesis, which may exert beneficial effects on glucose and energy homeostasis. Butyrate is also an essential component of endothelial cells which line the colon [17]. These cells consume large amounts of oxygen and generate an oxygen balance in the gut preventing an imbalance in the gut microbiota (dysbiosis).

Propionate is transferred to the liver where it regulates gluconeogenesis and satiety through the interaction with gut fatty acid receptors. Acetate, which is the most abundant SCFA, is an essential metabolite for the growth of bacteria [16]. It also reaches peripheral tissues where it may play a role in cholesterol metabolism and may also play a role in appetite regulation.

A number of trials have demonstrated that higher production of SCFA correlates with reduced risk of obesity and reduced insulin resistance. A variety of other specific products in the gut have been shown to directly play a role in human health outcomes [18–22]. For example, indole propionic acid is highly correlated with dietary fiber intake and is also a radical scavenger, which appears to reduce the incidence of type 2 diabetes [23].

24.3 MICROBIOTA BALANCE, DIVERSITY, AND HEALTH

Lower bacterial diversity is associated with inflammatory bowel disease, psoriatic arthritis, type 1 diabetes, eczema, obesity, type 2 diabetes, and arterial stiffness [21,22]. Diversity is thought to be a generally good indicator of gut health.

The recognition of the various vital functions of gut microbiota in work such as the Human Microbiome Project, conducted by the National Institutes of Health (NIH), has been developed to provide standard data regarding the human microbiome both in physiologic conditions and diseases.

This is known as the "microbicrobial core," which is fundamental to the health of the individual. Bacteria are the major components of the microbial core [24]. Up to 2,776 species of bacteria have been recognized in the human gut. The most common and extensive ones are the fermicutes (65%) followed by the bacteroidetes (23%) and actinobacterial (5%) [25,26].

Two terms are important to understand the role of microbiota in health and disease. The term eubiosis describes a favorable physiologic status of gut microbiota with so-called "good bacteria" that are capable of controlling "bad bacteria" [27,28]. The opposite situation, dysbiosis, is defined as a loss of this beneficial homeostatic balance [29]. Under eubiosis conditions, the gut bacteria perform a broad variety of functions essential for its health. These include the production of critical compounds such as SCFAs, which act as local and systemic signaling molecules with important health implications for health and disease conditions. The gut microbiota are also essential for the synthesis of vitamins such as vitamin K and any of the B complex, and even the metabolism of bile acids [30].

The term "taxonomic dysbiosis" relates to either quantitative or qualitative loss of the gut microbial composition, which is closely associated with reduced microbial diversity. This is typically an alternative Firmicutes-to-Bacteroidetes ratio, which has been reported in various pathologies including infections and noncommunicable diseases (NCDs) such as type 2 diabetes mellitus (T2DM) and obesity [31,21]. In these situations, a decrease in bacteria belonging to the phylum Bacteroidetes and an increase in non-favorable Firmicutes bacteria from the genus *Clostridium* has been reported [33–35].

There is a companion term entitled "metabolic dysbiosis." One of the most worrying effects of this type of dysbiosis is the presence of a component of the outer membrane of gram-negative bacteria in the bloodstream known as endotoxin or lipopolysaccharide (LPS), which is associated with chronic inflammation [36,37].

The functional role of the gut microbiome in humans has been shown using fecal microbiota transplantation. This procedure is effective in cases of severe drug-refractory *Clostridium difficile* infection and is routinely used for this purpose around the world [33].

24.4 THE EFFECTS OF FOOD AND DRUGS ON THE GUT MICROBIOTA

Specific foods and dietary patterns can all influence the abundance and types of bacteria in the gut which, in turn, can affect health. (See the subsequent section in this chapter concerning the effects of Western, Mediterranean, and vegan diets). Examples of foods that can impact on the gut include high-intensity sweeteners. There are some animal data to suggest negative effects from high-intensity sweeteners on the gut microbiota. For example, rats given sucralose for 12 weeks had higher proportions of Bacteroidetes clostridia and total anaerobic bacteria in their guts and significantly higher fecal pH than those without sucralose [38].

Food additives have also been shown to affect the gut microbiota in animals. Other areas of concern include various diets on gut health. For example, there are some strict vegan diets [39], raw food or "clean eating" diets, glucan-free diets [40], and lower fermentable oligosaccharides, disaccharides, monosaccharides, and polyols (FODMAP) diets to treat irritable bowel syndrome. It should be noted that gluten-free bread reduces microbiota dysbiosis in people with gluten-sensitive celiac disease. However, most people do not have celiac disease, and there are some data to suggest that gluten-free diets may increase the risk of heart disease, particularly since they reduce consumption of whole grains. A low-FODMAP diet has been shown in a number of randomized controlled trials to reduce symptoms of irritable bowel syndrome [41,42].

Medications may also result in changes in the gut microbiota composition. For example, laxatives may dramatically change the gut microbiota. In addition, commonly prescribed proton pump inhibitors can significantly change GI microbiota which may help explain higher rates of GI infection in people taking these drugs. Antibiotics clearly effect gut microbes [43,44]. Some studies have suggested an obesogenic effect of antibiotics in humans, even in tiny doses found in foods derived from animals. Conversely, dietary fiber intake, as already indicated, has a positive effect on gut microbiota composition and is related to better health.

24.5 MANIPULATING THE GUT MICROBIOTA THROUGH DIET

The gut microbiome exerts a very substantial relationship with the human diet. In fact, changes in the gut microbiota can occur within days of changing the diet. Most studies have shown that substantial changes can occur within two weeks. For example, in one study comparing African Americans and rural Africans who changed diets, the African Americans increased butyrate production 2.5 times while reducing the level of secondary bile acid within two weeks. Another study that compared shifts between plant- and animal protein–based diets showed these changes occurred in only five days. It should be noted, however, that healthy microbiota remain somewhat resistant to temporal changes in dietary interventions and can adapt so that homeostatic reactions restore the original community composition [1].

A variety of foods, food components, and supplements modulate the gut microbiota supporting the growth of bacteria that are considered favorable to health and well-being. These proposed health benefits include modulating the immune response and helping to control inflammation. Both probiotics and prebiotics may be considered in this context. (See the next two sections of this chapter.)

24.6 PROBIOTIC FOODS

Probiotics are defined as "live microorganisms that when administered in adequate amounts confer a health benefit on the host" [45]. Commonly used probiotics include *Lactobacillus* [46] and phytobacteria, although other bacteria in general and some yeast may also be used as probiotics. There is considerable debate about whether or not probiotics survive stomach acid and populate the intestines. Probiotics can be included in a variety of products including foods, dietary supplements, or drugs. Probiotics can affect health independently of the gut microbiota, which has direct effects on the host. One example is through immune modulation or the production of bioactive compounds. In a recent systemic review of probiotics, substantial evidence was obtained for beneficial effects in preventing diarrhea, acute enterocolitis, acute respiratory tract infections, pulmonary exacerbations in children with cystic fibrosis, and eczema in children [47–50].

Probiotics seem to improve a variety of cardiometabolic parameters including reduced high-sensitive C-reactive protein (CRP) in patients with type 2 diabetes. Probiotics are currently being researched as a component of personalized approaches in areas such as inflammation, cancer, lipid metabolism, and obesity [47–50].

Since there has been some controversy and debate about what constitutes probiotics, the International Scientific Association for Probiotic and Prebiotics issued a consensus statement in 2014 on the appropriate use of the term "probiotic" [51]. The consensus statement accepted the definition from the Food and Agricultural Organization of the United Nations and the World Health Organization (FAO/WHO), which defines probiotic as "live microorganisms which when administered in adequate amounts confer a health benefit on the host." This statement was reinforced in the consensus statement as relevant and appropriate for current and anticipated applications. The consensus statement went further and defined from various countries what constituted appropriate bacterial species to be included under the term "healthy probiotics." The details of these discussions is beyond the scope of this chapter; however, they are contained in the references for this consensus statement.

24.7 PREBIOTIC FOODS

Prebiotics were previously restricted to fructo-oligosaccharides and immunes that promote growth of beneficial bacteria, but the definition has now been broadened to include a "substrate that is selectively utilized by host microorganisms conferring a health benefit."

Oligosaccharides and polysaccharides remain the most commonly used prebiotics, and foods such as onions, artichokes, leeks, garlic, bananas, and asparagus have some of the highest potential to provide these prebiotics. Polyphenols in spices have been shown to affect gut microbiota and may be considered prebiotics. Both probiotics and prebiotics have been studied alone or in combination on immune infection and inflammatory conditions in humans. The effect of probiotics and prebiotics on influenza vaccination in older people has been investigated in a number of studies with variable findings according to the probiotic organism and prebiotic used [52].

24.8 THE EFFECTS OF VARIOUS DIETS ON THE MICROBIOTA

Diet is clearly described in the research and scientific literature as the most important factor that shapes gut microbiota and its relationship to chronic illness in general, inflammation, and the immune system. Other lifestyle factors, however, should not be omitted including exercise and circadian clocks (see the final section of this chapter). Diet rapidly effects gut microbiota composition, promoting the growth of certain bacterial groups over others as well as changing the intestinal pH, intestinal permeability, bacterial metabolites, and thus, inflammation. Macronutrients, particularly carbohydrates, are the best described, whereas protein and fat research is less well defined. Micronutrients are also important given that vitamin deficiencies alter interstitial permeability and immune response in the gut.

The immune system and microbiome interactions go together in diet. This will be discussed in detail in the next section. For now, it is important to emphasize that modern nutrition research focuses on dietary patterns as individual foods or nutrients. Thus, we will look at several diets and their effects on the microbiome.

In many ways, the Mediterranean diet (MedDiet) has become a model for healthy eating [53–55]. This diet is characterized by highly complex carbohydrates and fiber (found in fruits, vegetables, legumes, and cereal), polyunsaturated fatty acids with antiatherogenic and anti-inflammatory properties (found in olive oil and nuts), and bioactive compounds with antioxidant properties, flavonoids, phytosterols, terpenes, and polyphenols. In addition, this diet contains an abundance of micronutrients including vitamins and minerals. These will be discussed in more detail in a subsequent section of this chapter.

Vitamins and minerals help avoid malnutrition and immunodeficiencies. Nutrient-rich foods, such as those contained in the MedDiet, allow the body to repair inflammation triggered by nutrient-poor and high-calorie diets and contribute to attenuating cardiovascular risk factors. Adherence to the MedDiet also correlates with microbiota eubiosis and reestablishment of Bacteroidetes and certain beneficial *Clostridium* groups, while proteobacteria and bacillaceae species decrease [53]. Thus, the gut microbiota represents a good example of an individual's health status and also denotes adherence to a healthy diet such as MedDiet. Changes in the microbiota are speculated to play a significant role in why the MedDiet decreases the risk of cardiovascular disease.

It should be noted that while more research is available on the MedDiet than other heart-healthy diets, the likelihood remains that other heart-healthy diets which reduce the risk of heart disease and other chronic ailments, such as those recommended by the American Heart Association [56] and the *Dietary Guidelines for Americans 2020–2025* [57], are likely to result in similar beneficial changes in the gut microbiota. One other characteristic of these diets that is worth noting is the abundance of monounsaturated fats (MUFs), particularly in the MedDiet, and polyunsaturated fatty acids (PUFAs) and a very low consumption of saturated fatty acids. Both of these are important for both gut microbiota and the immune system.

In contrast to the MedDiet, the Western diet (WD) represents a global concern and is thought to be the key driver of the obesity pandemic and other NCDs including cancer, cardiovascular disease (CVD), osteoporosis, autoimmune disease, and T2DM, among others. The WD is characterized by a high content of unhealthy fats, refined grains, sugar, salt, alcohol, and other harmful elements along with reduced consumption of fruits and vegetables. This leads to critical changes in both the gut microbiota and the immune system, which can negatively affect gut integrity, thus promoting local and systemic chronic inflammation [58,59].

It is also worth noting that ultra-processed foods and drinks (UPFDs) such as those designated in that category by the NOVA Classification, are also thought to increase risk of comorbidities and mortality, although there is considerable debate about what constitutes an ultra-processed food and the role that they may play. In addition, reduced fiber contents of the WD generates further unfavorable alterations, particularly the reduction in production of SCFAs.

It is also worth noting that there is some research now that the vegan diet may also improve the gut microbiota. This diet, which contains no animal products, is rich in dietary fiber, polyphenols, and antioxidant vitamins. The vegan diet may serve as a marker for other vegetarian diets, which may also improve the microbiome [60]. There is considerable research that shows that vegan diets lower the risk of various chronic diseases including CVD, T2DM, cancer, and obesity. This diet, which includes high intake of fruits and vegetables, also has a low intake of both sodium and saturated fat.

There is some concern about micronutrients in the vegan diet, although plant-based diets such as the vegan diet clearly supply a wide array of vitamins including vitamin C and carotenoids, which are precursors of vitamin A and beta-carotene, while polyunsaturated vegetable oils contain significant amounts of lipid-soluble vitamin B. In contrast, there seem to be some deficiencies in the vegan diet concerning other vitamins such as vitamin B_{12} and vitamin D. Vitamin B_{12} is water soluble and commonly found in products of animal origin. Vitamin D is important for calcium absorption and bone mineralization. Low 25-hydroxy vitamin D concentrations have been documented in vegan societies, particularly in the winter and spring, or those living in high latitudes where there may be inadequate exposure to sunlight.

24.9 NUTRITION, IMMUNOSENESCENCE, INFECTIOUS DISEASE, AND THE MICROBIOME

The microbiome and the immune system are clearly bound together in a bidirectional relationship [61]. The immune system functions to protect the host individual from infectious agents that occur in the environment including pathogenic bacteria, viruses, fungi, parasites, and some other noxious insults. The immune system also plays an important role in surveillance and destruction of tumor cells, in clearing dying cells and cellular debris, in wound healing, and enabling tolerance of harmless environmental constituents like food and some bacteria to the host.

The immune response involves a variety of components and is distributed in many locations throughout the body. A detailed explanation of the immune system is beyond the scope of this chapter. Since physical barriers and lymphatic cells contribute to innate immunity, the GI tract may also be considered part of innate immunity. Many of the cell types that are involved in the immune system also play critical roles in the inflammatory response (see subsequent section).

There are two broad categories in the immune system. One is called innate immunity, and the other is called acquired immunity. Innate immunity involves a variety of physical barriers, soluble factors, and phagocytic cells such as neutrophils, eosinophils, and macrophages, whereas the acquired immune system plays a role in the specific recognition of molecules (antigens) and identifies an invading pathogen to distinguish it as being foreign to the host. Lymphocytes (class T and B lymphocytes) develop and mature in the bone marrow and are then released into circulation. Each lymphocyte carries multiple receptors for a single antigen. Thus, the acquired immune system is highly specific. In addition to interactions with T lymphocytes, B lymphocytes also produce immunoglobulins, which stimulate cellular immunity and phagocytosis. Typically, humoral immunity deals with extracellular pathogens such as bacteria. Some pathogens, however, including some viruses and certain bacteria, can enter host cells, meaning they escape humoral immunity. Instead, they are dealt with by cell-mediated immunity involving T lymphocytes.

The human gut is host for a significant number of bacteria and other microorganisms, which are referred to as gut microbiota. The large intestine has the greatest number and diversity of bacterial species, estimated at 10^{11}/gram of colonic contents. The gut wall is also the largest site of immune response, which is called gut-associated lymphoid tissue (GALT). It is estimated in humans that 70% of immune cells are associated with GALT. The key function of GALT is surveillance of microorganisms and other antigens in the gut lumen and mounting active responses to these. The human gut microbiota demonstrates a high degree of variability among individuals, which is a reflection of different exposures to environmental factors and their interaction with the host phenotype.

The human gut microbiome is strongly influenced by habitual diet. It is also impacted by aging. For example, with aging the abundance and diversity of healthy bacteria decline while bacteria including streptococci, staphylococci, enterococci, and enterobacteria increase. It is likely that the age-related changes in the microbiota are linked to immunosenescence and inflammation [62–64].

Nutrition plays a significant role in supporting the immune system. Foods and beverages provide macro- and micronutrients as well as bioactive compounds that contribute to the normal functioning of the immune system [61]. For example, macronutrients act as fuels for energy generation by immune cells and also provide building blocks for the biosynthesis involved in immune response such as amino acids, immunoglobins, cytokines, acute-phase proteins, etc.

Many micronutrients are regulators of molecular and cellular aspects of the immune system. Some micronutrients have specific antiinfection roles, e.g. zinc and vitamin D. Many nutrient and plant bioactives are involved in the protection of the host from the oxidative and inflammatory stress imposed by the immune response (e.g. vitamin C, vitamin E, cystine, zinc, copper, selenium, and flavonoids). Many food components contribute to creating diverse gut microbiota.

Aging is associated with changes in the immune system, including a decline in protective components (immunosenescence), which increase susceptibility to infectious disease, and a chronic elevation of low-grade inflammation (inflammaging), both of which increase the risk of multiple NCDs [62–64]. Many older people show changes in the gut microbiota. Age-related changes in immunocompetence, low-grade inflammation, and gut dysbiosis may be interlinked and may relay at least in part, to interrelated changes in nutrition.

24.10 MICRONUTRIENTS, THE IMMUNE SYSTEM, AND MICROBIOTA

Nutrient status and other dietary components can be used to favorably modulate immune cell function, inflammatory response, and infectious disease susceptibility and prognosis. Micronutrients are important in supporting the immune response and controlling inflammation. It has been suggested that micronutrient supplementation is beneficial to older adults. Among the micronutrients, the roles of vitamins A, C, D, and E as well as the minerals zinc, copper, iron, and selenium are the most explored.

Vitamin C contributes to supporting innate and adaptive immune responses as well as physical barriers that limit entering pathogens. Vitamin C is a potent antioxidant and plays an important role when granulocytes and macrophages produce reactive oxygen species (ROS) and promote apoptosis in infected host cells.

The Nobel Prize–winning chemist Linus Pauling suggested a high dose of vitamin C might decrease the incidence and duration of the common cold. However, subsequent research trials have not corroborated that concept.

There is some research that shows vitamin C supplementation in hospitalized older adults (at least 200 mg per day) who have acute respiratory tract infections and have very low vitamin C concentrations reduces respiratory symptom scores [65]. Thus, vitamin C supports many aspects of innate and acquired immunity in individuals who have vitamin C deficiency, which results in some benefit for older adults. This latter finding remains to be proven with larger investigations.

The precursor to the active form of vitamin D can be acquired from the diet or produced via ultraviolet B (UVB) irradiation of the skin. Subsequent hydroxylation reactions involving the enzymes 25-hydroxilate and 1-alpha-hydroxylate are located in the liver and kidney, respectively, and produce the active form 1-alpha 25-hydroxylated of vitamin D, also known as calcitriol. Some immune cells can also express 1-alpha-hydroxylated activity and can produce calcitriol. Many immune cell types express vitamin D receptors and respond to vitamin D. These include monocytes, macrophages, and T cell and B cells. Thus, vitamin D is now considered to be an important regulator of immune function and inflammation. Vitamin D also enhances epithelial integrity and plays a role in multiple cellular components of immunity.

Some observational studies have linked low concentrations of vitamin D to increased risk of viral acute respiratory infection. There has also been significant interest in vitamin D and COVID-19 [65,66]. A number of reports have documented associations between low vitamin D status and an increased susceptibility to, and severity of, COVID-19 [67]. In addition, a meta-analysis reported that vitamin D deficiency is associated with increased risk of severe COVID-19, hospitalization with COVID-19, and mortality from COVID-19. Thus, vitamin D has multiple effects on immunity, and supplementation of vitamin D may be useful to prevent or reduce the severity of respiratory diseases such as COVID-19. This may be particularly true in older adults where vitamin D intake and status are low.

Vitamin E, or tocopherol, is a potent lipid-soluble antioxidant that can mediate oxidative stress–induced damage to cellular lipids. Vitamin E also has anti-inflammatory activities which are independent from its antioxidant activities [68–70]. Vitamin E has been demonstrated to improve age-associated impairments in immune function in the elderly. Thus, vitamin E supports many aspects of innate and acquired immunity and also possess anti-inflammatory effects. To date, however, trials of vitamin E in relation to respiratory infections remain inconsistent, which may be the result of differences in dosage and characteristics of the participants studied. More research in this area is needed.

Zinc is required as a co-factor for enzymes involved in a number of processes including cell proliferation and differentiation, membrane integrity, and DNA and RNA synthesis [71,72]. Zinc status has been correlated with alterations in total immune cell numbers of B and T cells. Of note, zinc deficiency is prevalent in older individuals. For example, in one study in the United States, 30% of nursing home residents were zinc deficient. Zinc may also act on the buccal membranes of the oral cavity and nasopharyngeal tissues, suggesting individuals may also have a nonimmunologic mechanism which might influence the severity of the common cold. Zinc deficiency is thought to be a risk factor for pneumonia in older adults; however, trials of zinc in relationship to respiratory infection are inconsistent, perhaps relating to dose and formulation and characteristics of the participants studied.

24.11 NUTRITION, MICROBIOTA, AND INFLAMMATION

Inflammation is a component of innate immunity. The role of inflammation is to create an environment that is hostile to pathogens, initiate pathogen killing, and cause changes in the metabolism of the host. Multiple different cell types play roles in the inflammatory response, which also involves the production of and responses to a number of chemical mediators. The cardinal signs of inflammation are redness, swelling, heat, pain, and loss of function. These are all caused by cellular activation and chemical mediator release that occurs during the initiation and perpetuation of inflammatory responses.

Although inflammatory responses are important and designed to damage pathogens, the cellular activities and chemical mediators involved in inflammation can cause damage to host tissues [73]. Fortunately, inflammation is typically self-limiting and often resolves rapidly. This is because various inhibitory mechanisms are activated as inflammation runs its course. If these regulatory processes are lost, this can result in excessive, inappropriate, or ongoing inflammation, which can cause irreparable damage to host tissues, including pathology and disease. This was clearly demonstrated in the COVID-19 epidemic where hyperinflammation occurred and is thought to be one of the major underlying pathophysiologic features that cause severe disease and often mortality from COVID-19 [73].

It should be noted that while inflammation is necessary to coordinate the appropriate immune response to infection, aging results in a potential paradox ironically both raising grade inflammation, which is termed inflammaging, and decreasing the immune response.

As indicated in multiple chapters in this book, inflammation is now thought to play a key underlying role in multiple chronic metabolic diseases such as CVD, T2DM, obesity, metabolic syndrome, and cancer. Inflammation has been identified as a strong predictor of all-cause mortality in the elderly. This was clearly underscored with the age-related increases in COVID-19 in the elderly population. Once again, nutrition plays a critical role since nutrient-rich healthy diets such as the MedDiet lowers the risk of inflammation.

24.12 IMMUNE ENHANCEMENT THROUGH TARGETING THE GUT MICROBIOTA

A variety of food components and supplements can modulate the gut microbiota and support growth of bacteria that are considered favorable to health and well-being. These health benefits may also be a function of enhanced immune response and help to control inflammation.

Both probiotics and prebiotics can play an active role in supporting favorable microbiota [52]. In addition, probiotics can reduce the incidence, duration, and severity of diarrhea in children, suggesting they have beneficial effects on the GI tract. The gut microbiota may also play a role in determining infections initiated from the gut such as in the respiratory tract. This has caused some researchers to suggest that gut/lung access is important in maintaining respiratory health and may be positively modulated by probiotics.

24.13 DIET, STRESS, DEPRESSION, AND GUT MICROBIOTA

The brain and the gut have long been known to have an ongoing interaction through what is called the gut-brain axis. For example, psychological stress and depression can promote consumption of highly palatable foods, which can create inflammation and influence which gut bacteria thrive [74,75]. In addition, stress and depression can alter gut bacteria composition through stress hormones, inflammation, and autonomic alterations. In turn, the gut bacteria releases metabolites, toxins, and neurohormones that can alter eating behavior and mood.

Digestive disorders such as irritable bowel syndrome commonly coincide with mood disorders and may reflect dysfunctional composition of gut bacteria, viruses, and fungi and ensuing chronic inflammation. Thus, manipulating the gut microbiota by healthy diets such as MedDiet, DASH, and perhaps the use of probiotics can all reduce inflammation and reduce the likelihood of chronic disease. As already indicated earlier in this chapter, WD as well high-stress lifestyles can promote adverse gut bacteria and balance called dysbiosis. It has been suggested that dysbiosis may alter food cravings, metabolism, stress reactivity, and mood, which further compromise immune function and health.

24.14 GUT MICROBIOTA AND COVID-19

Considerable research links the gut and the lungs. COVID-19 mortality is largely related to hyperinflammation and damage to the lungs. Of interest, the COVID-19 RNA was found in feces of infected patients [64]. It is well known that intestinal epithelial cells, particularly the enterocytes of the small intestine, express ACE-2 receptors. This is similar to expression of these receptors in the lung. Substantial research demonstrates that respiratory virus infection causes changes in the gut microbiota. Diet and other environmental factors, as well as genetics, play an important role in shaping gut microbiota which can influence immunities.

We also know that gut microbiota diversity is decreased with old age, and COVID-19 has been mainly fatal in elderly patients, which further suggests the role that gut microbiota may play in this disease. Improving gut microbiota by eating a low-inflammatory diet such as the MedDiet and perhaps supplementation, including either prebiotics or probiotics, may play a meaningful role to minimize the impact of COVID-19 in elderly individuals and immune-compromised patients. Further research is needed in this area.

A recent study with 42,935 participants aged 55–99 drawn from two ongoing cohort studies, the Nurses Heath Study II and the Health Professionals Follow-up Study, evaluated dietary quality using the Alternative Healthy Eating Index (AHEI) 2010 and the Alternative Mediterranean Score (AMED) and found that individuals who had healthier diets as represented by high AHEI 2010 and AMED scores were associated with less likelihood of SARS-COV-2 infection. In the addition the analysis of COVID-19 severity in participants with a healthier diet had a lower likelihood of severe infection and were less likely to be hospitalized due to COVID-19. These associations were no longer significant after controlling for body mass index (BMI) and preexisting medical conditions. The investigators concluded that diet may be an important modifiable risk for COVID-19 infection as well its severity. As already indicated, this suggests that there may be a link between nutrition, microbiome, and COVID-19 [76–78].

24.15 GUT MICROBIOTA AND OBESITY

Emerging research suggests that gut microbiota may play a role in the development and progress of obesity. Studies in overweight and obese people show a dysbiosis characterized by lower bacterial diversity [79,80]. Gut microbiota dysbiosis may also promote diet-induced obesity and metabolic complications by a variety of mechanisms including immune dysfunction, altered systemic inflammation, and altered gut hormone regulation. Given the underlying role of gut microbiota in immunity and inflammation, it is not surprising that obesity, which has a significant component of inflammation, may also be affected by these factors.

24.16 MICROBIOTA AND GASTROINTESTINAL SYMPTOMS

As already indicated, the brain and the gut are well known to have significant interaction through the gut-brain axis. Many people have experienced that negative emotions and stress can perturb GI motility. It has also been shown that individuals who have dysbiosis have an increased risk of irritable bowel syndrome [81–83]. Furthermore, probiotics have been utilized as an important adjunct to treatment for children who have diarrhea [33]. It is not surprising that there are multiple interactions between the symptoms from the GI tract and the microbiota. Certainly, healthy nutrition plays an important role in this area.

24.17 OTHER LIFESTYLE MEDICINE AND MODALITIES AND THEIR IMPACT ON MICROBIOTA

In addition to the important role that healthy nutrition plays on gut microbiota, other lifestyle modalities such as weight management, regular physical activity, not smoking cigarettes, getting adequate sleep, and stress reduction all play significant roles in interactions with the gut microbiota [1]. Many of these factors lower inflammation and thereby lower chronic disease, which can have a very significant bidirectional impact on the gut microbiota.

24.18 CONCLUSIONS

The microbiome, which represents the collective microorganisms that are found in the human gut, plays key roles in many aspects of human health including immune, metabolic, and neuro-behavioral traits. Nutrition plays a very important role in modulating issues related to how the microbiome interacts with the immune system and inflammation.

The MedDiet has been shown to promote a healthy balance of gut bacteria and decrease the risk of inflammation. The components of the MedDiet include multiple fruits and vegetables, fiber, and abundant monounsaturated fat and polyunsaturated fats, all of which can play a significant role in creating a healthier gut microbiota.

Many researchers feel that the microbiome is best thought of as a virtual organ in the body. It has been estimated there are over 100 trillion microorganisms (most of them bacteria but also viruses fungi, and protozoa) that exist in the human GI tract. Emerging research has linked gut microbiota in significant ways to various chronic diseases. The good news is that healthy nutritional practices which are so important for lowering the risk of chronic disease in general also can play a significant role in creating a healthy gut microbiome.

Clinical Applications

- Clinicians should discuss with their patients the role of healthy eating and its impact on gut microbiota.
- The gut microbiome consists of over 100 trillion microorganisms (most of which are bacteria but also viruses, fungi, and protozoa) which exist in the human GI tract.
- Researchers have suggested that the microbiome is best thought of as a virtual organ.

REFERENCES

1. Rinninella E, Raoul P, Cintoni M, et al. What is the healthy gut microbiota composition? A changing ecosystem across age, environment, diet, and diseases. Microorganisms. 2019;10;7(1):14.
2. Thursby E, Juge N. Introduction to the human gut microbiota. Biochem J. 2017;16;474(11): 1823–1836.
3. Ley R, Turnbaugh P, Klein S, et al. Microbial ecology: Human gut microbes associated with obesity. Nature. 2006;21;444(7122):1022–1023.
4. Wilson K, Situ C. Systematic review on effects of diet on gut microbiota in relation to metabolic syndromes. J Clin Nutr Metab. 2017;1:2.
5. Gill S, Pop M, Deboy R, et al. Metagenomic analysis of the human distal gut microbiome. Science. 2006;312:1355–1359.
6. Luckey T. Introduction to intestinal microecology. Am J Clin Nutr. 1972;25:1292–1294.
7. Li D, Wang P, Wang P, et al. The gut microbiota: A treasure for human health. Biotechnol Adv. 2016;15;34(7):1210–1224.
8. Carrera-Bastos P, Fontes-Villalba M, O'Keefe J, et al. The western diet and lifestyle and diseases of civilization. Res Rep Clin Cardiol. 2011;2:15–35.
9. Centritto F, Iacoviello L, di Giuseppe R, et al. Dietary patterns, cardiovascular risk factors and C-reactive protein in a healthy Italian population. Nutr Metable Cardiovasc Dis. 2009;19(10):697–706.
10. Claesson M, Jeffery I, Conde S, et al. Gut microbiota composition correlates with diet and health in the elderly. Nature. 2012;9;488(7410):178–184.
11. Conlon M, Bird A. The impact of diet and lifestyle on gut microbiota and human health. Nutrients. 2014;24;7(1):17–44.
12. Cotillard A, Kennedy S, Kong L, et al. Dietary intervention impact on gut microbial gene richness. Nature. 2013;29;500(7464):585–588.
13. Clifford M. Diet-derived phenols in plasma and tissues and their implications for health. Planta Med. 2004;70(12):1103–1114.
14. Marchesi J, Adams D, Fava F, et al. The gut microbiota and host health: A new clinical frontier. Gut. 2016;65(2):330–339.
15. Kurokawa K, Itoh T, Kuwahara T, et al. Comparative metagenomics revealed commonly enriched gene sets in human gut microbiomes. DNA Res. 2007;31;14(4):169–181.
16. Fernandes J, Su W, Rahat-Rozenbloom S, et al. Adiposity, gut microbiota and faecal short chain fatty acids are linked in adult humans. Nutr Diabetes. 2014;30;4(6):e121.
17. Hamer H, Jonkers D, Venema K, et al. Review article: The role of butyrate on colonic function. Aliment Pharmacol Ther. 2008;15;27(2):104–119.

18. Laterza L, Rizzatti G, Gaetani E, et al. The gut microbiota and immune system relationship in human graft-versus-host disease. Mediterr J Hematol Infect Dis. 2016;8:e2016025.
19. Flint H, Scott K, Louis P, et al. The role of the gut microbiota in nutrition and health. Nat Rev Gastroenterol Hepatol. 2012;9:577–589.
20. Arumugam M, Raes J, Pelletier E, et al. Enterotypes of the human gut microbiome. Nature. 2011;473:174–180.
21. Toshitaka O, Kumiko K, Hirosuke S, et al. Age-related changes in gut microbiota composition from newborn to centenarian: A cross-sectional study. BMC Microbiol. 2016;16:90.
22. Guigoz Y, Doré J, Schiffrin E. The inflammatory status of old age can be nurtured from the intestinal environment. Curr Opin Clin Nutr Metab Care. 2008;11:13–20.
23. Moore W, Holdeman L. Human fecal flora: The normal flora of 20 Japanese-Hawaiians. Appl Microbiol. 1974;27(5):961–979.
24. Singh R, Chang H, Yan D, et al. Influence of diet on the gut microbiome and implications for human health. J Transl Med. 2017;8:15(1):73.
25. Flint H, Duncan S, Scott K. Interactions and competition within the microbial community of the human colon: Links between diet and health. Environ Microbiol. 2007;9(5):1101–1111.
26. Walker A, Ince J, Duncan S, et al. Dominant and diet-responsive groups of bacteria within the human colonic microbiota. ISME J. 2011;5(2):220–230.
27. Lundin A, Bok C, Aronsson L, et al. Gut flora, toll-like receptors and nuclear receptors: A tripartite communication that tunes innate immunity in large intestine. Cell Microbiol. 2008;10(5):1093–1103.
28. Lee Y, Mazmanian S. Has the microbiota played a critical role in the evolution of the adaptive immune system? Science. 2010;24;330(6012):1768–1773.
29. Belkaid Y, Hand T. Role of the microbiota in immunity and inflammation. Cell. 2014;27;157(1):121–141.
30. Ou J, DeLany J, Zhang M, et al. Association between low colonic short-chain fatty acids and high bile acids in high colon cancer risk populations. Nutr Cancer. 2012;64(1):34–40.
31. Qin J, Li Y, Cai Z, et al. A metagenome-wide association study of gut microbiota in type 2 diabetes. Nature. 2012;490:55–60.
32. Turnbaugh P, Ley R, Mahowald MA, et al. An obesity-associated gut microbiome with increased capacity for energy harvest. Nature. 2006;444:1027–1031.
33. Lau C, Chamberlain R. Probiotics are effective at preventing Clostridium difficile-associated diarrhea: A systematic review and meta-analysis. Int J Gen Med. 2016;22;9:27–37.
34. Sun X, Hirota S. The roles of host and pathogen factors and the innate immune response in the pathogenesis of clostridium difficile infection. Mol Immunol. 2015;63(2):193–202.
35. Greenblum S, Turnbaugh P, Borenstein E. Metagenomic systems biology of the human gut microbiome reveals topological shifts associated with obesity and inflammatory bowel disease. Proc Natl Acad Sci USA. 2012;10;109(2):594–599.
36. Lucas López R, Grande Burgos M, Gálvez A, et al. The human gastrointestinal tract and oral microbiota in inflammatory bowel disease: A state of the science review. APMIS. 2017;125(1):3–10.
37. Schicho R, Marsche G, Storr M. Cardiovascular complications in inflammatory bowel disease. Curr Drug Targets. 2015;16(3):181–188.
38. Suez J, Korem T, Zeevi D, et al. Artificial sweeteners induce glucose intolerance by altering the gut microbiota. Nature. 2014;9;514(7521):181–186.
39. Wu G, Compher C, Chen E, et al. Comparative metabolomics in vegans and omnivores reveal constraints on diet-dependent gut microbiota metabolite production. Gut. 2016;65(1):63–72.
40. Bonder M, Tigchelaar E, Cai X, et al. The influence of a short-term gluten-free diet on the human gut microbiome. Genome Med. 2016;21;8(1):45.

41. Bhattarai Y, Muniz Pedrogo D, Kashyap P. Irritable bowel syndrome: A gut microbiota-related disorder? Am J Physiol Gastrointest Liver Physiol. 2017;312:52–62.
42. Carroll I, Chang Y, Park J, et al. Luminal and mucosal-associated intestinal microbiota in patients with diarrhea-predominant irritable bowel syndrome. Gut Pathog. 2010;2:19.
43. Pérez-Cobas A, Artacho A, Knecht H, et al. Differential effects of antibiotic therapy on the structure and function of human gut microbiota. PLoS One. 2013;8:e80201.
44. Iizumi T, Battaglia T, Ruiz V, et al. Gut microbiome and antibiotics. Arch Med Res. 2017;48:727–734.
45. Hill C, Guarner F, Reid G, et al. The International Scientific Association for Probiotics and Prebiotics consensus statement on the scope and appropriate use of the term probiotic. Nat Rev Gastroenterol Hepatol. 2014;11:506–514.
46. Hickson M, D'Souza A, Muthu N, et al. Use of probiotic Lactobacillus preparation to prevent diarrhoea associated with antibiotics: Randomised double blind placebo controlled trial. BMJ. 2007;14;335(7610):80.
47. He T, Priebe M, Zhong Y, et al. Effects of yogurt and bifidobacteria supplementation on the colonic microbiota in lactose-intolerant subjects. J Appl Microbiol. 2008;104(2):595–604.
48. del Campo R, Garriga M, Pérez-Aragón A, et al. Improvement of digestive health and reduction in proteobacterial populations in the gut microbiota of cystic fibrosis patients using a lactobacillus reuteri probiotic preparation: A double blind prospective study. J Cyst Fibros. 2014;13(6):716–722.
49. Liu J, Zhang Y, Zhang J, et al. Probiotic yogurt effects on intestinal flora of patients with chronic liver disease. Nurs Res. 2010;59(6):426–432.
50. Kwak D, Jun D, Seo J, et al. Short-term probiotic therapy alleviates small intestinal bacterial overgrowth, but does not improve intestinal permeability in chronic liver disease. Eur J Gastroenterol Hepatol. 2014;26(12):1353–1359.
51. Gibson G, Hutkins R, Sanders M, et al. Expert consensus document: The International Scientific Association for Probiotics and Prebiotics (ISAPP) consensus statement on the definition and scope of prebiotics. Nat Rev Gastroenterol Hepatol. 2017;14(8): 491–502.
52. Lei W, Shih P, Liu S, et al. Effect of probiotics andprebiotics on immune response to influenza vaccination in adults: A systematicreview and meta-analysis of randomized controlled trials. Nutrients. 2017;27;9(11):1175.
53. De Filippis F, Pellegrini N, Vannini L, et al. High-level adherence to a Mediterranean diet beneficially impacts the gut microbiota and associated metabolome. Gut. 2016;65(11): 1812–1821.
54. Tosti V, Bertozzi B, Fontana L. Health benefits of the Mediterranean diet: Metabolic and molecular mechanisms. J Gerontol A Biol Sci Med Sci. 2018;2;73(3):318–326.
55. Bailey M, Holscher H. Microbiome-mediated effects of the Mediterranean diet on inflammation. Adv Nutr. 2018;1;9(3):193–206.
56. Lichtenstein A, Appel L, Vadiveloo M, et al. 2021 Dietary guidance to improve ardiovascular health: A scientific statement from the American Heart Association. Circulation. 2021;7;144(23):e472–e487.
57. Pendyala S, Walker J, Holt P. A high-fat diet is associated with endotoxemia that originates from the gut. Gastroenterology. 2012;142(5):1100–1101.e2.
58. Pussinen P, Havulinna A, Lehto M, et al. Endotoxemia is associated with an increased risk of incident diabetes. Diabetes Care. 2011;34(2):392–397.
59. Pussinen P, Havulinna A, Lehto M, et al. Endotoxemia is associated with an increased risk of incident diabetes. Diabetes Care. 2011;34(2):392–397.
60. Wu G, Chen J, Hoffmann C, et al. Linking long-term dietary patterns with gut microbial enterotypes. Science. 2011;334(6052):105–108.

61. Corrêa-Oliveira R, Fachi J, Vieira A, et al. Regulation of immune cell function by short-chain fatty acids. Clin Transl Immunology. 2016;22;5(4):e73.
62. Tanaka M, Nakayama J. Development of the gut microbiota in infancy and its impact on health in later life. Allergol Int. 2017;66:515–522.
63. Tidjani Alou M, Lagier J, Raoult D. Diet influence on the gut microbiota and dysbiosis related to nutritional disorders. Hum Microbiome J. 2016;1:3–11.
64. Yatsunenko T, Rey F, Manary M, et al. Human gut microbiome viewed across age and geography. Nature. 2012;486:222–227.
65. Penkert R, Rowe H, Surman S, et al. Influences of vitamin A on vaccine immunogenicity and efficacy. Front Immunol. 2019;10:1576.
66. Grant W, Lahore H, McDonnell S, et al. Evidence that vitamin D supplementation could reduce risk of influenza and COVID-19 infections and deaths. Nutrients. 2020;12:988.
67. Laird E, Rhodes J, Kenny R. Vitamin D and inflammation: Potential implications for severity of Covid-19. Ir Med J. 2020;113:81.
68. Buendia P, Ramirez R, Aljama P, et al. Klotho prevents translocation of NFkappaB. Vitam Horm. 2016;101:119–150.
69. Tan P, Sagoo P, Chan C, et al. Inhibition of NF-kappa B and oxidative pathways in human dendritic cells by antioxidative vitamins generates regulatory T cells. J Immunol. 2005;174:7633–7644.
70. Xuan N, Trang P, Van Phong N, et al. Klotho sensitive regulation of dendritic cell functions by vitamin E. Biol Res. 2016;49:45.
71. Black R. Zinc deficiency, infectious disease and mortality in the developing world. J Nutr. 2003;133(5 Suppl 1):1485S–1489S.
72. Bhutta Z. Iron and zinc deficiency in children in developing countries. BMJ. 2007;20;334 (7585):104–105.
73. Iddir M, Brito A, Dingeo G, et al. Strengthening the immune system and reducing inflammation and oxidative stress through diet and nutrition: Considerations during the COVID-19 crisis. Nutrients. 2020;27;12(6):1562.
74. Collins S, Surette M, Bercik P. The interplay between the intestinal microbiota and the brain. Nat Rev Microbiol. 2012;10(11):735–742.
75. Bailey M, Dowd S, Galley J, et al. Exposure to a social stressor alters the structure of the intestinal microbiota: Implications for stressor-induced immunomodulation. Brain Behav Immun. 2011;25(3):397–407.
76. Dhar D, Mohanty A. Gut microbiota and Covid-19- possible link and implications. Virus Res. 2020;285:198018.
77. Butler M, Barrientos R. The impact of nutrition on COVID-19 susceptibility and long-term consequences. Brain Behav Immun. 2020;87:53–54.
78. Zabetakis I, Lordan R, Norton C, et al. COVID-19: The inflammation link and the role of nutrition in potential mitigation. Nutrients. 2020;19;12(5):1466.
79. Ley R, Turnbaugh P, Klein S, et al. Microbial ecology: Human gut microbes associated with obesity. Nature. 2006;21;444(7122):1022–1023.
80. Million M, Angelakis E, Paul M, et al. Comparative meta-analysis of the effect of lactobacillus species on weight gain in humans and animals. Microb Pathog. 2012;53(2):100–108.
81. Joossens M, Huys G, Cnockaert M, et al. Dysbiosis of the faecal microbiota in patients with Crohn's disease and their unaffected relatives. Gut. 2011;60(5):631–637.
82. Sokol H, Pigneur B, Watterlot L, et al. Faecalibacterium prausnitzii is an anti-inflammatory commensal bacterium identified by gut microbiota analysis of Crohn disease patients. Proc Natl Acad Sci USA. 2008;28;105(43):16731–16736.
83. Marasco G, Di Biase AR, Schiumerini R, et al. Gut microbiota and celiac disease. Dig Dis Sci. 2016;61(6):1461–1472.

25 Lifestyle Habits and Practices to Reduce Risk Factors for Heart Disease, Diabetes, Obesity, Metabolic Syndrome, Dementia, and Cancer

Key Points

- Nutrition is a key component of risk reduction and treatment of chronic disease.
- Nutrition should optimally be placed in the context of other lifestyle modalities including physical activity, weight management, avoidance of tobacco, and healthy sleep.
- Clinicians should be aware of the synergistic effects of other lifestyle practices on healthy nutrition.

25.1 INTRODUCTION

While this book focuses on nutrition, there are a number of other lifestyle medicine–related habits and actions which complement nutrition and also exert profound effects on short- and long-term health and quality of life.

Nutrition plays a key role in lifestyle habits and practices and affects virtually every chronic disease. There is strong evidence for a role of nutrition in cardiovascular disease (CVD) [1–5], type 2 diabetes mellitus (T2DM) [6–9], obesity [10–13], and cancer [14–20], among many other conditions. The dietary guidelines [21] and consensus statements [22] from a variety of organizations have all recognized the key role for nutrition both in the prevention and treatment of various diseases. More specific details on this will be found later in this chapter and also in multiple other chapters of this book.

It is important to place nutrition in the context of lifestyle medicine. An overwhelming body of scientific and medical literature supports the concept that daily habits and actions exert enormous impact on short- and long-term health and quality of life. This includes regular physical activity, maintenance of a healthy body weight, not smoking cigarettes, following sound nutrition and other health-promoting

DOI: 10.1201/9781003452607-25

practices, getting healthful sleep, and engaging in positive social interactions with other people.

I had the privilege of authoring the first multiauthored, academic textbook in lifestyle medicine. This was published in 1999 and coined the term "lifestyle medicine" in the academic literature, which we defined as "The discipline of studying how daily habits and practices impact on both prevention and treatment of disease, often in conjunction with pharmaceutical or surgical therapy to provide an important adjunct to overall health" [23].

Many other mainstream medical organizations have now adopted the concept of lifestyle medicine. For example, the American Heart Association changed the name of one of its councils from the "Council on Nutrition and Physical Activity and Metabolism" to the "Council on Lifestyle and Cardiovascular Health" in 2013 [24]. Also, both the American College of Preventive Medicine and the American Academy of Family Practice have established working groups or educational tracks in the area of lifestyle medicine.

Importantly, a rising healthcare organization, the American College of Lifestyle Medicine (ACLM), which is devoted to providing a home for individuals who wish to emphasize lifestyle medicine in their practices, has grown remarkably in the last decade. There are now over 11,000 members of ACLM [25]. ACLM has fostered initiatives to develop curricula and encourage education of medical students and physicians at every level of training in lifestyle medicine. One of the priorities of this organization has been to establish certification boards in lifestyle medicine. One certification is already available as well as study materials to take the board of lifestyle medicine.

In addition, a peer-reviewed academic journal has been established, the *American Journal of Lifestyle Medicine* (AJLM), which exists as a forum for individuals exchanging academic information from all around the world in this growing field. AJLM currently has over 21,000 subscribers and in 2023 had over 290,000 downloads of full text articles [26].

Lifestyle medicine is an appropriate term for this discipline. First of all, "lifestyle" focuses on habits and actions in individuals' daily lives and their relationship to health, disease prevention, and treatment. Second, it is clearly "medicine" based on an enormous body of evidence supporting the health benefits of daily habits and actions. In this chapter, we will examine some of the other aspects of lifestyle medicine, in addition to nutrition, which form the pillars of the field of lifestyle medicine.

25.2 PHYSICAL ACTIVITY

Regular physical activity is a key consideration of overall health in the prevention and/or treatment of various diseases. Regular physical activity has been specifically demonstrated to reduce the risk of CVD, T2DM, metabolic syndrome, obesity, and certain types of cancer. The important role of physical activity has been underscored by its prominent role in evidence-based guidelines and consensus statements from virtually every organization that deals with metabolic disease [27].

The 2018 Physical Activity Guidelines for Americans Advisory Committee Scientific Report provides an important, evidence-based compendium of multiple benefits that physical activity carries [28]. Not only does regular physical activity lower the risk of various diseases, but it also powerfully improves the quality of life by improving sleep, general feelings of well-being, and daily functioning. Physical activity also has been shown to be a key factor to prevent or minimize excessive weight gain in adults. Physical activity has been demonstrated to lower the risk of dementia and improve other aspects of cognitive functioning and other conditions. Regular physical activity also improves osteoarthritis and hypertension.

Unfortunately, physicians are not as actively involved in counseling for physical activity as they should be. It has been estimated that only 40% of physicians regularly counsel their patients on the importance of regular physical activity [29]. Other studies have shown that physicians' own physical activity behavior predicts the likelihood that they will recommend physical activity to their patients.

The American College of Sports Medicine has launched a significant program entitled Exercise Is Medicine (EIM) with the goal of expediting the ability of physicians to provide evidence-based recommendations for physical activity [30]. EIM also recommends that healthcare providers record physical activity as a vital sign during patients' visits and finish each counseling session with an exercise "prescription."

25.3 NUTRITION

Of course, nutrition is featured in multiple chapters in this book. There is no question that nutrition plays a vital role in lifestyle habits and practices and affects virtually every chronic disease. These include CVD, diabetes, obesity, cancer, and many other conditions [21,22,31]. The dietary guidelines and consensus statements from a variety of organizations have been quite consistent with each other and have all recognized the key role for healthy nutrition in both the prevention and treatment of chronic disease.

These consensus statements are similar to each other and consistently recommend a dietary pattern high in fruits and vegetables, whole grains (particularly high fiber), nonfat dairy, seafood, legumes, and nuts. These guidelines also recommend that those who consume alcohol (among adults) do so in moderation. The guidelines are also consistent in recommending diets lower in red and processed meats, refined grains, sugar-sweetened foods, and saturated and trans fats. Importantly, all of the guidelines emphasize the importance of balancing calories and also regular physical activity as strategies for maintaining a healthy weight, which also reduces the risk for chronic diseases.

Healthy nutrition also plays a very significant role in metabolism and exerts multiple significant impacts on the microbiome. In addition, healthy nutrition is very important for cognition [32] and overall metabolic health. All of these issues will be dealt with in separate chapters in this book.

As will be emphasized throughout this, book dietary guidelines over the past two decades have moved from specifically recommending certain nutrients to a greater application on dietary patterns. Unfortunately, despite decades of dietary advice, only a significant minority of Americans are following these guidelines. For example, only 12% of Americans eat the recommended servings of fruits and only 7% eat the recommended servings of vegetables [33]. Even for people who have high blood pressure, less than 20% of individuals follow the DASH diet [34].

The *Dietary Guidelines for Americans 2020–2025* focus on integrating available science and food pattern modeling to develop the Healthy U.S.-Style Dietary Pattern, which will be discussed in a subsequent chapter. It should be noted that many of the foods in the Western diet (WD) are, in and of themselves, highly inflammatory. This includes saturated fats, red meat, refined grains, and alcohol. In contrast, healthy diets such as the DASH diet [35], the Mediterranean diet [36] (Med Diet), and the Healthy U.S.-Style [21] Dietary Pattern all are much lower in inflammatory potential.

A major problem in the area of nutrition is that physicians typically do not feel that they have adequate education in this area. Only one in five medical schools have courses in nutrition [37]. Unfortunately, 90% of cardiologists who were polled said they did not have adequate knowledge of nutrition, although 95% of them indicated that they felt it was important for them offer nutrition counseling to patients [38]. In the United States, 67% of physicians try to provide nutrition counseling. However, this counseling is mostly general with guidance about following a varied diet [39]. It is noteworthy that only 21% of patients feel they received effective communication in the area of nutrition from their physician.

25.4 WEIGHT MANAGEMENT

Overweight and obesity are extremely prevalent around the world. In the United States, over 72% of men and women are either overweight or obese [40]. Worldwide, it has been estimated that there are over 3 billion individuals who are either overweight or obese. While multiple pharmaceutical agents are available to help in the treatment of obesity as well as bariatric surgery, lifestyle measures serve as a cornerstone for obesity treatment and for creating an energy deficit to achieve weight loss. It should be noted that obesity has been shown to be a chronic inflammatory disease, and this is likely to be the underlying etiology that connects it to CVD, T2DM, and even some cancers. Nutrition and physical activity are the cornerstone modalities to achieve a caloric deficit. Nutrition is featured as one of the key steps in the obesity management guidelines from the American Heart Association/American College of Cardiology (AHA/ACC) and The Obesity Society (TOS).

25.5 TOBACCO PRODUCTS

There is overwhelming evidence from multiple sources that cigarette smoking and exposure to smoke increase the risk of multiple chronic diseases including CVD and stroke, T2DM, and cancer [41]. In the early 20th century, cigarette smoking was more prevalent in men than in women. However, women have rapidly caught up with men. The risks of cigarette smoking in women are equivalent to men. Substantial benefits come from reduction of risk of CVD and cancer to individuals who stop smoking cigarettes, and these benefits occur in a very brief period of time [42].

Unfortunately, after years of significant declines in cigarette smoking, the prevalence of cigarette smoking has leveled off at approximately 15% of adults currently smoking cigarettes.

It should also be noted that secondhand smoke increases the risk of multiple chronic diseases, since it contains numerous carcinogens, particularly in indoor environments where it can last for a number of hours after cigarettes have been smoked [43].

25.6 ALCOHOL

Alcohol consumption is extremely common in the United States. However, drinking too much alcohol can harm your health. Excessive alcohol use led to more than 140,000 deaths and 3.6 million years of potential life lost each year in the United States from 2015 to 2019, shortening the lives of those who died by an average of 26 years [44–48]. Excessive drinking was responsible for one in five deaths among individuals ages 20–49 years. There has been considerable debate about the amount of alcohol that is safe to be consumed. Recent studies from several researchers have suggested that no amount of alcohol is safe. However, the general recommendation has been that adults of the legal drinking age can chose to drink in moderation and limit intake to two drinks per day for men and one drink or fewer per day for women. Recent data have suggested that these levels of alcohol consumption may lower the risk of heart disease and diabetes.

Those who argue against consumption of any level of alcohol focus on the fact that alcohol consumption can lead to high blood pressure, CVD, stroke, liver disease, and digestive problems, as well as cancer of the breast, mouth, throat, esophageal, larynx, liver, colon, and rectum. The immune system is also weakened by excessive alcohol consumption. Mental health problems, including depression and anxiety, and social problems, including family and job-related problems and unemployment, are all associated with excessive drinking.

25.7 SLEEP

Disordered sleep patterns are extremely common. This is an issue both for children and adolescents, as well as adults [49,50]. Poor sleep patterns in childhood tend to persist into adulthood and often develop into chronic sleep disruption patterns. In addition, short sleep duration has been shown to influence a variety of important hormones including leptin, ghrelin, insulin, cortisol, and growth hormones. In one research study, when sleep patterns were shortened, disruption of diurnal eating patterns occurred and also an increase of energy-dense foods consumed. Sleep timing is also associated with dietary habits.

Disturbed sleep is associated with a wide variety of chronic disorders including CVD, where it accounts for 30–40% of risks. Other metabolic conditions, inflammatory conditions, and even cancer diagnoses are associated with disruption of sleep. Inadequate sleep is also associated with weight gain as well as mood disorders. For this reason, it is important that clinicians focus on sleep as a component of overall healthy lifestyle medicine assessment.

For most individuals, seven to nine hours of sleep is appropriate. Sleep duration of less than six hours or more than nine hours are both associated with adverse health consequences and chronic disease. A wide variety of lifestyle medicine interventions can assist in improving duration and quality of sleep such as controlling temperature in the bedroom. Mindful meditation and cognitive therapy have also been demonstrated to improve quality and duration of sleep. Of note, the AHA added healthy sleep as the eighth component of its framework to reduce the risk of CVD entitled "Life's Essential 8" to underscore the importance of sleep in heart health.

25.8 STRESS, ANXIETY, AND DEPRESSION

Stress is extremely common in the modern, fast-paced world [51]. It has been estimated that one-third of the adult population in the United States experiences enough stress in their daily lives to have an adverse impact on their home or work performance. Anxiety and depression are also very common. Lifestyle measures such as regular physical activity may provide effective amelioration for aspects of all three of these conditions.

In the past decade the concept of "positive psychology" also has emerged, which shows that individuals who express gratitude, forgiveness, and other strategies may also achieve significant stress reduction and amelioration of anxiety and depression [52]. Obtaining adequate amounts of sleep is also important to help control or reduce these conditions.

25.9 POSITIVE LIFESTYLE, ALTRUISM, AND SOCIAL CONNECTIONS

Interacting with other human beings is essential to having a long and happy life. Volunteering has been shown to also yield multiple health benefits. An interesting study was recently published in book form from the Harvard Longitudinal Study [53]. The book, entitled *The Good Life*, basically reports that of all the things an individual could do to bring happiness to their life, the interaction with other individuals is the most important. Conversely, a recent article suggested that social isolation and loneliness carried significant health risks. This is particularly true of individuals over the age of 65. These factors were particularly emphasized in the response to the COVID-19 pandemic.

25.10 LIFESTYLE MEDICINE AND CHRONIC DISEASE

As already indicated, lifestyle medicine practices significantly impact on both preventing and treating chronic disease. This is an important topic which will be dealt with in a subsequent chapter in this book. Certainly, nutrition is one of the key modalities in reduction in the risk of chronic disease.

25.11 BEHAVIORAL STRATEGIES AND ADHERENCE

In essence, all of the lifestyle medicine modalities, including nutrition, physical activity, and others, are ones where individuals are asked to make changes in their behavior. There are multiple constructs available to outline the most effective ways of helping people make behavioral changes. This topic is beyond the scope of the current chapter. However, there are multiple good resources available to assist in this topic including the third and fourth editions of the *Lifestyle Medicine* textbook that I edit [54,55]. Of note, the AHA has felt that adhering to behavioral strategies is so important that they have issued a separate scientific statement on this. This is in response to the fact that there is still low adherence to many of the recommendations that have been traditionally made by the AHA to promote heart health [56].

25.12 LIFESTYLE MEDICINE AROUND THE WORLD

Lifestyle medicine has become a global initiative. The leading organization in this is the Lifestyle Medicine Global Alliance, which was founded in 2015 with the goal of uniting lifestyle medicine organizations around the world and sharing globally the best practices and educational resources [57]. There are now over 25 lifestyle medicine programs which are found in every continent of the world. The goal is to bring the message of lifestyle medicine as an effective and cost-efficient way for lowering the risk of noncommunicable diseases (NCDs) around the world.

25.13 LIFESTYLE MEDICINE AND PLANETARY HEALTH

Lifestyle medicine plays a central role in the treatment and amelioration of many of the NCDs that the World Health Organization (WHO) has identified in its global NCD initiative [58]. The WHO estimates that NCDs are responsible for over 71% of mortality each year around the world.

In addition, it is important to note that the nutritional practices in lifestyle medicine can play a significant role in planetary health [59]. The last 20 years of research in lifestyle medicine and planetary health have demonstrated that there is no longer any serious debate in the scientific community that global warming is a threat to all humanity.

One important aspect of heart-healthy nutrition in lifestyle medicine is that it can help reduce methane gas. Methane comes from cows and other domestic animal waste. In addition, land use for animal husbandry is very inefficient and costly. Methane is a primary contributor to the formation of ground-level ozone, a hazardous air pollutant and greenhouse gas. It has been estimated that methane causes over 1 million premature deaths every year and that methane is 80 times more potent at global warming than carbon dioxide. More than half of U.S. grain and nearly 40% of world grains are fed to livestock rather than being consumed directly by humans. It takes about 10 times as much energy to generate a meat-based diet as does a plant-based diet. Many people are unaware that animal agribusiness generates more global warming due to greenhouse gases than all forms of transportation combined. This provides another compelling reason to consume a plant-based diet.

25.14 CONCLUSIONS

While this book focuses almost entirely on nutrition, it is important to place nutrition in the context of other lifestyle modalities, all of which can act synergistically to lower the risk of chronic disease and improve both short- and long-term life and quality of life. Included in these modalities are regular physical activity, weight management, avoidance of tobacco and alcohol, healthy sleep, stress reduction, and positive lifestyle/altruism and social connections. Placing nutrition in the context of an overall positive approach to lifestyle measures can contribute to optimal health. This is an area where clinicians can play a very important role.

Clinical Applications

- Nutrition acts synergistically with other lifestyle modalities including physical activity, weight management, avoidance of tobacco and alcohol, healthy sleep, stress reduction, positive lifestyle/altruism, and social connections.
- Clinicians should assess all of these issues when dealing with patients and recommend a variety of other lifestyle measures in addition to healthy nutrition.
- Healthy nutrition can also help ameliorate greenhouse gases and global warming.

REFERENCES

1. Rippe JM. Lifestyle strategies for risk reduction, prevention and treatment of cardiovascular disease. Am J Lifestyle Med. 2018;13(2).
2. Lloyd-Jones DM, Hong Y, Labarthe D, et al. Defining and setting national goals for cardiovascular health promotion and disease reduction: The American Heart Association's strategic impact goal through 2020 and beyond. Circulation. 2010;121:586–613.
3. Goff C, Lloyd-Jones D, Bennett G, et al. 2013 ACC/AHA guideline on the assessment of cardiovascular risk. A report of the American College of Cardiology/American Heart Association Task Force on Practice Guidelines. Circulation. 2014;129:S49–S73.
4. Whelton PK, Carey RM, Aronow WS, et al. 2017 ACC/AHA/ABC/ACPM/AGS/APHA/ASH/ASPC/NMA/PCNA guideline for the prevention, detection, evaluation, and management of high blood pressure in adults: A report of the American College of Cardiology/American Heart Association Task Force on Clinical Practice Guidelines. Hypertension. 2018;71(6).
5. US Department of Health and Human Service National Heart, Lung and Blood Institute. National Institutes of Health. Third report of the expert panel on detection, evaluation, and treatment of high blood cholesterol in adults (adult treatment panel III), Washington, DC, 2004. Circulation. 2002;106(25):3143–3421.
6. Colberg SR, Sigal RJ, Yardley JE, Riddell MC, Dunstan DW, Dempsey PC, et al. Physical activity/exercise and diabetes: A position statement of the American Diabetes Association. Diabetes Care. 2016;39(11):2065–2079.
7. Garber AJ, Handelsman Y, Grunberger G, et al. Consensus statement by the American Association of Clinical Endocrinologists and American College of Endocrinology on the comprehensive type 2 diabetes management algorithm: 2020 executive summary. Endocr Pract. 2020;26(1):107–139.
8. American Dietetic Association. General Practice Guidelines. https://professional.diabetes.org/content-page/practice-guidelines-resources (Accessed October 23, 2023).
9. Powers MA, Bardsley J, Cypress M, et al. Diabetes self-management education and support in type 2 diabetes: A joint position statement of the American Diabetes Association, the American Association of Diabetes Educators, and the Academy of Nutrition and Dietetics. J Acad Nutr Diet. 2015;115(8):1323–1334.

10. The Diabetes Prevention Program (DPP) Research Group; The Diabetes Prevention Program (DPP): Description of lifestyle intervention. Diabetes Care. 2002 Dec 1;25(12):2165–2171.
11. Berger SE, Huggins GS, McCaffery JM, Lichtenstein AH. Comparison among criteria to define successful weight-loss maintainers and regainers in the Action for Health in Diabetes (Look AHEAD) and Diabetes Prevention Program trials. Am J Clin Nutr. 2017;106(6):1337–1346.
12. Jakicic J, Rogers R, Collins K. Exercise management of the obese patient. In Rippe JM (ed). Lifestyle Medicine, 3rd edition. Boca Raton: CRC Press, 2019.
13. Shai I, Schwarzfuchs D, Henkin Y, et al. Weight loss with a low-carbohydrate, Mediterranean, or low-fat diet. NEJM. 2008;359:229–241.
14. Global Burden of Disease Cancer Collaboration. Global, regional, and national cancer incidence, mortality, years of life lost, years lived with disability, and disability-adjusted life-years for 29 cancer groups, 1990 to 2017: A systematic analysis for the global burden of disease study. JAMA Oncol. 2019;5(12):1749–1768.
15. Lauby-Secretan B, Scoccianti C, et al. Body fatness and cancer—viewpoint of the IARC Working Group. N Engl J Med. 2016;375(8):794–798.
16. Al-Amri A. Prevention of breast cancer. J Fam Community Med. 2005;12(2):71–74.
17. World Cancer Research Fund International. Cancer Preventability Estimates for Diet, Nutrition, Body Fatness, and Physical Activity. www.wcrf.org/dietandcancer/recommendations (Accessed July 1, 2018).
18. Rock C, Doyle C, Demark-Wanefried W, et al. Nutrition and physical activity guidelines for cancer survivors. CA Cancer J Clin. 2012;62(4):243–274.
19. Berger N. Obesity and cancer pathogenesis. Ann NY Acad Sci. 2014;1311:57–76.
20. Brown J, Winters-Stone K, Lee A. Cancer, physical activity, and exercise. Compr Physiol. 2012;2(4):2775–2809.
21. U.S. Department of Health and Human Services. *Dietary Guidelines for Americans, 2020–2025*, 9th edition. December 2020. DietaryGuidelines.gov (Accessed October 17, 2023).
22. Lichtenstein AH, Appel LJ, Vadiveloo M, et al, on behalf of the American Heart Association Council on Lifestyle and Cardiometabolic Health; Council on Arteriosclerosis, Thrombosis and Vascular Biology; Council on Cardiovascular Radiology and Intervention; Council on Clinical Cardiology; and Stroke Council. 2021 Dietary guidance to improve cardiovascular health: A scientific statement from the American Heart Association. Circulation. 2021;144:e472–e487.
23. Rippe JM. Lifestyle Medicine, 1st edition. Blackwell Science, 1999.
24. American Heart Association. www.heart.org/ (Accessed October 17, 2023).
25. American College of Lifestyle Medicine. https://lifestylemedicine.org/ (Accessed October 17, 2023).
26. American Journal of Lifestyle Medicine. https://journals.sagepub.com/home/ajl (Accessed March 30, 2024).
27. Gorelick PB, Furie KL, Iadecola C, et al. Defining optimal brain health in adults: A presidential advisory from the American Heart Association/American Stroke Association. Stroke. 2017;48:e284–e303.
28. Physical Activity Guidelines Advisory Committee. 2018 Physical Activity Guidelines Advisory Committee. 2018 Physical Activity Guidelines Advisory Committee Scientific Report. Washington, DC: U.S. Department of Health and Human Services, 2018.
29. Kennedy MA. What physicians need to know, do and say to promote physical activity. In Rippe JM (ed). Lifestyle Medicine, 3rd edition. Boca Raton: CRC Press, 2019.
30. Exercise is Medicine. www.exerciseismedicine.org/ (Accessed March 30, 2024).

31. Clark AM, Raine K, Raphael D. The American Cancer Society, American Diabetes Association, and American Heart Association joint statement on preventing cancer, cardiovascular disease, and diabetes: Where are the social determinants? Diabetes Care. 2004;27(12):3024. Epub 2004/11/25.
32. Chapman S, Robertson I, Zientz J, et al. The neuroscience of brain health. In Rippe JM (ed). Lifestyle Medicine, 4th edition. Boca Raton: CRC Press, 2024.
33. Archer E, Pavela G, Lavie CJ. The inadmissibility of what we eat in America and NHANES dietary data in nutrition and obesity research and the scientific formulation of national dietary guidelines. Mayo Clin Proc. 2015;90(7):911–926.
34. National Center for Health Statistics. National Health and Nutrition Examination Survey (NHANES). www.cdc.gov/nchs/data/factsheets/factsheet_nhanes.htm (Accessed October 17, 2023).
35. Obarzanek E, Sacks FM, Vollmer WM, et al. Effects on blood lipids of a blood pressure-lowering diet: The Dietary Approaches to Stop Hypertension (DASH) trial. Am J Clin Nutr. 2001;74(1):80–89.
36. Konstantinidou V, Ruiz LAD, Ordovás JM. Personalized nutrition and cardiovascular disease prevention: From Framingham to PREDIMED. Adv Nutr Int Rev J. 2014;5(3):368S–371S.
37. McGovern JP. As White House conference approaches, now is the time for a national plan to address the link between hunger, nutrition education, and health. Am J Clin Nutr. 2022;116:841–842.
38. Devries S, Agatston A, Aggarwal M, et al. A deficiency of nutrition education and practice in cardiology. Am J Med. 2017;130(11):1298–1305.
39. Aggarwal M, Devries S, Freeman AM, et al. The deficit of nutrition education of physicians. Am J Med. 2018;131(4):339–345.
40. Rippe J, Foreyt JP. COVID-19 and obesity: A pandemic wrapped in an epidemic. Am J Lifestyle Med. 2021;15(4):364–365.
41. US Centers for Disease Control and Prevention. The Health Consequences of Smoking: 50 Years of Progress: A Report of the Surgeon General. Atlanta, VA 2014.
42. Creamer MR, Wang TW, Babb S, Cullen KA, Day H, Willis G, et al. Tobacco product use and cessation indicators among adults—United States, 2018. MMWR Morb Mortal Wkly Rep. 2019;68(45):1013–1019.
43. Jha P, Ramasundarahettige C, Landsman V, et al. 21st-century hazards of smoking and benefits of cessation in the United States. N Engl J Med. 2013;368(4):341–350.
44. Marmoy M, Brunner E. Alcohol and cardiovascular disease: The status of the U-shaped curve. BMJ. 1991;303:565–568.
45. Ronksley P, Brien S, Turner B, et al. Association of alcohol consumption with selected cardiovascular disease outcomes: A systematic review and meta-analysis. BMJ. 2011;342:d671.
46. Mukamal K, Maclure M, Muller J, et al. Binge drinking and mortality after acute myocardial infarction. Circulation. 2005;112:3839–3845.
47. Costanzo S, di Castelnuovo A, Donati MB, et al. Cardiovascular and overall mortality risk in relation to alcohol consumption in patients with cardiovascular disease. Circulation. 2010;4:1951–1959.
48. Corrao G, Bagnardi V, Zambon A, et al. A meta-analysis of alcohol consumption and the risk of 15 diseases. Prev Med. 2004;38:613–619.
49. Consensus Conference Panel, Watson NF, Badr MS, et al. Joint consensus statement of the American academy of sleep medicine and sleep research society on the recommended amount of sleep for a healthy adult: Methodology and discussion. Sleep. 2015;38(8):1161–1183. Epub 2015/07/22.

50. Institute of Medicine, Committee on Sleep Medicine and Research, Board of Health Sciences Policy. Sleep Disorders and Sleep Deprivation: An Unmet Public Health Problem. Washington, DC: National Academic Press, 2006.
51. Steptoe A, Kivimaki M. Stress and cardiovascular disease: An update on current knowledge. Annu Rev Public Health. 2013;34:337–354.
52. Lichtman JH, Froelicher ES, Blumenthal JA, et al. Depression as a risk factor for poor prognosis among patients with acute coronary syndrome: Systematic review and recommendations: A scientific statement from the American Heart Association. Circulation. 2014;129(12):1350–1369.
53. Waldinger R, Schulz M. The Good Life: Lessons from the World's Longest Scientific Study of Happiness. New York: Simon & Schuster, 2023.
54. Rippe JM. Lifestyle Medicine, 3rd edition. Boca Raton: CRC Press, 2019.
55. Rippe JM. Lifestyle Medicine, 4th edition. Boca Raton: CRC Press, 2024.
56. Choudhry NK, Kronish IM, Vongpatanasin W, et al. Medication adherence and blood pressure control: A scientific statement from the American Heart Association. Hypertension. 2022;79(1):e1–e14.
57. Lifestyle Medicine Global Alliance. https://lifestylemedicineglobal.org/ (Accessed March 30, 2024).
58. World Health Organization Global Noncommunicable Diseases Compact 2020–2030. www.who.int/initiatives/global-noncommunicable-diseases-compact-2020-2030#:~:text=It%20is%20a%20high-profile%20flagship%20initiative%20of%20the,policies%20on%20the%20prevention%20and%20control%20of%20NCDs. (Accessed March 30, 2024).
59. Willett W, Rockstrom J, Loken B, et al. Food in the anthropocene: The EAT-Lancet commission on healthy diets from sustainable food systems. Lancet. 2019;393(10170):447–492.

26 Healthy Plant-Based Diets
Mediterranean, AHA, DASH, Healthy U.S.-Style Dietary Pattern, Vegetarian, and Vegan

Key Points

- There are profound linkages between diet and health.
- Multiple plant-based diets have been shown to lower the risk of chronic disease. These diets include the DASH diet, the Mediterranean diet, the Healthy U.S.-Style Dietary Pattern, the Nordic diet, and various vegetarian diets.
- Not all plant-based diets are created equal. Recent research has delineated "healthy" dietary plant-based patterns as distinguished from "unhealthy" plant-based dietary patterns.
- There are profound linkages between healthy plant-based diets for individuals and populations and overall planetary health.

26.1 INTRODUCTION

Multiple different organizations including the American Heart Association (AHA) [1], *Dietary Guidelines for Americans 2020–2025* (DGA 2020–2025) [2], the World Health Organization (WHO) [3], American Diabetes Association (ADA) [4], and many others have all recommended healthy dietary patterns which are very consistent with each other.

All of these recommendations provide guidance that is summarized in the following statement from the DGA 2020–2025:

> Within the body of evidence, higher intake of vegetables and fruits consistently have been identified as characteristics of healthy eating patterns; whole grains have been identified as well, although with slightly less consistency. Other characteristics of healthy eating patterns have been identified with less consistency including fat free and low fat dairy, seafood, legumes and nuts, lowering intakes of meats including processed meats, sugar sweetened foods, particularly beverages, and refined grains have been identified as characteristics of healthy eating patterns.

Multiple dietary patterns fit within the framework of healthy eating patterns including the Healthy U.S.-Style Dietary Pattern [2], as well as the Dietary Approach

DOI: 10.1201/9781003452607-26

to Systolic Hypertension (DASH) [5], Mediterranean [6], Nordic [7], vegetarian, and vegan diets. These will be discussed individually in this chapter, along with other healthy eating patterns. In addition to enhancing individual health and lowering the risk of various chronic diseases, healthy dietary patterns also interact in very favorable ways with planetary health [8–11]. Recent evidence has also suggested that not all plant-based eating patterns are the same. In fact, some research has categorized some plant-based eating patterns as "healthy" plant-based patterns versus "unhealthy" plant-based patterns [12].

26.2 WHAT IS A PLANT-BASED DIET?

Plant-based diets consist of a diverse family of dietary patterns [10]. They are fundamentally defined in terms of low frequency of consumption of animal foods. For example, vegetarian diets are a subset of plant-based diets that exclude intake of some or all animal foods entirely. Vegan diets exclude consumption of all animal products. Lacto-vegetarians consume dairy products but no other animal foods, and lacto-ovo vegetarians consume eggs and dairy products, while excluding other animal foods. Pesco-vegetarians or pescatarians consume fish in addition to eggs and dairy but exclude poultry and red meat from their diet. Some studies have also examined semi-vegetarian diets, such as flexitarian diets, which are sometimes defined as excluding just red meat, while other plant-based diets emphasize infrequent intake of poultry and red meat.

Instead of defining plant-based diets as the complete exclusion of some or all animal foods, as found in vegetarianism, recent research has focused on gradations of adherence to predominantly plant-based diets. An early attempt to do this was defined by Martinez-Gonzales et al. in what was called a "Pro Vegetarian Diet Score," which positively weighed plant foods and negatively weighed animal foods. These researchers conceptualized this as a progressive approach to vegetarianism, which incorporated progressively increased portions of plant-derived foods and concomitant reduction in animal-derived foods. This definition is more widely applicable to recommendations of moderate dietary changes, which may make it easier to adopt and adhere to than the more extreme recommendations such as complete exclusion of animal foods.

Multiple healthy plant-based diets fit into this broader definition, which will be discussed in this chapter including the Healthy U.S.-Style Dietary Pattern, DASH diet, Mediterranean diet, Nordic diet, and others. This broader definition has also given rise to research that has distinguished between "healthy" plant-based diets and "unhealthy" plant-based diets. While both of these are plant-based, one pattern has been clearly shown in research to lower the risk of cardiometabolic disease, while the other has not. It is this broader definition of "healthy" plant-based diets that will be largely followed in this chapter.

26.3 HEALTHY PLANT-BASED DIETS

A variety of plant-based diets will fit within the category of "healthy" plant-based diets:

- **The Healthy U.S.-Style Dietary Pattern** [2]—As in all the healthy dietary patterns, the Healthy U.S.-Style Dietary Pattern focuses on nutrient-dense foods and beverages including abundant fruits and vegetables, whole grains, low-fat dairy, nuts, seeds, and soy products as well as seafood. It allows red meats to be consumed in small quantities and also poultry and eggs as part of the protein food category. The Healthy U.S.-Style Dietary Pattern is found on Figure 26.1.

- **The Dietary Approaches to Stop Hypertension (DASH) Diet**—This diet contains 60% carbohydrates, protein at 15–20%, and fat at 20–30% [5]. This diet also emphasizes eating considerable amounts of fresh fruits and vegetables, low-fat dairy products, whole grains, fish, poultry, beans, seeds, and nuts and limits the consumption of red meat, sugar-containing drinks, and sodium. It is balanced in nutrients and high in fiber and low in saturated fats. This diet provides potassium, magnesium, and calcium at levels close to the 75th percentile for U.S. consumption. It allows sodium content at approximately the average consumed in the diet of 3,000 milligrams per day. In the initial trials in individuals with hypertension (systolic blood pressure ≥140 mm/Hg and diastolic pressure >90 mm/Hg or

CALORIE LEVEL OF PATTERN[a]	1,600	1,800	2,000	2,200	2,400	2,600	2,800	3,000
FOOD GROUP OR SUBGROUP[b]	Daily Amount of Food From Each Group (Vegetable and protein foods subgroup amounts are per week.)							
Vegetables (cup eq/day)	2	2 ½	2 ½	3	3	3 ½	3 ½	4
	Vegetable Subgroups in Weekly Amounts							
Dark-Green Vegetables (cup eq/wk)	1 ½	1 ½	1 ½	2	2	2 ½	2 ½	2 ½
Red & Orange Vegetables (cup eq/wk)	4	5 ½	5 ½	6	6	7	7	7 ½
Beans, Peas, Lentils (cup eq/wk)	1	1 ½	1 ½	2	2	2 ½	2 ½	3
Starchy Vegetables (cup eq/wk)	4	5	5	6	6	7	7	8
Other Vegetables (cup eq/wk)	3 ½	4	4	5	5	5 ½	5 ½	7
Fruits (cup eq/day)	1 ½	1 ½	2	2	2	2	2 ½	2 ½
Grains (ounce eq/day)	5	6	6	7	8	9	10	10
Whole Grains (ounce eq/day)	3	3	3	3 ½	4	4 ½	5	5
Refined Grains (ounce eq/day)	2	3	3	3 ½	4	4 ½	5	5
Dairy (cup eq/day)	3	3	3	3	3	3	3	3
Protein Foods (ounce eq/day)	5	5	5 ½	6	6 ½	6 ½	7	7
	Protein Foods Subgroups in Weekly Amounts							
Meats, Poultry, Eggs (ounce eq/wk)	23	23	26	28	31	31	33	33
Seafood (ounce eq/wk)	8	8	8	9	10	10	10	10
Nuts, Seeds, Soy Products (ounce eq/wk)	4	4	5	5	5	5	6	6
Oils (grams/day)	22	24	27	29	31	34	36	44
Limit on Calories for Other Uses (kcal/day)[c]	100	140	240	250	320	350	370	440
Limit on Calories for Other Uses (%/day)	6%	8%	12%	11%	13%	13%	13%	15%

FIGURE 26.1 Healthy U.S.-Style Dietary Pattern for adults ages 19–59, with daily or weekly amounts from food groups, subgroups, and components.

Source: U.S. Department of Agriculture and U.S. Department of Health and Human Services. U.S. Department of Agriculture and U.S. Department of Health and Human Services. *Dietary Guidelines for Americans, 2020–2025*. 9th Edition. December 2020. Available at DietaryGuidelines.gov.

both), this diet showed a reduction in systolic and diastolic blood pressure of 11.4 and 5.55 mm/Hg, respectively. A subsequent trial further reduced the sodium to 1,500 milligrams per day and resulted in further reductions in blood pressure in individuals with hypertension. Unfortunately, it is estimated that only 20% of individuals with high blood pressure follow the DASH diet.

- **Mediterranean Diet**—The Mediterranean diet (MedDiet) contains 35–40% carbohydrates, 12–20% protein, and fat at the level of 35–50% [6]. The Mediterranean diet emphasizes eating plant-based foods such as fruits, vegetables, whole grains, legumes, nuts, olives, and nontropical vegetable oils. It is high in dietary fat mainly because of the monounsaturated fats in olive oil and also allows moderate fish and poultry consumption and is low in red meats. A subsequent trial of the Mediterranean diet further enhanced the amount of either olive oil or nuts in the intervention arm, the PREDIMED (PREevención con DIeta MEDiterránea) Trial [6]. This trial increased the amount of olive oil to ≥4 tablespoons per day in one arm of the study. In another arm of the study increased amounts of nuts were recommended, consumption was one daily serving of 30 grams per day composed of 15 grams of walnuts, 7.5 grams of almonds, and 7.5 grams of hazelnuts. This diet allows wine ≥7 glasses per week in habitual wine drinkers. It discourages sugar-sweetened beverages, commercial bakery goods, breads, fats, and red meat and processed foods. The PREDIMED study showed a 30% reduction in cardiovascular risk in the arm that contained extra-virgin olive oil and 28% reduction in risk in the arm that contained added nuts.
- **The Nordic Diet**—The Nordic diet contains 45–60% carbohydrates, protein 10–20%, and fat 15–40% [7]. The Nordic Diet emphasizes whole, local, seasonal products and contains considerable fruits and vegetables, fish, and other lean proteins as well as whole grains, nuts, seeds, rye breads, fish, seafood, low-fat dairy, herbs, spices, and grape seed (canola) oil and moderate game meats as well as free range eggs, cheese, and yogurt and is low in other red meats and animal fats, added sugars and processed meats, food additives, and refined fast foods. The Nordic diet pattern is somewhat comparable to the Mediterranean diet since it emphasizes traditional, locally grown, and seasonal foods. However, in the case of the Nordic countries, it was developed to address concerns about obesity, taking into account local food culture, environmental aspects, and sustainability. The Nordic Diet is also based on utilizing locally grown foods to minimize the transport of food stuffs, which minimizes the negative impact of transportation on the environment. Local foods also enhance biodiversity. Food sourced from the wild countryside minimizes the use of fertilizers and pesticides. Since Nordic countries are surrounded by water, the Nordic diet also emphasizes high-quality fish and shellfish. Wild fish are recommended over farm-fed fish because of improved nutritional characteristics.
- **The Vegetarian Diet**—The macronutrient composition of the typical vegetarian diet includes carbohydrates at 51–55%, protein at 12–14%, and fat 30–33% [13]. The typical vegetarian diet consists of grains, vegetables,

fruits, sugars, oils, eggs (ovo-vegetarian), and dairy (lacto-vegetarian) and generally not more than one serving per month of meat or seafood. Meat-based protein sources are replaced by a mix of plant-based proteins (legumes, fruits, and vegetables).

- **Pescatarian Diet**—The macronutrient composition of the pescatarian diet is carbohydrates 50–53%, protein at 14%, and fat at 15–33%. The pescatarian diet is similar to the lacto-ovo-vegetarian diet with the addition of fish and seafood. Wheat-based protein sources are replaced by a mix of seafood, fruits, and vegetables.
- **The Flexitarian Diet**—The macronutrient composition of the flexitarian diet is carbohydrates 52%, protein at 13%, and fat at 35% [14]. This diet is similar to the pescatarian diet. It emphasizes eating plant-based foods such as fruits, vegetables, legumes, and whole grains but allows meat or other animal products (poultry, fish, and dairy) in moderation. It limits sugars, sweets, and processed foods in general. It is designed to give people a way to move forward in a more comfortable approach to more vegetarian eating.
- **Vegan Diet**—The macronutrient composition of the vegan diet is carbohydrates 55–58%, protein at 12–14%, and fat at 28–30%. The vegan diet replaces all animal-based protein sources with a mix of plant-based proteins (legumes, fruits, and vegetables) and excludes eggs and dairy products.

26.4 HEALTHY VERSUS UNHEALTHY PLANT-BASED DIETS

Recent research has focused on the issue of specific components of plant-based diets and whether or not they lower the risk of various chronic diseases. Studies of plant-based diets define these as basically "vegetarian" diets that exclude some or all animal foods. In previous research on these diets, all plant foods were treated equally, even though it is clear that certain plant foods such as refined grains and sugar-sweetened beverages are associated with increased cardiometabolic risks.

To overcome these limitations, researchers used the nutrition information available through the Nurses' Health Study and Male Health Professionals Study which gave them a total of over 125,000 individuals [15]. The researchers divided plant food groups into "healthy" food groups and "less healthy" food groups. Healthy food groups were given positive scores, and less healthy food groups were given reverse scores.

The healthy food groups category contained the following food groups: Whole grains, fruits, vegetables, nuts, legumes, vegetable oils, tea, and coffee. The less healthy plant-based diet food groups included fruit juices, refined grains, potatoes, sugar-sweetened beverages, sweets, and desserts. Both the "healthy" and "unhealthy" plant-based diet excluded animal products, dairy, eggs, fish or seafood, meat, and various animal-based foods such as pizza, chowder, or creamed soup.

By following these distinctions, it was shown that the "healthy" plant-based diet showed significant reduction in the risk of coronary heart disease (CHD), whereas the "unhealthy" plant-based diet was associated with higher CHD risk. A number of studies have now confirmed that within the spectrum of plant-based diets there are diets that are "healthy" and "less healthy."

26.5 EFFECTS OF HEALTHY PLANT-BASED DIETS ON CHRONIC DISEASE RISK

- **Cardiovascular Disease**—Convincing evidence supports the intake of healthy nutritional patterns to lower the risk of cardiovascular disease. In particular, positive, healthy plant-based diets are central to treating dyslipidemia and also play a significant role in lowering the risk of high blood pressure as well as helping to control weight. All of the benefits of healthy plant-based diets have been shown in multiple studies. Perhaps most prominent are the Healthy American Heart Association Diets, the DGA 2020–2025 Healthy U.S.-Style Dietary Pattern, the MedDiet, and the DASH diet, all of which have been shown to lower the risk of cardiovascular disease.
- **Type 2 Diabetes**—Healthy plant-based diets have been demonstrated to reduce the risk of type 2 diabetes mellitus (T2DM) [16]. In particular, the foods contained in the healthy plant-based diets have been shown to substantially lower the risk of T2DM. In contrast, the unhealthy plant-based diet did not lower the risk of T2DM. In fact, it actually slightly raised it.
- **Obesity and Weight Gain**—Healthy plant-based diets have been demonstrated to decrease adult weight gain both in men and women and, in particular, overweight individuals [17,18]. Healthy plant-based diets also are associated with decreased risk of obesity, although these data should be treated with some caution, since people who followed healthy plant-based diets are also likely to follow other health-promoting behaviors such as increased physical activity, which may impact on the likelihood of developing obesity.
- **Cancer**—Prospective cohort studies have examined mortality and overall cancer incidence among vegetarians [19]. A recent meta-analysis and systematic review of seven cohort studies totaling 124,706 participants demonstrated that vegetarians have an overall 18% reduction in risk of cancer compared to nonvegetarians. Since many of the risk factors for cancer are similar to those for heart disease, it is reasonable to speculate that plant-based healthy nutritional patterns also are likely to lower the risk of cancer.
- **Chronic Kidney Disease (CKD)**—An analysis conducted on 14,686 middle-aged adults in the Atherosclerosis Risk in Communities Study (ARIC) showed that diets that were consistent with the healthy plant-based diet index significantly reduced the risk of CKD and also were associated with decrease in decline of glomerular filtration rate [20].
- **Brain Health**—The effects of healthy plant-based eating patterns on the brain are still a matter of debate [21]. A recent systematic review showed that the healthy plant-based diets lowered the risk of obesity and systemic inflammation in healthy participants. However, they did not demonstrate a positive impact on cognitive functions, mental, or neurologic health. Thus, this issue remains in debate and will require further studies to address these issues.
- **All-Cause Mortality**—Data from over 12,000 individuals in the ARIC study showed that diets higher in plant foods and lower in animal foods were associated with both the lower risk of cardiovascular and morbidity and mortality as well as all-cause mortality.

26.6 HEALTHY DIETS AND PLANETARY HEALTH AND SUSTAINABILITY

Personal and population health and planetary health are closely interrelated, which makes them vulnerable to similar issues [9–12]. On a personal health level, chronic diseases are increasingly driven by poor dietary quality and overconsumption of calories. The global food production system is also draining the planet's resources and jeopardizing the environment and future food security. The typical Western diet, which contains high amounts of animal products, is not only associated with chronic disease but also with adverse planetary impacts. For example, in one study that examined actual diets and evaluated their relationship to greenhouse gas (GHG) emission, GHG emissions were twice as high in meat eaters as compared to vegans.

The environmental impact of the Western diet has threatened the sustainability of food production on the planet. For example, food production systems affect a variety of natural resources. The global food production system is responsible for over 70% of freshwater usage and 30% of human-generated GHG emissions as well as 80% of deforestation [11].

Food production is also the largest contributor to loss of biodiversity. In addition, large phosphorous flows from agricultural fields have led to an increased degradation of fresh water and hypoxic zones in both fresh water and salt water. These issues are becoming increasingly common both in chronic disease research and also in research related to planetary warming.

There is increasing understanding that aligning food patterns that are healthy and nutritionally sound will not only support human health but are more environmentally sustainable. For example, the Food and Agriculture Organization (FAO) of the United Nations has identified the MedDiet as an example one of the most sustainable diets because of its smaller portions and emphasis on plant-based dietary diversity. The EAT-Lancet Commission on Healthy Diets and Sustainable Food Systems [11] concluded that unhealthy and unsustainably produced foods pose a global risk for people on the planet, with more than 820 million people currently having insufficient food and many more consuming an unhealthy diet, which contributes to death and morbidity.

Global food production represents the largest pressure caused by humans on the Earth and threatens local ecosystems and stability of the Earth. The EAT-Lancet Commission further concluded that current dietary trends, combined with projected population growth to about 10 billion in the year 2050, will exacerbate risks to people in the planet. Furthermore, the goal burden of noncommunicable diseases will worsen the effects of food production on GHG emissions, nitrogen, and phosphorous pollution. Biodiversity loss and water and land use will reduce the stability of the Earth's systems. Transformation to healthy diets from sustainable food systems is also essential to achieve the UN Sustainable Development Goals.

The EAT-Lancet Commission concluded that scientific targets for healthy diets and sustainable food production are urgently required. Transformation into healthy diets will require significant changes, including a 50% reduction in global consumption of unhealthy foods such as red meat and sugar and a greater than 100% increase in the consumption of healthy foods such as nuts, fruits, vegetables, and legumes.

26.7 EVIDENCE-BASED GUIDANCE ON DIETARY PATTERNS TO PROMOTE CARDIOMETABOLIC HEALTH

The AHA, in their 2021 Dietary Guidance to Improve Cardiovascular Health, listed evidence supporting dietary patterns to promote cardiometabolic health. This guidance listed a total of ten different recommendations [1]. These include the following:

- Adjust energy intake and expenditure to achieve and maintain a healthy body weight.
- Eat plenty of fruits and vegetables.
- Choose foods mostly made with whole grains rather than refined grains.
- Choose healthy sources of protein (this includes choosing mostly protein from plants such as legumes and nuts).
- Use liquid plant oils rather than tropical oils.
- Choose minimally processed foods instead of ultra-processed foods.
- Minimize intake of foods and beverages with added sugar.
- Choose and prepare foods with little or no salt.
- If you do not drink alcohol, do not start. If you choose to drink alcohol, limit intake.
- Adhere to these premises regardless of wherever food is prepared or consumed.

26.8 ROLE OF SPECIFIC COMPONENTS OF THE HEALTHY DIETARY PATTERNS TO LOWER THE RISK OF CVD

Fat quality is an important component of heart-healthy diets, and the AHA emphasizes either polyunsaturated fats or monosaturated fats as opposed to saturated fats to help lower low-density lipoprotein cholesterol (LDL-C) [22]. In addition, healthy plant-based diets contain abundant dietary fibers, which have been associated in multiple studies to lower risk of CVD, T2DM, obesity, and certain forms of cancer. Currently in the United States, both men and women consume less than half of the recommended amount of fiber in the diet. Healthful plant-based diets are also likely to be low in energy density due to the low saturated fat content and high fiber content, which should help with weight loss and long-term weight maintenance. In addition, plant foods such as whole grains, fruits, vegetables and vegetable oil, nuts, tea, coffee, and cocoa are also rich in polyphenols, which are natural bioactive compounds produced by plants. Numerous individual polyphenols are important for scavenging and neutralizing free radicals and nitrogen species and protecting against oxidative stress.

A healthful plant-based diet is also replete with numerous other antioxidant nutrients such as vitamin C, E, and beta-carotene. The potassium also found in healthy plant-based diets helps reduce blood pressure and lower stroke risk. Magnesium found in healthy plant-based diets also is associated with improved cardiometabolic outcomes because of its effects on glucose metabolism and insulin sensitivity as well as anti-inflammatory and vasodilatory properties.

In contrast, dietary factors that are abundant in animal foods have been associated with increased risk of CVD. For example, heme iron, which is found mainly in animal foods such as red meat, poultry, and seafood, is associated with higher risk of CVD in several prospective studies. Other nutrients in processed meats such as sodium, nitrates, and nitrites may also increase the risk of CVD through raised blood pressure and endothelial dysfunction.

26.9 HEALTHY DIETARY PATTERNS AND EXERCISE PERFORMANCE

While healthy plant-based diets have clearly been demonstrated to lower the risk of chronic disease and contain environmental health benefits, historically animal derived proteins have been viewed as an important component of athletes' diets. This raises the question of whether or not vegetarian or vegan diets will support athletic performance. Recent reviews have suggested that plant-based diets compared to omnivorous diets do not result in any decrease in strength, anaerobic, or aerobic exercise performance [23]. Thus, plant-based diets appear to be a viable option for adequately supporting athletic performance, while contributing to overall lower risk of chronic disease and improving environmental health. There is still not enough evidence to determine whether or not vegetarian or vegan dietary patterns may result in decreased performance at the very highest levels of training or athletic endeavors.

26.10 THE MICROBIOME AND HEALTHY PLANT-BASED DIETS

The gut microbiome is increasingly being studied as a potential pathway through which a healthy plant-based diet may influence cardiovascular risk. While research in this area is in its infancy, the microorganisms that reside in the human gut can potentially influence cardiovascular health through a variety of mechanisms. One example is trimethylamine N-oxide (TMAO) pathways. Compounds derived mainly from animal foods such as red meat, poultry, and seafood are broken down to generate trimethylamine (TMA), which is then further broken down into TMAO in the liver. TMAO has been associated with high-risk cardiovascular events over and above the traditional risk factors [24]. TMAO may adversely affect cardiac health due to its effects in cholesterol and cholesterol metabolism, inflammation, thrombotic, and atherosclerotic pathways.

Plant-based diets differ from animal-based diets with respect to many microbial-dependent metabolic pathways including increased metabolism of fiber and polyphenols and decreased metabolism of bile acids and amino acids, which may help mediate inverse association between plant-based diets and cardiovascular endpoints. Further studies are currently in progress and will be needed to elucidate how the microbiome is impacted by healthy plant-based diets.

26.11 HEALTHY PLANT-BASED DIETS AND HEALTH EQUITY

In the United States, cardiovascular disease (CVD) remains the leading cause of death and disability [25]. Nutrition and dietary quality are responsible for a greater percentage of CVD-related morbidity and mortality than any other modifiable risk factors. Some population groups experience substantial greater burden of CVD than others. For example, CVD disproportionately effects non-Hispanic Blacks and individuals of low socioeconomic status (SES). While these differences are multifactorial, poor dietary scores play a leading role. For example, non-Hispanic Blacks and Hispanics have a greater prevalence of poor dietary scores as measured by the Healthy Eating Index (HEI) than non-Hispanic Whites and non-Hispanic Asians.

A heart-healthy diet is the cornerstone of atherosclerotic CVD prevention and treatment. Thus, incremental improvements in diet quality can have a meaningful cardiovascular benefit. To address these disparities in nutritional risk factors will require great effort because of the reality that food choices are complex. For example, racial segregation is a contributing factor to disparities in CVD risk based both in SES and nutritional factors. An unfavorable nutritional environment disproportionately affects some racial and ethnic groups. The availability, price, and quality of foods available in a neighborhood relative to healthy or less healthy foods directly impact dietary quality. Living in a food desert, as defined by the Centers for Disease Control and Prevention as an area of limited access to affordable fruits, vegetables, and whole grains; low-fat milk; and other foods, may make it difficult to follow a healthy diet. In addition, food access, defined as proximity to supermarkets, also significantly impacts diet quality.

Food deserts disproportionately impact individuals in terms of low income, low educational attainment, and racial/ethnic minorities. In addition, low-income areas and communities have a higher proportion of racial and ethnic minorities and also have a greater density of fast food outlets and convenience stores, which have minimal healthy food offerings. These areas have been described as "food swamps," where nutrient-poor, energy-dense food availability swamps healthy food options.

In addition, there are economic barriers, such as food insecurity, attributable to factors including food pricing and income level. For all of these reasons, it will be essential to adopt aggressive public policy changes to improve dietary quality and healthy dietary patterns in currently underserved populations. Programs such as the Healthy Eating Incentive Pilot Project showed that a 30% incentive for fruit and vegetable purchases could result in increased fruit and vegetable consumption for Supplemental Nutrition Assistance Program (SNAP) participants, which could result in over 300,000 CVD deaths being averted [25]. While there are multiple and complicated issues related to current disparities in healthy eating patterns, all these issues merit urgent action. Multilevel interventions with the dietary components needed to address disparities associated with CVD will be required.

26.12 HEALTHY PLANT-BASED NUTRITION AND OTHER LIFESTYLE MEDICINE MODALITIES

All of the major organizations that recommend a healthy plant-based diet also emphasize the importance of other positive health-related behaviors, including increased physical activity and weight management. Thus, for clinicians it is important to not only emphasize healthy plant-based diets but also to put these patterns in the context of an overall approach to lifestyle habits to lower the risk of chronic disease.

26.13 PRECISION PREVENTION

Recent research has continued to focus on optimizing the role of healthy nutritional patterns to enhance health and lower the risk of chronic disease [26,27]. An important initiative in this area focuses on how differences among individuals in disease risk and biological response to diet make it difficult to answer the question of what is best for each individual to eat. This emphasis involves moving beyond a "one size fits all" dietary prescription for optimal health and disease prevention.

A major effort in this area is entitled "precision nutrition," which aims to understand the health effects of the complex interplay among genetics, the microbiome, antibiotic and probiotic use, metabolism, food environment, and physical activity as well as economic, social, and other behavioral characteristics.

The National Institutes of Health (NIH) is leading this effort in 2020–2030. Its strategic plan has an initial investment of $150 million over six years to further explore the area of precision nutrition [26]. This area intends to harness the power of genotyping, bioinformatics, and artificial intelligence in combination with implementation and behavioral sciences. It is hoped that these strategies will help reduce the socioeconomic, racial, and ethnic disparities in dietary intake and chronic disease outcomes. While this area holds great promise, current focus should remain on public health nutrition strategies as described in this chapter.

26.14 CONCLUSIONS

Multiple healthy dietary patterns have been demonstrated to lower the risk of chronic disease. These include the Healthy U.S.-Style Dietary Pattern, the DASH diet, the Mediterranean diet, the Nordic diet, and various vegetarian diets. All of these diets are consistent in recommending increased intake of fruits and vegetables and whole grains and nontropical plant oils, while decreasing the amounts of red meats, refined grains, sugar, saturated fats, and sodium.

Clinical Applications

- Healthy dietary patterns are consistent in recommending increased fruits and vegetables and whole grains, while minimizing red meat, processed meats, refined grains, sugar-sweetened beverages, and ultra-processed foods.
- Not all plant-based diets are created equal. Recent research has made a distinction between "healthy" plant-based diets and "unhealthy" plant-based diets depending on their specific contributions of various foods within these two different categories.
- Healthy individual dietary patterns are also inextricably linked to overall planetary health.
- Clinicians should be aware of the multiple different healthy dietary patterns so that they can counsel patients on how to achieve improved health by following such plans.
- Currently available healthy dietary plans include the Healthy U.S.-Style Dietary Pattern, the DASH diet, the Mediterranean diet, the Nordic diet, and various vegetarian plans.

REFERENCES

1. Lichtenstein A, Appel L, Vadiveloo M, et al. Dietary guidance to improve cardiovascular health: A scientific statement from the American Heart Association. Circulation. 2021;144(23):e472–e487.
2. U.S. Department of Health and Human Services. *Dietary Guidelines for Americans, 2020–2025*, 9th edition. December 2020. DietaryGuidelines.gov. (Accessed October 17, 2023).
3. World Health Organization. Global Noncommunicable Diseases Compact 2020–2030. www.who.int/initiatives/global-noncommunicable-diseases-compact-2020-2030#:~:text=It%20is%20a%20high-profile%20flagship%20initiative%20of%20the,policies%20on%20the%20prevention%20and%20control%20of%20NCDs. (Accessed October 18, 2023).
4. American Diabetes Association. Professional practice committee for the standards of medical care in diabetes—2015. Diabetes Care. 2014;38(Suppl 1):S88–S89.
5. Obarzanek E, Sacks F, Vollmer W, et al. Effects on blood lipids of a blood pressure-lowering diet: The Dietary Approaches to Stop Hypertension (DASH) trial. Am J Clin Nutr. 2001;74(1):80–89.
6. Konstantinidou V, Ruiz L, Ordovás J. Personalized nutrition and cardiovascular disease prevention: From framingham to PREDIMED. Adv Nutr Int Rev J. 2014;5(3):368S–371S.
7. Mithril C, Dragsted L, Meyer C, et al. Guidelines for the new nordic diet. Public Health Nutr. 2012;15(10):1941–1947.
8. Tilman D, Clark M. Global diets link environmental sustainability and human health. Nature. 2014;515:518–522.
9. Nelson M, Hamm M, Hu F, et al. Alignment of healthy dietary patterns and environmental sustainability: A systematic review. Adv Nutr. 2016;15;7(6):1005–1025.
10. Hemler E, Hu F. Plant-based diets for personal, population, and planetary health. Adv Nutr. 2019;10(Suppl 4):S275–S283.
11. Willett W, Rockström J, Loken B, et al. Food in the anthropocene: The EAT-Lancet Commission on healthy diets from sustainable food systems. Lancet. 2019;2;393(10170):447–492.
12. Satija A, Bhupathiraju S, Spiegelman D, et al. Healthful and unhealthful plant-based diets and the risk of coronary heart disease in U.S. adults. J Am Coll Cardiol. 2017;25;70(4):411–422.
13. Mozaffarian D, Appel L, Van Horn L. Components of a cardioprotective diet: New insights. Circulation. 2011;123(24):2870–2891.
14. The Cleveland Clinic. What Is the Flexitarian Diet? https://health.clevelandclinic.org/what-is-the-flexitarian-diet/ (Accessed October 18, 2023).
15. Satija A, Hu F. Plant-based diets and cardiovascular health. Trends Cardiovasc Med. 2018;28(7):437–441.
16. Toumpanakis A, Turnbull T, Alba-Barba I. Effectiveness of plant-based diets in promoting well-being in the management of type 2 diabetes: A systematic review. BMJ Open Diabetes Res Care. 2018;30;6(1):e000534.
17. Bassuk S, Manson J. Lifestyle and risk of cardiovascular disease and type 2 diabetes in women: A review of the epidemiologic evidence. Am J Life Med. 2008;2:191–213.
18. Fung T, Pan A, Hou T, et al. Long-term change in diet quality is associated with body weight change in men and women. J Nutr. 2015;145(8):1850–1856.
19. Huang T, Yang B, Zheng J, et al. Cardiovascular disease mortality and cancer incidence in vegetarians: A meta-analysis and systematic review. Ann Nutr Metab. 2012;60(4):233–240.

20. Carrero J, González-Ortiz A, Avesani C, et al. Plant-based diets to manage the risks and complications of chronic kidney disease. Nat Rev Nephrol. 2020;16(9):525–542.
21. Medawar E, Huhn S, Villringer A, et al. The effects of plant-based diets on the body and the brain: A systematic review. Transl Psychiatry. 2019;12;9(1):226.
22. Rimm E, Appel L, Chiuve S, et al. American Heart Association Nutrition Committee of the Council on Lifestyle and Cardiometabolic Health; Council on Epidemiology and Prevention; Council on Cardiovascular Disease in the Young; Council on Cardiovascular and Stroke Nursing; and Council on Clinical Cardiology. Seafood long-chain Ω-3 polyunsaturated fatty acids and cardiovascular disease: A science advisory from the American Heart Association. Circulation. 2018;3;138(1):e35–e47.
23. Lynch H, Johnston C, Wharton C. Plant-based diets: Considerations for environmental impact, protein euality, and exercise performance. Nutrients. 2018;10(12):1841.
24. Guasch-Ferré M, Satija A, Blondin S, et al. Meta-analysis of randomized controlled trials of red meat consumption in comparison with various comparison diets on cardiovascular risk factors. Circulation. 2019;9;139(15):1828–1845.
25. Etherton-Kris P, Peterson K, Velarde G. Barriers, opportunities, and challenges in addressing disparities in diet-related cardiovascular disease in the United States. J Am Heart Assoc. 2020;9(7):e014433.
26. National Heart, Lung, and Blood Institute. The Science of Precision Prevention to Reduce Disparities in Cardiovascular Health, December 5–7, 2022. www.nhlbi.nih.gov/events/2022/science-precision-prevention-reduce-disparities-cardiovascular-health
27. Wang D, Hu F. Precision nutrition for prevention and management of type 2 diabetes. Lancet Diabetes Endocrinol. 2018;6(5):416–426.

27 Nutrition for the Elderly

Key Points

- A number of age-related changes occur that may make healthy eating more challenging in the elderly.
- Particular nutrients of concern in the elderly are calcium, vitamin D, protein, potassium, and fiber.
- Malnutrition is common and not diagnosed frequently enough in the elderly. Screening tools are available to help clinicians make the proper diagnosis.

27.1 INTRODUCTION

The population of individuals over the age of 65 is the most rapidly growing of all age groups. It is also one where nutrition plays a particularly important role in lowering the risk or assisting in the treatment of various chronic diseases. This is not to say that nutrition is unimportant for other life stages; however, it becomes critically important in the elderly population, since people over the age of 65 face significant nutritional and health challenges and often are battling chronic illnesses.

In 2015, there were approximately 46 million individuals living in the United States over the age of 65. This number is expected to double to approximately 98 million by the year 2060, at which time it will represent 24% of the total population [1].

Individuals over the age of 65 are expected to work longer and obtain a higher level of education than prior generations. Among the chronic conditions that individuals over the age of 65 are likely to encounter, obesity is perhaps the most prominent. Obesity is associated with other chronic diseases including cardiovascular disease (CVD), type 2 diabetes mellitus (T2DM), metabolic syndrome, and cancer. In addition, the COVID-19 pandemic illustrated that individuals over the age of 65 are particularly vulnerable to infectious diseases.

As the population of individuals over the age of 65 increases, an important need exists for specific nutrition guidance to allow these individuals to achieve and maintain optimal physical health and cognitive function. Numerous research studies have shown that within this population, older adults who score in the higher categories for dietary quality and physical activity measures have the best survival rates [1–4]. This chapter will focus largely on unique nutritional needs over the age of 65, as well as other important issues related to lifestyle such as physical activity, healthy weight maintenance, avoiding tobacco products, moderating alcohol intake, achieving adequate sleep, reducing stress, and maintaining positive relationships. These other lifestyle medicine issues also play very important roles in the health and quality of life in individuals over the age of 65.

DOI: 10.1201/9781003452607-27

27.2 AGING CHANGES RELEVANT TO NUTRITION IN INDIVIDUALS OVER THE AGE OF 65

Numerous changes become manifest particularly in individuals over the age of 65 [1–4]. For example, sensory changes in taste perception, including decreases in salt taste and alterations in sweet and sour tastes, occur, although these changes have not been shown to affect dietary intake. Sense of smell also decreases with age, but again this has not been shown to impact nutrition in individuals over the age of 65. In addition, individuals over the age of 65 consistently demonstrate lower caloric intakes, which means that these individuals must focus even more attention on nutrient-dense foods and healthy nutritional patterns in order to maintain decreased risk of chronic illnesses. Lower intakes may be due to impaired swallowing. Tooth loss or decay may result in decreased masticatory ability, which can also affect food intake [5,6].

Multiple body composition changes occur with aging, most prominently a decrease in lean body mass and increase in body fat. These may also contribute to caloric intake decreases with age. For example, the second National Health and Nutrition Examination Survey (NHANES) showed that men between the ages of 23 and 34 years consume on average 2,700 kcals per day, but this decreases to 1,800 kcals per day at ages 65–74 [7]. Elderly women consume even fewer calories, ranging between 1,300 and 1,600 kcals per day.

Nutrient absorption may also be diminished, including such important vitamins as vitamin B_{12}, because of impaired gastrointestinal absorption.

As has been discussed in multiple chapters in this book, healthy nutritional habits play a critically important role in both reducing the risk of and treating chronic diseases. This is particularly important in individuals over the age of 65 for all of the reasons already outlined and because of the fact that individuals in this age range are more susceptible to chronic illnesses or often already have more chronic illnesses and conditions compared to younger individuals.

27.3 CURRENT RECOMMENDATIONS

The Recommended Dietary Allowance (RDA) for various nutrients is issued by the Food and Nutrition Board of the Institute of Medicine. Starting in the 1990s, it has become more precise for individuals over the age of 50 [8–15]. Current Dietary Reference Intakes (DRIs) are further categorized according to age and include separate categories for individuals aged 51–70 and greater than 70 years [16]. DRIs for most nutrients including vitamin A, vitamin C, vitamin E, vitamin K and a variety of other vitamins do not differ between adults over the age of 65 and over the age of 50.

In contrast, nutrient recommendations for vitamin D, calcium, and vitamin B_6 are higher for older adults [17]. DRIs for vitamin D increase from 600 IU/day for females and males between the ages of 51 and 70 years of age to over 800 IU/day for both males and females over the age of 70 years. DRIs for calcium decrease from 1,210 mg per day for males and females between the ages of 51 and 70 years to 1,200 mg/day for both females and males over the age of 70. DRIs for vitamin B_6 increase from 1.6 mg/day to 1.4 mg/day for females and males, respectively, between 51 and

70 years of age to 1.7 mg/day and 1.5 mg/day for males and females, respectively, over the age of 70 years.

Even though DRIs for most nutrients do not increase with advancing age with the exception of vitamin D, calcium, and vitamin B_6, it may be increasingly difficult for individuals in this age range to achieve the recommended intakes as they advance in years. This is due in part to a decrease in energy needs associated with lower levels of physical activity and loss of mean muscle mass and higher proportion of fat mass resulting in a lower basal metabolic rate [18,19]. Thus, nutrient needs must be met within the context of reduced food intake and low energy requirement. This emphasizes the importance of selecting nutrient-dense foods (high nutrient content per calories).

A graphic that summarizes the key points related to dietary modification for older adults has been developed to provide specific guidance and is termed MyPlate for Older Adults. This graph is found in Figure 27.1. The differences between this graphic and the MyPlate Food Guide for a younger population rests in its emphasis of nutrient-dense foods per age category and illustrations of foods that are particularly convenient for older adults (e.g. bags of frozen vegetables) as well as a greater emphasis on fluids and incorporation of suggestions for regular physical activity as an integral part of the icon. The knife and fork on the side of the plate encourage focusing on enjoying food while eating it [20].

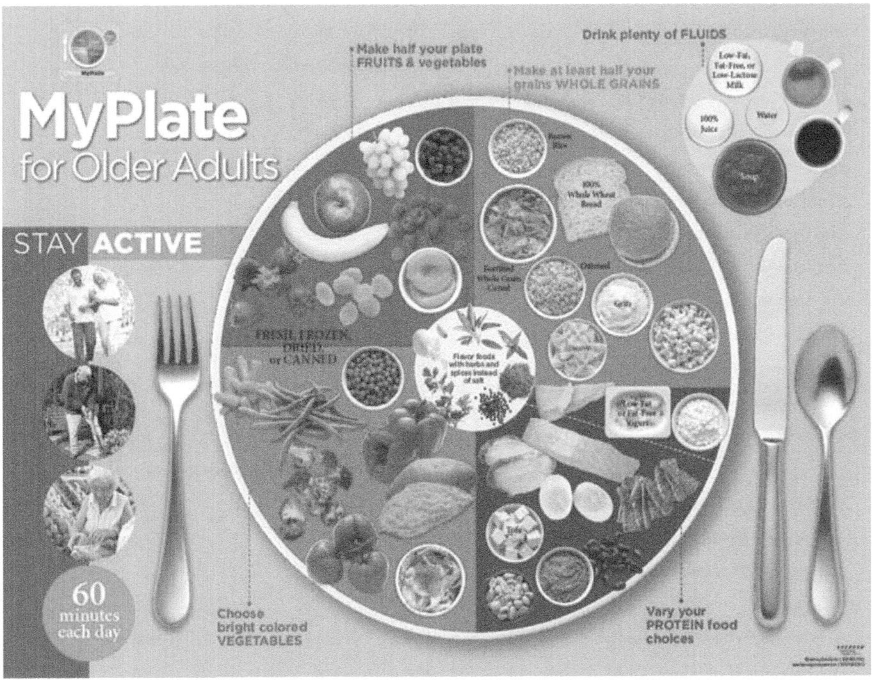
MyPlate
for Older Adults
STAY ACTIVE
60 minutes each day
Make half your plate FRUITS & vegetables
Make at least half your grains WHOLE GRAINS
Drink plenty of FLUIDS
Choose bright colored VEGETABLES
Vary your PROTEIN food choices

FIGURE 27.1 MyPlate for older adults.

Source: USDA. MyPlate. U.S. Department of Agriculture. Based on the *Dietary Guidelines for Americans, 2020–2025.*

27.4 HEALTHY DIETARY PATTERNS

Throughout this book, the emphasis has been based on healthy dietary patterns. This reflects current scientific understandings of nutrition and underscores the fact that foods are eaten in an overall pattern. Thus, it is the overall dietary pattern that should be emphasized.

Older adults are encouraged to follow the recommendations of the types of foods and beverages that make up a healthy dietary pattern, which are described in Chapter 26. These healthy dietary patterns may include the Mediterranean dietary pattern (MedDiet) [21], the Dietary Approaches to Stop Hypertension (DASH) diet [22], multiple diets recommended by the American Heart Association (AHA) [23], and the Healthy U.S.-Style Dietary Pattern developed by the Dietary Guidelines for American (DGAs) 2020–2025 [24]. The nutrient composition of the Healthy U.S.-Style Dietary Pattern for older adults is found in Figure 27.2 [25].

CALORIE LEVEL OF PATTERN[a]	1,600	1,800	2,000	2,200	2,400	2,600
FOOD GROUP OR SUBGROUP[b]	Daily Amount of Food From Each Group (Vegetable and protein foods subgroup amounts are per week.)					
Vegetables (cup eq/day)	**2**	**2 ½**	**2 ½**	**3**	**3**	**3 ½**
	Vegetable Subgroups in Weekly Amounts					
Dark-Green Vegetables (cup eq/wk)	1 ½	1 ½	1 ½	2	2	2 ½
Red & Orange Vegetables (cup eq/wk)	4	5 ½	5 ½	6	6	7
Beans, Peas, Lentils (cup eq/wk)	1	1 ½	1 ½	2	2	2 ½
Starchy Vegetables (cup eq/wk)	4	5	5	6	6	7
Other Vegetables (cup eq/wk)	3 ½	4	4	5	5	5 ½
Fruits (cup eq/day)	**1 ½**	**1 ½**	**2**	**2**	**2**	**2**
Grains (ounce eq/day)	**5**	**6**	**6**	**7**	**8**	**9**
Whole Grains (ounce eq/day)	3	3	3	3 ½	4	4 ½
Refined Grains (ounce eq/day)	2	3	3	3 ½	4	4 ½
Dairy (cup eq/day)	**3**	**3**	**3**	**3**	**3**	**3**
Protein Foods (ounce eq/day)	**5**	**5**	**5 ½**	**6**	**6 ½**	**6 ½**
	Protein Foods Subgroups in Weekly Amounts					
Meats, Poultry, Eggs (ounce eq/wk)	23	23	26	28	31	31
Seafood (ounce eq/wk)	8	8	9	9	10	10
Nuts, Seeds, Soy Products (ounce eq/wk)	4	4	5	5	5	5
Oils (grams/day)	**22**	**24**	**27**	**29**	**31**	**34**
Limit on Calories for Other Uses (kcal/day)[c]	**100**	**140**	**240**	**250**	**320**	**350**
Limit on Calories for Other Uses (%/day)	7%	8%	12%	12%	13%	5

FIGURE 27.2 Healthy U.S.-Style Dietary Pattern for Adults Ages 60 and Older, with Daily or Weekly Amounts from Food Groups, Subgroups, and Components. https://www.dietaryguidelines.gov/sites/default/files/2021-03/Dietary_Guidelines_for_Americans-2020-2025.pdf

As already indicated, calorie needs are generally lower for females compared to males, particularly those who are older, smaller, and less physically active. Females aged 60 and older require about 1,600–2,200 calories per day and males 60 and older approximately 2,000–2,600 calories per day. The Healthy U.S.-Style Dietary Pattern provides a flexible framework for older adults to follow a healthy dietary pattern and also meets the guidelines' key recommendations. The flexibility allows a variety of food and beverage choices so individuals can customize their choices in each food group based on lifestyle, traditions, culture, and other individual needs.

27.5 CURRENT INTAKES AND HEALTHY EATING INDEX SCORE

The average Healthy Eating Index score (on a scale of 0–100) for people over the age of 60 is 63 [25,26]. Older adults can improve their Healthy Eating Index by increasing consumption of fruits, vegetables, whole grains, and dairy and ensuring that their protein intake meets recommendations. Reducing intake of added sugars, saturated fats, and sodium will also create additional benefits for heathy nutrition. Older adults should pay particular attention when choosing nutrient-dense options within each food group while consuming appropriate portion sizes since calorie needs decline with age.

The good news is that the Healthy Eating Index score for individuals over the age of 65 is slightly higher than the Healthy Eating Index for adults between the ages of 19 and 59. Both men and women are close to the recommended amount of daily consumption of protein, which is good news. Unfortunately, most of that protein consumption in both men and women over the age of 65 comes from meat, poultry, and eggs, and recommended consumption of seafood for both men and women is less than half of the recommended servings of seafood per week.

The bad news is that it is far too low, which suggests that there is considerable room to move to improve the overall healthy dietary pattern for individuals over the age of 65.

Both the total intakes of fruits and vegetables are lower than recommended levels. The average intake of total vegetables for men is 3 servings and for women approximately 2.5 servings per day, both of which are below recommended levels. For fruits, the average for both men and women is one serving per day [25]. Once again, these are below the recommended levels, which for both men and women are two servings per day. In the areas that should be limited, in the area of added sugars, 54% of men and 58% of women over the age of 60 exceed the recommended limit of more than 10% of total energy. In the area of saturated fat, 80% of males and 70% of females exceed the recommended limit of 10% of total energy from saturated fat. In the area of sodium, the recommended limit is 2,300 mg. This is exceeded by 94% of males, who average 3,800 mg per day. The recommended level is also exceeded by females, who consume an average of 2,800 mg per day.

27.6 NUTRIENTS OF CONCERN

According to the DGAs 2020–2025, for older adults a number of nutrients of concern exist. Nutrients of concern are divided into two categories—some of the concern is overconsumption and some of the concern is for underconsumption [25]. Current public health concerns include underconsumption of vitamin D, calcium, potassium, fiber, and iron (although iron is not a concern for older adults). The nutrients of concern for overconsumption are sodium and saturated fat.

- Calcium and Vitamin D
  Vitamin D and the mineral calcium are interrelated, which makes the discussion of them together logical. Vitamin D is required for bone synthesis, collagen metabolism, and maintenance of normal plasma calcium levels [27]. The active form of vitamin D produced by the kidney, which is necessary for calcium absorption, is 1,25-vitamin D, dihydroxy vitamin D_3, or calcitriol. 25-Hydroxy vitamin D_3 is produced by the liver, and a second hydroxylation occurs in the kidney.

  Many elderly (up to 50% in some studies) have inadequate vitamin D intakes. Some of this deficit relates to lack of sunlight exposure and dairy product avoidance because of lactose intolerance. Also decreased intestinal vitamin D absorption often occurs in the elderly. Recommendations for vitamin D intake in the elderly or those who consume inadequate amounts of dairy products, or do not absorb vitamin D, or who have scant sunlight exposure may require supplementation to meet the RDA [28–30]. The RDA for vitamin D is 5 micrograms or 200 international units (IU) per day. Many experts believe the elderly should take at least 20 micrograms or 400 IU per day.

  There is no consensus on how much sunlight is necessary for vitamin D, but estimates range from a minimum of 10 minutes two times per week to maximum of 30 minutes per day.

  The vast majority of calcium in the body resides in the bone and teeth. Bone mass declines with age, particularly in White females. This decrease is associated with osteoporosis and increased fracture risk. Calcium supplementation of 1,000 mg daily without estrogen, but with exercise, slows bone loss particularly in postmenopausal women. The RDA for the over-51 age group is currently 800 mg. Many experts believe that this level is too low for postmenopausal females and recommend at least 1,000 mg per day. Calcium supplements are contraindicated in patients with a history of calcium kidney stones, primary hyperthyroidism, sarcoidosis, or renal hypercalciuria.
- Protein Requirements
  Consuming enough protein is important to prevent the loss of lean muscle mass which occurs naturally with aging [31]. About 50% of women and 30% of men age 71 or older fall short of protein recommendations. As already indicated, most older adults meet or exceed weekly recommendations for meat, poultry, and eggs. Seafood, dairy, and fortified soy alternatives, as well as bean, peas, and lentils, are underconsumed despite the fact that these provide important nutrients that support healthy dietary patterns. The current U.S. dietary recommendation or RDA is 0.8 grams protein/kg per day, which appears adequate for older adults. Healthy, free-living

adults typically consume 1 gram/kg of protein per day, which many experts believe should be the recommended allowance. Since individuals over the age of 65 experience a decline in overall energy intake, there is also a decline in protein intake. Protein should be 12–14% of total energy intake, which would result in about 1 gram/kg/per day.

- Potassium
  Potassium has multiple important roles within the body. It is involved with proper cardiac function and skeletal and smooth muscle contraction. Dietary sources of potassium include fish and plant foods including legumes, vegetables, and fruits. Higher fruit and vegetable intakes have been associated with a number of positive health outcomes including bone health, blood pressure control, and lower risk of metabolic syndrome, stroke, and CVD [32].
- Vitamin B_{12}
  Vitamin B_{12} is important for good health and represents a concern for some older adults because the ability to absorb this nutrient tends to decrease with age. Certain medicines can also decrease its absorption. Older adults are encouraged to meet recommendations for protein foods which are also a source of vitamin B_{12}. Vitamin B_{12} can also be found in foods fortified with this vitamin such as breakfast cereals. It is also possible to obtain vitamin B_{12} dietary supplements. Before using supplements of vitamin B_{12}, an individual should speak with their healthcare provider to determine if such supplementation is appropriate.
- Fiber
  Fiber plays multiple beneficial roles in the human body. Whole vegetables and fruits are good sources of dietary fiber, as are whole grains and whole grain products. For this reason, older adults should be encouraged to consume more fruits and vegetables in their natural state rather than in the juice form [40]. They should also be encouraged to choose whole grain products rather than refined or processed grain products. In general, fiber supplements are not routinely recommended.
- Sodium
  Small amounts of dietary sodium along with potassium may help maintain normal blood pressure as well as adequate muscle and nerve function [32]. High amounts of dietary sodium are associated with hypertension. The major source of dietary sodium is commercially prepared foods, while only a small percentage comes from salt added at the table. Recently a significant increase in the availability of reduced salt products has occurred. Both the AHA and the DGAs 2020–2025 recommend no more than 2,300 mg of sodium per day. As already indicated, this amount is typically significantly exceeded by both men and women in all age groups and is especially a problem in older adults who experience a high likelihood of high blood pressure.
- Saturated Fat
  Higher intakes of saturated fat are associated with an increased risk of developing CVD when compared to intake of unsaturated fat—both

monounsaturated and polyunsaturated. As previously indicated in this chapter, both men and women over the age of 60 consume too much saturated fat in the diet. Animal fats are a major source of dietary saturated fats, as are tropical oils. Tropical oils include palm and coconut. Dairy products may also be a major source of saturated fat. Thus low-fat and fat-free dairy products should be chosen if they are readily available. If choosing red meats, lean cuts of meats and limiting frequency and portion size should be observed.

- Added Sugar
  High levels of added sugar have been associated with the risk of multiple chronic diseases including CVD, obesity, and T2DM [24]. Approximately half of added sugar in the diet comes from sugar-sweetened beverages, while 31% comes from snacks and sweets, and the rest comes from a combination of other foods that are often less obvious. Listing the amount of added sugar was made a mandatory requirement in the revised nutrition facts label.
- Alcohol
  The DGAs do not recommend starting alcohol consumption for any reason. Older adults can choose to drink or not to drink alcohol in moderation [24]. Limiting intake of two drinks or fewer per day for men and one drink or fewer per day for women when alcohol is consumed is recommended. Older adults experience the effects of alcohol more quickly than they did when they were younger. This puts older adults at a higher risk for falls, car crashes, and other injuries. Alcohol use may also have a greater impact on comorbid health conditions that are more frequent in older adults than in younger adults. Finally, alcoholic beverages are a significant source of calories. The average adult who consumes alcohol consumes approximately 9% of calories from alcohol (approximately 200–300 calories per day) on days when alcohol is consumed, which may make weight management more difficult.

27.7 SPECIAL DIETARY CONSIDERATIONS FOR OLDER ADULTS

Maintaining optimal nutritional status for older adults must take into account a variety of physiologic and psychological factors. Paying attention to these factors is critical for ensuring optimal health outcomes.

- **Organ Systems**—The way the body handles nutrients can change with advancing age. These changes are mostly due to alterations in the function of organ systems, which can ultimately impact on health outcomes [33–39]. Some of the biologic changes can contribute to altered nutrient status in older adults and are found in Table 27.1. In addition to the factors already discussed, the increased use of prescription and nonprescription medications as well as the overall diminished capacity of the liver to metabolize drugs can compromise nutrient utilization [40]. Therefore, these factors should be considered by every clinician when dealing with people over the age of 65.

TABLE 27.1
Potential Biologic Changes Contributing to Altered Nutrient Status in Older Adults

System	Change
Digestive system	↓ Hydrochloric acid secretion
	↓ Digestive juice secretion (pancreas and small intestine)
	↓ Absorptive capacity (malabsorption)
	↓ Muscles tone large intestine (↓ gastrointestinal motility)
	↑ Chronic blood loss due to ulcers and hemorrhoids
Liver	↓ Hepatic and biliary function
	↓ Rate detoxification
Heart	↓ Cardiac output
↓ Strength and flexibility of blood vessels	Kidneys
↓ Blood flow	↓ Glomerular filtration
Senses	↓ Acuity vision and hearing
↓ Taste (loss taste buds, mainly salt and sweet)	
↓ Smell	Skin
↓ Synthesis vitamin D	Body composition
↓ Lean muscle mass	
↑ Fat mass	↓ Mobility
↓ Dexterity	Immune system
↓ T cell-mediated function	↑ Susceptibility to infection and malignancy
Pharmacokinetics	↑ Prescription and nonprescription drug use
↑ Chronic drug therapy	
↓ Capacity to metabolize drugs	Mouth
↓ Salivary secretion	↑ Altered bite pattern due to tooth loss

Source: Lichtenstein A. Optimal Nutrition Guidance for Older Adults. In Rippe (ed) Lifestyle Medicine, 3rd Edition. CRC Press, Boca Raton, FL. 2019. Use with permission.

- **Taste and Smell**—Individuals over the age of 65 often experience diminished taste and smell, which can lead to poor appetite and decrease the desire to eat and enjoy a variety of foods. Tastebud acuity may decrease primarily with respect to salty and sweet food items, which results in greater sensitivity to acid and bitter food items [41]. Also, a diminished sense of smell is frequently observed in older adults. It has been demonstrated that older adults with poor odor perception can result in lower nutrient intakes than those with good odor perception [42–44].
- **Vision, Dexterity, and Mobility**—Diminished vision, dexterity, and mobility can make food acquisition and preparation difficult which, in turn, may severely alter the variety and quality of foods consumed. Examples include difficulty opening jars or cans or packaged goods because of arthritis or diminished strength. Accommodations for older adults may include kitchen reorganization or utilization of packaging that allows double or

triple servings and minimal preparation such as bags of frozen vegetables or fruits. Older adults may not automatically take advantage of newer packaging items of common foods such as precut fruit or prewashed greens and may require guidance in this area. This may be done either by their physician or registered dietitian nutritionist.

- **Social Factors**—In addition to physical capacity decreases associated with the aging process, there may also be changes in the social environment for older adults which can impact on nutritional status. Some of these are listed in Table 27.2. For example, possible death or disability of a spouse or other family member with whom an individual shared prepared meals in common can lead to social isolation and diminished desire to prepare well-balanced and varied meals. Older adults may also experience deterioration in mental or economic status and may be faced with having to adapt to a new living environment. All of these factors can result in dramatic changes in mealtimes, food preparation, and foods available. Chronic disease can further limit food choices. Depression may also accompany the aging process, with individuals without adequate support to make necessary adaptations [45]. Older adults are at increased risk of alcohol abuse. All of these factors may contribute to poor food consumption patterns.
- **Physiologic Changes**—Various chronic diseases that are nutrient related become more prevalent in later years. These include CVD, cancer, T2DM, hypertension, osteoporosis, disorders in dentition, and declines in immune

TABLE 27.2
Psychosocial Factors Contributing to Compromised Food Intake in Older Adults

Factor	Change
Companionship	↑ Loss of spouse
↑ Social isolation	
↑ Loss of companions	↓ Social interaction secondary to ↓ mobility
Mental state	↑ Depression
↑ Mental deterioration (dementia)	
↑ Alcoholism	↑ Loneliness
↑ Chronic disease	Economic
↑ Fixed income (poverty)	
↓ Choice and availability	↓ Quantity needs
↓ Variety	Nutrition knowledge
↑ Susceptibility to food fads	↑ Susceptibility to nutrient supplement claims
Housing	↑ Change in status (loss of home)
↓ Independence	

Source: Lichtenstein A. Optimal Nutrition Guidance for Older Adults. In Rippe (ed) Lifestyle Medicine, 3rd Edition. CRC Press, Boca Raton, FL. 2019. Used with permission.

function. Some of the goals of nutritional recommendations for older adults are designed to help delay the onset of chronic disease, while in other instances they are intended to treat or accommodate the disorder.

- Dentition—Changes in oral health and dentition are frequently associated with older aged individuals [46,47]. In fact, some studies have shown that the number of teeth that remain is the strongest dental association with the ability to consume a varied diet [6]. Chewing and swallowing fibrous foods may be difficult with poor dentition. Salivary secretions also decrease with increasing age; thus, it is important for the clinician to carefully discuss dentition with all older patients.
- Cardiovascular Disease—The rate of CVD is clearly associated with age [48]. For this reason, the DGAs 2020–2025 recommends dietary patterns that are rich in fruits and vegetables, whole grains, legumes, fat-free and low-fat dairy products, fish, and lean meat. These recommendations are made for dietary changes for all adults as they age and may be particularly important for people over the age of 65.
- Osteoporosis—Osteoporosis (bone loss) is significantly associated with the aging process. Osteoporosis is estimated to affect 200 million woman worldwide, which represents approximately one-tenth of women aged 60, one-fifth of women aged 70, two-fifths of women aged 80, and two-thirds of women aged 90. Even in men it is estimated that a lifetime risk of experiencing an osteoporotic fracture over the age of 50 is 27% [49]. Detailed description of osteoporosis plus nutritional and other lifestyle related strategies to ameliorate it are found in Chapter 23.
- Sarcopenia—Sarcopenia is common in individuals over the age of 65 [50]. Sarcopenia is the progressive loss of muscle, which also accompanies decreases in strength. Since muscle and bone are in direct communication with each other, sarcopenia also contributes to osteoporosis. There is an approximately 8% decline in muscle mass per decade between the ages of 40 and 70 years, and this increases to 15% every decade thereafter. Five to thirteen percent of 60- to 70-year-olds and 11%–15% of individuals over the age of 80 have sarcopenia. Sarcopenia is related to some degree to decreased physical activity, although there are certain other causes such as neuro and cytokine factors which can stimulate sarcopenia. More details about sarcopenia may be found in Chapter 23.
- Glucose Intolerance/Type 2 Diabetes—The incidence of both glucose intolerance and T2DM increases with age [51,52]. This increased incidence is strongly associated with weight gain in later years. As discussed in detail in Chapter 20, lifestyle interventions including proper nutrition have been shown to prevent or significantly delay the onset of T2DM particularly in individuals with glucose intolerance [53–55]. These lifestyle factors include regular physical activity, weight loss (if necessary), and dietary modification consisting of healthy nutritional standards which are consistent with those recommended for lowering the risk of heart disease.
- Hypertension—The incidence of hypertension increases with age [48]. According to Framingham data, individuals at the age of 65 who have

normal blood pressure still have a greater than 90% chance of having high blood pressure as they move into their 70s and 80s [56]. Multiple trials have shown that dietary modification is helpful in treating hypertension in all age groups. The DASH diet pattern, which has been discussed in multiple chapters, is rich in vegetables, fruits, and fat-free and low-fat dairy products and decreases blood pressure in a variety of individuals. If this pattern is further combined with sodium restriction, further decreases in blood pressure will occur.

- Immune Function—Immune function decreases with age [57,58]. There is some evidence that vitamin E supplementation may be beneficial in reducing the incidence of respiratory infections in older individuals living in residential settings. Moreover, the "Western diet," which is high in processed foods, red meat, processed meats, and carbohydrates, has been shown to increase inflammation in the human body, and this, in turn, is associated with decreased immune function. These factors may have contributed to some older adults experiencing excessive hospitalization and mortality during the COVID-19 pandemic. (See subsequent section.)
- Cancer—The incidence of cancer of all types increases with age. A large body of research supports the idea that diet is associated with cancer [59]. Some specific cancers have been associated with various dietary components including alcohol intake (laryngeal cancer) and fat intake, (breast, colon, and prostate). The general dietary guidelines to reduce the risk of cancer are similar to the recommendations to decrease the risk of CVD including the consumption of more fruits and vegetables, whole grains, etc.
- Dehydration—The thirst mechanism decreases in individuals over the age of 65, and for this reason older adults may be more susceptible to dehydration [60–62]. Mean intakes of beverages in adults over the age of 60 have been shown to be decreased by up to two fewer cups of fluid a day. Most of this decrease is due to drinking less water. For this reason, older adults should be counseled to drink plenty of water to prevent dehydration and aid in the digestion of food and absorption of nutrients. The amount of water that is contained in foods such as fruits, vegetables, and soups contributes to hydration status and is a contributor to total fluid intake.

27.8 MALNUTRITION

Nutrition is a key factor in the aging process and a significant contributor to future health, helping to maintain good health, and reducing the risk of chronic disease. Malnutrition in the elderly significantly increases an individual's risk of developing generally poor health and chronic disease [63–66]. Malnutrition is quite common and significantly underdiagnosed in the elderly population. Malnutrition can be used to describe an overall state of poor nutritional status. This may include undernutrition and overnutrition of macronutrients and/or micronutrients. According to the American Society of Parenteral and Enteral Nutrition (ASPEN) and the Academic of Nutrition and Dietetics, a minimum of two of the following six criteria must be fulfilled in order to diagnosis an individual as being malnourished [67]. They are low energy intake, weight loss, loss of muscle mass, loss of subcutaneous fat, fluid accumulation, and reduced hand grip strength.

As the life expectancy has increased, so have chronic health problems which can be prevented or delayed or improved by maintaining a healthy diet. It has been estimated that approximately 15% of community dwelling elderly people are malnourished. Among those who are hospitalized, in some research studies an estimated 60%–80% of geriatric hospitalized patients are malnourished [63].

There are a number of risk factors for reduced nutritional intake and body weight. These have been called "the anorexia of aging" where energy intake is reduced, and the likelihood increases that elderly individuals will become malnourished. Factors that may contribute include sarcopenia, cachexia (characterized by involuntary loss of fat free mass caused by catabolism), and decreased sensory function (e.g. loss of taste, smell). A variety of health problems can accompany malnutrition including nutrient deficiencies, osteoporosis, and immune dysfunction, as well as increased risk of various chronic diseases such as CVD and T2DM.

Given the negative health-related impact of malnutrition, it is important to diagnosis this condition as soon as possible so that effective nutritional intervention can begin. The need to carry out additional screening as part of a regular check-up is important in all patients, but particularly in the elderly and those in whom malnutrition may be present. Malnutrition and risk of malnutrition are significantly underdiagnosed. In fact, in multiple studies up to one-quarter of nutritionally at-risk patients who were in contact with healthcare professionals did not receive nutritional intervention. A variety of assessment methods are now available both to diagnose malnutrition in the elderly and to provide an overall nutritional assessment. (See the next section.)

Several other factors are particularly important in the area of malnutrition. First, the level of protein consumption plays a critical role in whether or not an individual develops sarcopenia. It has been argued that elderly patients should consume at least as much or more protein as younger people in order to prevent lean muscle loss and decreased metabolism [50,66].

In addition, several studies have shown that social and economic factors are particularly prevalent in elderly individuals with malnutrition. In one meta-analysis, the increased likelihood of malnutrition was associated with low educational level; being single, widowed, or divorced; living alone; or having a low income level. Therefore, these factors should also be assessed in every elderly patient.

The COVID-19 pandemic also played a role in many health factors, particularly in the elderly population [68]. People over the age of 65 were significantly more likely to be hospitalized or die from COVID-19 than were younger individuals. Part of the increased risk appears to relate to malnutrition. In one study in Wuhan, China, 27.5% of hospitalized patients were in the group of malnutrition risk and 52.7% were in the malnutrition group. This fact underscores the importance of assessing nutrition in hospitalized patients and the role that malnutrition may play in adverse comes from the COVID-19 pandemic.

27.9 NUTRITIONAL ASSESSMENT IN THE ELDERLY

A variety of screening instruments are available to provide nutritional assessment in the elderly. These include the Many Nutritional Assessment (MNA) [69], the Malnutrition Screening Tool (MUST) [70], the Geriatric Nutritional Risk Index (GNRI) [71], and the Nutritional Risk Screening 2002 (NRS-2002) [72].

- **Many Nutritional Assessment (MNA)**—The MNA is the most widely used and recommended research method for assessing nutrition and malnutrition in the elderly. It is made up of four components including anthropometric measurements, general assessment, dietary assessment, and self-assessment. The form most often used for the MNA is found in Figure 27.3. As shown in Figure 27.3, the score varies from 24 points or greater, which is well nourished; 17–23.5 points, which is at risk of malnutrition; and less than 17 points is malnourished.
- **Malnutrition Screening Tool (MUST)**—The MUST is a nutritional and screening tool that involves three primary considerations: current body mass index (BMI), weight loss over time, and presence of acute disease that could significantly decrease the individual's intake for more than five days. It has been developed for and applied to adults in all healthcare settings. If patients on this instrument are assessed at a medium risk for malnutrition, their nutritional status must be undertaken. Treatment should be initiated for those at high risk for malnutrition.
- **Geriatric Nutritional Risk Index (GNRI)**—GNRI is an indicator of risk of elderly individuals developing nutrition-related health problems. It is derived from the general Nutritional Risk Index (NRI) but is specifically targeted toward the elderly population. It involves consideration of serum albumin levels, current body weight, and optimal body weight to assess nutritional status. GNRI has been shown to predict mortality in hospitalized elderly patients but has not been validated for the community-living elderly population. GNRI values are calculated using the following equation: GNRI = [1.489 × serum albumin (g/l)] + {41.7 × (current weight/ideal weight)]. A GNRI greater than 98 suggests no risk for nutrition-related health problems. An index between 92 and 98 indicates low risk, an index between 82 and 91 indicates a moderate risk, and an index less than 82 indicates major risk of nutrition-related complications.
- **Nutritional Risk Screening 2002 (NRS-2002)**—The NRS-2002 is a screening tool that takes into consideration an individual's current BMI (>20.5 kg/m^2), their recent weight loss, any recent decrease in food intake, and the severity of illness. This particular instrument is rarely used to diagnose malnutrition.

27.10 NUTRITIONAL-RELATED KNOWLEDGE AND ATTITUDES

An interesting research project across five European countries demonstrated that nutrition-related knowledge and attitudes were necessary to make dietary changes in terms of healthier dietary patterns [73]. The scores of the Nutrition Related

MINI NUTRITIONAL ASSESSMENT (MNA) AND PERCENTAGES OF SUBJECTS WITH MEAN NUTRIENT INTAKES LESS THAN TWO-THIRDS THE 1991 FRENCH RDA (CHI-SQUARE ANALYSIS)

			MNA status						
			Malnourished <17 points		At risk of malnutrition 17–23.5 points		Well-nourished ≥24 points		
	French RDA	2/3 RDA	*n*	%	*n*	%	*n*	%	Pearson chi-square *P*
Energy (kJ/d)	6280–8790	5020/6280	18	33	15	35	1	2	<0.0001
kJ/d per kg body weight	125	84	7	13	8	19	3	6	0.1465
Protein (g/d)	60	40	6	11	7	16	0	0	0.0137
g/d per kg body weight	1	0.67	4	7	5	12	1	2	0.1577
Fiber (g/d)	20	13	40	73	24	56	11	21	<0.0001
Calcium mg/d	1200	800	30	55	23	54	7	13	<0.0001
Iron mg/d	10	6.7	18	33	13	30	1	2	0.0001
Vitamin A μg RE/d	800	533	18	33	15	35	9	17	0.0894
Vitamin B1 mg/d	1.3	0.9	47	86	38	88	29	55	0.0001
Riboflavin mg/d	1.5	1	14	26	11	26	3	6	0.0113
Vitamin B6 mg/d	2	1.3	39	71	30	70	17	32	<0.0001
Vitamin C mg/d	80	53	16	29	17	39	1	2	<0.0001

FIGURE 27.3 Mini Nutritional Assessment (MNA) and percentages of subjects with mean nutrient intakes less than two-thirds the 1991 french RDA (CHI-Square Analysis)

Source: Vellas B, Guigoz Y, Garry PJ, Nourhashemi F, Bennahum D, Lauque S, et al. The mini nutritional assessment (MNA) and its use in grading the nutritional state of elderly patients. Nutrition. 1999;15(2):116–22. Used with permission.

Knowledge (NRK) and Nutrition Related Attitudes (NRA) were associated with a lower BMI and higher physical activity level. This supports the concept that physician counseling in the area of nutrition is particularly important to the elderly population to enhance knowledge and improve attitudes about nutrition.

27.11 MICROBIOME

Increasing research is being accomplished on the role of the microbiome in overall health. In one study of nursing home patients, a microbiome that was thought to be balanced and helpful was reduced in patients, and this reduction in microbiome diversity was associated with frailty and poor nutrition. In this study, as individuals became malnourished, short-chain fatty acid–producing organisms declined and dysbiotic material species increased [74]. While this area of research is new, it may carry significant potential for nutrition in the elderly moving forward.

27.12 OTHER LIFESTYLE-RELATED FACTORS CONTRIBUTING TO PROPER NUTRITION IN THE ELDERLY

Several studies have shown that long-term physical activity results in improved nutrition in the elderly. The synergy between physical activity and nutrition has been demonstrated in multiple population groups [75]. This synergy provides further impetus for clinicians to recommend physical activity to individuals over the age of 65 as well as younger individuals.

27.13 SUPPORTING HEALTHY EATING

As in other life stages, healthy eating for older adults should be supported by professionals, family, and friends to achieve beneficial dietary patterns. This must account for factors such as cost, preferences, traditions, and access. In addition, other factors should be considered such as enjoyment of food, abilities to chew and swallow food, and food safety. A variety of resources are available through the federal government to support healthy eating throughout all life stages and are particularly important in the elderly [25].

27.14 CONCLUSIONS

A variety of factors impact on nutrition in the elderly due to decreased core food consumption in individuals typically over the age of 65. It is particularly important to emphasize nutrient-dense foods and healthy eating habits. In addition, malnutrition is more common in the elderly population, which should be assessed in all patient encounters with individuals over the age of 65.

Clinical Applications

- The elderly population in the United States currently has 46 million people and is expected to double by the age of 2060. There are unique nutritional challenges for the elderly due to the aging process.

- Malnutrition is underdiagnosed in the elderly, and screening tools are available to assist in the diagnosis.
- Clinicians should pay particular attention to healthy nutrition in the elderly in order to lower the risk of chronic disease and improve quality of life.

REFERENCES

1. Lichtenstein A. Optimal nutrition guidance for older adults. In Rippe (ed). Lifestyle Medicine, 3rd edition. Boca Raton: CRC Press, 2019.
2. Hoffman N. Diet in the elderly. Needs and risks. Med Clin N Am. 1993;77(4):745–756.
3. Bruins M, Van Dael P, Eggersdorfer M. The role of nutrients in reducing the risk for noncommunicable diseases during aging. Nutrients. 2019;11(1).
4. de Groot L, van Staveren W, Burema J. Survival beyond age 70 in relation to diet. Nutr Rev. 1996;54(7):211–212.
5. U.S. Department of Health and Human Services, Health.gov, DeSilva D, Anderson-Villaluz D. Nutrition as we age: Healthy eating with the dietary guidelines. Nutrition as We Age: Healthy Eating with the Dietary Guidelines—News & Events | health.gov. (Accessed January 25, 2024).
6. Okamoto N, Amano N, Nakamura T, et al. Relationship between tooth loss, low masticatory ability, and nutritional indices in the elderly: A cross-sectional study. BMC Oral Health. 2019;19(1):110.
7. Paulose-Ram R, Graber J, Woodwell D, et al. The National Health and Nutrition Examination Survey (NHANES), 2021–2022: Adapting data collection in a COVID-19 environment. Am J Public Health. 2021;111(12):2149–2156.
8. IOM. How Should the Recommended Dietary Allowances Be Revised? Washington, DC: National Academy of Sciences, 1994.
9. IOM. Dietary Reference Intakes: Calcium, Phosphorus, Magnesium, Vitamin D and Fluoride. Washington, DC: National Academy of Sciences, 1997.
10. IOM. Dietary Reference Intakes: Thiamin, Riboflavin, Niacin, Vitamin B6, Folate, Vitamin B_{12}, Pantothenic Acid, Biotin and Choline. Washington, DC: National Academy of Sciences, 1998.
11. IOM. Dietary Reference Intakes: Vitamin C, Vitamin E, Selenium and Carotenoids. Washington, DC: National Academy of Sciences, 2000.
12. IOM. Dietary Reference Intakes: Vitamin A, Vitamin K, Arsenic, Boron, Chromium, Copper, Iodine, Iron, Manganese, Molybdenum, Nickel, Silicon, Vanadium and Zinc. Washington, DC: National Academy of Sciences, 2001.
13. IOM. Dietary Supplements: A Framework for Evaluating Safety. Committee on the Framework for Evaluating the Safety of Dietary Supplements. Washington, DC: National Academy of Sciences, 2004.
14. IOM. Dietary Reference Intakes: Energy, Carbohydrate, Fiber, Fat, Fatty Acids, Cholesterol, Protein and Amino Acids. Washington, DC: National Academy of Sciences, 2005.
15. IOM. Dietary Reference Intakes, Water, Potassium, Sodium, Chloride and Sulfate. Washington, DC: National Academy of Sciences, 2005.
16. Otten J, Hellwig J, Linda D, IOM. Dietary Reference Intakes: The Essential Guide to Nutrient Requirements. Washington, DC: National Academy of Sciences, 2006.
17. IOM. Dietary Reference Intakes for Calcium and Vitamin D. 2010. www.iomedu/Reports/2010/Dietary-Reference-Intakes-for-Calcium-and-Vitamin-Daspx
18. Williamson D. Descriptive epidemiology of body weight and weight change in U.S. adults. Ann Intern Med. 1993;119(7 Pt 2):646–649.

19. Bruins M, Van Dael P, Eggersdorfer M. The role of nutrients in reducing the risk for noncommunicable diseases during aging. Nutrients. 2019 Jan 4;11(1).
20. Lichtenstein A, Rasmussen H, Yu W, et al. Modified mypyramid for older adults [Erratum appears in J Nutr. 2008 Jul;138(7):1400]. J Nutr. 2008;138(1):5–11.
21. Estruch R, Ros E, Salas-Salvado J, et al. Primary prevention of cardiovascular disease with a mediterranean diet. N Engl J Med. 2013;368(14):1279–1290.
22. Sacks F, Svetkey L, Vollmer W, et al. Effects on blood pressure of reduced dietary sodium and the Dietary Approaches to Stop Hypertension (DASH) diet. DASH-Sodium Collaborative Research Group. N Engl J Med. 2001;344(1):3–10.
23. Lichtenstein A, Appel L, Vadiveloo M, et al. 2021 Dietary guidance to improve cardiovascular health: A scientific statement from the American Heart Association. Circulation. 2021;144(23):e472–e487.
24. Malik V, Schulze M, Hu F. Intake of sugar-sweetened beverages and weight gain: A systematic review. Am J Clin Nutr. 2006;84(2):274–288.
25. *Dietary Guidelines for Americans, 2020–2025*. Older Adults. Chapter 6. Page 121. www.dietaryguidelines.gov/resources/2020-2025-dietary-guidelines-online-materials. (Accessed January 25, 2024).
26. USDA Food and Nutrition Service. U.S. Department of Agriculture. Healthy Eating Index (HEI). Healthy Eating Index (HEI) | Food and Nutrition Service (usda.gov). (Accessed January 25, 2024).
27. Moore C, Murphy M, Keast D, et al. Vitamin D intake in the United States. J Am Diet Assoc. 2004;104(6):980–983.
28. MacLaughlin HM. Aging decreases the capacity of human skin to produce vitamin D3. J Clin Invest. 1985;76(4):1536–1568.
29. Holick M. Sunlight and vitamin D. for bone health and prevention of autoimmune diseases, cancers, and cardiovascular disease. Am J Clin Nutr. 2004;80(6 Suppl):1678S–1688S.
30. Holick M. Vitamin deficiency. N Engl J Med. 2007;357(3):266–281.
31. Wolfe R, Miller S, Miller K. Optimal protein intake in the elderly. Clin Nutr. 2008;27(5):675–684.
32. Sacks F, Svetkey L, Vollmer W, et al. Effects on blood pressure of reduced dietary sodium and the Dietary Approaches to Stop Hypertension (DASH) diet. DASH-Sodium Collaborative Research Group. N Engl J Med. 2001;344(1):3–10.
33. Panagiotakos D, Pitsavos C, Skoumas Y, et al. The association between food patterns and the metabolic syndrome using principal components analysis: The ATTICA study. J Am Diet Assoc. 2007;107(6):979–987.
34. Perez-Cornago A, Travis R, Appleby P, et al. Fruit and vegetable intake and prostate cancer risk in the European Prospective Investigation into Cancer and Nutrition (EPIC). Int J Cancer. 2017;141(2):287–297.
35. Takachi R, Inoue M, Sugawara Y, et al. Research group for the development and evaluation of cancer prevention strategies in Japan. Fruit and vegetable intake and the risk of overall cancer in Japanese: A pooled analysis of population-based cohort studies. J Epidemiol. 2017;27(4):152–162.
36. Erkkila A, Booth S, Hu F, et al. Phylloquinone intake and risk of cardiovascular diseases in men. Nutr Metab Cardiovasc Dis. 2007;17(1):58–62.
37. Steffen L, Folsom A, Cushman M, et al. Greater fish, fruit, and vegetable intakes are related to lower incidence of venous thromboembolism: The longitudinal investigation of thromboembolism etiology. Circulation. 2007;115(2):188–195.
38. Pearson-Stuttard J, Bandosz P, et al. Reducing US cardiovascular disease burden and disparities through national and targeted dietary policies: A modelling study. PLoS Med. 2017;14(6):e1002311.

39. Stefler D, Pikhart H, Kubinova R, et al. Fruit and vegetable consumption and mortality in Eastern Europe: Longitudinal results from the health, alcohol and psychosocial factors in Eastern Europe study. Eur J Prev Cardiol. 2016;23(5):493–501.
40. U.S. Department of Agriculture and U.S. Department of Health and Human Services. *Dietary Guidelines for Americans, 2020–2025*, 9th edition. December 2020. Dietary Guidelines.gov. 2020; www.dietaryguidelines.gov/resources/2020-2025-dietary-guidelines-online-materials.
41. Lipson L, Bray G. Nutritional Aspects of Aging. Vol. I, Chen LH (ed). Boca Raton: CRC Press, 1986.
42. Griep M, Collys K, Mets T, et al. Sensory detection of food odour in relation to dental status, gender and age. Gerodontology. 1996;13(1):56–62.
43. Griep M, Verleye G, Franck A, et al. Variation in nutrient intake with dental status, age and odour perception. Eur J Clin Nutr. 1996;50(12):816–825.
44. Griep M, Mets T, Collys K, et al. Risk of malnutrition in retirement homes elderly persons measured by the "mini-nutritional assessment". J Gerontol A Bio Sci Med Sci. 2000;55(2):M57–M63.
45. James W, Nelson M, Ralph A, et al. Socioeconomic determinants of health. The contribution of nutrition to inequalities in health. BMJ. 1997;314(7093):1545–1549.
46. Papas A, Joshi A, Giunta J, et al. Relationships among education, dentate status, and diet in adults. Spec Care Dentist. 1998;18(1):26–32.
47. Papas A, Palmer C, Rounds M, et al. The effects of denture status on nutrition. Spec Care Dentist. 1998;18(1):17–25.
48. AHA Centers for Health Metrics and Evaluation. Heart Disease and Stroke Statistics, 2018. https://healthmetrics.heart.org/at-a-glance-heart-disease-and-stroke-statistics-2018/
49. The Osteoporosis Foundation. www.osteoporosis.foundation/facts-statistics (Accessed January 30, 2024).
50. Giglio J, Kamimura M, Lamarca F, et al. Association of sarcopenia with nutritional parameters, quality of life, hospitalization, and mortality rates of elderly patients on nemodialysis. J Ren Nutr. 2018;28(3):197–207.
51. Ford E, Ajani U, Croft J, et al. Explaining the decrease in U.S. deaths from coronary disease, 1980–2000. N Engl J Med. 2007;356(23):2388–2398.
52. Ford E, Li C, Zhao G, et al. Prevalence of the metabolic syndrome among U.S. adolescents using the definition from the International Diabetes Federation. Diabetes Care. 2008;31(3):587–589.
53. Tuomilehto J, Lindstrom J, Eriksson J, et al. Prevention of type 2 diabetes mellitus by changes in lifestyle among subjects with impaired glucose tolerance. N Engl J Med. 2001;344(18):1343–1350.
54. Knowler W, Barrett-Connor E, Fowler S, et al. Reduction in the incidence of type 2 diabetes with lifestyle intervention or metformin. N Engl J Med. 2002;346(6):393–403.
55. Sakane N, Sato J, Tsushita K, et al. Prevention of type 2 diabetes in a primary healthcare setting: Three-year results of lifestyle intervention in Japanese subjects with impaired glucose tolerance. BMC Public Health. 2011;11:40–49.
56. Chobanian A, Bakris G, Black H, et al. The seventh report of the joint national committee on prevention, detection, evaluation, and treatment of high blood oressure: The JNC 7 report. JAMA. 2003;289(19):2560–2572.
57. Meydani S, Wu D. Nutrition and age-associated inflammation: Implications for disease prevention. J Parenter Enteral Nutr. 2008;32(6):626–629.
58. Meydani S, Wu D. Age-associated inflammatory changes: Role of nutritional intervention. Nutr Rev. 2007;65(12 Pt 2):S213–S216.

59. Schwedhelm C, Boeing H, Hoffmann G, et al. Effect of diet on mortality and cancer recurrence among cancer survivors: A systematic review and meta-analysis of cohort studies. Nutr Rev. 2016;74(12):737–748.
60. Albert S, Nakra B, Grossberg G, et al: Vasopressin response to dehydration in Alzheimer's disease. J Am Geriatr Soc. 1989;37:843–847.
61. Helderman J, Vestal R, Rowe J, et al: The response of arginine vasopressin to intravenous ethanol and hypertonic saline in man: The impact of aging. J Gerontol. 1978;33:39.
62. Rowe J, Shock N, DeFronzo R. The influence of age on the renal response to water deprivation in man. Nephron. 1976;17:270.
63. Stratton R, Hackston A, Longmore D, et al. Malnutrition in hospital outpatients and inpatients: Prevalence, concurrent validity and ease of use of the 'malnutrition universal screening tool' ('MUST') for adults. Br J Nutr. 2004;92(5):799–808.
64. Corcoran C, Murphy C, Culligan E, et al. Malnutrition in the elderly. Sci Prog. 2019;102(2):171–180.
65. Besora-Moreno M, Llaurado E, Tarro L, et al. Social and economic factors and malnutrition or the risk of malnutrition in the elderly: A systematic review and meta-analysis of observational studies. Nutrients. 2020;12(3).
66. van der Pols-Vijlbrief R, Wijnhoven H, Schaap L, et al. Determinants of protein-energy malnutrition in community-dwelling older adults: A systematic review of observational studies. Ageing Res Rev. 2014;18:112–131.
67. Anderson A, Harris T, Tylavsky F, et al. Dietary patterns and survival of older adults. J Am Diet Assoc. 2011;111(1):84–91.
68. Li T, Zhang Y, Gong C, et al. Prevalence of malnutrition and analysis of related factors in elderly patients with COVID-19 in Wuhan, China. Eur J Clin Nutr. 2020;74(6):871–875.
69. Vellas B, Guigoz Y, Garry P, et al. The Mini Nutritional Assessment (MNA) and its use in grading the nutritional state of elderly patients. Nutrition. 1999;15(2):116–122.
70. Poulia K, Yannakoulia M, Karageorgou D, et al. Evaluation of the efficacy of six nutritional screening tools to predict malnutrition in the elderly. Clin Nutr. 2012;31(3):378–385.
71. Bouillanne O, Morineau G, Dupont C, et al. Geriatric Nutritional Risk Index: A new index for evaluating at-risk elderly medical patients. Am J Clin Nutr. 2005;82(4):777–783.
72. Sasaki M, Miyoshi N, Fujino S, et al. The Geriatric Nutritional Risk Index predicts postoperative complications and prognosis in elderly patients with colorectal cancer after curative surgery. Sci Rep. 2020;10(1):10744.
73. Jeruszka-Bielak M, Kollajtis-Dolowy A, Santoro A, et al. Are nutrition-related knowledge and attitudes reflected in lifestyle and health among elderly people? A study across five European countries. Front Physiol. 2018;9:994.
74. Haran J, Bucci V, Dutta P, et al. The nursing home elder microbiome stability and associations with age, frailty, nutrition and physical location. J Med Microbiol. 2018;67(1):40–51.
75. Fiorilli G, Buonsenso A, Centorbi M, et al. Long term physical activity improves quality of life perception, healthy nutrition, and daily life management in elderly: A randomized controlled trial. Nutrients. 2022;14(12).

28 Childhood Nutrition

Key Points

- Healthy nutrition starts in infancy.
- Establishing lifelong patterns of healthy nutrition, including increased fruit and vegetable consumption as well as whole grains, is particularly appropriate for children between the ages of 2 and 18. These guidelines are consistent with adult guidelines for healthy eating.
- For infants, the DGA 2020–2025 recommends the consumption of human milk for six months. If human milk is not available, infant formula may be utilized as long as it is fortified with iron. Infant formula is regulated by the Food and Drug Administration (FDA).
- Healthy nutrition throughout life is a key consideration for lowering the risk of chronic diseases, which are often manifest in adulthood.
- Childhood obesity has dramatically increased in the United States in the past two decades. Establishing healthy nutritional patterns is one highly effective strategy for lowering the risk of obesity and other chronic illnesses.

28.1 INTRODUCTION

Healthy nutrition throughout childhood is very important to establish lifelong eating patterns to lower the risk of chronic disease and maintain good health and vitality [1–4]. In contrast, poor eating habits contribute to the increasing prevalence of obesity in children and also cardiovascular disease (CVD) [5–13], type 2 diabetes mellitus (T2DM), and hypertension [14–22]. Moreover, around the world malnutrition is a significant health risk for children of all ages [23,24]. In the United States, hunger and malnutrition, as well as issues related to health equity, also apply significantly to children [25,26]. All of these issues will be discussed in this chapter.

This chapter will be divided according to age. While general nutritional principles apply to children of all ages, there are some specific issues that are related to the nutritional needs and requirements of children at various ages.

28.2 INFANTS AND TODDLERS

Multiple areas of nutrition play critically important roles during the period from birth to a child's second birthday [25]. This is a time for growth and development. It is also a key time for establishing healthy dietary patterns that may influence behaviors and health throughout the entire life course. This is also a time when nutrients critical for brain development and growth must be provided in adequate amounts. Of course, children in this age group consume very small quantities of foods, so it is important to pay close attention to nutritional concerns.

DOI: 10.1201/9781003452607-28

The Dietary Guidelines for Americans (DGAs) 2020–2025 make a number of important recommendations for the period of time between birth and two years [25]. Specifically, for the first six months the DGAs recommend feeding infants human milk. If human milk is not available, infants should be fed an iron-fortified commercial infant formula (this will be labeled "with iron"). Formula is regulated by the FDA and is based on the standards that ensure nutrient content and safety. Infant formulas are designed to meet the nutritional needs of infants but are not needed beyond the age of 12 months. If human milk is utilized, it is important to take precautions to refrigerate and store it safely. This is also true of prepared infant formula. In addition, infants should be provided with supplemental vitamin D beginning soon after birth.

At about six months infants can be introduced to nutrient-dense complementary foods. Introducing complementary foods before the age of four months is not recommended, but at around the age of six months complementary foods are necessary to ensure adequate nutrition and also expose the baby to flavors, textures, and different kinds of food. Infants should also be given appropriate foods to help prevent choking. This is a good time to also introduce potentially allergenic foods with other complementary foods. Infants who are fed human milk should receive foods that are rich in iron and zinc. Safety and proper handling and storage of human milk or formula are mandatory. Thorough handwashing is essential to feed human milk or preparing to feed human milk or formula. When utilizing powdered infant formula, a safe water source is essential, as is following instructions on the label. Freshly expressed human milk should be refrigerated within four hours and up to four days. Prepared infant formula can be refrigerated up to 24 hours.

It is important not to use a microwave to warm human milk or infant formula. Warming of human milk or infant formula can take place by placing the bottle in warm water or under warm running tap water. Thoroughly wash all infant feeding items including bottle and nipples. It is also recommended that infants avoid foods and vegetables with added sugar and should consume only limited amounts of foods and beverages that are higher in sodium. Once the baby is weaned from human milk or infant formula, this is the time to transition to a healthy dietary pattern.

The time at which infants are ready to begin eating solid foods will depend on where they are in the developmental stage. This will typically occur between four and six months and involves being able to control the head and neck, sitting up alone or with support, bringing objects to the mouth, trying to grasp small objects such as toys or food, and swallowing food rather than pushing it back or out onto the chin. As already indicated, steps should be taken to decrease potential choking foods. This typically involves offering foods at the appropriate size and consistency that allow the infant to eat and swallow easily. It is essential to ensure that an adult is supervising feeding during mealtimes and not putting infant cereal or other solid foods in the infant bottle. When introducing foods to potentially allergenic foods [26], this can occur at age four to six months but should be done in consultation with the infant's healthcare provider, particularly in the area of feeding the infant peanut-containing foods.

Specific guidelines are available from the National Institutes of Health (NIH) about how to prevent peanut allergies in children. In addition to introducing iron-rich foods between the ages of 6 and 11 months, if the infant has been fed with human milk, vitamin D, choline, and potassium should also be included in complementary foods. Protein foods including meats, poultry, eggs, seafood, nuts, seeds, and soy products are good sources of iron, zinc, protein, choline, and long-chain polyunsaturated fatty acids. Long-chain fatty acids such as omega-3 and omega-6 are important for rapid brain development that occurs during the first two years of life. A number of dietary components should be eliminated. These include, as already mentioned, added sugar and foods that are higher in sodium. Infants also should not be given any foods containing raw or cooked honey, which may contain the *Clostridium botulinum* organism.

It is also important to establish a healthy beverage pattern. Small amounts of water can be given to infants with the introduction to complementary foods. Infants should not consume cow milk or fortified soda beverages before the age of 12 months to replace human milk or infant formula. Before the age of 12 months, 100% fruit or vegetable juice should not be given to infants. Furthermore, caffeinated beverages should not be given to children younger than the age of two.

28.3 HEALTHY DIETARY PATTERN DURING A TODDLER'S SECOND YEAR OF LIFE

Toddlers consuming less human milk and infant formula is not recommended. Calories and nutrients should predominantly be met from the healthy dietary pattern of age-appropriate foods and beverages [25]. The Healthy US-Style Dietary Pattern for toddlers ages 12 through 23 months who no longer consume human milk or infant formula is found in Figure 28.1. As indicated, the diets are portioned according to how many calories the infant is consuming between 700 and 1,000 calories. The appropriate caloric level is based on age, sex, and weight. Specific information concerning this can be found on the usda.gov website listed under the table.

Current intakes for infants aged 12–23 months are generally consistent with those recommended with regard to total vegetables, total fruits, total grains, and total protein foods [27]. Dairy is currently consumed at levels that are somewhat higher than recommended. With regard to foods that are recommended to be limited, the average infant is currently consuming 104 kcals from added sugars. As already indicated, this category is recommended to be avoided. The average infant is currently consuming 1,586 mg of sodium, which is somewhat above the recommended limit of 1,200 mg.

The DGA 2020–2025 provides some recommendations to support healthy eating for infants from birth to age 23 months. One of the key recommendations is called "responsive feeding," which is defined as emphasizing and responding to hunger and fullness displayed by the infant and young child. More information concerning this may be found at the DGA 2020–2025. The recommendation also suggests that parents utilize resources from the U.S. Department of Agriculture (USDA) to support healthy growth and development during infancy and toddlerhood.

There are a number of federally supported programs that can promote a healthy dietary pattern in households with limited income. These include the Special Supplemental Nutrition Program for Women, Infants and Children (WIC), the Child and Adult Care Food Program (CACFP), and the Supplemental Nutrition Assistance

CALORIE LEVEL OF PATTERN[a]	700	800	900	1,000
FOOD GROUP OR SUBGROUP[b,c]	Daily Amount of Food From Each Group[d] (Vegetable and protein foods subgroup amounts are per week.)			
Vegetables (cup eq/day)	⅔	¾	1	1
	Vegetable Subgroups in Weekly Amounts			
Dark-Green Vegetables (cup eq/wk)	1	⅓	½	½
Red and Orange Vegetables (cup eq/wk)	1	1 ¾	2 ½	2 ½
Beans, Peas, Lentils (cup eq/wk)	¾	⅓	½	½
Starchy Vegetables (cup eq/wk)	1	1 ½	2	2
Other Vegetables (cup eq/wk)	¾	1 ¼	1 ½	1 ½
Fruits (cup eq/day)	½	¾	1	1
Grains (ounce eq/day)	1 ¾	2 ¼	2 ½	3
Whole Grains (ounce eq/day)	1 ½	2	2	2
Refined Grains (ounce eq/day)	¼	¼	½	1
Dairy (cup eq/day)	1 ⅔	1 ¾	2	2
Protein Foods (ounce eq/day)	2	2	2	2
	Protein Foods Subgroups in Weekly Amounts			
Meats, Poultry (ounce eq/wk)	8 ¾	7	7	7 ¾
Eggs (ounce eq/wk)	2	2 ¾	2 ½	2 ½
Seafood (ounce eq/wk)[e]	2-3	2-3	2-3	2-3
Nuts, Seeds, Soy Products (ounce eq/wk)	1	1	1 ¼	1 ¼
Oils (grams/day)	9	9	8	13

FIGURE 28.1 Healthy U.S.-Style Dietary Pattern for toddlers ages 12 through 23 months who are no longer receiving human milk or infant formula, with daily or weekly amounts from food groups, subgroups, and components.

Source: *Dietary Guidelines for Americans, 2020–2025*, page 64.

Program (SNAP). The government-supported nutrition programs are particularly important for the 14% of families with children who experience food insecurity and may struggle to have access to foods needed to support a healthy dietary pattern.

28.4 CHILDREN AND ADOLESCENTS AGED 2–18 YEARS

During this period of time, the life stage is characterized by transitions and the formation of dietary patterns [28]. Current intake patterns among children and adolescents are inadequate and the physical activity is lower than it should be, both of which contribute to overweight and obesity. At this life stage there is also a potential to develop risk factors for chronic disease such as CVD and T2DM later in life. It is important to focus on this stage because dietary patterns established during this life stage tend to continue into adult years.

The youngest children are fully reliant on others to provide meals and snacks. As they move into school age and through adolescence, they begin to have more autonomy in terms of foods that are selected. This can create both opportunities and challenges. Current data on the youngest children show some erosion of the components of a dietary healthy pattern that may have been established during the infant and toddler stages. Unfortunately, dietary quality worsens through childhood and into adolescence, and the pattern drifts further from recommendations from the DGAs.

- Healthy Dietary Patterns
  The healthy dietary pattern involving more fruits and vegetables and whole grains that is recommended for adults is also recommended for children 2–18 years old. Moreover, calorie needs vary and are typically higher in males than in females. During adolescence, calorie intakes also must support diverse growth trajectories. In ages 2–4, females typically require 1,000–1,400 calories per day and males require 1,000–1,600 calories per day. At ages 5–8 females require 1,200–1,800 calories per day and males 1,200–2,000 calories per day.

  Unfortunately, childhood overweight and obesity have dramatically increased in the United States. Currently 41% of children and adolescents are either overweight or have obesity [5–13]. The prevalence of these conditions is higher in Hispanic and non-Hispanic Black children and adolescents compared to non-Hispanic Asians and Whites. Overweight and obesity had slowed somewhat in the decade prior to the COVID-19 pandemic but rapidly increased during this epidemic, particularly affecting low-income and minority groups. Overweight and obesity predispose youth to higher risk for serious health concerns later in life. In addition, children with obesity also are at increased risk for health concerns including high blood pressure, elevated cholesterol, and impaired glucose tolerance. This puts them at increased risk for both CVD and T2DM often occurring in teenage years and on into adulthood. In addition, there are significant psychological issues such as anxiety and depression and social concerns such as bullying and stigma that are more likely in children and adolescents with overweight or obesity.

  Clearly nutritional issues carry a significant role in overweight and obesity, although these conditions are multifactorial. Emphasizing nutrient-dense foods and beverage choices as well as encouraging regular physical activity represent key interventions to combat overweight and obesity. According to the Physical Activity Guidelines for American 2018 (PAGA 2018), over 60% of children and adolescents do not achieve the recommended level of physical activity, and this decreases significantly as children move into adolescence [29]. The Healthy U.S.-Style Dietary Pattern for children ages 2–8 is found in Figure 28.2. As in adults, emphasis is placed on fruits and vegetables, whole grains, and protein foods while limiting calories from other sources.

  Unfortunately, current intakes are not consistent with recommendations from the DGA 2020–2025 and deteriorate during the period between the ages of 2 and 18. Between the ages of 2 and 4 children have

CALORIE LEVEL OF PATTERN[a]	1,000	1,200	1,400	1,600	1,800	2,000
FOOD GROUP OR SUBGROUP[b]	**Daily Amount of Food From Each Group** (Vegetable and protein foods subgroup amounts are per week.)					
Vegetables (cup eq/day)	**1**	**1 ½**	**1 ½**	**2**	**2 ½**	**2 ½**
	Vegetable Subgroups in Weekly Amounts					
Dark-Green Vegetables (cup eq/wk)	½	1	1	1 ½	1 ½	1 ½
Red and Orange Vegetables (cup eq/wk)	2 ½	3	3	4	5 ½	5 ½
Beans, Peas, Lentils (cup eq/wk)	½	½	½	1	1 ½	1 ½
Starchy Vegetables (cup eq/wk)	2	3 ½	3 ½	4	5	5
Other Vegetables (cup eq/wk)	1 ½	2 ½	2 ½	3 ½	4	4
Fruits (cup eq/day)	**1**	**1**	**1 ½**	**1 ½**	**1 ½**	**2**
Grains (ounce eq/day)	**3**	**4**	**5**	**5**	**6**	**6**
Whole Grains (ounce eq/day)	1 ½	2	2 ½	3	3	3
Refined Grains (ounce eq/day)	1 ½	2	2 ½	2	3	3
Dairy (cup eq/day)	**2**	**2 ½**	**2 ½**	**2 ½**	**2 ½**	**2 ½**
Protein Foods (ounce eq/day)	**2**	**3**	**4**	**5**	**5**	**5 ½**
	Protein Foods Subgroups in Weekly Amounts					
Meats, Poultry, Eggs (ounce eq/wk)	10	14	19	23	23	26
Seafood (ounce eq/wk)[c]	2-3[d]	4	6	8	8	8
Nuts, Seeds, Soy Products (ounce eq/wk)	2	2	3	4	4	5
Oils (grams/day)	**15**	**17**	**17**	**22**	**22**	**24**
Limit on Calories for Other Uses (kcal/day)[e]	**130**	**80**	**90**	**150**	**190**	**280**
Limit on Calories for Other Uses (%/day)	13%	7%	6%	9%	10%	14%

FIGURE 28.2 Healthy U.S.-Style Dietary Pattern for children ages 2–8, with daily or weekly amounts from food groups, subgroups, and components.

Source: *Dietary Guidelines for Americans, 2020–2025*, page 74.

a Healthy Eating Index (HEI) of 61, but by the time they've reached the ages of 14–18, it has declined to 51. The current intake of added sugars, saturated fat, and sodium, even for children ages 2–4 are too high, with 61% of males and 57% of females exceeding the recommendations for added sugar and 87% of males and 88% of females exceeding the recommended limit for saturated fat, while 97% of males and 95% of females exceed the recommended 1,200 mg/day of sodium [30]. These unfortunate intakes continue to remain far too high all the way through the age of 18.

The Healthy U.S.-Style Dietary Pattern for children and adolescents ages 9–13 is found in Figure 28.3 while the Healthy U.S.-Style Dietary Pattern for adolescents ages 14–18 is found in Figure 28.4. In both instances, the same basic recommendations are made for the Healthy U.S.-Style Dietary Pattern including an emphasis on fruits and vegetables, beans, peas, lentils, whole grains, and protein-containing foods. The only differences are slightly lower calories are recommended for 9- to 13-year-olds and also 14- to 18-year-olds compared with recommendations for adults.

CALORIE LEVEL OF PATTERN[a]	1,400	1,600	1,800	2,000	2,200	2,400	2,600
FOOD GROUP OR SUBGROUP[b]	Daily Amount of Food From Each Group (Vegetable and protein foods subgroup amounts are per week.)						
Vegetables (cup eq/day)	**1 ½**	**2**	**2 ½**	**2 ½**	**3**	**3**	**3 ½**
	Vegetable Subgroups in Weekly Amounts						
Dark-Green Vegetables (cup eq/wk)	1	1 ½	1 ½	1 ½	2	2	2 ½
Red & Orange Vegetables (cup eq/wk)	3	4	5 ½	5 ½	6	6	7
Beans, Peas, Lentils (cup eq/wk)	½	1	1 ½	1 ½	2	2	2 ½
Starchy Vegetables (cup eq/wk)	3 ½	4	5	5	6	6	7
Other Vegetables (cup eq/wk)	2 ½	3 ½	4	4	5	5	5 ½
Fruits (cup eq/day)	**1 ½**	**1 ½**	**1 ½**	**2**	**2**	**2**	**2**
Grains (ounce eq/day)	**5**	**5**	**6**	**6**	**7**	**8**	**9**
Whole Grains (ounce eq/day)	2 ½	3	3	3	3 ½	4	4 ½
Refined Grains (ounce eq/day)	2 ½	2	3	3	3 ½	4	4 ½
Dairy (cup eq/day)	**3**	**3**	**3**	**3**	**3**	**3**	**3**
Protein Foods (ounce eq/day)	**4**	**5**	**5**	**5 ½**	**6**	**6 ½**	**6 ½**
	Protein Foods Subgroups in Weekly Amounts						
Meats, Poultry, Eggs (ounce eq/wk)	19	23	23	26	28	31	31
Seafood (ounce eq/wk)[c]	6	8	8	8	9	10	10
Nuts, Seeds, Soy Products (ounce eq/wk)	3	4	4	5	5	5	5
Oils (grams/day)	**17**	**22**	**24**	**27**	**29**	**31**	**34**
Limit on Calories for Other Uses (kcal/day)[d]	**50**	**100**	**140**	**240**	**250**	**320**	**350**
Limit on Calories for Other Uses (%/day)	4%	6%	8%	12%	11%	13%	13%

FIGURE 28.3 Healthy U.S.-Style Dietary Pattern for children and adolescents ages 9–13, with daily or weekly amounts from food groups, subgroups, and components.

Source: *Dietary Guidelines for Americans, 2020–2025*, page 81.

28.5 SPECIAL CONSIDERATIONS

Guidelines for healthy nutrition already described for the general U.S. population also apply to children and adolescents. The same nutrients of concern for adults are also of concern for children and adolescents—namely, calcium, vitamin D, potassium, and dietary fiber. The DGAs provide the foundation for healthy dietary patterns in adulthood and help to lower the risk of chronic disease later in life.

Some of the categories of foods to limit or avoid included sugar-sweetened beverages and processed foods that often contain considerable amounts of both saturated fat and sodium. Throughout childhood and adolescence, consumption of dairy and fortified soy alternatives can make a contribution to a healthy dietary pattern. Nutrient-dense options within the dairy group are unsweetened and fat-free and low-fat (1%) milk, yogurt, and cheese, as well as fortified beverages. These alternatives provide protein and a variety of nutrients that are typically underconsumed in childhood. Dairy foods are an important source of protein and vitamin D, which are important to adolescents' support, development, and increase in bone mass.

CALORIE LEVEL OF PATTERN[a]	1,800	2,000	2,200	2,400	2,600	2,800	3,000	3,200
FOOD GROUP OR SUBGROUP[b]	**Daily Amount of Food From Each Group** (Vegetable and protein foods subgroup amounts are per week.)							
Vegetables (cup eq/day)	**2 ½**	**2 ½**	**3**	**3**	**3 ½**	**3 ½**	**4**	**4**
	Vegetable Subgroups in Weekly Amounts							
Dark-Green Vegetables (cup eq/wk)	1 ½	1 ½	2	2	2 ½	2 ½	2 ½	2 ½
Red and Orange Vegetables (cup eq/wk)	5 ½	5 ½	6	6	7	7	7 ½	7 ½
Beans, Peas, Lentils (cup eq/wk)	1 ½	1 ½	2	2	2 ½	2 ½	3	3
Starchy Vegetables (cup eq/wk)	5	5	6	6	7	7	8	8
Other Vegetables (cup eq/wk)	4	4	5	5	5 ½	5 ½	7	7
Fruits (cup eq/day)	**1 ½**	**2**	**2**	**2**	**2**	**2 ½**	**2 ½**	**2 ½**
Grains (ounce eq/day)	**6**	**6**	**7**	**8**	**9**	**10**	**10**	**10**
Whole Grains (ounce eq/day)	3	3	3 ½	4	4 ½	5	5	5
Refined Grains (ounce eq/day)	3	3	3 ½	4	4 ½	5	5	5
Dairy (cup eq/day)	**3**	**3**	**3**	**3**	**3**	**3**	**3**	**3**
Protein Foods (ounce eq/day)	**5**	**5 ½**	**6**	**6 ½**	**6 ½**	**7**	**7**	**7**
	Protein Foods Subgroups in Weekly Amounts							
Meats, Poultry, Eggs (ounce eq/wk)	23	26	28	31	31	33	33	33
Seafood (ounce eq/wk)	8	8	9	10	10	10	10	10
Nuts, Seeds, Soy Products (ounce eq/wk)	4	5	5	5	5	6	6	6
Oils (grams/day)	**24**	**27**	**29**	**31**	**34**	**36**	**44**	**51**
Limit on Calories for Other Uses (kcal/day)[c]	**140**	**240**	**250**	**320**	**350**	**370**	**440**	**580**
Limit on Calories for Other Uses (%/day)	8%	12%	11%	13%	13%	13%	15%	18%

FIGURE 28.4 Healthy U.S.-Style Dietary Pattern for adolescents ages 14–18, with daily or weekly amounts from food groups, subgroups, and components.

Source: *Dietary Guidelines for Americans, 2020–2025*, page 84.

The difference between the recommended food group amounts and the current intake is greater for adolescents aged 14–18 than in any other age group across the lifespan. This makes adolescents at greater risk for dietary inadequacy than other age groups. This is particularly problematic since this creates nutritional risks at a time of rapid growth and development.

28.6 SUPPORTING HEALTHY EATING

Many changes occur during childhood including physical, mental, and emotional changes. It is important for people involved in the lives of children and adolescents to help establish and maintain healthy dietary patterns as well as supporting healthy weight to lower the risk of chronic disease [28].

Parents, guardians, and caregivers have a primary role in supporting healthy eating, particularly in early childhood. It should be emphasized that children's dietary patterns often resemble those of the household, which highlights the importance of the environment to establish a healthy eating pattern. It is particularly important that children be exposed to healthy eating when they experience changes in their daily routines such as spending time at childcare or school settings. A good example of this is providing nutrient-dense foods and vegetables, carrot sticks, etc., during snack time.

During adolescence as the individuals transitions to increasing autonomy, the influence of peers plays a significant role in food choices, and more foods and beverages are consumed outside the home. This might lead to a preference for convenience foods that are not nutrient dense. Parents, guardians, and caregivers can continue to support healthy eating by providing convenient access to nutrient-dense foods. In schools and community settings, healthy eating can be encouraged by creating an environment that makes healthy choices the norm.

28.7 EFFECTIVE NUTRITION EDUCATION PROGRAMS

Providing effective nutrition education programs is very important to help both children and parents understand and implement healthy nutritional practices [31,32]. Research in this area has shown that successful interventions involve a multicomponent approach that is age appropriate and conducted for an adequate duration (greater than or equal to six months). It is also important to engage parents and ensure proper alignment between stated objectives of the intervention and desired outcomes. Engaging parents on a face-to-face basis was particularly important, particularly in elementary schools. In secondary school, nutrition education interventions often add policy and environmental changes and emphasize age-appropriate activities just as done in successful elementary school programs.

Preschool programs that are successful also emphasize face-to-face parental engagement and feature hands-on activities with parents and children interacting in activities such as preparing fruit and vegetable snacks.

28.8 CARDIOVASCULAR RISK AND DIET IN CHILDREN

Nutrition plays a significant role in lowering the risk of CVD in children. Strong evidence exists that the atherosclerotic process begins in early childhood and progresses slowly into adulthood [14–22]. This ultimately leads to coronary heart disease (CHD), which remains the leading cause of death in the United States. Many risk factors are important for the development of CVD, including family history of CVD, obesity, elevated blood pressure, dyslipidemia, diabetes, and cigarette smoking. In addition, diets high in saturated fat and trans fat and excessive energy intake, as well as physical inactivity, are lifestyle-related behaviors that can increase the risk of CVD. Many risk factors that have been previously considered to be largely found in adults are now increasingly being found in children. Many of these are driven by obesity and poor diet.

Dietary factors that can contribute to excessive energy intake relative to energy expenditure include regular intake of sugar-sweetened beverages (SSBs) [33], greater intake of fast foods, increased intake of dietary fats and added sugars, and larger portions of food. Some observational research also indicates that low intake of dairy and calcium-rich foods may also increase obesity risk. Skipping breakfast has been shown to be a dietary behavior associated with obesity. Increased intake of fruits and vegetables may be associated with decreased risk of obesity in children. Family meals [34], especially those with positive family and parent-level interpersonal dynamics, including positive food communication and positive reinforcement, are associated with reduced risk of childhood overweight and obesity.

Foods that are high in total calories, sugars, salt, and fat and low in nutrients are often highly advertised and marketed through the media and are typically targeted to children and adolescents. This can influence food choices and increase overall caloric intake. There is some emerging research that formula-fed infants may be at higher risk for increased weight compared to breastfed infants. In addition, low access to healthy foods may also have an unfavorable impact on food choices and eating behaviors. It is also possible that food insecurity is related to pediatric overweight and obesity.

Dyslipidemia is often associated with obesity and has become an increasing problem in children. Nutrition plays a vital role in treating dyslipidemia in children as well as adults. The current pediatric dietary guidelines for treating children identified with dyslipidemia includes a two-step approach called the Cardiovascular Health and Integrative Lifestyle Diet or CHILD-1 and CHILD-2 [35]. The nutritional components of CHILD-1 and CHILD-2 diets for low-density lipoprotein cholesterol (LDL-C) and non–high-density lipoprotein cholesterol (HDL-C) reduction are summarized in Table 28.1. CHILD-1 is appropriate for all children over the age of two and, for the most part, consistent with the 2025 DGAs. This pattern is considered the first-line approach to managing LDL-C and non–HLD-C levels in children. In children who have persistently high elevated LDL-C and non–HLD-C after three to six months of compliance with CHILD-1, CHILD-2 is recommended. The nutritional components of CHILD-1 and CHILD-2 are found in Table 28.1.

TABLE 28.1
Nutritional Intervention Approaches in the Cardiovascular Health Integrated Lifestyle Diet-1 and -2 for Lowering Lipids in Children over Two Years of Age

Nutrient Target for Lowering LDL	CHILD-1	CHILD-2
Total dietary fat	25–30% of calories	25–30% of calories
Saturated fat	<10 % of daily calories	<7 % of daily calories
Trans fat	Avoided	Avoided
Monounsaturated fat	Up to 10–15% of calories	Up to 10–15% of calories
Polyunsaturated fat	Up to 10% of calories	Up to 10% of calories
Cholesterol	300 mg or less	200 mg or less
Dietary fiber	Child's age + 5 g up to 14 g/1,000 calories	Child's age + 5 g up to 14 g/1,000 calories
Simple carbohydrates	Reduction of sugar-sweetened beverages	Reduction of sugar-sweetened beverages

Source: Adapted from Faulkner C, Couch S, Hemingway J. Cardiovascular risk and Diet in Children. In Rippe JM: Lifestyle Medicine, 3rd ed. CRC Press. (Boca Raton), 2019. Used with permission.

In addition, weight management is recommended for children with a body mass index (BMI) of greater than or equal to the 85th percentile. High blood pressure is also becoming increasingly common in children. Reducing salt intake plays an important role in children, as in adults, to aid in lowering blood pressure. As already indicated, the median sodium intake for children and adolescents in the United States currently exceeds the current guidelines from the DGA 2020–2025. In the United States, an average of 83% of total sodium consumption comes from pre-prepared foods purchased from grocery stores and restaurants. Pizza, breads and rolls, and processed meats and poultry are the greatest sources of sodium in children. Therefore, it is important to teach parents and their children how to read nutrition facts panels on product labels for sodium content and to choose products that have lower sodium. Foods cooked from scratch are naturally lower in sodium than most instant or boxed meals and takeout foods.

28.9 NUTRITION AND EARLY CHILDHOOD EDUCATION

Childcare outside of the home is relatively common in the United States. Over half of children aged two to five years attend some form of out-of-home childcare and spend approximately 30 hours per week or more in this care [36,37]. Thus, parents and early childhood education (ECE) providers share the responsibility for feeding children. For this reason, providers of ECE should pay close attention to the nutritional quality of foods and beverages served, as well as the mealtime environments [38]. Other factors that may impact on issues such as childhood obesity include physical activity, sleep, and stress while at childcare. Important tips for how to improve nutrition during the ECE are available from the Academy of Nutrition and Dietetics in their Position Statement on the Benchmarks for Nutrition in Childcare [38]. This may be found in the references at the end of this chapter.

28.10 VEGAN NUTRITION FOR MOTHERS AND CHILDREN

Over the past decade, the number of individuals following vegan diets has increased [37]. A completely plant-based diet is suitable during pregnancy, infancy, and childhood provided that it is well planned. It is particularly important to pay attention to nutrients that may be critical such as protein, fiber, omega-3 fatty acids, iron, zinc, iodine, calcium, vitamin D, and vitamin B_{12}. Recommendations made by a panel of experts from the Scientific Society for Vegetarian Nutrition (SSVN) provide useful information for good nutrition for children who live in a family that practices a vegan nutritional plan [39]. This information may be found in the references at the end of this chapter.

28.11 COVID-19 AND CHILD FOOD AND NUTRITION INSECURITY

The COVID-19 pandemic had significant adverse effects on food, nutrition, and health security for a variety of particularly vulnerable groups including young children and pregnant and lactating women and further exacerbated social and health inequities [40–43]. This was partially due to economic insecurities as well as disruption in food supply chains. A variety of recommendations have been made to try to mitigate the effects that COVID-19 has had on childhood food insecurity. Specific recommendations include the following:

1. Adopt and continue school feeding and other food assistance programs to continue with the provision of meals to quarantined families with children, adolescents, and pregnant and lactating women.
2. Develop equitable, effective rapid response systems to prevent or mitigate food insecurity based on complex, adaptive system frameworks.
3. Monitor and use surveillance systems to effectively identify and target the provision of healthy and nutritious foods to families who are particularly socioeconomically vulnerable. This is particularly true for families where women are pregnant or lactating and where young children are present.

28.12 DEVELOPING HEALTHY FOOD PREFERENCES IN PRESCHOOL CHILDREN

It is important to find ways of increasing fruit and vegetable intake in early childhood. Research in this area suggests that taste exposure interventions yield the best outcomes [32]. Visual exposure and experiential learning also show some success. This is important since developing eating habits in the early years of life often extend into adulthood. Children learn about their food likes and dislikes by direct contact with food such as through tasting, feeling, seeing, and smelling and also by observing the food in the environment, for example, the eating behaviors of others. Developing early exposure and food preferences for healthy nutritional foods such as vegetables can be an effective strategy for lowering the risk of obesity in later childhood years and adulthood.

28.13 MALNUTRITION, WASTING, OVERWEIGHT, STUNTING, AND HUNGER

Malnutrition is a broad term that includes undernutrition, wasting, stunting, underweight, and inadequate vitamins or minerals as well as overweight [23,24], obesity, and resulting diet-related noncommunicable diseases. Globally in 2020, 149 million children under five years old were estimated to be stunted (too short for age), 45 million were estimated to be wasted (too thin for height), and 38.9 million were overweight or obese.

According to the World Health Organization (WHO), approximately 45% of deaths among children under the age of five years are linked to undernutrition. These mostly occur in lower- to middle-income countries. In addition, malnutrition can result in inadequate intake of vitamins and minerals. These nutritional components are essential to enable the production of enzymes, hormones, and other substances essential for proper growth and development.

Reducing stunting in children is a significant equity consideration for achieving global nutrition targets that the WHO has established for 2025. In the United States about one in eight children are at risk for hunger. Black and Latino children are more likely to face hunger than White children because of systemic racial injustice and inequities. According to the USDA in 2021, 22% of Black children were food insecure and 18.5% of Latino children were food insecure. This means that there are an estimated 12 million children struggling with hunger in the United States. This is an unacceptable level of food insecurity in the world's most affluent country.

28.14 CONCLUSIONS

Nutrition during childhood is critically important to lower the risk of chronic disease. Healthy nutrition starts at the beginning of life and is an important issue for infants and toddlers. The DGA 2020–2025 recommends human milk be consumed during the first six months of life. If human milk is not available, infant formula may be utilized. If infant formula is utilized, infants should be fed an iron-fortified commercial infant formula. Infant formulas are regulated by the FDA. In addition, children should be exposed to a variety of different foods after the age of six months, which allows for taste preferences to be developed, which in turn may contribute to lifelong eating patterns.

For children between the ages of 2 and 18, the general guidance on healthy eating for adults should be maintained. This involves consuming a diet with increased fruits and vegetables and whole grains and reducing the quantities of red meat or processed meats, sugar, salt, and refined grains. The Healthy U.S.-Style Dietary Pattern is appropriate for children between the ages of 2 and 18 with adjustments made for the number of calories consumed at any given age given the size and gender of each child. Typically, female children consume fewer calories than males.

Excellent information for establishing healthy nutrition patterns for children from infants through the age of 18 can be found, listed by age group, in the 2020–2025 DGA.

Clinical Applications

- Establishing healthy nutrition during infancy and childhood is critically important for improving lifelong nutritional habits.
- Healthy nutritional habits are essential for lowering the risk of obesity, CVD, and diabetes.
- The recommended components of healthy nutrition for children aged 2–18 include increased fruits and vegetable consumption as well as whole grains. Added sugars, salt, and refined grains, as well as processed foods and red meat, should be minimized.
- Nutrients at risk for childhood are similar to those for adults and include calcium, vitamin D, fiber, and potassium.
- Since food is typically provided by a parent or caretaker, discussions should take place with the entire family.
- Childhood obesity has risen dramatically in the past two decades in the United States. Proper caloric consumption should be discussed with the entire family.

REFERENCES

1. Benjamin-Neelon S. Position of the Academy of Nutrition and Dietetics: Benchmarks for nutrition in child care. J Acad Nutr Diet. 2018;118(7):1291–1300.
2. U.S. Department of Agriculture and U.S. Department of Health and Human Services. *Dietary Guidelines for Americans, 2020–2025*, 9th edition. December 2020. DietaryGuidelines.gov. 2020.
3. Das J, Lassi Z, Hoodbhoy Z, et al. Nutrition for the next generation: Older children and adolescents. Ann Nutr Metable. 2018;72(Suppl 3):56–64.
4. Clark H, Coll-Seck A, Banerjee A, et al. A future for the world's children? A WHO-UNICEF-Lancet commission. Lancet. 2020;22;395(10224):605–658.
5. Moore J, Haemer M. Childhood obesity. In Rippe JM (ed). Lifestyle Medicine, 4th edition. Boca Raton: CRC Press, 2024.
6. Ogden C, Carroll M, Lawman H, et al. Trends in obesity prevalence among children and adolescents in the United States, 1988–1994 through 2013–2014. JAMA. 2016;7;315(21):2292–2299.
7. Ogden C, Carroll M, Kit B, et al. Prevalence of childhood and adult obesity in the United States, 2011–2012. JAMA. 2014;311(8):806–814.
8. Wang Y, Cai L, Wu Y, et al. What childhood obesity prevention programmes work? A systematic review and meta-analysis. Obes Rev. 2015;16(7):547–565.
9. Vine M, Hargreaves M, Briefel R, et al. Expanding the role of primary care in the prevention and treatment of childhood obesity: A review of clinic- and community-based recommendations and interventions. J Obes. 2013;2013:172035.
10. Skinner A, Skelton J. Prevalence and trends in obesity and severe obesity among children in the United States, 1999–2012. JAMA Pediatr. 2014;168:561.
11. Barlow S, Expert Committee. Expert committee recommendations regarding the prevention, assessment, and treatment of child and adolescent overweight and obesity: Summary report. Pediatrics. 2007;120(Suppl 4):S164–S192.
12. Kelly A, Barlow S, Rao G, et al. Severe obesity in children and adolescents: Identification, associated health risks, and treatment approaches: A scientific statement from the American Heart Association. Circulation. 2013;128:1689–1712.
13. US Preventive Services Task Force, Grossman D, Bibbins-Domingo K, et al. Screening for obesity in children and adolescents: US Preventive Services Task Force recommendation statement. JAMA. 2017;317:2417.
14. Faulkner C, Couch S, Hemingway J. Cardiovascular risk and diet in children. In Rippe JM (ed). Lifestyle Medicine, 4th edition. Boca Raton: CRC Press, 2024.
15. Berenson G, Srinivasan S, Bao W, et al. Association between multiple cardiovascular risk factors and atherosclerosis in children and young adults. The Bogalusa Heart Study. N Engl J Med. 1998;338(23):1650–1656.
16. McMahan C, Gidding S, Malcom G, et al. Pathobiological determinants of atherosclerosis in Youth Research Group. Pathobiological determinants of atherosclerosis in youth risk scores are associated with early and advanced atherosclerosis. Pediatrics. 2006;118(4):1447–1455.
17. Raitakari O, Juonala M, Kähönen M, et al. Cardiovascular risk factors in childhood and carotid artery intima-media thickness in adulthood: The cardiovascular risk in young finns study. JAMA. 2003;290(17):2277–2283.
18. Kavey R, Simons-Morton D, de Jesus J (supple eds). Expert panel on integrated guidelines for cardiovascular health and risk reduction in children and adolescents: Summary report. Pediatrics. 2011;128(5):S213–S256.

19. Caranti D, Tock L, Prado W, et al. Long-term multidisciplinary therapy decreases predictors and prevalence of metabolic syndrome in obese adolescents. Nutr Metable Cardiovasc Dis. 2007;17:e11–e13.
20. Sinha R, Fisch G, Teague B, et al. Prevalence of impaired glucose tolerance among children and adolescents with marked obesity. N Engl J Med. 2002;346:802–810.
21. Kit B, Kuklina E, Carroll M, et al. Prevalence of and trends in dyslipidemia and blood pressure among US children and adolescents, 1999–2012. JAMA Pediatr. 2015;169:272–279.
22. Baker-Smith C, Gidding S. Diagnosis, management and treatment of systemic hypertension in youth. In Rippe JM (ed). Lifestyle Medicine, 4th edition. Boca Raton: CRC Press, 2024.
23. World Health Organization. Reducing stunting in children: Equity considerations for achieving the global nutrition targets 2025. Reducing Stunting in Children: Equity Considerations for Achieving the Global Targets 2025 (who.int) (Accessed January 18, 2024).
24. World Health Organization. Malnutrition. Malnutrition (who.int) (Accessed January 18, 2024).
25. *Dietary Guidelines for Americans, 2020–2025*, Infants and Toddlers. Chapter 2. Page 51. www.dietaryguidelines.gov/ (Accessed January 18, 2024).
26. Togias A, Cooper S, Acebal M. Addendum Guidelines for the Prevention of Peanut Allergy in the United States: Report of the National Institute of Allergy and Infectious Diseases-Sponsored Expert Panel. www.niaid.nih.gov/sites/default/files/addendum-peanut-allergy-prevention-guidelines.pdf (Accessed January 18, 2024).
27. *Dietary Guidelines for Americans, 2020–2025*, Current Intakes: Ages 12 Through 23 Months. Chapter 2, Page 65. www.dietaryguidelines.gov/ (Accessed January 19, 2024).
28. *Dietary Guidelines for Americans, 2020–2025*, Children and Adolescents. Chapter 3, Page 70. www.dietaryguidelines.gov/ (Accessed January 19, 2024).
29. Dietary Guidelines for Americans, 2018. https://health.gov/our-work/nutrition-physical-activity/dietary-guidelines. (Accessed January 19, 2024).
30. *Dietary Guidelines for Americans, 2020–2025*, Analysis of What We Eat in America, NHANES 2015–2016, Ages 2–18, Day 1 Intake, Weighted. Healthy Eating Index Scores Across Childhood and Adolescence. Chapter 3, Page 75.
31. Murimi M, Moyeda-Carabaza A, Nguyen B, et al. Factors that contribute to effective nutrition education interventions in children: A systematic review. Nutr Rev. 2018 Aug 1;76(8):553–580.
32. Nekitsing C, Hetherington M, Blundell-Birtill P. Developing healthy food preferences in preschool children through taste exposure, sensory learning, and nutrition education. Curr Obes Rep. 2018;7(1):60–67.
33. Academy of Nutrition and Dietetics Evidence Analysis Library (EAL). 2015 Pediatric Weight Management Evidence-Based Nutrition Practice Guideline. 2015. pqnew139.pdf (andeal.org) (Accessed February 1, 2024).
34. Berge J, Rowley S, Trofholz A, et al. Childhood obesity and interpersonal dynamics during family meals. Pediatrics. 2014;134(5):923–932.
35. Van Horn L, Vincent E. The CHILD-1 and DASH diets: Rationale and translational applications. Pediatric Annals. 2013:42:372–374.
36. US Census Bureau. Childcare: An Important Part of American Life. www.census.gov/library/visualizations/2013/comm/child_care.html (Accessed January 19, 2024).
37. The Federal Interagency Forum on Child and Family Statistics. America's Children: Key National Indicators of Well-Being. Washington, DC: US Government Printing Office, 2015.

38. American Academy of Pediatrics, American Public Health Association, National Resource Center for Health and Safety in Child Care and Early Education. Caring for Our Children: National Health and Safety Performance Standards; Guidelines for Early Care and Education Programs. 4th edition. Itasca, IL: American Academy of Pediatrics, 2019.
39. Baroni L, Goggi S, Battaglino R, et al. Vegan nutrition for mothers and children: Practical tools for healthcare providers. Nutrients. 2018;20;11(1):5.
40. Pérez-Escamilla R, Cunningham K, Moran V. COVID-19 and maternal and child food and nutrition insecurity: A complex syndemic. Matern Child Nutr. 2020;16(3):e13036.
41. Osendarp S, Akuoku J, Black R, et al. The COVID-19 crisis will exacerbate maternal and child undernutrition and child mortality in low- and middle-income countries. Nat Food. 2021;2(7):476–484.
42. Roberton T, Carter E, Chou V, et al. Early estimates of the indirect effects of the COVID-19 pandemic on maternal and child mortality in low-income and middle-income countries: A modelling study. Lancet Glob Health. 2020;8(7):e901–e908.
43. Masonbrink A, Hurley E. Advocating for children during the COVID-19 school closures. Pediatrics. 2020;146(3).

29 Nutrition and Women's Health

Key Points

- Healthy nutrition as recommended by the *Dietary Guidelines for Americans 2020–2025* and other prestigious medical organizations should be recommended to all women.
- Typically, women currently follow the traditional Western diet, which is an unhealthy diet.
- Women should be recommended to consume more fruits and vegetables and whole grains, while avoiding foods high in sugar, fat, and excess sodium.
- All of these issues apply equally well to women of all life stages and particularly for women who are pregnant or lactating.

29.1 INTRODUCTION

Healthy nutrition is critically important for women at every stage of their lives. This chapter will focus largely on health considerations for adult women between the ages of 19 and 59. The issues related to healthy nutrition and healthy dietary patterns, however, apply also equally well to children and older women and, indeed, boys and men as well.

Some nuanced differences exist in these other groups. These other issues are dealt with in separate chapters in this book.

In addition to general issues related to nutrition in adult women, there is also a section in this chapter devoted to nutrition during pregnancy and lactating. The current chapter will also briefly delineate issues related to nutrition during the preconception period. Other lifestyle medicine modalities will also be outlined such as physical activity, weight maintenance, and avoiding tobacco products, all of which factor into the overall health of women. Other sections of this chapter will focus on key issues related to how nutrition plays a role in reducing the risk of cardiovascular disease (CVD) as well as diabetes and osteoporosis in women.

During the adult years individuals go through a variety of changes which are characterized by increased responsibilities, including starting or completing an education and training and managing work and family, all the while planning for transitioning to older adulthood. The complex tasks of this period in adult women's lives can create real or perceived barriers for healthy eating. In addition, constraints on available time and financial resources may make it challenging for women to adopt and maintain a healthy dietary patten.

To further complicate matters, many individuals enter the adult life stage with an unhealthy dietary pattern already established from childhood and adolescence. This

DOI: 10.1201/9781003452607-29

can make the transition into healthy eating much more challenging. Women, in particular, are often the individuals who shop for and prepare food for the entire family, so establishing healthy eating habits for a woman herself also plays an important role for establishing healthy dietary patterns both for her husband or partner and children.

In addition, over half of adult women live with one or more chronic diseases [1]. These diseases are often related to poor-quality diets as well as physical inactivity and adult weight gain. The average adult woman gains a pound a year after the age of 20 [2], which also creates issues related to weight management. All of these issues will be addressed in this chapter.

29.2 HEALTHY DIETARY PATTERNS

As discussed in multiple chapters in this book, modern nutrition research focuses on dietary patterns. In contrast, in previous decades more emphasis was placed on individual nutrients or individual foods. A consensus among nutrition professionals exists now that the overall dietary pattern is the key to either healthy or unhealthy nutrition. A large body of research demonstrates that multiple dietary patterns are associated with improved health and reduced risk of chronic disease. These include the Healthy U.S.-Style Dietary Pattern which will be a focus of this chapter [3]. Other healthy diets include the Mediterranean diet (MedDiet) [4], multiple diets recognized by the American Heart Association [5], and the Dietary Approach to Stop Hypertension (DASH) diet [6]. All of these diets are consistent in emphasizing increased consumption of fruits and vegetables and whole grains, low-fat dairy products, fish, and liquid, nontropical oils such as olive oil. In addition to cardiovascular benefits, all of these dietary patterns lower the risk of gaining weight and becoming obese.

The Healthy U.S.-Style Pattern for adults between ages 19 and 59 is listed in Figure 29.1. This table is divided according to calorie level. Calorie levels typically decline during adulthood due to changes in metabolism that accompany aging. Level of physical activity, body composition, and presence of chronic disease are additional factors that affect calorie needs.

In general terms, females between the ages of 19 and 30 require approximately 1,800–2,400 calories a day. Calorie needs for women between the ages of 31 and 59 range between 1,600–2,200 calories a day. It should be emphasized that at all calorie levels nutrient-dense foods and beverages are recommended. These are foods and beverages that provide vitamins, minerals, and other health-promoting components and have little added sugars, saturated fat, or sodium. Components of a healthy diet fit into the category of nutrient-dense foods, which includes vegetables, fruits, whole grains, seafood, eggs, beans, peas, and lentils as well as unsalted nuts and seeds, fat-free or low-fat dairy products, and lean meats or poultry when prepared with little or no added sugars, salt, and sodium.

29.3 CURRENT INTAKES

As already indicated in the chapter on the Western diet (WD) [7], many women consume the standard American diet, which is unhealthy. The WD contains too much

CALORIE LEVEL OF PATTERN[a]	1,600	1,800	2,000	2,200	2,400	2,600	2,800	3,000
FOOD GROUP OR SUBGROUP[b]	Daily Amount of Food From Each Group (Vegetable and protein foods subgroup amounts are per week.)							
Vegetables (cup eq/day)	2	2 ½	2 ½	3	3	3 ½	3 ½	4
	Vegetable Subgroups in Weekly Amounts							
Dark-Green Vegetables (cup eq/wk)	1 ½	1 ½	1 ½	2	2	2 ½	2 ½	2 ½
Red & Orange Vegetables (cup eq/wk)	4	5 ½	5 ½	6	6	7	7	7 ½
Beans, Peas, Lentils (cup eq/wk)	1	1 ½	1 ½	2	2	2 ½	2 ½	3
Starchy Vegetables (cup eq/wk)	4	5	5	6	6	7	7	8
Other Vegetables (cup eq/wk)	3 ½	4	4	5	5	5 ½	5 ½	7
Fruits (cup eq/day)	1 ½	1 ½	2	2	2	2	2 ½	2 ½
Grains (ounce eq/day)	5	6	6	7	8	9	10	10
Whole Grains (ounce eq/day)	3	3	3	3 ½	4	4 ½	5	5
Refined Grains (ounce eq/day)	2	3	3	3 ½	4	4 ½	5	5
Dairy (cup eq/day)	3	3	3	3	3	3	3	3
Protein Foods (ounce eq/day)	5	5	5 ½	6	6 ½	6 ½	7	7
	Protein Foods Subgroups in Weekly Amounts							
Meats, Poultry, Eggs (ounce eq/wk)	23	23	26	28	31	31	33	33
Seafood (ounce eq/wk)	8	8	8	9	10	10	10	10
Nuts, Seeds, Soy Products (ounce eq/wk)	4	4	5	5	5	5	6	6
Oils (grams/day)	22	24	27	29	31	34	36	44
Limit on Calories for Other Uses (kcal/day)[c]	100	140	240	250	320	350	370	440
Limit on Calories for Other Uses (%/day)	6%	8%	12%	11%	13%	13%	13%	15%

FIGURE 29.1 Healthy U.S.-Style Dietary Pattern for adults ages 19–59, with daily or weekly amounts from food groups, subgroups, and components.

Source: Chapter 4. U.S. Department of Agriculture and U.S. Department of Health and Human Services. U.S. Department of Agriculture and U.S. Department of Health and Human Services. *Dietary Guidelines for Americans, 2020–2025*. 9th Edition. December 2020. Available at DietaryGuidelines.gov. 2020.

red meat, saturated fat, added sugar and salt, and refined grains. While the average diet for adult women is slightly more healthy than for men, it is still far below what it should be.

The percentage of females who exceed the recommended limit of 10% of added calories from sugar is 66%. In the area of saturated fat, 71% of women exceed the recommended limit of 10%. In the area of sodium, the average women consumes 3,642 milligrams. Eighty-four percent of women exceed the recommended limit of 2,300 milligrams of sodium per day. In addition, the average women currently consumes only slightly more than one serving of vegetable a day and consumes less than 1 ounce of whole grain, both of which are far below recommended levels. While total protein foods in women are within the recommended average, unfortunately, most of this comes from meats, poultry, and eggs. The average female consumes less than half of the recommended servings of seafood. These current intake levels are consistent both for ages 19–30 and 31–59 among women.

29.4 SPECIAL CONSIDERATIONS

As described in Chapter 8, the Dietary Guidelines for Americans (DGAs) 2020–2025 recommend focusing on dietary changes to increase intakes of fiber, calcium, and vitamin D, while decreasing intake of added sugars, saturated fat, and sodium. The issue of how much alcohol that both men and women are consuming in the United States is also important to consider.

- **Dietary fiber**—Dietary patterns that do not meet the recommended intakes of fruits, vegetables, and whole grains result in low intakes of dietary fiber [8]. More than 90% of women do not meet recommended intakes of dietary fiber. This results from the fact that 85% of women do not consume the recommended amounts of fruits, vegetables, and whole grains. The low consumption of fiber is particularly important during adulthood since this is a period of time where there is often the onset or progression of diet-related chronic diseases. Dietary fiber reduces the risk of CVD and diabetes.
- **Calcium and vitamin D**—Calcium and vitamin D are important for both men and women at any age [9–11]. At most, women do not consume adequate amounts of these nutrients. Close to 60% of women over the age of 19 do not consume enough calcium, and more than 90% do not consume enough vitamin D [3]. Dietary sources of calcium and vitamin D include low-fat dairy foods, fortified soy alternatives, and seafood, all of which are being underconsumed by females between the ages of 19 and 59. Calcium consumption is particularly important during the period when peak bone mass is accruing for both men and women (ages 19–30). It is also important for women in the postmenopausal period when rapid bone remodeling occurs. A healthy dietary pattern that includes calcium-rich foods such as low-fat milk and yogurt and fortified soy alternatives and fish such as salmon can help adult women better meet recommendations. Vitamin D aids in the absorption of calcium, and choosing foods that are fortified with vitamin D including milk, fortified soy beverages, and some whole grain cereals can help females meet these needs. While the body can make vitamin D from exposure to the sun, many individuals have difficulty producing sufficient vitamin D from sunlight exposure alone [12,13].
- **Saturated fat**—As already indicated, over 70% of adult females exceed the recommend percentage of total calories from saturated fat [3]. This is unfortunate since saturated fat is associated with increased risk of CVD. The prevalence of CVD increases with age. High low-density lipoprotein (LDL) cholesterol becomes more prevalent between the ages of 60 and 69 in women. The top sources of saturated fats for women include deli sandwiches, burgers, tacos, burritos, grilled cheese, and hot dogs [14]. Strategies for lowering saturated fat include using lean meats or low-fat cheese to prepare foods and substituting beans in place of meats for a protein source. Utilizing sources of unsaturated fat such as olive oil, avocados, nuts, and

seeds as well as canola oil, saffron, soybean, and sunflower oil instead of butter can also reduce intakes of saturated fat.

- **Sodium**—As already indicated, over 80% of females consume more sodium than the recommended limits from the DGA 2020–2025 of 2,300 milligrams per day. The average female in the United States is consuming over 3,600 milligrams per day. This is important since the prevalence of high blood pressure increases throughout adult life, and over 50% of females between the ages of 40 and 59 have high blood pressure [3]. Increased sodium consumption is clearly associated with high blood pressure. This is particularly important because hypertension is a significant risk factor for both CVD and stroke. Decreasing the amount of sodium can make a big difference in lowering the prevalence of hypertension. Sodium is found in many prepared foods and beverages where it is often added during commercial processing. Reducing sodium by not adding salt during food preparation can make a start in lowering the amount of sodium consumption. Since females are often the individuals who prepare food for the family, this can also make a big difference in the prevalence of high blood pressure in men as well.
- **Added sugars**—As already indicated, over 60% of women exceed the recommended amount of added sugar in the diet of 10% of total energy [3]. This increase in added sugar is particularly concerning since added sugar has been associated with excess calorie intake and weight gain. Sugar-sweetened beverages (SSBs) contribute over 40% of the daily intake of added sugars. SSBs should be replaced with beverage options that contain no added sugars such as water. About 30% of added sugar comes from desserts and sweet snacks, candies, and sweetened breakfast cereals. The remaining 30% of added sugars comes from a variety of food categories. By understanding where added sugar comes from in the total diet, food choices can be made to minimize the amount of added sugars.
- **Alcoholic beverages**—Alcoholic beverages are not a component of the USDA Dietary Pattern. Calories from alcoholic beverages are considered "discretionary." Regular consumption of alcoholic beverages can make it challenging for adults to meet the food group and nutrient needs while not consuming excess calories.

The majority of adults, both males and females, currently consume alcoholic beverages. Over 60% of the adult females between the ages of 21 and 59 report alcoholic beverage consumption in the past month, and approximately half of those report binge drinking, sometimes multiple times a month [3]. Among adults who chose to drink alcoholic beverages, the average intake of calories from these beverages alone exceeds the caloric limit available after food group recommendations are met. Multiple sources have recommended that for adult males who drink, intake should be limited to no more than two alcoholic beverages per day. Females should be limited to one drink or less a day [15–17]. More details concerning this are found in Chapter 8.

29.5 UNIQUE NUTRITIONAL NEEDS OF WOMEN

Women have some unique nutritional needs, including needing more of certain vitamins and minerals, particularly during pregnancy (see subsequent sections) and after menopause. These unique nutritional needs include the following:

- **Calories**—Women typically need fewer calories than men. This is because women typically have less muscle and more body fat than men and are usually smaller. As already indicated in Figure 29.1, adult women on average need between 1,600 and 2,400 calories a day. Women who are more physically active need more calories. Formulas are available to help women compute the actual number of calories needed. The most commonly employed formula for this is called the Mifflin–St. Jeor Formula [18]. This combines basic metabolic rate (BMR) along with level of physical activity. The formula for BMR is as follows:

  Men: BMR (kcal/day) = (10 × weight in kg) + (6.25 × height in cm – (5 × age in years) + 5

  Women: BMR (kcal/day) = (10 × weight in kg) + (6.25 × height in cm – (5 × age in years) – 161

  The activity factor multipliers are as follows. These BMR must be multiplied by these activity factors to approximate physical activity level and compute the total number of calories needed:

  Little to no exercise: BMR × 1.2
  Light exercise 1–3 days per week: BMR × 1.375
  Moderate exercise 3–5 days per week: BMR × 1.55
  Heavy exercise 6–7 days per week: BMR × 1.725
  Very heavy exercise twice per day, extra-heavy workouts: BMR × 1.9
- **Vitamins and minerals**—Calcium [10,11], iron [19], and folic acid [11] are particularly important for women.
- **Reproductive health**—Different nutritional needs are present for women during different stages of life [20–22], for example, during pregnancy and breastfeeding (see subsequent section in this chapter) and after menopause.
- **Health problems**—Women are more likely to have some health problems related to nutrition than men such as celiac disease and lactose intolerance and vitamin and mineral deficiencies such as iron deficiency anemia.
- **Metabolism**—Women may process some substances differently and burn fewer calories at rest and during exercise than do men. This is largely a function of hormonal differences as well as differences in lean muscle mass.

29.6 CHANGING NUTRITIONAL NEEDS BY LIFE STAGE

Nutrition and regular exercise are the cornerstones of good health and optimum energy at every stage of women's lives [3,23]. It is important, however, to understand that certain vitamins and minerals are especially important at particular stages of life.

- **Nutrition for girls in childhood and early teens**—At this stage of life growing girls need a diet of abundant in fruits, vegetables, whole grains, and low-fat dairy products as well as lean sources of proteins. Two nutrients are of particular importance.

  Calcium—Calcium is particularly important during adolescence and early adulthood when bones are absorbing calcium. Calcium and vitamin D are often paired in fortified food such as milk [10,11]. This is because the body needs vitamin D in order to absorb calcium (see more detail concerning this in Chapter 23 on osteoporosis). Most experts recommend 1,300 milligrams of calcium a day for girls ages 9–19. Natural sources of calcium such as low-fat dairy products are an excellent choice because they also contain vitamin D and protein, both of which are required for calcium absorption. Milk, yogurt, and cheese contribute most of the calcium in our diet. Some vegetables are also good sources of calcium such as broccoli, kale, and Chinese cabbage. Many foods are supplemented with calcium including some brands of orange juice and tofu. The daily intake for vitamin D is 600 IU per day for most children and healthy adults [13].

  Iron—Iron is essential for healthy blood cells and is particularly important when girls begin to menstruate [19]. During each menstrual period a women loses small amounts of iron. Approximately 10% of American women are iron deficient, and about 5% have iron deficiency anemia. Symptoms of low iron can include fatigue, impaired immunity, and poor performance at school or work. When girls begin to menstruate, they need about 8 milligrams a day in iron. Between the ages of 14 and 18, recommended intake increases to 15 milligrams per day. A variety of foods can contribute iron including beef, turkey, chicken, halibut, tuna, bean, lentils, and breakfast cereals.

- **Nutrition for women during childbearing years**—A number of nutrients are particularly important to women especially during the stage of life when they are capable of becoming pregnant. These include the following:

  Folic acid—This form of B vitamins helps prevent neural tube defects. Many foods are now fortified with folic acid [10,11]. Leafy greens are also a good source of folic acid. Some physicians recommend that women who are pregnant take a supplement that includes folic acid to make sure they are getting the recommended 400–800 micrograms per day [24].

  B1^{2}—Just as with folic acid, B_{12} is central for healthy nervous system development and function [24]. Vegans and vegetarians may fall short on B_{12} since it is typically consumed in animal protein and to a lesser degree in dairy. Teenagers and adult women need 2.4 mcg, and these levels rise to 2.6 mcg and 2.8 mcg for lactating women.

  Choline—Some evidence exists that low choline levels are associated with increased risk of neural tube defects. Recommended levels have not been established; however, it is easy to get choline in the diet from such sources as eggs which are an excellent source of choline [25]. Other choline-rich food sources include milk, liver, and peanuts.

Omega-3 fatty acids—Omega-3s are essential fatty acids including eicosapentaenoic acid (EPA) and docosahexaenoic acid (DHA). They are important for many different aspects of health including building healthy brain and nerve cells [26]. These omega-3s have been shown to reduce the risk of heart disease, which remains the number one killer of women. Olive oil and fish contain multiple omega-3s. Omega-3s are thought to play an important role in why the Mediterranean diet reduces the risk of heart disease in both men and women.

Vitamin D—As already indicated, vitamin D is an important nutrient for building healthy bones and remains important for women during childbearing years [11].

Calcium—Consuming enough calcium is important for women throughout the adult years. Current recommendations include aiming for between 1,000 and 1,300 milligrams of calcium a day [10].

Iron—As already indicated, iron is a critical nutrient for building healthy red blood cells. In addition, during pregnancy the amount of blood cells almost doubles, which increases the demand for iron [19].

Fluids—Fluid needs increase as women age. This is because the kidneys are less efficient at removing toxins as individuals age. In addition, thirst signals often are impaired as people age, so it is important to emphasize drinking enough fluids, particularly in the form of water [27].

29.7 SUPPORTING HEALTHY EATING

It is important for individuals to receive support to make healthy choices to build healthy dietary patterns [3]. At the current time, national food expenditures suggest that the purchase of prepared food is a regular habit for most adults. These expenditures outpace food purchased for household meal preparation.

Since women are often responsible for food shopping and food preparation in the family, an opportunity exists for improving healthy nutrition through the preparation of healthy meals. When adults prepare meals for themselves, they can focus on choosing nutrient-dense options which contribute to food group goals with little or no added sugars and saturated fats and less sodium. Preparing meals at home may require learning new skills such as meal planning and preparation. Women who are parents, guardians, or caregivers of children or adolescents also provides an opportunity to teach valuable cooking skills and model behaviors that support healthy dietary patterns throughout life. It is important to be mindful of portion sizes while still achieving a healthy dietary pattern. Health promotion activities that center on increasing consumer knowledge and access to healthy options will help provide support for adults in consuming a healthier dietary pattern.

Physicians and other healthcare professionals can play an important role in supporting adult healthy eating patterns. An increasing number of medical schools are now offering programs to teach physicians skills like cooking and meal planning

[28] which, in turn, should help adults understand such issues as label reading and enhance cooking skills. On a community level, supporting farmers' markets, community gardens, and other related educational programming efforts is also important in an area where both men and women can make an important contribution.

29.8 OBESITY

According to the most recent data over 65% of U.S. women are overweight or obese. Over 40% of women are obese (body mass index [BMI] ≥30 mg/kg) [29]. Obesity is associated with an increased risk of developing CVD, type 2 diabetes mellitus (T2DM), and certain types of cancer.

Nutritional interventions are critically important for effective weight loss. Effective weight loss also requires a commitment to long-term lifestyle change. Typical weight loss programs include decreasing the amount of calories consumed by about 500 kcals per day. It is particularly important to emphasize that nutrient-dense foods should be selected.

29.9 PHYSICAL ACTIVITY

Both the Physical Activity Guidelines for Americans 2018 and the American College of Sports Medicine emphasize the importance of obtaining regular physical activity. Recommendations are consistent for 150 minutes of moderate-intensity physical activity or 75 minutes of vigorous physical activity on a weekly basis. Only 28% of U.S. women meet this physical activity criteria, and 41% of women engage in low-intensity physical activity [1]. Nutritional concerns for physically active individuals will be handled in Chapter 30. In general terms, physically active individuals have the same recommendations for healthy eating as do inactive individuals, although people who are physically active have more latitude to consume more calories than people who are inactive.

29.10 NUTRITION AND CARDIOVASCULAR DISEASE IN WOMEN

It is important to understand that coronary heart disease (CHD) is as prevalent in women as it is in men, although it tends to appear on average approximately ten years later. Unfortunately, once women develop CHD, they have a significantly worse prognosis than men. Among women aged older than 40, 43% die within five years after the first myocardial infarction [30]. Recommendations for healthy nutrition to lower the risk of CHD are basically the same between men and women. These are summarized in the 2021 Dietary Guidelines to Improve Cardiovascular Health: A Scientific Statement from the American Heart Association [5]. These recommendations basically follow the premises of the healthy diets such as the Healthy U.S.-Style Diet, MedDiet, and DASH diet. These will all be discussed in more detail in the chapter on nutrition and cardiovascular disease.

29.11 NUTRITION AND DIABETES

Nutrition plays a critical role in lowering the risk of diabetes and also in treating diabetes if it already exists. Proper nutrition is important for healthy weight loss, which has been shown to be a key component of reducing the risk of prediabetes advancing to diabetes [31]. Nutrition for individuals who already have diagnosis of diabetes plays a critically important role, where it typically prescribed as medical nutrition therapy (MNT) [32,33]. This is discussed in more detail in Chapter 22.

29.12 WOMEN'S SPECIFIC CONCERNS

- **Nutrition and Bone Health**—Consuming adequate amounts of calcium and vitamin D together with regular weight-bearing exercise are all important for lowering the risk of osteoporosis [9]. Osteoporosis is a significant problem for women, particularly after menopause. These issues are discussed in more detail in the chapter on osteoporosis.
- **Women Who Are Pregnant or Lactating**—Nutrition plays an extremely important role during special phases of life of pregnancy and lactation for women [34]. Following a healthy dietary pattern is particularly important for women at this life stage since increasing calorie and nutrient intakes is necessary to support the growth and development of the baby and also are important to maintain the mother's health. In addition, a healthy dietary pattern both before and during pregnancy can improve pregnancy outcomes. Thus, following a healthy dietary pattern both before and during pregnancy and lactation can not only affect the health outcome of the mother but also the child at every subsequent life stage. A healthy dietary pattern includes changing calorie and nutrient needs during pregnancy and lactation. This is important for a variety of reasons, including achieving and maintaining a healthy weight before pregnancy and gaining weight within gestational weight gain guidelines. In addition, monitoring caloric and nutrient needs is essential for returning to a healthy weight during the postpartum period. Nutritional issues such as the intake of seafood, alcohol, and caffeinated beverages all are very important, as are dealing with such issues as nausea, vomiting, and food aversions, as well as food cravings, which may complicate optimum healthy nutritional patterns.
- **Preconception Nutrition**—A women who is healthy at the time of conception is more likely to have a successful pregnancy and a healthy child than one who is unhealthy [35]. Strong links exist between health before pregnancy and both maternal and child health outcomes. Poor nutrition and obesity are particularly prevalent in women of reproductive age. Furthermore, typical diets fall far short of nutritional recommendations. Micronutrient supplementation started during pregnancy can correct some of the maternal nutritional deficiencies. The effect on child health outcomes, however, remains disappointing. It is particularly important to consider nutritional planning, particularly if pregnancy is anticipated and desired. Other issues such as reducing cigarette smoking, alcohol consumption, and obesity are all important for preconception health. This is particularly true of diet and nutrition. This is an area where health professionals should be alerted to ways of identifying women who are planning pregnancy and helping to assist in this often underemphasized area of preconception health.

- **Healthy Dietary Patterns**—Women who are pregnant or lactating should be counseled to follow the types of foods and beverages that make up a healthy dietary pattern as described earlier in this chapter. As found in Figure 29.2 (on page 111 of the Dietary Guidelines for Americans), the healthy dietary pattern during pregnancy is similar to one for women in general. Increased calories are necessary, however, given the increased needs to support both mother and fetus. Estimated calorie needs during pregnancy and lactation for a women who begins the pregnancy at a healthy weight are found in Figure 29.3 (page 112 of the Dietary Guidelines for Americans).
- **Weight Management**—Weight management during pregnancy and lactation is complicated. It is important for a woman to seek advice from a healthcare provider on the best way to achieve her goals [36]. Women should be encouraged to achieve and maintain a healthy weight before becoming pregnant and follow gestational weight gain guidelines developed by

CALORIE LEVEL OF PATTERN[a]	1,800	2,000	2,200	2,400	2,600	2,800
FOOD GROUP OR SUBGROUP[b]	Daily Amount of Food From Each Group (Vegetable and protein foods subgroup amounts are per week.)					
Vegetables (cup eq/day)	**2 ½**	**2 ½**	**3**	**3**	**3 ½**	**3 ½**
	Vegetable Subgroups in Weekly Amounts					
Dark-Green Vegetables (cup eq/wk)	1 ½	1 ½	2	2	2 ½	2 ½
Red & Orange Vegetables (cup eq/wk)	5 ½	5 ½	6	6	7	7
Beans, Peas, Lentils (cup eq/wk)	1 ½	1 ½	2	2	2 ½	2 ½
Starchy Vegetables (cup eq/wk)	5	5	6	6	7	7
Other Vegetables (cup eq/wk)	4	4	5	5	5 ½	5 ½
Fruits (cup eq/day)	**1 ½**	**2**	**2**	**2**	**2**	**2 ½**
Grains (ounce eq/day)	**6**	**6**	**7**	**8**	**9**	**10**
Whole Grains (ounce eq/day)	3	3	3 ½	4	4 ½	5
Refined Grains (ounce eq/day)	3	3	3 ½	4	4 ½	5
Dairy (cup eq/day)	**3**	**3**	**3**	**3**	**3**	**3**
Protein Foods (ounce eq/day)	**5**	**5 ½**	**6**	**6 ½**	**6 ½**	**7**
	Protein Foods Subgroups in Weekly Amounts					
Meats, Poultry, Eggs (ounce eq/wk)	23	26	28	31	31	33
Seafood (ounce eq/wk)[c]	8	8	9	10	10	10
Nuts, Seeds, Soy Products (ounce eq/wk)	4	5	5	5	5	6
Oils (grams/day)	**24**	**27**	**29**	**31**	**34**	**36**
Limit on Calories for Other Uses (kcal/day)[d]	**140**	**240**	**250**	**320**	**350**	**370**
Limit on Calories for Other Uses (%/day)	8%	12%	11%	13%	13%	13%

FIGURE 29.2 Healthy U.S.-Style Dietary Pattern for women who are pregnant or lactating, with daily or weekly amounts from food groups, subgroups, and components.

Source: Chapter 5. U.S. Department of Agriculture and U.S. Department of Health and Human Services. U.S. Department of Agriculture and U.S. Department of Health and Human Services. *Dietary Guidelines for Americans, 2020–2025*. 9th Edition. December 2020. Available at DietaryGuidelines.gov. 2020.

Estimated Change in Calorie Needs During Pregnancy and Lactation for Women With a Healthy[a] Prepregnancy Weight

Stage of Pregnancy or Lactation	Estimated Change in Daily Calorie Needs Compared to Prepregnancy Needs
Pregnancy: 1st trimester	+ 0 calories
Pregnancy: 2nd trimester	+ 340 calories
Pregnancy: 3rd trimester	+ 452 calories
Lactation: 1st 6 months	+ 330 calories[b]
Lactation: 2nd 6 months	+ 400 calories[c]

[a] These estimates apply to women with a healthy prepregnancy weight. Women with a prepregnancy weight that is considered overweight or obese should consult their healthcare provider for guidance regarding appropriate caloric intake during pregnancy and lactation.

[b] The EER for the first 6 months of lactation is calculated by adding 500 calories/day to prepregnancy needs to account for the energy needed for milk production during this time period, then subtracting 170 calories/day to account for weight loss in the first 6 months postpartum.

[c] The EER for the second 6 months of lactation is calculated by adding 400 calories/day to prepregnancy needs to account for the energy needed for milk production during this time period. Weight stability is assumed after 6 months postpartum.

NOTE: Estimates are based on Estimated Energy Requirements (EER) set by the Institute of Medicine. Source: Institute of Medicine. *Dietary Reference Intakes for Energy, Carbohydrate, Fiber, Fat, Fatty Acids, Cholesterol, Protein, and Amino Acids*. Washington, DC: The National Academies Press; 2005.

FIGURE 29.3 Estimated change in calorie needs during pregnancy and lactation for women with a healthy pre-pregnancy weight.

Source: Chapter 5. U.S. Department of Agriculture and U.S. Department of Health and Human Services. U.S. Department of Agriculture and U.S. Department of Health and Human Services. *Dietary Guidelines for Americans, 2020–2025*. 9th Edition. December 2020. Available at DietaryGuidelines.gov. 2020.

the National Academy of Science during the pregnancy. These guidelines are found in Figure 29.4. It should be noted that about half of women retain 10 pounds or more, and nearly one in four women retain 20 pounds or more at 12 months postpartum. This weight retention results in about one in seven women advancing from the healthy weight classification before pregnancy to overweight classification postpartum. Furthermore, women who are overweight or obese at the start of pregnancy frequently exceed gestational weight gain recommendations during pregnancy. Such weight gain increases the likelihood of excess postpartum weight retention. Effective weight management goals may improve pregnancy outcomes such as increasing the likelihood of delivering a healthy-weight infant, while improving long-term health for both mother and child. These issues should be discussed and implemented, along with advice from a healthcare provider.

- **Current Intakes**—While the Healthy Eating Index (HEI) score for women who are pregnant or lactating is slightly higher than all adult women, the HEI score is still below what is recommended by the DGA 2020–2025 [37]. Seventy percent of women who are pregnant exceed the recommended limit of 10% of total calories from added sugar, while 51% of women who are lactating exceed this recommendation [38]. With regard to saturated fat, 75% of pregnant women exceed the recommended 10% of total energy from saturated fats and 77% of lactating women exceed the total from saturated fat. With regard to sodium, 88% of pregnant women exceed the recommended sodium limit recommended by DGA 2020–2025, as do 97% of

Weight Gain Recommendations for Pregnancy[a]

Pre-pregnancy Weight Category	Body Mass Index	Range of Total Weight Gain (lb)	Rates of Weekly Weight Gain[b] in the 2nd and 3rd Trimesters (mean [range], lbs)
Underweight	Less than 18.5	28-40	1 [1-1.3]
Healthy Weight	18.5-24.9	25-35	1 [0.8-1]
Overweight	25-29.9	15-25	0.6 [0.5-0.7]
Obese	30 and greater	11-20	0.5 [0.4-0.6]

[a] **Reference:** Institute of Medicine and National Research Council. 2009. *Weight Gain During Pregnancy: Reexamining the Guidelines*. Washington, DC: The National Academies Press. **doi.org/10.17226/12584**.

[b] Calculations assume a 1.1 to 4.4 lb weight gain in the first trimester.

FIGURE 29.4 Weight gain recommendations for pregnancy.

Source: Institute of Medicine and National Research Council. 2009. Weight Gain During Pregnancy: Reexamining the Guidelines. Washington, DC: The National Academies Press. doi.org/10.17226/12584.

lactating women. One major reason for these relatively unhealthy dietary parameters is that women are far below the recommended servings of vegetables, consuming about 1–1/2 cup equivalents per day. In addition, pregnant or lactating women are well below recommended whole grain consumption. The average woman consumes about an average of 1 cup of whole grain equivalent either during pregnancy or lactation, which is about 1% of the recommended amount from DGA 2020–2025. For all of these reasons, women who are either pregnant or lactating can benefit from making dietary changes to better align with healthy dietary patterns.

- **Special Considerations**—Nutritional conditions for general female population in the United States also apply to women who are pregnant or lactating. Nutrients of health concern, namely calcium, vitamin D, potassium, and dietary fiber, that apply to women of all life stages are also of concern for women who are pregnant. There are, however, some special nutrient and dietary considerations specifically related to pregnancy, as listed next. It is important to eat a diet containing ample folate/folic acid, iron, iodine, and vitamin D without excessive intakes.

  Folate/folic acid—The U.S. Preventative Services Task Force (USPSTF) recommends that all women who are planning or capable of becoming pregnant take a daily supplement containing 400–800 micrograms of folic acid [11]. This folic acid supplementation is in addition to the amount of folate found in the foods in a normal healthy eating pattern. Folate is found typically in dark green vegetables and beans, peas, and lentils. All enriched grains (e.g. bread, pasta, rice and cereal, and some corn masa flours) are fortified with folic acid.

Iron—Iron needs increase during pregnancy compared to pre-pregnancy. For women who are lactating before menstruation returns, iron needs fall and then return to pre-pregnancy levels once menstruation resumes [19]. Iron deficiency effects about one in ten women who are pregnant and one in four women during the third trimester. Nutritional sources of iron include foods enriched or fortified with iron which include whole wheat breads and ready-to-eat cereals. It may be necessary for a woman who is pregnant to take a supplement containing iron, which should be done in consultation with her physician.

Iodine—Iodine needs increase substantially during pregnancy and lactation [24]. This micronutrient is important for neurocognitive development of the fetus. Nutritional sources of iodine include dairy products, eggs, seafood, or the use of iodized table salt. It should be noted that women who are pregnant or lactating should not be encouraged to start using table salt if they do not use this already.

Choline—Choline needs increase during pregnancy and lactation. This is important to replenish maternal stores and support growth and development of the child's brain and spinal cord [25]. Meeting choline needs can be accomplished by consuming dairy and protein food groups such as eggs, meats, and some seafood as well as beans, peas, and the lentil subgroups.

Seafood—Consuming seafood during pregnancy is recommended since it is associated with measures of cognitive development in young children. The recommendation is to consume 8–12 ounces of a variety of seafood a week [37]. It is also important to avoid certain types of seafood consumption to limit ethyl mercury exposure. This is particularly important during pregnancy. For this reason, pregnant women should eat less of certain species of seafood such as shark, swordfish, or king mackerel, which should be avoided during pregnancy.

Alcoholic beverages—Women who are or may be pregnant should not drink alcohol [37]. Unfortunately, about one woman in ten who is pregnant reported consuming alcohol during an average month with an average of two or more drink equivalents per day if alcohol is consumed. It is not safe for women to drink any type or amount of alcohol during pregnancy. Women who drink alcohol and become pregnant should stop drinking alcohol immediately.

Caffeine—Many women consume caffeine during pregnancy or lactation. Caffeine passes from the mother to the infant in small amounts of breast milk, but usually does not adversely affect the infant provided that the mother consumes low to moderate amounts [37]. This would be the equivalent of 300 milligrams or less per day, which is about two to three cups of coffee. This is a topic to discuss with the individual's physician.

- **Food Safety**—Women who are pregnant or lactating or more susceptible than the general population to the effect of foodborne illnesses such as listeriosis [37]. It is essential to take special care to keep food safe and not eat foods that increase the risk of foodborne illnesses. During pregnancy women should eat only meals containing seafood, meats, poultry, or eggs that have been cooked at a recommended safe minimum internal temperature. They should also not consume unpasteurized juice or milk or soft cheeses made from unpasteurized milk. Deli and luncheon meats and hot dogs should be reheated to steaming hot or 165°F to kill *Listeria*, the bacteria that causes listeriosis.
- **Physical Activity during Pregnancy and Postpartum as Recommended by the American College of Obstetrics and Gynecology** [39]–Physical activity during pregnancy can be beneficial to both mother and baby. Healthy women without contraindications should perform at least 150 minutes of moderate-intensity aerobic activity a week. Women who have habitually performed vigorous-intensity activity may continue to do so during pregnancy. These issues should be discussed with their healthcare provider to make any adjustments that may be necessary in physical activity patterns during pregnancy.

  In the postpartum period, physical activity remains important and can increase cardiorespiratory fitness, improve mood, and reduce the symptoms of postpartum depression. Physical activity can also help to achieve a healthy weight and, when combined with caloric restriction, helps promote weight loss. When starting physical activity, either during pregnancy or postpartum, women should start slow and build up to more activity over time. The ultimate goal is to aim for at least 150 minutes of moderate-intensity aerobic activity per week. More information on physical activity during pregnancy and postpartum is available through the Physical Activity Guidelines for Americans 2018.
- **Vegetarian or vegan dietary patterns**—Women who are following vegetarian or vegan dietary patterns during pregnancy of lactation may need to take special care to ensure nutrient adequacy. This may include making sure they get adequate iron and vitamin B_{12} [37]. Choline is also important to assure [35]. This may be achieved by following the recommended intake in the dairy and protein groups. Seafood during pregnancy is recommended and associated with variable measures of cognitive development in young children.

29.13 CONCLUSIONS

Health and nutrition play a vital role throughout every life stage for women. While specifics may change according to life stage, the overall recommendation remains to follow healthy dietary patterns throughout every life stage. This is particularly true for women who are pregnant or lactating. All of these issues should be discussed with every woman the clinician sees.

Clinical Applications

- Women at all life stages should follow a healthy dietary pattern that is consistent with the Healthy U.S.-Style Dietary Pattern described by the DGA 2020–2025 and other prestigious organizations.
- Following healthy guidelines is particularly important for women who are pregnant or lactating, but is very important at all life stages.
- Healthy nutrition is important to lower the risk of both heart disease and diabetes in women.
- Heart disease is the leading cause of death in women in the United States.
- Every clinical encounter should include recommendations for following healthy nutrition for women, which includes more fruits and vegetables and whole grains, while avoiding excess sugar, saturated fat, and sodium.

REFERENCES

1. Physical Activity Guidelines Advisory Committee. 2018 Physical activity guidelines advisory committee. 2018 Physical Activity Guidelines Advisory Committee Scientific Report. Washington, DC: U.S. Department of Health and Human Services, 2018.
2. Bassuk S, Manson J. Lifestyle and risk of cardiovascular disease and type 2 diabetes in women: A review of the epidemiologic evidence. Am J Lifestyle Med. 2008;2(3):191–213.
3. U.S. Department of Agriculture and U.S. Department of Health and Human Services. *Dietary Guidelines for Americans, 2020–2025*, 9th edition. December 2020. DietaryGuidelines.gov. 2020. www.dietaryguidelines.gov/resources/2020-2025-dietary-guidelines-online-materials
4. Estruch R, Ros E, Salas-Salvado J, et al. Primary prevention of cardiovascular disease with a mediterranean diet. N Engl J Med. 2013;368(14):1279–1290.
5. Lichtenstein A, Appel L, Vadiveloo M, et al. 2021 Dietary guidance to improve cardiovascular health: A scientific statement from the American Heart Association. Circulation. 2021;144(23):e472–e487.
6. Sacks F, Svetkey L, Vollmer W, et al. Effects on blood pressure of reduced dietary sodium and the Dietary Approaches to Stop Hypertension (DASH) diet. DASH-Sodium Collaborative Research Group. N Engl J Med. 2001;344(1):3–10.
7. Cordain L, Eaton S, Sebastian A, et al. Origins and evolution of the western diet: Health implications for the 21st century. Am J Clin Nutr. 2005;81(2):341–354.
8. Anderson K, Pauly K, Shapiro D, et al. Optimal nutrition for women. In Tollefson, Eriksen, and Pathak (eds). Improving Women's Health Across the Lifespan. Boca Raton: CRC Press, 2021.
9. Gagne L, Maizes V. Osteoporosis. In Rakel D (ed). Integrative Medicine, 4th edition. Philadelphia, PA: Elsevier, 2018.
10. Heaney R, Weaver C. Calcium absorption from kale. Am J Clin Nutr. 1990;51(4):656–657.
11. Nutrition Working Group, O'Connor DL, Blake J, Bell R, Bowen A, Callum J, et al. Canadian consensus on female nutrition: Adolescence, reproduction, menopause, and beyond. J Obstet Gynaecol Can. 2016;38(6):508–554 e18.
12. Bjelakovic G, Gluud L, Nikolova D, et al. Vitamin D supplementation for prevention of mortality in adults. Cochrane Database Syst Rev. 2014;(1):CD007470.

13. Holick M, Binkley N, Bischoff-Ferrari H, et al. Evaluation, treatment, and prevention of vitamin D deficiency: An endocrine society clinical practice guideline. J Clin Endocrinol Metab. 2011;96(7):1911–1930.
14. Rippe JM, Lifestyle strategies for risk factor reduction, orevention, and treatment of cardiovascular disease. Am J Lifestyle Med. 2018;2;13(2):204–212.
15. Baliunas D, Taylor B, Irving H, et al. Alcohol as a risk factor for type 2 diabetes: A systematic review and meta-analysis. Diabetes Care. 2009;32(11):2123–2132.
16. Ronksley P, Brien S, Turner B, et al. Association of alcohol consumption with selected cardiovascular disease outcomes: A systematic review and meta-analysis. BMJ. 2011;342:d671.
17. Brien S, Ronksley P, Turner B, et al. Effect of alcohol consumption on biological markers associated with risk of coronary heart disease: Systematic review and meta-analysis of interventional studies. BMJ. 2011;342:d636.
18. Mifflin M, St Jeor S, Hill L, et al. A new predictive equation for resting energy expenditure in healthy individuals. Am J Clin Nutr. 1990;51(2):241–247.
19. Qi L, van Dam R, Rexrode K, et al. Heme iron from diet as a risk factor for coronary heart disease in women with type 2 diabetes. Diabetes Care. 2007;30(1):101–106.
20. Centers for Disease Control and Prevention. Infertility FAQ. Content Source: Division of Reproductive Health, National Center for Chronic Disease Prevention and Health Promotion. Reproductive Health | CDC (Accessed January 11, 2024).
21. Chavarro J, Rich-Edwards J, Rosner B, et al. Diet and lifestyle in the prevention of ovulatory disorder infertility. Obstet Gynecol. 2007;110(5):1050–1058.
22. Gaskins A, Chavarro J. Diet and fertility: A review. Am J Obstet Gynecol. 2018;218(4):379–389.
23. U.S. Department of Health & Human Services. OASH Office on Women's Health. Healthy eating and women. Healthy Eating and Women | Office on Women's Health (womenshealth.gov) (Accessed January 11, 2024).
24. Kominiarek M, Rajan P. Nutrition recommendations in pregnancy and lactation. Med Clin N Am. 2016;100(6):1199–1215.
25. Wiedeman A, Barr S, Green T, et al. Dietary choline intake: Current state of knowledge across the life cycle. Nutrients. 2018;10(10).
26. Gaby A. Omega-3 fatty acids. Nutritional Medicine, 2nd edition. Concord: Fritz Perlberg Publishing, 2017.
27. Nelms M, Sucher K, Lacey K, et al. Nutrition Therapy and Pathophysiology, 3rd edition. Boston: Cengage Learning, 2016.
28. AAMC, Association of American Medical Colleges. Doctors in the kitchen. Doctors in the Kitchen | AAMC (Accessed January 11, 2024).
29. U.S. Department of Health & Human Services. OASH Office on Women's Health. Weight and obesity. Weight and Obesity | Office on Women's Health (womenshealth.gov) (Accessed January 11, 2024).
30. Rippe J. Women and cardiovascular disease. In Rippe (ed). Integrating Lifestyle Medicine in Cardiovascular Health and Disease Prevention. Boca Raton: CRC Press, 2023.
31. Knowler W, Barrett-Connor E, Fowler S, et al. Reduction in the incidence of type 2 diabetes with lifestyle intervention or metformin. N Engl J Med. 2002;346(6):393–403.
32. Rippe J. Diabetes, prediabetes, and metabolic syndrome. In Rippe J (ed). Manual of Lifestyle Medicine. Boca Raton: CRC Press, 2021.
33. Diabetes Prevention Program Research Group, Knowler W, Fowler S, et al. 10-year follow-up of diabetes incidence and weight loss in the Diabetes Prevention Program Outcomes Study. Lancet. 2009;374(9702):1677–1686.
34. Franz M, MacLeod J, Evert A, et al. Academy of Nutrition and Dietetics nutrition practice guideline for type 1 and type 2 diabetes in adults: Systematic review of evidence for

medical nutrition therapy effectiveness and recommendations for integration into the nutrition care process. J Acad Nutr Diet. 2017;117(10):1659–1679.
35. Stephenson J, Heslehurst N, Hall J, et al. Before the beginning: Nutrition and lifestyle in the preconception period and its importance for future health. Lancet. 2018;391(10132):1830–1841.
36. Koletzko B, Godfrey K, Poston L, et al. Nutrition during pregnancy, lactation and early childhood and its implications for maternal and long-term child health: The Early Nutrition Project Recommendations. Ann Nutr Metab. 2019;74(2):93–106.
37. Women who are pregnant or lactating. In *Dietary Guidelines for Americans, 2020–2025.* Chapter 5 Page 107. *Dietary Guidelines for Americans, 2020–2025.*
38. Chapter 5. U.S. Department of Agriculture and U.S. Department of Health and Human Services. *Dietary Guidelines for Americans, 2020–2025*, 9th edition. December 2020. DietaryGuidelines.gov. 2020. www.dietaryguidelines.gov/resources/2020-2025-dietary-guidelines-online-materials.
39. The American College of Obstetricians and Gynecologists. Physical activity and exercise during pregnancy and the postpartum period. Physical Activity and Exercise During Pregnancy and the Postpartum Period | ACOG (Accessed January 11, 2024).

30 Nutrition for Physically Active People and Athletes

Key Points

- Physical activity is important for good health.
- Basic nutrition for physically active adults and children is similar to that for individuals who do not participate in physical activity. However, there is increased latitude for caloric consumption
- Fluid balance is critically important both for children and adults participating in physical activity and athletics.

30.1 INTRODUCTION

Regular physical activity is a key lifestyle habit that can lower the risk of multiple chronic diseases [1,2]. As a result, regular physical activity should be a component of every counseling session for physicians for their patients. Many individuals also participate in athletic contests. In addition, many adults have children who participate in athletic contests or who need guidance for physical activity or athletic endeavors. In all of those situations, nutrition is a key consideration. This chapter will focus attention on various aspects of nutrition, both for physical activity and for participation in athletic activities both for adults and children. A key consideration that is often underestimated in nutrition is the role of fluids for hydration, which will be a central focus of this chapter [3,4].

30.2 NUTRITION FOR PHYSICALLY ACTIVE ADULTS

In general, recommendations for nutrition for physically active adults are similar to those for healthy nutrition for all adults. There are, however, a few minor differences that should be noted [5,6].

By engaging in regular physical activity, adults have somewhat more latitude in terms of the number of calories that they can consume without gaining weight. As indicated in other chapters in this book, metabolism is the process by which the food individuals consume is converted into the energy that is essential for all of life's processes. There are two general components for metabolism that indicate how much energy adults can consume. These components are basal metabolic rate (BMR) and physical activity. There are also some minor contributions in energy consumption from metabolism required to digest food, although in the broadest sense BMR and

DOI: 10.1201/9781003452607-30

TABLE 30.1
Mifflin–St. Jeor Equation

Formula
Females: (10 * weight [kg]) + (6.25 * height [cm]) – (5*age [years]) – 161
Males: (10 * weight [kg]) + (6.25 * height [cm]) – (5 * age [years]) + 5
Multiply by scale factor for activity level:
Sedentary * 1.2
Lightly active * 1.375
Moderately active * 1.55
Active * 1.725
Very active * 1.9

Source: Mifflin MD, St Jeor ST, Hill LA, Scott BJ, Daugherty SA, Koh YO. A new predictive equation for resting energy expenditure in healthy individuals. Am J Clin Nutr. 1990;51(2):241–247.

physical activity are the key components for how many calories individuals can consume while maintaining a stable weight.

BMR can be estimated by a calculation that is called the Mifflin–St. Jeor equations. They are listed in Table 30.1. [7]. BMR accounts for 60–80% of total energy expenditure (TEE) and encompasses the energy required to perform basic metabolic functioning.

As can be seen in these equations, men have a somewhat higher BMR than women. This is a result of men being generally larger than women and having more muscle mass. When physical activity is accounted for, the BMR is multiplied by an activity factor that approximates physical activity level [8]. The following are general activity factor multipliers:

Little or no exercise: BMR × 1.2
Light exercise 1–3 days per week: BMR × 1.375
Moderate exercise 3–5 days per week: BMR × 1.55
Heavy exercise 6–7 days per week: BMR × 1.725
Very heavy exercise twice per day, including extra-heavy workouts: BMR × 1.9

As can be seen in these calculations, physical activity allows for increased caloric consumption. Many people have the misconception that they can perform enough physical activity to lose weight; however, the vast majority of research in this area indicates that increased physical activity alone is not sufficient to result in significant weight loss [9]. Regular physical activity is, however, a key component of the maintenance of weight loss or lowering the risk of gaining weight in the first place. It should also be noted that in some instances physical activity will increase appetite, while in others it decreases appetite. Each individual will have to experiment with this to determine how regular physical activity impacts on their appetite.

30.3 NUTRITION AND ATHLETIC PERFORMANCE

Increasingly adults desire to participate in athletic performance events either in such periodic events as running in marathons or 10K runs or walks or recreational or professional athletic contests or tournaments. This may impact on how an individual prepares with meals and fluids both prior to and following participation in athletic contests [5,6,10,11].

It may be tricky to manage meal planning around an athletic event. The timing of meals is very important both for adults and children (see subsequent section on children's athletics). It is important for an athlete of any age to discover foods they like and that maximize their performance. Individuals should not experiment with new foods or new routines on the day of competition. In general, an individual should consume a meal a minimum of three hours before an event to allow for proper digestion and minimize the incidence of gastrointestinal upset during exercise. Meals should consist of carbohydrates, proteins, and fats. Fiber should be limited. High-fat meals should be avoided before exercise because the fat can delay gastric emptying and make an athlete feel sluggish and thereby adversely affect performance [5,6,10,11]. For early morning practices or events, having a snack or meal one to two hours before exercise followed by a full breakfast after the event will help ensure sufficient energy to maximize performance.

Fluids, particularly water, are a critically important nutrient for athletes. Athletic performance may be affected by what, how much, and when an athlete drinks. Since this is so important, it will be handled in a subsequent section on physical activity and fluid replacement.

In addition, many people have questions about what should be consumed in recovering from an athletic event. In general, recovery foods should be consumed within 30 minutes of exercise and again within an hour or two after exercise to help reload muscles with glycogen and allow for proper recovery. These foods should include protein and carbohydrates. Some good examples include graham crackers with peanut butter, juice, yogurt with fruit or perhaps a sports drink, fruit, and perhaps cheese. These recommendations apply equally as well to adults and children. There is also some recent research that suggest that milk and other dairy products can be part of a recovery regimen to provide protein.

30.4 PHYSICAL ACTIVITY AND FLUID REPLACEMENT

- General Considerations

  The ability to regulate body water content, particularly of tissues within a relatively narrow range, is a defining characteristic of all animal life. This regulation must be achieved in the face of continuous but variable loss of water and salts from the body [3,4,12]. Humans can survive for several weeks without food, but deprivation of water for even a few days can be fatal, with survival time dictated largely by the rate of water loss. This was seen dramatically in the 2023 horrendous earthquakes in Turkey.

  Water comprises 50–70% of body mass, which makes it the most abundant component in the human body except for the very obese [3,4]. This means that the average 70-kg male has 40–42 liters of water. Females normally have a lower percentage of water content than males of the same size, largely because women typically have less muscle and muscle contains a large amount of water [12–14].

If water amount increases or decreases by more than 10%, a variety of substantial health risks can occur, but regulatory and behavioral mechanisms normally intervene long before this point is reached. Euhydration is considered when the body is at normal hydration levels, which is about 0.2% decrease in the normal amount of water in temperate conditions and within 0.5% in heat or during exercise. Individuals are considered to be hypohydrated (reduced by body water) or hyperhydrated (increased body water) if they lie outside these limits [15–17]. Both of these conditions, if sufficiently severe, can impair all aspects of physiologic function and in extreme cases may prove fatal.

Physical activity poses a number of challenges in both water and salt homeostasis because of increased rates of water and salt (particularly sodium and chloride) loss. These efforts are magnified as activity level, ambient temperature, and environmental humidity increase. Thus, those who are physically active, whether on a recreational or occupational basis, must be aware of their body's need for water and salt and should not ignore or consciously override physiologic signals.

- Water Balance

Water balance occurs when water intake matches water losses. Water balance fluctuates during the course of a day. Over a 24-hour period water balance is generally maintained without any particular conscience effort to take water or other fluids [18–22]. For sedentary individuals in temperate environments daily water turnover is about 2–3 liters [3,4]. The main avenue of water loss is via urine. Additional losses occur via respiration, sweating, and fecal loss. Individuals exercising in hot conditions may lose this amount of water in an hour, but sweating is essential to limit the rise of core temperature in these situations. Urine production is regulated by a number of hormones that respond to intravascular volume and osmolality. These include arginine vasopressin (AVP), aldosterone, and atrial natriuretic peptide (ANP).

Thirst and habit are major drivers of fluid intake. It should be noted that generally thirst is considered a poor indicator of short-term deviations in body water. The thirst response, however, is sufficient to restore body water levels for longer periods of time. The average daily water intake is 2.0 liters for the average adult female and 2.5 liters for the average adult male. For physically active individuals who lose volumes of water via sweating, which is exacerbated by a hot environment, fluid intake may be much more than these average amounts.

In many physical activities sweat rate may be 0.5–1.5 liters per hour. In well-trained or very large athletes, a sweat rate may reach or exceed 3–4 liters per hour.

- Sweating, Water Balance, and Water Turnover

During physical activity or exercise, metabolic demand increases, which generates heat, which must be dissipated to avoid large increases in core temperature. This is achieved largely through an increase in sweat rate [16,23,24]. Sweat consists of water, minerals, and organic compounds. Thus, as sweat rate increases during physical activity, what is lost is not just water. The main electrolytes lost through sweat are sodium and chloride in concentrations with approximately 15–80 mmols/liter.

There are large variations in sweat loss, so there is no single hydration strategy suitable for all physically active individuals, and hydration advice must be tailored to the individual in question.

Body water turnover is approximately 5–10% of total body water content per day for sedentary individuals living in a temperate environment but can increase to 20–40% if prolonged exercise is undertaken in hot environments. Most people don't recognize that highly trained individuals actually sweat more than lesser trained individuals because they are more efficient at lowering their core body temperature.

- Hydration Status and Performance

  Small changes in body water content throughout the day have no measurable effects on physiologic function, but large changes clearly exert an impact. High levels of debate exist concerning when the amount of water reduction in the body affects physiologic function [25–27]. It has been suggested that reduction of body water of 3–4% is necessary to induce detrimental effects in muscle function. Some studies, however, have suggested that even smaller degrees of hypohydration can be detrimental to muscle function. Even mild levels of hypohydration can have been shown to negatively affect cognition.

  In one study, hypohydration of approximately 1.5% body mass loss resulted in reduced cognitive aspects such as visual vigilance and visual working memory compared to euhydrated states. In one study, the volunteers who had been studied after a period of hypohydration which resulted in a reduction of body mass of 1.1% resulted in more minor driving errors than the same task under normal fluid drinking guidelines.

  These studies suggest that even very mild levels of hypohydration can have a negative impact on cognition. Studies have been done in racecar drivers and fighter pilots that have demonstrated that a 2% decrease in body mass from water loss can result in measurable cognitive decline. For this reason, adequate hydration is considered a high priority for the U.S. Air Force.

- Hydration for Recreational Activity

  As already indicated in multiple chapters in this book, physical activity produces multiple health benefits. In addition, cardiorespiratory fitness is an independent risk factor for a number of disease states. Thus, physical activity is routinely prescribed to improve health. As already noted in this chapter, physical activity by itself does not appear to induce large degrees of short-term weight loss. However, it is key, along with caloric restriction, for maintaining weight loss and preventing weight regain. Even small amounts of hypohydration can result in ratings of perceived exertion increasing in individuals [4–6]. Considerable research shows that starting exercise in a hypohydrated state or allowing hypohydration to occur during exercise results in increased perception of effort [25–27].

- Implications for Drinking Strategies
  Considerable research has been done in an attempt to determine optimum strategies for hydration during exercise performance [28–30]. Since a large variation among physically active individuals exists with regard to sweat rate, one strategy does not fit all people. Two main drinking strategies have been promoted for physically active individuals. One of these strategies is to advise individuals to drink only when thirsty. The other is *ad libitum* where individuals are allowed to drink when they want. It is not clear that one strategy is better than the other.

  Hypohydration commonly occurs following exercise, and a large body of research relates to post-exercise rehydration strategy. If only a single moderate exercise session is completed during the day, there is no need for an aggressive rehydration strategy since normal regulatory process covered in food intake ensures that water balance will be maintained over a 24-hour period. If several exercise sessions are performed during the day, post-exercise rehydration status may be needed to ensure that the second session is not started while hypohydrated. This typically is translated into the advice to drink 1.5 liters of fluid for every 1.0 liter of net fluid deficit at the end of the first exercise session. Since sodium and chloride are also lost in sweat, additional sodium in a rehydration solution has been shown to improve effectiveness and maintain fluid balance during the recovery period. If food is ingested during recovery, plain water is adequate, particularly if the meal contains adequate electrolytes.
- Hydration as Part of a Healthy Lifestyle
  As already indicated, adequate water levels are critically important for athletic performance. For physically active members of the general public, however, and for individuals whose occupations involve manual work, it is also important to recognize the importance of adequate hydration. As already indicated, regulatory physiologic mechanisms will maintain adequate water balance, and small amounts of hypohydration are likely to cause relatively mild symptoms. Some investigators have suggested that adequate hydration lowers the incidence of urinary tract infection in women and, in general, improves kidney health, although much more work is needed in this area.

  It should be noted that the aging process results in blunted thirst response which, in turn, yields an increasing risk of hypohydration in older individuals [31–33]. Hypohydration is thought to lead to infection in elderly populations and is particularly prominent during heatwaves in countries or cities where there is not adequate air conditioning. For example, in Europe in 2003 there were reports of temperatures that were several degrees higher than in the period of June–September 2003 compared to that time frame in other years which resulted in 7.6% more deaths in Munich, 10.4% more deaths in all of Europe, 26.8% more deaths in Rome, and 33.6% in Milan than in comparable three-month periods with lower temperatures.

  Conversely, acute increases in body water, while less common than hypohydration, can also be hazardous [34,35]. Overhydration (hyperhydration) can result from ingestion of water in excess of the amount needed to maintain euhydration. Overhydration can result in serious health consequences in healthy individuals and can even be fatal. In severe cases, this can result in symptoms associated with water intoxication, including headache, nausea, confusion, and changes in behavior leading to central nervous system dysfunction, coma, and even death. For example, it was reported that 13% of finishers of the Boston Marathon in 2002 experienced hyperhydration, although none of these individuals showed clinical symptoms. Occasional cases have been reported where mentally ill individuals have become water intoxicated, and also excessive water ingestion hyperhydration may also occur during weight loss plans and in social competition involving large volumes of fluid intake.

- Hydration Assessment
  A variety of technical ways exist to assess hydration biomarkers [36,37]. As a general rule of thumb for the average physically active individual, however, perhaps the easiest rough estimate of hydration status is to take the first morning body weight (BW) measurements. For a well-hydrated person who is in water and energy balance, a first morning (after urinating) nude BW will be stable and fluctuate by less than 1%. At least three consecutive morning nude measurements should be made to establish a baseline which approximates euhydration. In men consuming food and fluid *ad libitum* and women may need more BW measurements to establish a baseline value because menstrual cycle influences body weight status. For example, some menstrual phases can increase body water by greater than 2 kg. Lastly, the first morning BW is influenced by changes in eating and bowel habits. Acute changes in BW during exercise can be used to calculate sweating rates and changes in hydration status that occur in different environments.

30.5 HEALTH CONSIDERATIONS

While physical activity and exercise are important health-promoting behaviors, individuals should be aware that significant dehydration or hyperhydration can result in significant adverse consequences.

- Heat Illnesses
  Dehydration increases the risk for heat exhaustion and for heat stroke [25,38,39]. Dehydration was present in approximately 17% of heat stroke hospitalizations in the U.S. Army over a 22-year period. Skeletal muscle cramps are believed to be associated with dehydration as well as electrolyte deficits and muscle fatigue and are common in non-heat-acclimatized American football players. For example, muscle cramps may occur in early summer practice sessions, tennis matches (particularly when played in hot temperatures), long cycling races, late or tropical marathons, soccer, and beach volleyball. Muscle cramps can also occur in winter activities such as cross country skiing and in ice hockey, particularly in goalies who wear heavy equipment. Persons susceptible to muscle cramps are believed to be perfuse sweaters who experience large sodium loss.

Rhabdomyolysis (a symptom caused by release of skeletal muscle contents) may be observed in novel strenuous overexertion and can increase the consequences of dehydration [40,41]. In one study of U.S. soldiers hospitalized with serious heat illness who had experienced large fluid and electrolyte losses, 25% had rhabdomyolysis and 13% had acute renal failure.

As already indicated, it is also possible, although much less likely, to consume enough water to result in hyponatremia, which typically occurs when sodium levels fall rapidly to less than 130 mmol/liter (normal is 140–145]. In individuals participating in marathons, symptomatic hyponatremia tends to occur in individuals who run slowly, sweat less, and consume excessive water and other hypotonic fluids before, during, and after the race. This also occasionally occurs in American football and tennis players who drink too much water to treat or try to prevent heat cramps or when a cramping player is given hypotonic fluid intravenously.

30.6 MODIFYING FACTORS

- Sex

  Women typically have lower sweating rates and electrolyte losses than men [12,13,14]. This is primarily due to their smaller body size and lower metabolic rates for certain exercise tasks. It has also been suggested that women turn water over more quickly than men due to differences in AVP, which is typically somewhat reduced in women, which may result in elevated renal water and electrolyte depletion.

  Women appear to be at greater risk than men to develop hyponatremia when competing in marathons and ultimate marathon races. Greater risk in women for hyponatremia has not been firmly established.
- Age

  Older individuals (age greater than 65 years) are typically adequately hydrated. There is, however, an age-related blunting of thirst response to water deprivation, making older individuals more susceptible to becoming dehydrated. Older individuals also have slower water and sodium excretion, which can lead to fluid retention and potentially increases in blood pressure. For all these reasons, older individuals should be encouraged to carefully rehydrate during and after exercise while considering the risk of excess water.

  On the other side of the spectrum, prepubescent children have lower sweating rates than adults. This is typically a result of smaller body mass and lower metabolic rate. Electrolyte content is similar or slightly lower in children and adults.
- Diet

  Regular meal consumption is critical to ensure full hydration on a day-to-day basis. Eating food promotes fluid intake and retention and helps with replenishing sodium and potassium losses, which are typically accomplished for both men and women during meals. Diet macronutrient consumption does not measurably alter daily fluid needs for individuals. As already indicated, however, the basic recommendations for healthy plant-based diets are important for women and are particularly valuable in replacing potassium.

Caffeine consumption has been a source of controversy related to physical activity at high levels. For the average individual, a relatively small doses (up to two to three cups of coffee per day) will likely not increase urine output or cause dehydration. The influence of caffeine consumption on urine output during exercise, or in dehydrated individuals, does not appear to change urine output and induce dehydration during exercise.

Whether or not supplementation with caffeine can acutely enhance exercise performance remains controversial [42]. Performance enhancement has been shown in many, but not all, studies. Aerobic endurance appears to be the form of exercise where more benefits ensue from caffeine use, although the magnitude of these effects differs between individuals. Typical consumption of coffee up to three to four cups of coffee per day may slightly improve exercise performance, High doses of caffeine (e.g. more than five cups of coffee in a day), however, are associated with side effects and do not appear to elicit any improvement in performance.

The commonly used timing for caffeine supplementation is typically 60 minutes pre-exercise. Optimal timing of caffeine ingestion seems to depend on the source of caffeine. For example, chewing gum with caffeine in it may require shorter waiting time from consumption to start an exercise session. It should be noted that in addition to coffee, tea, and cocoa, caffeine is also added to many foods beverages and novelty products. Over 95% of caffeine consumption comes from beverages including coffee, soft drinks, and tea.

Controversy exists about whether caffeine should be legal in sports. The International Olympic Committee (IOC) recognizes that caffeine is frequently used by athletes because of reported performance-enhancing effects. Caffeine is on the list of banned substances by the IOC and the World Anti-Doping Association, but the levels for doping offenses are quite high, exceeding a cutoff of 15 micrograms per milliliter initially, but in 1985 this was reduced to 12 microgram per milliliter [42]. The cut-off guide was chosen to differentiate what was considered to be apparently use of caffeine for the purpose of sport performance rather than common dietary or social coffee drinking patterns.

In addition, alcohol can act as a diuretic (particularly in high doses) and can increase urine output. If alcohol is consumed in moderation, then rehydration is particularly important.

30.7 FLUID REPLACEMENT

- Before Exercise

The goal of prehydrating is to start physical activity in the state of euhydration with normal plasma electrolyte levels [28–30]. Enhancing the palatability of ingested fluid is one way to help fluid consumption [43]. Before, during, and after exercise, palatability is influenced by flavor, temperature, and sodium content. Flavor preference varies between individuals and culture. Prehydrating with beverages should be initiated at least several hours before starting a physical activity session to enable fluid absorption and allow urine output to return to a normal level.

- During Exercise
  The goal of drinking during exercise is to prevent excessive dehydration, which has typically been defined as greater than 2% BW loss through water deficit. In addition, drinking fluids during exercise is useful to reduce the likelihood of excessive changes in electrolyte balance [44,45]. Some research has suggested that a possible starting point for marathon runners who are euhydrated to start is that they drink *ad libitum* 0.4–0.8 liters per hour, although this varies considerably depending on the size of the individual and how warm the ambient environment is.
  The Institute of Medicine (IOM) has provided guidance for composition for "sports beverages" for individuals performing physical activity in hot weather [46]. The IOM recommends that these types of fluid replacement beverages might contain between 20 and 30 mEq per liter of sodium and 2–5 mEq per liter of potassium and 5–10% of carbohydrates. Consuming carbohydrates can be beneficial to sustain exercise intensity during high-intensity exercise events lasting longer than one hour or less intense exercise events lasting for longer periods. Carbohydrate consumption at a rate of 40–60 grams per hour has been demonstrated to maintain glucose levels and sustain exercise performance. If consumed as part of a beverage, carbohydrate concentration should not exceed 8%.
- After Exercise
  The goal of hydration after exercise is to fully replace any fluid and electrolyte deficit. Individuals who are attempting to achieve rapid and complete recovery from dehydration should drink approximately 1.5 liters of fluid for each kilogram of body weight lost [28,30,47]. These fluids should optimally be consumed over time with sufficient electrolytes to maximize fluid retention.

30.8 SPORT NUTRITION FOR YOUNG ATHLETES

Parents and guardians are often in a position of helping provide proper nutrition for children and adolescent athletes. Considerations include obtaining proper growth and performing optimal performance in sports [6,10]. As always, a healthy plant-based diet is appropriate for children and adolescents and will provide an appropriate amount of macronutrients and micronutrients, which are essential to provide enough energy for growth and activity. Fluids are also particularly important for hydration—both for growth and athletic performance.

- Energy Requirements
  Balancing energy intake with energy expenditure is essential to prevent energy deficit or excess [6]. Before puberty, hormonal nutritional and energy requirements are similar for boys and girls. Energy requirements after the age of 10 become different for boys compared to girls because

of their typically larger size. From ages 4–10 typical daily energy requirements for both males and females vary between 1,800 and 2,000 calories. From ages 11–14 typical male energy requirements are 2,500 calories per day and females 2,200 calories per day. For individuals 15–18, males typically consume 3,000 calories and females 2,200. Extra calories are needed during growth spurts and to replenish energy used during athletic endeavors. These may vary considerably. For example, 60 minutes of playing soccer for a young girl might consume 270 calories, and for a 60-kg boy playing soccer for 60 minutes, an average calorie expenditure might be as high as 936 according to some published research.

- Macronutrients
  Recommendations for carbohydrates, proteins, and fats are no different for children than for adults [6,10]. Carbohydrates are the most important fuel for athletes because they provide glucose used to generate energy. Proteins are essential to build and repair muscle, hair, nails, and skin. Fat is necessary to absorb fat-soluble vitamins (A, D, E, and K) and to provide essential fatty acids, protect vital organs, and provide insulation.
- Micronutrients
  Micronutrient requirements do not differ for children from adults [6,10]. However, it is important for children and adolescents to consume proper amounts of calcium, vitamin D, and iron. Calcium and vitamin D are essential for bone health, and iron is important for oxygen delivery to bodily tissues. During adolescence, more iron is required to support growth as well as increase blood volume and lean muscle mass. Typical amounts of iron needed for both boys and girls up to age 13 should be approximately 8 mg per day; adolescents 14–18 years old require more iron—up to 11 mg per day for males and 15 mg per day for females. Iron depletion is common in athletes because of diets poor in meat, fish, and poultry and increased iron losses in urine, feces, sweat, and menstrual blood. Athletes who are vegetarian, and particularly female athletes and distant runners, should be screened periodically for iron status. Iron-rich foods to recommend include eggs, leafy green vegetables, fortified grains, and lean meats.
- Fluids
  As already indicated, fluids, particularly water, are important nutrients for athletes of all ages [38,48]. Adequate fluid hydration is important to regulate body temperature and replace sweat losses during exercise. Proper hydration recommendations during, before, and after exercise for athletes is found in Table 30.2 [4].
- Recovery Foods
  Recovery foods and beverages may be consumed within 30 minutes of exercise and again one to two hours after exercise to help reload muscles with glycogen and allow for proper recovery [28,30,47]. These foods should include both protein and carbohydrates.
- Meal Planning
  It is important to manage meal planning around athletic events. General guidelines include eating meals a minimum of three hours before an event

TABLE 30.2
Recommendations for Minimal Fluid Intake During and After Exercise in Child Athletes, Based on the Calculation of 13 mL/kg of Fluid During Exercise and 4 mL/kg after Exercise

Body Weight, kg	Fluid Replacement during Exercise, mL/h	Fluid Replacement after Exercise, mL/h
25	325	100
30	390	120
35	455	140
40	520	160
45	585	180
50	650	200
55	715	220
60	780	240

Source: Adapted from American College of Sports Medicine Position Stand: Exercise and fluid replacement. Med Sci Sports Exerc 2007;39(2):377–90.

to allow for proper digestion and minimize incidence of gastrointestinal upset during exercise. Meals should include carbohydrate, protein, and fat, and fiber should be limited. Pregame snacks or liquid meals should be ingested one to two hours before an event. During an event, sports drinks, fruit, yogurt, or granola bars can be adjusted to help refuel and keep energy levels high.

30.9 SPORTS DRINKS AND ENERGY DRINKS FOR CHILDREN AND ADOLESCENTS

The American Academy of Pediatrics has issued a statement emphasizing that sports drinks and energy drinks are significantly different products, and the term should not be used interchangeably [46]. An increasing use of sports and energy drinks in children and adolescents has often resulted in both appropriate and inappropriate use. Sports drinks are beverages that may contain carbohydrates, minerals, electrolytes, and flavoring and are intended to replenish water and electrolyte loss through sweating and exercise. In contrast, energy drinks contain substances that act as non-nutrient stimulants such as caffeine, guarana, taurine, ginseng, and creatine. The American Academy of Pediatrics stated that caffeine and other stimulant substances contained in energy drinks have no place in the diet of children and adolescents. Furthermore, excessive intake of caloric sports drinks can substantially increase the risk of overweight or obesity in children and adolescents. It is important for physicians and parents to discuss appropriate use of sports drinks for the elite athlete and discourage the use of energy drinks.

30.10 SPECIAL CONSIDERATIONS: WEIGHT STATUS AND EATING DISORDERS

During adolescence the prevalence of eating disorders increases. In some sports such as wrestling or martial arts, competitions are placed in certain weight classes. Other sports such as gymnastics and dance place a strong emphasis on lean physique. For these reasons, adolescent athletes may need additional guidance to ensure they are consuming a sufficient amount of nutrients in order to meet [49–51] demands being placed on their body as well as overall health considerations. Scheduling an appointment with a dietitian may be helpful. Coaches, too, can play an important role in recognizing eating disorders.

Promoting a healthy environment for sports competition is also very important. Youth sports should be seen as an opportunity to encourage physical activity and a healthy food environment. In several studies, team snacks provided by parents during games were often unhealthy including French fries, chips, candies, and cookies [52]. Beverages were most likely diet soda, water, or sugar-sweetened sports drinks. Drinks consumed in dugouts during games were often sugar sweetened. Unfortunately, food consumed by spectators in one study found that 85% of food purchased comes from the concession stand and 73% of these items were unhealthy (French fries, chips, candy, cookies, and ice cream). It is important for parents to be vigilant to make sure the sporting environment is nutritionally healthy.

30.11 CONCLUSIONS

Physical activity is an important health-promoting behavior. Generally, nutritional recommendations for physical activity and athletics are similar to healthy plant-based diets in general. Special consideration should be given to food consumption. Dehydration can occur when total body weight is diminished by 2% through decreases in water. Health considerations are particularly important for children participating in athletic events.

Clinical Applications

- All patients should be counseled to increase physical activity
- Nutritional recommendations for physically active adults should include a healthy plant-based diet.
- Fluid recommendations during physical activity depend on the age, sex, and size of the individual and should be discussed during every clinical visit.
- Children and adolescents who participate in athletics should be counseled concerning proper fluid replacement, both before exercise, during exercise, and after exercise.

REFERENCES

1. Physical Activity Guidelines Advisory Committee. 2018 Physical Activity Guidelines Advisory Committee Scientific Report. Washington, DC: U.S. Department of Health and Human Services 2018, 2018.

2. Rippe J. Lifestyle Medicine: Increasing Physical Activity: A Practical Guide. Boca Raton: CRC Press, 2020.
3. Evans G, James L, Maughan R, et al. Effects of an active lifestyle on water balance and water requirements. In Rippe JM (ed). Lifestyle Medicine, 4th edition. Boca Raton: CRC Press, 2024.
4. American College of Sports Medicine, Sawka MN, Burke LM, Eichner ER, et al. American College of Sports Medicine position stand. Exercise and fluid replacement. Med Sci Sports Exerc. 2007;39(2):377–390.
5. Herrmann J. Nutrition for Physical Activity and Athletics. Oklahoma Cooperative Extension Service. Division of Agricultural Sciences and Natural Resources. Stillwater, OK: U.S. Department of Agriculture, the Director of Cooperative Extension Service, Oklahoma State University. April 2021.
6. Boulos R, Davee A. Nutritional considerations for young athletes. In Rippe J (ed). Nutrition in Lifestyle Medicine. Nutrition and Health. Cham: Humana Press, 2017.
7. Mifflin M, St Jeor S, Hill L, et al. A new predictive equation for resting energy expenditure in healthy individuals. Am J Clin Nutr. 1990.51(2):241–247.
8. Liguori G. ACSM's Guidelines for Exercise Testing and Prescription, 11th edition. Philadelphia: Wolters Kluwer, 2021.
9. Rippe J, Foreyt J. Lifestyle Medicine: Obesity Prevention and Treatment: A Practical Guide. Boca Raton: CRC Press, 2021.
10. Purcell L, Canadian Paediatric Society, Paediatric Sports and Exercise Medicine Section. Sport nutrition for young athletes. Paediatr Child Health. 2013;18(4):200–205.
11. Rodriguez N, DiMarco N, Langley S, American Dietetic Association; Dietitians of Canada; American College of Sports Medicine: Nutrition and Athletic Performance. Position of the American Dietetic Association, Dietitians of Canada, and the American College of Sports Medicine: Nutrition and athletic performance. J Am Diet Assoc. 2009;109(3):509–527.
12. Avellini B, Kamon E, Krajewski J. Physiological responses of physically fit men and women to acclimation to humid heat. J Appl Physiol. 1980;49:254–261.
13. Sawka M, Toner R, Francesconi P, et al. Hypohydration and exercise: Effects of heat acclimation, gender, and environment. J Appl Physiol. 1983;55:1147–1153.
14. Shapiro Y, Pandolf B, Avellini N, et al. Physiological responses of men and women to humid and dry heat. J Appl Physiol. 1980;49:1–8.
15. Casa D, Clarkson P, Roberts W. American College of Sports Medicine roundtable on hydration and physical activity: Consensus statements. Curr. Sports Med Rep. 2005; 4:115–127.
16. Cheuvront S, Haymes M, Sawka M. Comparison of sweat loss estimates for women during prolonged high-intensity running. Med Sci Sports Exerc. 2002;34:1344–1350.
17. Institute of Medicine. Water. In Dietary Reference Intakes for Water, Sodium, Chloride, Potassium and Sulfate. Washington, DC: National Academy Press, 2005: 73–185.
18. Ayus C, Varon J, Arieff A. Hyponatremia, cerebral edema, and noncardiogenic pulmonary edema in marathon runners. Ann Intern Med. 2002;132:711–714.
19. Baker L, Munce T, Kenney W. Sex differences in voluntary fluid intake by older adults during exercise. Med Sci Sports Exerc. 2005;37:789–796.
20. Bar-Or O. Temperature regulation during exercise in children and adolescents. In Gisolf C, and Lamb D (eds). Perspectives in Exercise Science and Sports Medicine, Vol 2, Youth, Exercise and Sport. Indianapolis: Benchmark Press, 1989: 335–367.
21. Barr S, Costill D. Water: Can the endurance athlete get too much of a good thing. J Am Diet Assoc. 1989;89:1629–1632.

22. Bartok C, Schoeller D, Sullivan J, et al. Hydration testing in collegiate wrestlers undergoing hypertonic dehydration. Med Sci Sports Exerc. 2004;36:510–517.
23. Cheuvront S, Carter III R, Montain S, et al. Influence of hydration and air flow on thermoregulatory control in the heat. J Therm Biol. 2004;29:532–540.
24. Sawka M, Wenger C, Pandolf K. Thermoregulatory responses to acute exercise-heat stress and heat acclimation. In Blatteis D, and Fregly M (eds). Handbook of Physiology, Environmental Physiology. New York: Oxford University Press for the American Physiological Society, 1996: 157–186.
25. Sawka M, Young A, Latzka W, et al. Human tolerance to heat strain during exercise: Influence of hydration. J Appl Physiol. 1992;73:368–375.
26. Mustafa K, Mahmoud N. Evaporative water loss in African soccer players. J Sports Med Phys Fitness. 1979;19:181–183.
27. Wyndham C, Strydom N. The danger of an inadequate water intake during marathon running. S Afr Med. 1969;43:893–896.
28. Maughan R, Leiper J, Shirreffs M. Restoration of fluid balance after exercise-induced dehydration: Effects of food and fluid intake. Eur J Appl Physiol. 1996;73:317–325.
29. Ray M, Bryan M, Ruden T, et al. Effect of sodium in a rehydration beverage when consumed as a fluid or meal. J Appl Physiol. 1998;85:1329–1336.
30. Shirreffs S, Maughan R. Volume repletion after exercise-induced volume depletion in humans: Replacement of water and sodium losses. Am J Physiol. 1998;274:F868–F875.
31. Leaf A. Dehydration in elderly. N Engl J Med. 1984;311:791–792.
32. Mack G, Weseman C, Langhans G, et al. Body fluid balance in dehydrated healthy older men: Thirst and renal osmoregulation. J Appl Physiol. 1994;76:1615–1623.
33. Rolls B, Phillips P. Aging and disturbances of thirst and fluid balance. Nutr Rev. 1990; 48:137–144.
34. Freund B, Montain J, Young A, et al. Glycerol hyperhydration: Hormonal, renal, and vascular fluid responses. J Appl Physiol. 1995;79:2069–2077.
35. Greenleaf J, Looft-Wilson E, Wisherd J, et al. Hypervolemia in men from fluid ingestion at rest and during exercise. Aviat Space Environ Med. 1998;69:374–386.
36. Consolazio F, Johnson R, Pecora L. The computation of metabolic balances. In Physiological Measurements of Metabolic Function in Man. New York: McGraw-Hill, 1963: 313–339.
37. Mitchell J, Nadel E, Stolwijk J. Respiratory weight losses during exercise. J Appl Physiol. 1972;32:474–476.
38. McArdle B. Physiology of man in the desert. Nature. 1948;161:744.
39. McLellan T, Cheung S, Latzka W, et al. Effects of dehydration, hypohydration, and hyperhydration on tolerance during uncompensable heat stress. Can J Appl Physiol. 1999;24:349–361.
40. Brown T. Exertional rhabdomyolysis. Early recognition is key. Phys Sports Med. 2004;32:15–20.
41. Sayers S, Clarkson P. Exercise-induced rhabdomyolysis. Curr Sports Med Rep. 2002;1: 59–60.
42. Guest N, VanDusseldorp T, Nelson M, et al. International Society of Sports Nutrition Position Stand: Caffeine and exercise performance. J Int Soc Sports Nutr. 2021;2;18(1):1.
43. Engell D, Hirsch E. Environmental and sensory modulation of fluid intake in humans. In Ramsey D, and Booth D (eds). Thirst: Physiological and Psychological Aspects. Berlin: Springer-Verlag, 1999: 382–402.
44. Montain S, Cheuvront S, Carter III R, et al. Human water and electrolyte balance with physical activity. In Bowman B, and Russell R (eds). Present Knowledge in Nutrition, Washington, DC: International Life Sciences Institute, 2006.

45. Montain S, Cheuvront S, Sawka M. Exercise-associated hyponatremia: Quantitative analysis for understand the aetiology. Br J Sports Med. 2006;40:98–106.
46. Schneider M, Benjamin H. Sports drinks and energy drinks for children and adolescents: Are they appropriate? Committee on Nutrition and the Council on Sports Medicine and Fitness. Pediatrics. 2011;27(6):1182–1189.
47. Maughan R, Leiper J. Effects of sodium content of ingested fluids on post-exercise rehydration in man. Eur J Appl Physiol. 1995;71:311–319.
48. Shirreffs S, Taylor A, Leiper J, et al. Post-exercise rehydration in man: Effects of volume consumed and drink sodium content. Med Sci Sports Exerc. 1996;28:1260–1271.
49. Stice E, Marti C, Rohde P. Prevalence, incidence, impairment, and course of the proposed DSM-5 eating disorder diagnoses in an 8-year prospective community study of young women. J Abnorm Psychol. 2013;122(2):445–457.
50. Favaro A, Ferrara S, Santonastaso P. The spectrum of eating disorders in young women: A prevalence study in a general population sample. Psychosom Med. 2003;65(4):701–708.
51. Boisseau N, Vera-Perez S, Poortmans J. Food and fluid intake in adolescent female judo athletes before competition. Pediatr Exerc Sci. 2005;17:62–71.
52. Thomas M, Nelson T, Harwood E, et al, Exploring parent perceptions of the food environment in youth sport. J Nutr Educ Behav. 2012;44(4):365–371.

31 Lifestyle Nutrition
Components of a Healthy Heart Diet

Key Points

- While modern nutritional research has emphasized the importance of healthy dietary patterns, individual foods within these patterns have either been demonstrated to yield health benefits or are key components of healthy diets.
- This chapter focuses on the six major food groups identified by the *Dietary Guidelines for Americans 2020–2025.*
- In addition, red meat should be consumed in limited amounts.
- Added sugar, salt, and sources of saturated fatty acids should also be consumed in limited quantities.
- While alcohol is not included in the healthy dietary patterns, there seems to be little or no harm in women consuming up to one alcoholic beverage a day, and men up to two alcoholic beverages a day. Individuals who do not consume alcoholic beverages should not start. Individuals who consume more than the recommended limit are susceptible to an increased variety of chronic diseases.

31.1 INTRODUCTION

While throughout this book, we follow the modern nutritional practice of focusing on healthy dietary patterns, it is important to recognize that a healthy dietary pattern is made up of groupings of food [1,2]. There are many ways to consume a healthy eating pattern, and, as already indicated, there are multiple approaches to healthy eating. The major healthy eating patterns all include vegetables, fruits, grains, dairy, protein foods, and nontropical oil which are consumed at appropriate calorie levels and with limited amounts of saturated fats, added sugars, and sodium.

One example of how to put this guidance in practice is provided by the Healthy U.S.-Style Dietary Pattern. Since calorie needs change based on age, sex, height, weight, and level of physical activity, patterns developed in the Dietary Guidelines for Americans (DGA) 2020–2025 have been developed at a variety of calorie levels. In Figure 31.1 foods are shown based on the six groups established by the DGA 2020–2025. These are based on a 2,000-calorie diet. As indicated, the number of calories consumed in order to maintain a healthy weight will vary according to age, sex, body size, level of physical activity, etc. Further information related to this may be found in the DGA 2020–2025.

DOI: 10.1201/9781003452607-31

FOOD GROUP OR SUBGROUP[a]	Daily Amount[b] of Food From Each Group (Vegetable and protein foods subgroup amounts are per week.)
Vegetables (cup eq/day)	**2 ½**
	Vegetable Subgroups in Weekly Amounts
Dark-Green Vegetables (cup eq/wk)	1 ½
Red and Orange Vegetables (cup eq/wk)	5 ½
Beans, Peas, Lentils (cup eq/wk)	1 ½
Starchy Vegetables (cup eq/wk)	5
Other Vegetables (cup eq/wk)	4
Fruits (cup eq/day)	**2**
Grains (ounce eq/day)	**6**
Whole Grains (ounce eq/day)	≥ 3
Refined Grains (ounce eq/day)	< 3
Dairy (cup eq/day)	**3**
Protein Foods (ounce eq/day)	**5 ½**
	Protein Foods Subgroups in Weekly Amounts
Meats, Poultry, Eggs (ounce eq/wk)	26
Seafood (ounce eq/wk)	8
Nuts, Seeds, Soy Products (ounce eq/wk)	5
Oils (grams/day)	**27**
Limit on Calories for Other Uses (kcal/day)[c]	**240**
Limit on Calories for Other Uses (%/day)	12%

It should be noted that there are studies of certain specific foods which suggest that individual foods can either increase or decrease the risk of various chronic diseases. The good news is that many of these food items are contained in the healthy plant based dietary patterns.

NOTE: The total eating pattern should not exceed Dietary Guidelines limits for intake of added sugars, saturated fats, and alcohol and would be within the Acceptable Macronutrient Distribution Ranges for calories and protein, carbohydrate, and total fats. Most calorie patterns do not have enough calories available after meeting food groups needs to consume 10% of calories from added sugars and 10% of calories from saturated fats and stay within calorie limits. Values are rounded. See the 2020-2025 Dietary Guidelines for all calorie levels of the Patterns.

Food group amounts shown in cup equivalents (cup eq) or ounce equivalents (ounce eq). Oils are shown in grams. Quantity equivalents for each food group are:

Vegetables, Fruits (1 cup eq): 1 cup raw or cooked vegetable or fruit; 1 cup vegetable or fruit juice; 2 cups leafy salad greens; ½ cup dried fruit or vegetable.

Grains (1 ounce eq): ½ cup cooked rice, pasta, or cereal; 1 ounce dry pasta or rice; 1 medium (1 ounce) slice bread, tortilla, or flatbread; 1 ounce of ready-to-eat cereal (about 1 cup of flaked cereal).

Dairy (1 cup eq): 1 cup milk, yogurt, or fortified soymilk; 1½ ounces natural cheese such as cheddar cheese or 2 ounces of processed cheese.

Protein Foods (1 ounce eq): 1 ounce lean meats, poultry, or seafood; 1 egg; ¼ cup cooked beans or tofu; 1 tbsp nut or seed butter; ½ ounce nuts or seeds.

FIGURE 31.1 Healthy U.S.-Style Dietary Pattern at the 2,000-calorie level, with daily or weekly amounts from food groups, subgroups, and components.

Source: U.S. Department of Health and Human Services and U.S. Department of Agriculture. 2020–2025 Dietary Guidelines for Americans. 9th Edition. 2020:164.

31.2 INDIVIDUAL FOOD ITEMS

The DGA 2020–2025 [1] lists specific fruits and vegetables, as indicated here:

Fruits and Vegetables—Diets that emphasize consumption of fruits and vegetables have been routinely shown to produce substantial improvement in risk factors for coronary heart disease (CHD), including lipid levels, blood pressure, insulin resistance, inflammatory biomarkers, and weight control. Lowering the risk of heart disease through healthy dietary patterns has been shown in both cohort studies and randomized controlled trials (RCTs). Research is currently underway to determine which specific types of fruits and vegetables are most beneficial to lower chronic disease.

- **Fruits**
  This category includes:
  All fresh, frozen, canned, and dried fruits and 100% fruit juices: for example, apples, Asian pears, bananas, berries (e.g. blackberries, blueberries, currants, huckleberries, kiwifruit, mulberries, raspberries, and strawberries); citrus fruit (e.g. calamondin, grapefruit, lemons, limes, oranges, and pomelos); cherries, dates, figs, grapes, guava, jackfruit, lychee, mangoes, melons (e.g. cantaloupe, casaba, honeydew, and watermelon); nectarines, papaya, peaches, pears, persimmons, pineapple, plums, pomegranates, raisins, rhubarb, sapote, and soursop starfruit and tamarind.
- **Vegetables**
  This category includes:
  - *Dark Green Vegetables:* All fresh, frozen, and canned dark green leafy vegetables and broccoli, cooked or raw: For example, amaranth leaves, bok choy, broccoli, chamnamul, chard, collards, kale, mustard greens, poke greens, romaine lettuce, spinach, taro leaves, turnip greens, and watercress.
  - *Red and Orange Vegetables:* All fresh, frozen, and canned red and orange vegetables or juice, cooked or raw: For example, calabaza, carrots, red or orange bell peppers, sweet potatoes, tomatoes, 100% tomato juice, and winter squash such as acorn, kabocha, or pumpkin.
  - *Lentils:* All cooked from dry or canned beans, peas, chickpeas, and lentils: For example, black beans, black-eyed peas, bayo beans, chickpeas (garbanzo beans), edamame, kidney beans, lentils, lima beans, mung beans, pigeon peas, pinto beans, and split peas. Does not include green beans or green peas.
  - *Starchy Vegetables:* All fresh, frozen, and canned starchy vegetables: For example, breadfruit, burdock root, cassava, corn, jicama, lotus root, lima beans, plantains, white potatoes, salsify, taro root (dasheen or yautia), water chestnuts, yam, and yucca.
  - *Other Vegetables:* All other fresh, frozen, and canned vegetables, cooked or raw: For example, asparagus, avocado, bamboo shoots, beets, bitter melon, brussels sprouts, cabbage (green, red, napa, savoy), cactus pads (nopales), cauliflower, celery, chayote (mirliton), cucumber, eggplant, green beans, kohlrabi, luffa, mushrooms, okra, onions, radish, rutabaga, seaweed, snow peas, summer squash, tomatillos, turnips, and winter melons.
- **Whole Grains and Dietary Fiber**
  Whole grains are those containing the endosperm, bran (outer layer of whole grain), and germ in relative proportions as they exist in the intact grain [3]. Refined grains, in contrast, contain only the endosperm. Dietary fiber consists of the remnants of the edible plant lignin, polysaccharides, and

associated substances that are resistant to ingestion by the human gastrointestinal tract and enzymes. There are two major types of fiber: Insoluble fiber (including cellular lignins), which is found in some vegetables and some fruits and grains, and soluble fiber, which includes pectin, fruits, guar gum, and mucilage.

Eating whole grains decreases total cholesterol by 7–10 mg/dL and low-density lipoprotein cholesterol (LDL-C) cholesterol by 6.9 mg/dL according to a recent Cochran analysis [4]. The American Heart Association Dietary Guidelines [2] as well as the National Cholesterol Education Program (ATP III and IV) [5,6] all include recommendations to increase fiber [8–11]. Whether or not fiber is a supplement rather than in food can similarly decrease risk factors for CVD is controversial. The Dietary Reference Intakes (DRI) [7] and Academy of Nutrition and Dietetics [12] recommend 25 grams of fiber for adult women and 38 grams for men. Unfortunately, most of the United States averages less than half of the recommended amount of fiber in the diet [12].

- *Whole grains:* All whole grain products and whole grains used as ingredients: For example, amaranth, barley (not pearled), brown rice, buckwheat, bulgur, millet, oats, popcorn, quinoa, dark rye, whole-grain cornmeal, whole wheat bread, whole wheat chapati, whole grain cereals and crackers, and wild rice.
- *Refined grains:* All refined grain products and refined grains used as ingredients: For example, white breads, refined grain cereals and crackers, corn grits, cream of rice, cream of wheat, barley (pearled), masa, pasta, and white rice. Refined grain choices should be enriched.

- **Fish**

A variety of healthy substances including unsaturated fat, vitamin D, selenium, and long-chain omega-3 polyunsaturated fatty acids (PUFAs) are all contained in fish and other seafood [13]. Some studies have suggested that fish oil may have direct antiarrhythmic effects [14,15]. Fish oil has been shown to lower triglyceride levels [16], systolic and diastolic blood pressure, and resting heart rate [17,18]. For all of these physiologic benefits, regular fish consumption is associated with lower risk of CVD and risk of cardiac death, and for this reason the American Heart Association (AHA) dietary recommendations include consumption of two fish meals (preferably oily fish) per week [2]. It is uncertain whether the benefits of eating fish can be reproduced by consuming fish oil supplements.

Seafood examples that are lower in methylmercury include anchovy, black sea bass, catfish, clams, cod, crab, crawfish, flounder, haddock, hake, herring, lobster, mullet, oyster, perch, pollock, salmon, sardine, scallops, shrimp, sole, squid, tilapia, freshwater trout, light tuna, and white fish.

It should be noted that in the Nordic diet, which is one of the plant-based healthy diets, the recommendation is to eat "wild" fish rather than "farmed" fish, because wild fish contain more nutrients. Furthermore, factory-fed fish are fed grains, which makes them less healthy for the planet [19].

- Nuts
  Both tree nuts and peanuts are nutrient-dense foods that are high in unsaturated fats and other bioactive compounds and contain high-quality vegetable protein, fiber, minerals, tocopherols, phytosterols, and phenolic compounds [20–22]. Epidemiologic studies have consistently shown a negative association between nut consumption and CVD risk [23,24]. Consumption of nuts can lower LDL-C concentration by approximately 10 mg/dL without significantly changing high-density lipoprotein cholesterol (HDL-C) levels [25,26]. Triglyceride (TG) levels have also been shown to be reduced by greater than 20 mg/dL in individuals with elevated blood cholesterol who consume nuts, although not in individuals with normal TG levels [25,26].
  Nuts and seeds include all nuts (tree nuts and peanuts), nut butters, seeds (e.g. chia, flax, pumpkin, sesame, and sunflower), and seed butters (e.g. sesame or tahini and sunflower). Soy includes tofu, tempeh, and products made from soy flour, soy protein isolate, and soy concentrate. Nuts should be unsalted.
- Meat
  Dietary patterns that include lower consumption of red meat have been consistently demonstrated to lower CVD risk [23,27]. Various constituents of red meat including saturated fatty acids (SFAs) may raise cholesterol levels. In processed meats sodium has also been shown to increase risk factors for CVD. The consumption of red meats and processed meats has also been associated with weight gain, which may also increase the risk of CVD.
  Meats include beef, goat, lamb, pork, and game meat (e.g. bison, moose, elk, deer). Poultry includes chicken, Cornish hens, duck, game birds (e.g. ostrich, pheasant, and quail), goose, and turkey. Organ meats include chitterlings, giblets, gizzard, liver, sweetbreads, tongue, and tripe. Eggs include chicken eggs and other birds' eggs. Meats and poultry should be lean or low fat [1].
- Dairy Products
  Dairy products are rich in minerals such as calcium, potassium, magnesium, protein (casein), whey, and vitamins (riboflavin and vitamin B_{12}) and may help in lowering the risk of CVD [28–31]. Some concern remains, however, about saturated fat in full-fat dairy products. For this reason, most dietary guidelines recommend low-fat dairy products rather than full-fat dairy products. Recent research has suggested that the matrix in dairy products may make the SFAs in them less hazardous to CVD risk than other SFAs [32]. The DGA 2020–2025 recommend adults consume three cups of low-fat milk or the equivalent on a daily basis. This is much greater than the average serving of one cup per day currently consumed by adults in the United States. Children and adolescents also consume lower than the

recommended levels. The health effects of other dairy products such as yogurt, cheese, and butter are subject to considerable research and require further study [33–35].

This category includes all fluid, dry, or evaporated milk, including lactose-free and lactose-reduced products and fortified soy beverages (soy milk), buttermilk, yogurt, kefir, frozen yogurt, dairy desserts, and cheeses (e.g. brie camembert, cheddar, cottage cheese, Colby, edam, feta, fontina, goad, gouda, gruyere, limburger, Mexican cheeses [queso anejo, queso asadero, queso chihuahua], Monterey, mozzarella, muenster, parmesan, provolone, ricotta, and Swiss) [1]. Most choices should be fat free or low fat. Cream, sour cream, and cream cheese are not included due to their low calcium content.

- Soy
  Protein found in soybeans is typically referred to as "soy" and is often used to replace animal protein in individual diets. Soybeans contain no cholesterol and are low in saturated fat and contain considerable protein. Soy is the only vegetable to contain all eight amino acids. The effects of soy on CVD risk have been inconsistent.
- Sugar-Sweetened Beverages (SSBs)
  Most studies related to SSBs have suggested increased consumption of SSBs increases the risk of heart disease, diabetes, and obesity [36,37]. Not all studies have supported these findings. The AHA recommends that adult males consume no more than 150 kcals/day in SSBs and adult females no more than 100 kcals/day from SSBs [38]. The DGAs 2020–2025 recommend no more than 10% of calories from added sugars [1]. Increased SSB consumption may be an indication for overall poor diet quality [39].
- Alcohol
  Alcohol consumption has been demonstrated in various studies to have both beneficial and adverse cardiovascular outcomes. Heavy alcohol consumption (three alcoholic drinks per day or more for men and two alcoholic drinks or more per day for women) is associated with increased risk of cardiomyopathy and higher rates of atrial fibrillation [40,41]. Alcohol consumption is also associated with a variety of other noncardiac adverse health consequences such as motor vehicle accidents.

  Moderate consumption of alcohol (up to two drinks per day for men and one drink per day for women) has been shown to lower the incidence of CVD and diabetes [42]. It is possible that moderate alcohol consumption raises HDL-C, while reducing systemic inflammation and improving insulin resistance.
- Coffee and Caffeine
  Coffee is consumed throughout the world and is the leading source of caffeine. Other sources of caffeine include primarily tea, cocoa products, cola beverages, and "energy drinks." It has been estimated that 80–90% of adults regularly consume caffeine-containing beverages. Coffee consumption has long been suspected to be a contributing factor for the development of CVD. However, data in the last few years have suggested no harm and possibly even a protective association between moderate coffee drinking and CVD mortality [43–45].

- Tea
  Tea is also widely consumed throughout the world. Most of the tea consumed in Western countries (78%) is black tea, while 20% is green tea, which is the most commonly consumed tea in Asian countries. Oolong tea (2%) is mainly consumed in Southern China. Some studies suggest that tea consumption may protect against the incidence and progression of CVD [46,47]. It has been speculated that these findings may result from improvement of endothelial function based on the interaction between tea phenolic components and nitric oxide (NO).
- Eggs
  For many years the public had been cautioned to limit egg consumption due to the high cholesterol content of egg yolks and the potential association with CVD. Recent research, however, has demonstrated that cholesterol in eggs has minimal effect on blood cholesterol. Furthermore, eggs are a good source of high-value protein and a variety of vitamins and minerals [48]. The DGA Guidelines 2020–2025 continue, however, to recommend the restriction of dietary cholesterol to less than 300 milligrams/day.
- Garlic
  Garlic preparations have been investigated for both prevention and treatment of CVD. Long-term observational studies for garlic are not available, however. Some studies have suggested that garlic may reduce platelet aggregation, but the effect on other CVD risk factors is controversial [49].
- Chocolate
  Chocolate is similar to green teas with regard to the content of polyphenols. It is important to recognize that chocolate and cocoa are not the same thing. Cocoa powder is used in the production of chocolate. However, fat and sugar are the major components of chocolate, which create a higher caloric content. For these reasons it is appropriate to potentially recommend cocoa rather than chocolate due to the increased calories from sugar and fat in chocolate [50].
- Salt and Sodium
  Various heart-healthy dietary plans are consistent in recommending a reduction of sodium. Dietary sodium may come in a variety of sources in the diet. A major source of sodium is processed food. As dietary sodium increases so does blood pressure [51,52].

  Numerous studies have shown that reduction of salt intake lowers the risk of CVD. For this reason, the AHA established an interim goal of 2,300 mg/day of sodium and less than 1,500 mg/day for individuals with hypertension [2]. The current average intake of sodium in the United States is 3.4 grams/day. Some studies have suggested that this level of sodium consumption does not increase the risk of CVD when compared to higher or lower intake, although this is controversial.
- Vitamin D
  Vitamin D consumption is associated with decreased risk of bone disease. At the current time there are insufficient data to recommend increased consumption of vitamin D as a strategy for lowering the risk of CVD [53].

- Antioxidant Vitamins E and C
  Some observational studies have suggested that antioxidant vitamins E and C were associated with lower risk of CVD. Randomized controlled trials (RCTs) in this area have been largely disappointing [54,55]. In fact, several studies have shown increased mortality with pre-existing, late-stage atherosclerosis and cancer in individuals receiving antioxidant supplements with vitamin E or C [54,55].

31.3 CONCLUSIONS

All throughout this book we have emphasized the modern nutritional understandings that overall dietary patterns are most important to emphasize rather than individual foods or nutrients. In this chapter we have focused on components of a healthy diet. It should be emphasized that these components fit within an overall healthy diet. It should also be emphasized that lower consumption of red meats, SSBs, and salt have also been emphasized as recommendations in all of the healthy dietary patterns.

Clinical Applications

- While clinicians should focus on overall healthy dietary patterns, in this chapter we have indicated a variety of foods based on six food groups identified by the DGA 2020–2025. Many of the components of these food groups are contained in healthy dietary patterns.
- Foods to limit include red meat and other sources of SFAs as well as added sugar and salt.
- Clinicians should discuss not only the overall dietary pattern but, if appropriate, also discuss components contained in most heart-healthy diets.
- The DGA 2020–2025 emphasized that brightly colored fruits and vegetables are typically more "nutrient dense" than lesser colored items and should be emphasized.

REFERENCES

1. U.S. Department of Agriculture and U.S. Department of Health and Human Services. *Dietary Guidelines for Americans, 2020–2025*, 9th edition. December 2020. Available at DietaryGuidelines.gov.
2. Lichtenstein A, Appel L, Vadiveloo M. 2021 dietary guidance to improve cardiovascular health: A scientific statement from the American Heart Association. Circulation. 2021;7;144(23):e472–e487.
3. Zhang G, Hamaker B. The nutritional property of endosperm starch and its contribution to the health benefits of whole grain foods. Crit Rev Food Sci Nutr. 2017;12;57(18):3807–3817.
4. Hartley L, May M, Loveman E, et al. Dietary fibre for the primary prevention of cardiovascular disease. Cochrane Database Syst Rev. 2016;7;2016(1).
5. National Cholesterol Education Program (NCEP) Expert Panel on Detection, Evaluation, and Treatment of High Blood Cholesterol in Adults (Adult Treatment Panel III). Third report of the National Cholesterol Education Program (NCEP) expert panel on detection, evaluation, and treatment of high blood cholesterol in adults (Adult Treatment Panel III) final report. Circulation. 2002;17;106(25):3143–3421.

6. National Heart, Lung, and Blood Institute. Cardiovascular Risk Reduction Guidelines in Adults: Cholesterol Guideline Update (ATP IV); Hypertension Guideline Update (JNC 8); Obesity Guideline Update (Obesity 2); Integrated Cardiovascular Risk Reduction Guideline. (Accessed October 25, 2023).
7. Trumbo P, Schlicker S, Yates A, et al. Food and nutrition board of the institute of medicine, the national academies. Dietary reference intakes for energy, carbohydrate, fiber, fat, fatty acids, cholesterol, protein and amino acids. J Am Diet Assoc. 2002;102(11):1621–1630.
8. Soliman G. Dietary fiber, atherosclerosis, and cardiovascular disease. Nutr. 2019;11:1155.
9. McRae M. Dietary fiber is beneficial for the prevention of cardiovascular disease: An umbrella review of meta-analyses. J Chiropr Med. 2017;16:289–299.
10. Ning H, Van Horn L, Shay CM, et al. Associations of dietary fiber intake with long-term predicted cardiovascular disease risk and C-reactive protein levels (from the National Health and Nutrition Examination Survey Data [2005–2010]). Am J Cardiol. 2014;113:287–291.
11. Kim Y, Je Y. Dietary fiber intake and total mortality: A meta-analysis of prospective cohort studies. Am J Epidemiol. 2014;180:565–573.
12. Dahl W, Stewart ML. Position of the academy of nutrition and dietetics: Health implications of dietary fiber. J Acad Nutr Diet. 2015;115:1861–1870.
13. Mozaffarian D, Rimm E. Fish intake, contaminants, and human health: Evaluating the risks and the benefits. JAMA. 2006;296:1885–1899.
14. Brouwer I, Raitt M, Dullemeijer C, et al. Effect of fish oil on ventricular tachyarrhythmia in three studies in patients with implantable cardioverter defibrillators. Eur Heart J. 2009;30:820–826.
15. Kowey P, Reiffel J, Ellenbogen K, et al. Efficacy and safety of prescription omega-3 fatty acids for the prevention of recurrent symptomatic atrial fibrillation: A randomized controlled trial. JAMA. 2010;304:2363–2372.
16. Eslick G, Howe P, Smith C, et al. Benefits of fish oil supplementation in hyperlipidemia: A systematic review and meta-analysis. Int J Cardiol. 2009;136:4–16.
17. Geleijnse J, Giltay E, Grobbee D, et al. Blood pressure response to fish oil supplementation: Metaregression analysis of randomized trials. J Hypertens. 2002;20:1493–1499.
18. Mozaffarian D, Geelen A, Brouwer I, et al. Effect of fish oil on heart rate in humans: A meta-analysis of randomized controlled trials. Circulation. 2005;112:1945–1952.
19. Lankinen M, Uusitupa M, Schwab U. Nordic diet and inflammation-a review of observational and intervention studies. Nutr. 2019;18;11(6):1369.
20. Kris-Etherton P, Hu F, Ros E, et al. The role of tree nuts and peanuts in the prevention of coronary heart disease: Multiple potential mechanisms. J Nutr. 2008;138:1746S–1751S.
21. King J, Blumberg J, Ingwersen L, et al. Tree nuts and peanuts as components of a healthy diet. J Nutr. 2008;138:1736S–1740S.
22. Ros E. Nuts and novel biomarkers of cardiovascular disease. Am J Clin Nutr. 2009;89: 1649S–1656S.
23. Mente A, de Koning L, Shannon H, et al. A systematic review of the evidence supporting a causal link between dietary factors and coronary heart disease. Arch Intern Med. 2009;169:659–669.
24. Kelly J, Sabate J. Nuts and coronary heart disease: An epidemiological perspective. Br J Nutr. 2006;96(suppl 2):S61–S67.
25. Banel D, Hu F. Effects of walnut consumption on blood lipids and other cardiovascular risk factors: A meta-analysis and systematic review. Am J Clin Nutr. 2009;90:56–63.
26. Kendall C, Josse A, Esfahani A, et al. Nuts, metabolic syndrome and diabetes. Br J Nutr. 2010;104:465–473.

27. Micha R, Wallace S, Mozaffarian D. Red and processed meat consumption and risk of incident coronary heart disease, stroke, and diabetes: A systematic review and meta-analysis. Circulation. 2010;121:2271–2283.
28. Ard J, Grambow SC, Liu D, et al. The effect of the PREMIER interventions on insulin sensitivity. Diabetes Care. 2004;27(2):340–347.
29. Elmer P, Obarzanek E, Vollmer W, et al. PREMIER Collaborative Research Group. Effects of comprehensive lifestyle modification on diet, weight, physical fitness, and blood pressure control: 18-month results of a randomized trial. Ann Intern Med. 2006;4;144(7):485–495.
30. Miller E 3rd, Erlinger T, Appel L. The effects of macronutrients on blood pressure and lipids: An overview of the DASH and OmniHeart trials. Curr Atheroscler Rep. 2006;8(6): 460–465.
31. Al-Solaiman Y, Jesri A, Mountford W, et al. DASH lowers blood pressure in obese hypertensives beyond potassium, magnesium and fibre. J Hum Hypertens. 2010;24(4):237–246.
32. Mozaffarian D, Cao H, King I, et al. Trans-palmitoleic acid, metabolic risk factors, and new-onset diabetes in U.S. adults: A cohort study. Ann Intern Med. 2010;153:790–799.
33. Tholstrup T, Hoy C, Andersen L, et al. Does fat in milk, butter and cheese affect blood lipids and cholesterol differently? J Am Coll Nutr. 2004;23:169–176.
34. Biong A, Muller H, Seljeflot I, et al. A comparison of the effects of cheese and butter on serum lipids, haemostatic variables and homocysteine. Br J Nutr. 2004;92:791–797.
35. Messina M. Soy and health update: Evaluation of the clinical and epidemiologic literature. Nutr. 2016;24;8(12):754.
36. Mozaffarian D, Hao T, Rimm E, et al. Changes in diet and lifestyle and long-term weight gain in women and men. N Engl J Med. 2011;364:2392–2404.
37. Wolff E, Dansinger M. Soft drinks and weight gain: How strong is the link? Medscape J Med. 2008;10(8):189.
38. Johnson RK, Appel LJ, Brands M, et al. Dietary sugars intake and cardiovascular health: A scientific statement from the American Heart Association. Circulation. 2009;120(11): 1011–1120.
39. Rippe J, Saltzman E. Sweetened beverages and health: Current state of scientific understandings. Adv Nutri. 2013;(4) 527–529.
40. Laonigro I, Correale M, Di Biase M, et al. Alcohol abuse and heart failure. Eur J Heart Fail. 2009;11:453–462.
41. Conen D, Tedrow U, Cook N, et al. Alcohol consumption and risk of incident atrial fibrillation in women. JAMA. 2008;300:2489–2496.
42. Rimm E, Williams P, Fosher K, et al. Moderate alcohol intake and lower risk of coronary heart disease: Meta-analysis of effects on lipids and haemostatic factors. BMJ. 1999;319:1523–1528.
43. Ding M, Bhupathiraju S, Chen M, et al. Caffeinated and decaffeinated coffee consumption and risk of type 2 diabetes: A systematic review and a dose-response meta-analysis. Diabetes Care. 2014;37:569–586.
44. Ding M, Bhupathiraju S, Satija A, et al. Long-term coffee consumption and risk of cardiovascular disease: A systematic review and a dose-response meta-analysis of prospective cohort studies. Circulation. 2014;129:643–659.
45. Steffen M, Kuhle C, Hensrud D, et al. The effect of coffee consumption on blood pressure and the development of hypertension: A systematic review and meta-analysis. J Hypertens. 2012;30:2245–2254.
46. Yang W, Wang W, Fan W, et al. Tea consumption and risk of type 2 diabetes: A dose-response meta-analysis of cohort studies. Br J Nutr. 2014;111:1329–1339.

47. Zhang C, Qin Y, Wei X, et al. Tea consumption and risk of cardiovascular outcomes and total mortality: A systematic review and meta-analysis of prospective observational studies. Eur J Epidemiol. 2015;30:103–113.
48. Zhang X, Lv M, Luo X, et al. Egg consumption and health outcomes: A global evidence mapping based on an overview of systematic reviews. Ann Transl Med. 2020;8(21):1343.
49. Bayan L, Koulivand P, Gorji A. Garlic: A review of potential therapeutic effects. Avicenna J Phytomed. 2014;4(1):1–14.
50. Katz D, Doughty K, Ali A. Cocoa and chocolate in human health and disease. Antioxid Redox Signal. 2011;15;15(10):2779–2811.
51. Mozaffarian D, Fahimi S, Singh G, et al. Global sodium consumption and death from cardiovascular causes. N Engl J Med. 2014;371(7):624–634.
52. Aburto N, Ziolkovska A, Hooper L, et al. Effect of lower sodium intake on health: Systematic review and meta-analyses. BMJ. 2013;346:f1326.
53. Ford J, MacLennan G, Avenell A, et al. RECORD Trial Group. Cardiovascular disease and vitamin D supplementation: Trial analysis, systematic review, and meta-analysis. Am J Clin Nutr. 2014;100(3):746–755.
54. Bjelakovic G, Nikolova D, Gluud L, et al. Mortality in randomized trials of antioxidant supplements for primary and secondary prevention: Systematic review and meta-analysis. JAMA. 2007;28;297(8):842–857.
55. Ye Y, Li J, Yuan Z. Effect of antioxidant vitamin supplementation on cardiovascular outcomes: A meta-analysis of randomized controlled trials. PLoS One. 2013;8(2):e56803.

32 Genetics, Epigenetics, and Precision Nutrition

Key Points

- Current recommendations both for diet and other lifestyle activities are based on population data.
- While good population-based data exist that following a healthy plant-based diet lowers the risk of heart disease, diabetes, and certain cancers, not all individuals will achieve the same level of benefits from these recommendations.
- While the general recommendations are still highly appropriate, the field of genetics, epigenetics, and precision nutrition offers an opportunity to make these recommendations more precise and personalized in the future.
- The fields of genetics, epigenetics, and their interrelationship with precision nutrition is in its infancy, so these areas are typically not applicable to current clinical practice, but offer great promise for the future.

32.1 INTRODUCTION

There are multiple interactions between genetics, epigenetics, and, ultimately, the emerging area of precision nutrition. While many of these concepts are not yet ready for clinical application, they hold enormous promise for the future of making nutritional choices evermore precise and personalized [1–8].

While the human genome is known to change minimally over thousands of years, nutrition can play a role in how various portions of the genome are activated. In addition, a number of nutritional practices can play a significant role in the area of epigenetics, which can significantly alter which portions of the genome are either activated or suppressed [4–7,9–14]. Both of these areas play a very significant role in the development of more precise nutrition, which holds enormous promise in the future by giving individuals specific recommendations based on their genetic profile for how various nutrients will interact with them in a way that can promote good health.

Moreover, the fields of genetics and epigenetics are beginning to unravel why certain nutritional practices are more effective than others for reducing risk of chronic diseases. For example, it is now thought that polymorphisms in genetic material may at least partially explain why some individuals are more sensitive to salt restriction than others when it comes to blood pressure control. In addition, great diversity exists related to how individuals respond to statins for cholesterol control. Genetic and epigenetic research offer the opportunity to potentially move nutrition from a population-based set of recommendations to more highly individualized and perhaps much more effective precise recommendations.

DOI: 10.1201/9781003452607-32

At the current time advances in this area do not suggest that current general recommendations, which are population based, are irrelevant. Quite the contrary. The current recommendations, as they have evolved, provide the fundamental groundwork for how we think about lifestyle habits and actions and their impact on health.

One intriguing aspect of the field of genetics, epigenetics, and precision nutrition reflects interactions with human microbiome. Recent research has suggested that the microbiome plays a very significant role in how nutrients are handled and forms the basis for a number of recommendations for healthy nutritional practices.

These areas are all enormously complex, and it is essential to remain humble about claims that are made in the area of nutrition and genetics. This caution is all the more important since advances in decoding the human genome have made what used to be a cumbersome and enormously expensive process much more efficient and able to be accomplished at a fraction of the cost from previous genetic analyses. These technical advances have led to a number of commercially marketed and readily available programs with claims for nutrition and health. At the current time these should be approached with considerable skepticism since the field is still in its infancy.

32.2 GENETICS AND NUTRITION

An abundant research literature demonstrates a nutrient-dependent regulation of the genome machinery. This is a two-way street. Nutrients can influence the development of a particular phenotype, but the response to a specific nutrient is determined by the individual's genotype. Therefore, the nutrient/gene interaction is complex and bidirectional.

Research has demonstrated that not all individuals respond to nutrient therapy in the same way and with the same intensity. In the past, this phenomena has created problems attempting to understand responses from nutrients and foods used based on population data. Individuals may be classified as "good," "poor," and "nonresponders" to such interventions. Current research has begun to explore an understanding of how genotype influences the response to nutrients with greater precision than in the past. This field is classified as nutrient-gene interactions.

- **Gene-nutrient interactions**—Enormous complexity exists in the area of how the human genome interacts with various nutrients. The human genome contains approximately 30,000 genes [15]. A part of this genome is involved in metabolic regulation. The link between nutrients and genes is bidirectional in the sense that food availability interacts with gene expression in response to nutrients dependent on genetic background. One example of this is that lipid- and carbohydrate-rich diets have been linked to obesity, non-insulin-dependent diabetes mellitus, and hyperlipidemia [16,17]. This represents an example of the body trying to keep cholesterol levels within a narrow concentration range by transcription control mechanisms through which excess cholesterol is converted to a variety of transcription factors, which limits the accumulation of excess cholesterol.
- **Vitamins, DNA stability, and gene expression**—Multiple different vitamins participate in DNA protection. Thus, dietary deficiencies might lead

to an increase in DNA damage, ultimately resulting in cellular dysfunction, which can occur with both aging and cancer [18]. For example, carotenoids, which are vitamin A precursors, have antioxidant properties and quench free radicals to lower DNA damage. Research evidence has emerged showing that carotenoids influence gene expression. Another example is vitamin B_{12} and folate, which are essential for DNA metabolism [5]. If folic acid deficiency exists, the base pair of uracil is incorporated into DNA instead of thymine, which may result in chromosomal breaks. Vitamin C has also been demonstrated to have strong antioxidant properties and modulates the expression of several genes. Vitamin D exerts in vitro antioxidant activity and stabilizes chromosomal structure. It has also been suggested that vitamin E increases the removal of damaged DNA. Thus, the role of multiple vitamins appears essential to maintaining genomic integrity.

- **Nutrient-specific regulation of gene expression**—A variety of nutrients have a role in controlling expression of genes and are involved in different biological systems. For example, amino acids can play a role in nutritional signals in modulation of expression of particular genes [5]. Fatty acids are involved in the regulation of biological process through the modulation of gene expression. Recently, the issue of carbohydrate regulation of gene expression has been a subject of research. The most-studied pathway in this area is one involving glucose [8,16,19]. Research now documents that a high glucose concentration induces the transcription of several genes in the glycolytic and lipogenic pathways, although much of the research in this area is at the level of cultured cells rather than in vivo research. Thus, numerous studies have now demonstrated the role of nutrients in the regulation of some of the processes of gene expression. It should be cautioned, once again, that this is an area where research is in its infancy.
- **Biological complexity of genes/diet interaction**—Enormous complexity exists in the area of how genes and diet interact. The Human Genome Project showed that there is substantial genetic heterogeneity within the human population [15]. Millions of singular nucleotide polymorphisms (SNPs) have been found to have a relationship with nutrition. These SNPs involve multiple genes, which may highly influence the individual response to multiple exposures, including diet. To further complicate research in this area, nutrition-related disorders have been reported to be the result of a mixture of nutrients with multiple genes, not a single gene. Thus, while the interaction between nutrition, metabolism, and gene expression is essential to maintain homeostasis, the field supplying specific research knowledge in this area is only beginning to be understood. This general area of research has been divided into two interrelated concepts: Nutritional genomics and nutritional genetics.
- **Nutritional genomics and nutritional genetics [20]**—As already noted, a bidirectional relationship exists between nutrition and the human genome. This relationship defines and marks gene expression and metabolic response which, in turn, may affect an individual's health conditions and

susceptibility to disease. In one direction, the genetic background of the individual can define the nutrient state and metabolic response as well as susceptibility to diet-dependent or related health disorders. Second, nutrients regulate the transcription factors that modify gene expression up or down, which adjusts the metabolic response at the molecular level.

The bidirectional interplay between nutrition and the human genome has led to two research sub-definitions, namely nutrigenetics and nutrigenomics. The science of nutrigenetics defines the risk of individuals to diseases, nutrient daily requirements, cellular metabolic response, and behavior toward the bioactive dietary components of nutritional therapy. Thus, nutragenetics defines the impact of gene variability on the interaction between nutrients and diseases.

In contrast, nutrigenomics is the study of the overall genome impact of nutrition, which explores the functional effect of various food components and includes the genome, transcriptome, proteome, and metabolome. There are four principles of nutritional genomics:

- Diet is considered to be a critical predisposing factor for many diseases.
- Diet ingredients change the structure or expression and consequently change the human genome.
- Variation in genotype between individuals may explain the relationship between health and disease.
- Genes that are dependent on dietary factors in their regulation may impact on the various aspects of chronic disease.

- **Nutrient gene-cancer interaction**—The overall diet is a mix of protective, carcinogenic, and immunogenic agents which are metabolized by enzymes in the biotransformation process. Genetic polymorphisms can modify these nutrients in a diet to change the risk of developing cancer. More than 25,000 different bioactive food ingredients exist in the human diet, and of these, 500 types of bioactive food ingredients have been proven to be possible as predisposing agents and may play a role in cancer pathogenesis, while others are not. A diet containing protective micronutrients as well as carcinogens can modulate the risk of cancer development, particularly in genetically susceptible individuals. (For more information in this area see Chapter 15 on nutrition and cancer) [18,20].
- **Current approaches in nutrition research**—Various nutritional deficiencies can compromise the immune response leading to increased susceptibility to infectious diseases, cancer, and suboptimal response to vaccination and other immunologic disorders. Recent studies suggest that increased needs for nutrients in times of stress may have an effect on both innate and adaptive immunity. Increased immune response metabolic demands may be linked to increased needs for specific dietary nutrients. This has led to research in the area of nutritional immunology and focused on such nutrients as vitamins E, A, and D as well as dietary factors that may regulate hormones. Some nutrients such as antioxidants are also important in the immune response. Thus, nutrition can play a significant role in various chronic diseases.

- **Nutrition and chronic disease**—Deficiencies that may be attributed to malnutrition can lead to both undernutrition and overnutrition. It is well known that obesity is associated with a variety of other chronic diseases such as cardiovascular disease (CVD), other forms of atherosclerosis, type 2 diabetes mellitus (T2DM) [2,8], hypertension, and infection-related mortality. Recent research has suggested that obesity creates an inflammatory state and may decrease the effectiveness of the immune system.
- **Oxidative stress and antioxidant defenses**—Reactive oxygen is needed in many metabolic and physiologic processes. Homeostatic equilibrium, however, is maintained by the antioxidant defenses which preserve health by controlling levels of these species. Unhealthy diets have been shown to generate oxidative stress which, in turn, has been shown to play an important role in the development of CVD, hypertension, atherosclerosis, myocardial infarction, diabetes, obesity, and cancer [21–23]. (See also Chapter 9 on nutrition and inflammation.) Antioxidants play a role in reducing the risk of a variety of chronic diseases which have inflammation as an underlying pathology.
- **Public health nutrition and genetics**—The role of nutrition interacting with the human genome may play a significant role in strategies used in public health nutrition. For example, interactions between nutrients and the genome may impact on global food security since over 800 million in the world population are food insecure. In addition, the role of nutrients on the genome may play a significant role in the presence of noncommunicable diseases (NCDs). This is particularly true since the Western diet has been demonstrated to be increasingly inappropriate to the health needs of those consuming it [24–26]. While at the current time public health applications of nutrigenomics are only in their infancy, this is an area where the interaction between nutrients and the genome is likely to play an ever-increasing role in public nutrition policy. This is particularly true in the area of global malnutrition, where increased efficacy of nutrition policy may be necessary to meet ongoing increasing needs of healthy nutrition for the entire population.

32.3 EPIGENETICS

The human genome changes exquisitely slowly—perhaps no more than 1% over a millennia. Given the stability of the human genome, why have such issues as obesity increased 40% over the last two decades? To some degree this can be explained by what some people have called the "obesogenic" environment, namely, increased consumption of calories, inflammation caused by the Western diet, and decreasing levels of physical activity. These habits and actions, however, fall short of completely explaining why various chronic diseases have increased so dramatically in the past 30–40 years. A partial answer may lie in the area of epigenetics.

- **The rise of the field of nutritional epigenetics**—Studies in epigenetics have dramatically increased in the past two decades and have fundamentally changed many assumptions about how the human genome functions.

Epigenetics refers to the control of gene expression via mechanisms that are not directly related to the DNA coding sequence [4,5,9,11,27]. Thus, cells in an organism may respond very differently, despite having the same genome. Epigenetics explores the process which modulate and regulate gene expression through a variety of epigenetic "marks." This is a term that applies to chemical compounds that are added to DNA or the histone proteins which help determine the shape of the DNA and are recognized by enzymes that either lay down or remove a specific mark [5,28–30]. Nutrition is a key consideration as a major factor determining these "marks." The marks, in turn, change the spatial confirmation of the DNA which may prevent binding of transcription factors or exposing it to allow upregulating or downloading cellular process.

Perhaps the most-studied mark in the field of epigenetics is DNA methylation [29–31]. This denotes the addition of methyl groups to the five carbons of cytosine, which act together with histone modifications to regulate gene expression. DNA methylation may act as a promoter to induce gene silencing of histone acetylation to the underlying euchromatin [9].

It is in the area of methylation, in particular, where nutrition plays such a critical role. DNA methylation occurs within a carbon metabolism pathway, which depends on several enzymes in the presence of dietary micronutrients as cofactors including the availability of folate, choline, and betaine through the diet. DNA methylation is primarily stable. Its regulation, however, is more dynamic than previously believed. Hence, the role of folate, choline, and betaine, all of which are fundamentally found in plants, can fundamentally change the way DNA is transcribed. This can, in turn, significantly influence the likelihood of developing chronic diseases such as CVD, cancer, and diabetes. These nutritional factors are dependent on both lifestyle and environmental factors, and this has given rise to the field of "environmental epigenetics," which refers to how environmental exposures affect epigenetic changes. While life experience, habits, and the environment can impact on the epigenome and health, nutrition is particularly prominent in this area.

- **Nutritional epigenetics in health and disease**—Nutrition is perhaps the most-studied and most-understood environmental epigenetic factor. For example, numerous associations have been observed between adverse prenatal nutritional conditions, postnatal health, and increased risk for disease [5,10–12]. An extreme example of this was the Dutch Famine Birth Cohort, which resulted from the Dutch famine in 1944 and1945. Research on this cohort led to the study of the effects of starvation during pregnancy and subsequent health and development outcomes in offspring including increased risk of T2DM, CVD, metabolic disease, and a decreased cognitive function in later life.

  The epigenetic differences in prenatal exposure to the famine have been attributed to a lower degree of methylation of genes implicated in insulin metabolism. There is evidence of transgenerational effects of poor maternal diet with respect to metabolic outcomes. Interestingly, poor food availability for men has also been demonstrated to result in transgenerational transmission all the way through grandchildren.

Various nutrients can act either directly by inhibiting epigenetic enzymes or altering availability of substrates necessary for these enzymatic reactions. This process, in turn, modifies expressions of critical genes impacting on overall health and longevity. In the area of nutrition, a number of studies have looked at folate metabolism and its relationship to DNA methylation [9]. Maternal methyl donor nutrient availability in early pregnancy is essential for proper fetal development and carries consequences for health and fetal disease susceptibility to cancer in children throughout life [10]. Other nutrients such as choline and betaine, which also are derived from plants, can also impact on DNA methylation. In addition, DNA methylation changes occur throughout the lifespan and, in particular, in an Asian population which may impact on overall longevity and susceptibility to various chronic diseases.

- **Nutritional epigenetics and cancer**—Both folic acid and vitamin B_{12} are epigenetically active ingredients which play a role in DNA methylation [18,20,31]. Low folate intake has been associated with hypomethylation and increased risk of colorectal and pancreatic cancer. In addition, diets that are rich in fruits and vegetables contain natural antioxidants which can also protect against cancer, which suggests that they also may carry epigenetic effects due to nutritional components in addition to folate. For example, green tea contains polyphenols which may also impact on DNA methylation. Other compounds in addition to folate, such as choline and betaine, also can impact on DNA methylation. Choline, which is often found in animal products such as egg yolks, cooked beef, chicken, veal and turkey, is also found in soy and is a methyl donor. Betaine, which is found in spinach, shellfish, and sugar beets, helps remove toxic by-products which involves a process of methylation.

  An intriguing body of information exists related to butyrate, which is a compound produced in the intestines when dietary fiber is fermented and plays a role in histone serialization, turning on "protective genes" and, at least in some animal models, generating increased lifespan. This is another area of intense investigation about how healthy plant-based diets which are typically high in fiber impact on the microbiome in ways that can reduce the risk of various chronic diseases including both cancer and CVD.
- **Maternal diet and gut microbiome linkage to obesity in offspring**—Nutrition is the most important environmental factor that can influence early development processes through regulation of epigenetic mechanisms during pregnancy and neonatal period [10,27,32]. Maternal diets are crucial for the establishment of epigenetic profiles in the fetus that carry profound effects on individual susceptibility to certain disorders in the offspring later in life. Several research studies have shown that maternal nutrition status is closely associated with obesity in progeny [10]. This strongly suggests that there is a significant role of maternal nutrition in disease susceptibility to chronic conditions such as obesity.

Factors that impact on the gut microbiota include fiber and folate that are more prominent in plant-based diets and in the typical Western diet and can significantly impact on gut bacteria, in particular. Bacteria in the Bacteroidaceae family are a major source of butyrate. Butyrate, as already indicated, interacts with histone acetylation, and turns on "protective genes," which may lower the risk of both cancer and CVD. Butyrate is a short-chain fatty acid (SCFA) which may also exert its health-promoting effects through anti-inflammatory functions.

- **Cancer control and prevention by nutrition and epigenetic approaches**—Cancer is both a genetic and epigenetic disease [18,20]. As already indicated, dietary components may play a major role in both cancer prevention and treatment. A variety of bioactive food components including tea polyphenols (found in green tea), genistein (from soybeans), folate, choline, and betaine, as already indicated, can play roles in regulating how genes interact with health. These effects may occur through DNA methylation and histone modification. In addition, these plant-based compounds may participate in the regulation of RNA-based mechanisms which interact with DNA methylation or histone modification and result in silenced or enhanced gene expression [5,9,12]. There is considerable research currently in progress which may carry significant implications for ongoing nutritional and epigenetic approaches to cancer control and prevention.
- **Food as exposure**—Given the wide variety of impacts on various components of the diet on epigenetics, some investigators have suggested that a new way of thinking about food is to consider "food as exposure" rather than just a source of nutrients [33]. The whole area of epigenetics is experiencing rapid development and may provide insights into how various components of the diet either enhance or reduce the likelihood of developing chronic diseases.

32.4 PRECISION NUTRITION

As research has continued to clarify issues related to nutrition and its role in both genetics and epigenetics, a corresponding increase has emerged in interest in a field that has been called "precision nutrition" [8,16,19,34,35].

Recommendations for nutrition have traditionally been based on population data. For example, recommendations concerning levels of blood pressure or healthy levels of cholesterol or even healthy levels of weight have all been based on population data. We know now, however, that there are significant polymorphisms concerning how different individuals respond to either lifestyle measures or pharmaceutical interventions in all of these areas. For this reason, there has been recent interest in exploring whether or not more precise recommendations can be made for individuals within a population group. Hence, the field of precision nutrition has emerged. This is also called "personal" nutrition.

- **Definition**—Personalized nutrition is intended to develop interventions to prevent or treat chronic disease risks based on a person's unique characteristics such as DNA, race, gender, health history, nutritional practices, and lifestyle habits in general [18,34,35]. The goal is to provide more effective ways to prevent or treat disease by providing more accurate and targeted strategies [8,36]. Precision nutrition assumes that each person may have a different response to specific foods and nutrients so that the best diet for one individual may look quite different from the best diet for another.

Precision nutrition also encompasses the microbiome. There are the trillions of bacteria in the human body which reside in the microbiome and that play a key role in various daily internal operations and responses to both nutrients and pharmaceutical agents. The types of bacteria that human beings house are unique to each individual. An individual's diet can determine which types of bacteria live in their digestive tract. The reverse is also true since the types of bacteria that are located in an individual's gut may also determine how certain foods are digested and what types of foods are most beneficial for each individual.

- **Framework for nutrition as a tool for precision medicine**—High-quality nutrition studies form the basis for recommendations that have been made by the American Heart Association (AHA), Dietary Guidelines for Americans (DGA) 2020–2025, and other prestigious organizations. These recommendations are based on research that has demonstrated that for the average person eating more vegetables, whole grains, and lean proteins, while eating less processed foods including added sugars and salt, and saturated fat, reduce the risk of various diseases.

  Preliminary studies in the area of precision nutrition have shown substantial variations in physiologic responses in the areas of glucose and triglycerides even if individuals are eating identical meals. The individual's microbiome is thought to contribute to variations in blood triglycerides after a meal. Nonfood factors such as sleep, physical activity, and time of meals also appear to play a role in causing variations in blood levels of glucose and triglycerides after meals [37]. Therefore, an individual may see additional benefits from following personalized nutritional guidance beyond general health recommendations.

  The goal of precision nutrition is to evaluate one's DNA, microbiome, and metabolic response to specific foods or dietary patterns to determine the most effective individualized eating plan or prevent or treat disease. Various frameworks to assist in developing the complex task of evaluating various foods and responses to individuals are currently being developed. It should be emphasized, however, that this whole area is in its infancy [38].
- **NIH Program in Precision Health**—The National Institutes of Health (NIH) has launched a program in "Nutrition in Precision Health" with the goal of recruiting a diverse total of 100,000 participants to help inform through research personalized nutrition recommendations [34,35]. The NIH is awarding $170 million over five years to a variety of clinics and centers around the country to work in this area. The NIH is utilizing an infrastructure called "All of Us" where genomics of participants are available and can be correlated, along with their electronic pulse record data. The intent is also to collect microbiomes and do metabolomics. As already

indicated, this field is only beginning and the field of nutrigenomics has made very few breakthroughs on single gene nutrient interactions, but there is considerable research underway sponsored by the NIH and some private investors to further this field.

- **Relationship of precision nutrition and other lifestyle factors and habits in disease management**—An example of this might be in the area of T2DM [8]. There is already abundant research that healthy lifestyle factors such as regular exercise, achieving and maintaining a healthy weight, and following a healthy nutritional diet plan based on population studies are the current keys to managing T2DM. However, with precision prevention, the goal will be to apply this general information to strategies involving whether or not there are individual variations in the effects of eating fruits and vegetables, having a high intake of dietary fat, etc., in the area of risk for developing T2DM. In addition, the goal will be to discover the types of gut bacteria that improve blood glucose control.
- **Applying precision nutrition to specific foods**—There are some examples of how the concept of precision nutrition may be helpful. A good example is coffee. Some people are unphased by drinking multiple cups of coffee during the day, while others are unable to get to sleep and remain agitated after only one cup [15]. Coffee beans are known to contain a variety of plant chemicals that may achieve health benefits, but many people cannot tolerate the side effects. Some research has already discovered genes specifically related to coffee intake. These genes may determine how fast or slow the caffeine in coffee is metabolized. These genes may also be associated with anti-inflammatory effects which are related to certain chronic diseases. Thus, precision nutrition can help an individual determine how they might respond to drinking coffee. This is one of many examples that are currently being explored.
- **Nutritional interventions for Alzheimer's disease**—Alzheimer's disease (AD) is a major source of morbidity and mortality in many countries around the world, and the disease burden from AD is expected to rise as the population ages. Currently, no disease-modifying agent is available, but recent research suggests that nutritional and lifestyle modifications can delay or prevent the onset of AD. Preventive nutritional interventions, however, are not universally applicable and may depend on the clinical profile of the individual patient [39]. This is another area which has potential applications for personalized nutrition [40].
- **The rise of consumer genomics as a component of overall personalized lifestyle recommendations**—The area of precision nutrition is also accompanied by other areas where lifestyle recommendations can benefit from more precise information. One example might be the area of regular physical activity. All the general guidelines for physical activity recommend participating in 150 minutes of moderate-intensity physical activity per week [41]. There may be considerable differences among individuals related to their response to this amount of physical activity. Some people can achieve the same benefits with much less activity; some will require more. Once

again, the ability of scientific research to help articulate these issues will be very important to make more precise lifestyle recommendations.

- **The rise of consumer genomics and digital health**—The ferment in the area of genetics and epigenetics and personalized nutrition has spawned a series of commercially available products that maintain they can help an individual obtain more precise nutritional and health information and benefits [42,43]. Since this field is still in its infancy, the best recommendation remains to treat any of these recommendations and commercially available platforms with great caution since there is a tendency on the part of companies marketing these materials to overstate potential benefits.

32.5 CONCLUSIONS

An explosion of interest in genetics and epigenetics has occurred as well as their potential role in providing more precision related to nutrition. The goal of this area is to go beyond population-based recommendations and apply more precise information to individuals with the intent of providing more effective recommendations in the area of nutrition. This approach is also being currently applied to other lifestyle activities such as physical activity. While this field remains at the early stages of research, it offers great promise for the future to make evermore precise and personalized recommendations both in the areas of nutrition and other lifestyle habits and practices.

Clinical Applications

- The genetic pool changes very slowly, often only a few percentage points over many thousands of years.
- Epigenetics is a rapidly emerging field of research that shows that various nutritional habits can impact on DNA methylation and significantly alter individual responses without changing the basic DNA.
- The fields of genetics and epigenetics are now being applied to make nutritional and other lifestyle recommendations more precise.
- This field is in its infancy, so clinicians should be very careful not to overpromise.
- Commercially available products in this area should be approached with caution since their marketing materials often exaggerate potential benefits.
- However, this field holds enormous opportunities in the future to make nutrition and other lifestyle recommendations even more precise.

REFERENCES

1. Darnton-Hill I, Margetts B, Deckelbaum R. Public health nutrition and genetics: Implications for nutrition policy and promotion. Proc Nutr Soc. 2004;63(1):173–185.
2. Raqib R, Cravioto A. Nutrition, immunology, and genetics: Future perspectives. Nutr Rev. 2009;67(Suppl 2):S227–S236.
3. Paoloni-Giacobino A, Grimble R, Pichard C. Genetics and nutrition. Clin Nutr. 2003;22(5):429–435.

4. Lorenzo P, Izquierdo A, Rodriguez-Carnero G, F et al. Epigenetic effects of healthy foods and lifestyle habits from the Southern European Atlantic diet pattern: A narrative review. Adv Nutr. 2022;13(5):1725–1247.
5. Tiffon C. The impact of nutrition and environmental epigenetics on human health and disease. Int J Mol Sci. 2018;19(11).
6. Choi S, Friso S. Epigenetics: A new bridge between nutrition and health. Adv Nutr. 2010; 1(1):8–16.
7. Remely M, Stefanska B, Lovrecic L, et al. Nutriepigenomics: The role of nutrition in epigenetic control of human diseases. Curr Opin Clin Nutr Metable Care. 2015;18(4):328–333.
8. Wang D, Hu F. Precision nutrition for prevention and management of type 2 diabetes. Lancet Diabetes Endocrinol. 2018;6(5):416–426.
9. Anderson O, Sant K, Dolinoy D. Nutrition and epigenetics: An interplay of dietary methyl donors, one-carbon metabolism and DNA methylation. J Nutr Biochem. 2012;23 (8):853–859.
10. Li Y. Epigenetic mechanisms link maternal diets and gut microbiome to obesity in the offspring. Front Genet. 2018;9:342.
11. Jiménez-Chillarón J, Díaz R, Martínez D, et al. The role of nutrition on epigenetic modifications and their implications on health. Biochim. 2012;94(11):2242–2263.
12. Pizzorusso T, Tognini P. Interplay between metabolism, nutrition and epigenetics in shaping brain DNA methylation, neural function and behavior. Genes. 2020;11(7).
13. Zhang Y, Kutateladze T. Diet and the epigenome. Nat Commun. 2018;9(1):3375.
14. Verma M. Cancer control and prevention by nutrition and epigenetic approaches. Antioxid Redox Signal. 2012;17(2):355–364.
15. Cornelis M, Byrne E, Esko T, et al. Genome-wide meta-analysis identifies six novel loci associated with habitual coffee consumption. Molecular Psychiatry. 2015;20(5):647–656.
16. Zeevi D, Korem T, Zmora N, et al. Personalized nutrition by prediction of glycemic responses. Cell. 2015;163(5):1079–1094.
17. De Toro-Martín J, Arsenault B, Després J, et al. Precision nutrition: A review of personalized nutritional approaches for the prevention and management of metabolic syndrome. Nutr. 2017;9(8):913.
18. Esteller M. Epigenetics in Cancer. N Engl J Med. 2008;13;358(11):1148–1159.
19. Berry S, Valdes A, Drew D, et al. Human postprandial responses to food and potential for precision nutrition. Nat Med. 2020;26(6):964–973.
20. Elsamanoudy A, Neamat-Allah M, Mohammad F, et al. The role of nutrition related genes and nutrigenetics in understanding the pathogenesis of cancer. J Micros Ultrastruct. 2016;4(3):115–122.
21. Mishra V. Oxidative stress and role of antioxidant supplementation in critical illness. Clin Lab. 2007;53(3–4):199–209.
22. Berger M, Shenkin A. Update on clinical micronutrient supplementation studies in the critically ill. Curr Opin Clin Nutr Metable Care. 2006;9(6):711–716.
23. Eaton S. The biochemical basis of antioxidant therapy in critical illness. Proc Nutr Soc. 2006;65(3):242–249.
24. Fabiani R, Minelli L, Bertarelli G, et al. A western dietary pattern increases prostate cancer risk: A systematic review and meta-analysis. Nutr. 2016;8(10).
25. de la Rocha C, Perez-Mojica J, Leon S, et al. Associations between whole peripheral blood fatty acids and DNA methylation in humans. Sci Rep. 2016;6:25867.
26. Fung T, Hu F, Fuchs C, et al. Major dietary patterns and the risk of colorectal cancer in women. Arch Intern Med. 2003;163(3):309–314.
27. Paparo L, di Costanzo M, di Scala C, et al. The influence of early life nutrition on epigenetic regulatory mechanisms of the immune system. Nutr. 2014;6(11):4706–4719.

28. Struhl K. Histone acetylation and transcriptional regulatory mechanisms. Genes Dev. 1998;12(5):599–606.
29. Finnin M, Donigian J, Cohen A, et al. Structures of a histone deacetylase homologue bound to the TSA and SAHA inhibitors. Nat. 1999;401(6749):188–193.
30. Kouzarides T. Histone acetylases and deacetylases in cell proliferation. Curr Opin Genet Dev. 1999;9(1):40–48.
31. Kuo M, Allis C. Roles of histone acetyltransferases and deacetylases in gene regulation. Bioessays: News Rev Mol Cell Dev Biol. 1998;20(8):615–626.
32. Greco E, Lenzi A, Migliaccio S, et al. Epigenetic modifications induced by nutrients in early life phases: Gender differences in metabolic alteration in adulthood. Front Genet. 2019;10:795.
33. Landecker H. Food as exposure: Nutritional epigenetics and the new metabolism. BioSocieties. 2011;6(2):167–194.
34. Collins F, Varmus H. A new initiative on precision medicine. N Engl J Med. 2015;372 (9):793–795.
35. Rodgers G, Collins F. Precision nutrition-the answer to "What to eat to stay healthy." JAMA. 2020;324(8):735–736.
36. Minich D, Bland J. Personalized lifestyle medicine: Relevance for nutrition and lifestyle recommendations. Sci World J. 2013;2013:129841.
37. Vallée Marcotte B, Cormier H, Guénard F, et al. Novel genetic loci associated with the plasma triglyceride response to an Omega-3 fatty acid supplementation. J Nutrigenet Nutrigenomics. 2016;9(1):1–11.
38. Simpson S, Le Couteur D, James D, et al. The geometric framework for nutrition as a tool in precision medicine. Nutr Healthy Aging. 2017;4(3):217–226.
39. Shah R. The role of nutrition and diet in Alzheimer disease: A systematic review. J Am Med Dir Assoc. 2013;14(6):398–402.
40. Schelke M, Hackett K, Chen J, et al. Nutritional interventions for Alzheimer's prevention: A clinical precision medicine approach. Ann N Y Acad Sci. 2016;1367(1):50–56.
41. Physical Activity Guidelines Advisory Committee. 2018 Physical Activity Guidelines Advisory Committee. 2018 Physical Activity Guidelines Advisory Committee Scientific Report. Washington, DC: U.S. Department of Health and Human Services, 2018.
42. 23andMe. 23andMe DNA Testing Kit for Health + Ancestry—23andMe (Accessed January 19, 2024).
43. CRI Genetics. Cellular Research Institute. DNA Testing Kit | Health, Ancestry and Traits | CRI Genetics (Accessed January 19, 2024).

33 Nutrition and Planetary Health

Key Points

- There is a strong relationship between diet and planetary health.
- Sustainable food production and healthy diets are also strongly linked.
- Unhealthy and unsustainably produced food produces a global risk to people and the planet.
- More than 800 million people have insufficient food, and many more consume unhealthy diets that contribute to premature death and morbidity.
- A significant transformation will be required to generate healthy diets around the world.
- Healthy diets which consist largely of fruits, vegetables, and whole grains compared with meat, sugar, and saturated fats found in unhealthy diets also have less adverse impact on planetary health.

33.1 INTRODUCTION

There is a strong relationship between the diet that is consumed around the world, particularly in high-income countries such as the United States, and planetary health [1–10]. The food system has been recognized as the major source of adverse environmental impact. For example, the food system is currently estimated to contribute between 19% and 29% of global greenhouse gas (GHG) emissions and account for approximately 70% of freshwater use [11,12]. For these reasons, a commitment to achieving reduced environmental impacts to dietary change is strong. This represents a strategy that many national food dietary pattern guidelines incorporate as a principle and component of global health and sustainability.

An expanding research literature describes and compares environmental outcomes based on different dietary patterns. Some of this literature has framed the environmental outcomes in the broader context of sustainable diets, which can also include social and economic aspects [13]. Other research has focused on combining environmental performance and nutritional heath indicators [7,14–21]. It is essential to understand that dietary strategies to reduce environmental impact must also be nutritionally complete and, in addition, support long-standing public health nutrition objectives. This area is extremely complex given the wide variety of foods eaten and the diversity of agricultural production methods.

A significant portion of this literature focuses on replacing animal-sourced foods with plant-based ones, which carries the dual opportunity to improve health and reduce premature mortality as well as reducing a variety of adverse environmental impacts.

DOI: 10.1201/9781003452607-33

Around the world it is estimated that 2 billion people consume primarily a meat-based diet [9] and an estimated 4 billion live primarily on a plant-based diet. To further compound the problem, the World Health Organization (WHO) has reported that more than 3 billion people around the world are malnourished [8,22–24]. In the United States, the population continues to grow rapidly. The U.S. population has doubled in the last 60 years and is projected to double again in the next 70 years. Currently, the U.S. food production system uses 50% of the total U.S. land area, approximately 80% of the fresh water [25–28], and consumes 17% of fossil energy use in the country. All of these figures suggest that the U.S. food system is not sustainable.

This chapter will explore various diets including those to be considered "healthy" and those considered to be "unhealthy" and their impact particularly related to planetary health.

33.2 WHAT CONSTITUTES A HEALTHY DIET?

Determining what constitutes a healthy diet is important for a variety of reasons. For example, dietary patterns are used to provide dietary guidance to a population, underscore counseling in clinical settings, and develop practices and policies to enhance diet, as well as monitor trends and dietary quality for an individual and the population [29].

Defining a global healthy diet remains challenging given the diversity of populations around the world. A general statement could be made that a healthy diet should optimize factors which are defined by the broadly by the WHO as being in the state of "complete, physical, mental and social well-being and not just the absence of disease" [30].

Within the focus of healthy diets individuals zero to two years old have unique requirements to support rapid growth and development, but they represent such a small portion of the total population that the impact on planetary health is small. Animal-sourced foods have important effects on human health and environmental sustainability and will be the focus of this chapter.

The EAT-Lancet Commission on Healthy Diets and Sustainable Food Systems defines a healthy diet as one using diverse food groups while taking into consideration nutritional adequacy. This general definition does not incorporate added fats, sugars, and salt, and those need to be considered as well. The healthy dietary pattern described by the EAT-Lancet Commission consists of ranges of intake for each food group which allows for flexible global applications [2]. These criteria allow for preferences and cultures from different populations. Incorporated into a healthy diet should be adequacy of energy and energy balance. The global average per capita energy intake has been estimated at 2,370 kcals/day. In addition, a healthy diet should contain adequate protein intake for adults which is considered 0.8 grams/kg body weight or 56 grams/day for 70 kilogram individual or about 10% of energy intake.

A number of studies have shown that poultry and red meat consumption (mainly pork) is inversely associated with all-cause mortality in Asian cohort studies. The inverse, however, is true in Europe and the United States. Red meat consumption in multiple dietary analyses has been repeatedly associated with total mortality and risks of other chronic diseases [31]. In addition, high intake of dairy products such as three servings per day of low-fat dairy has been promoted in the United States and other European countries as important for bone health and fracture prevention due to its high calcium intake [31]. However, data on the amount of calcium needed remains somewhat in dispute.

Fish intake has been associated with reduced risk of cardiovascular disease (CVD) largely due to its high content of omega-3 fatty acids. It must be noted, however, that mercury concentrations are high in some fish, including frequently consumed ones such as swordfish and tuna, which should be avoided by pregnant or lactating women.

Legumes have also been associated with lower risk of coronary heart disease and serve as an alternative, and perhaps healthier, source of protein than red meat [32,33]. Grains remain the largest source of energy in most diets around the world [21]. However, refining grains results in major loss of nutrients and fiber, which has important health implications. Increased consumption of fiber has been linked to lower risk of chronic diseases including CVD. Increased fruit and vegetable consumption has been a consistent recommendation for healthy diets, and a wide variety of evidence shows that fruit and vegetable consumption is important for the prevention of CVD particularly when consuming five servings or more per day [20].

High fruit and vegetable consumption is somewhat associated with reduced cancer incidence.

Added fats from animal sources, such as butter and lard, may comprise up to 30% of total energy in some diets around the world. Most dietary recommendations, however, suggest reducing or limiting total fat intake to decrease the risk of coronary heart disease (CHD) and cancer [34,35]. Both polyunsaturated and monounsaturated fats have been associated with lower risk of CVD. For example, the Mediterranean diet, as reported in the PREDIMED study, which is high in extra-virgin olive oil and a major source of monounsaturated fats, reduces the incidence of CVD and improves cognitive function [36]. In addition, low-fat diets have been widely promoted for weight loss and prevention of weight gain, although the data are not completely clear on this.

Sugar and other refined starches have been shown to be associated with multiple adverse metabolic effects, High intake of refined starches may further increase plasma triglyceride concentration as well as being associated with weight gain, type 2 diabetes mellitus (T2DM), and increased CVD mortality. For this reason, many national recommendations [37], as well as those from the WHO, recommend sugar intake be less than 10% of energy [38].

To summarize this complex literature, it appears that healthy diets feature protein sources primarily from plants [32], fat from mostly unsaturated plant sources, low intake of saturated fats, carbohydrates primarily from whole grains and less from refined grains, and less than 10% of energy from sugar. In addition, at least five servings of fruits and vegetables per day as well as moderate dairy consumption all represent key components of a healthy diet. These recommendations allow great flexibility and are compatible with a wide variety of food and agricultural systems, cultural traditions, and individual dietary preferences [29]. Indeed, these recommendations can be combined in various types of healthy nutritional patterns including vegetarian and vegan diets. This type of healthy diet is also associated with less adverse impact on planetary health, which will be considered further in subsequent sections of this chapter.

33.3 SUSTAINABLE FOOD PRODUCTION AND DIETS

An urgent imperative exists to develop sustainable food practices that, in addition, safeguard planetary health [31]. It has become widely recognized that sustainable food production and human well-being are inextricably intertwined. Most of the issue of sustainability focuses on the farm practices which includes reduction of nutrient leakage from fields (see subsequent section) and enhanced efficiency of water use by crops. Since the 1950s humans have been the dominating driver of change in food production, which is the largest source of environmental degradation and has the greatest adverse effect on planetary health. Thus, finding ways of making food production more sustainable is imperative. Sustainable food production needs to be accomplished in ways that safeguard the ecosystem of the Earth. From the farm perspective, sustainable food production is generally defined from a nutrient perspective emphasizing the need to reduce nutrient leakage of either nitrogen or phosphorous in the ground water in rivers.

It is also increasingly recognized that sustainable food production is necessary for global health considerations. This involves GHG emissions, land and water use, nitrogen and phosphorous applications, biodiversity loss, and chemical harm from herbicides and pesticides—all of which must fit into the definition of sustainable food production. The definition of sustainable food production requires setting boundaries for the effects of this production on climate systems, land systems, fresh water, biodiversity, and nutrient cycles of nitrogen and phosphorus [39,40]. These will all be handled in subsequent sections of this chapter.

Multiple reasons underscore why the current global food system is not sustainable. For example, there are 2 billion malnourished individuals and almost 800 million undernourished in the world while 1 billion are overweight or obese [2]. Of note, the majority of the poor and hungry are in food-producing nations. Moreover, a third of the food produce is lost or wasted.

The Food and Agriculture Organization (FAO) of the United Nations estimates that global food demand will increase by 60% by the year 2050 when compared to 2007 [41].

There is now considerable research pointing to synergies between heart-healthy diets and reduced environmental degradation. This also encompasses the notion of both sustainable food production and sustainable diets, which are inextricably linked to each other. The linkages between diet and food systems is strong. Diet involves a selection of foods eaten by an individual and chosen among those made available by the food system. Conversely, the sum of diets creates the overall food demand that directly impacts food systems. Thus, diets are both the result and driver of the food system.

Diets represent a good entry point in what can be done individually and collectively to improve food systems. This places the consumer at the center of the overall system, playing an intermediate role between food production and nutrition outcomes [42–45]. The High Level Panel of Experts (HLPE) on food security and nutrition defined a food system as the following: "A food systems gathers all the elements (environment, people, inputs, processes, infrastructures, institutions, etc. and activities that relate to the production, processing, and distribution, preparation, and consumption of food and the outputs of these activities including socio-economic and environmental outcomes" [46]. Within this definition, a sustainable diet plays a central role. The HLPE defined sustainable diets as follows: "A sustainable diet is a diet that contributes to food nutritional status and long-term good health of the individual/community that contributes to and is enabled by sustainable food systems thus incorporating long-term food security and nutrition."

Thus, sustainable food systems and sustainable diets are inextricably linked to each other. Within the definition, the key words are "food security and nutrition," as evidenced by the high levels of hunger and malnutrition on a global scale [46], the food system is not fulfilling this function. Components of sustainable food production system will be discussed in subsequent sections of this chapter.

33.4 CLIMATE CHANGE

Emissions from human activities drive GHG, which cause climate change and lead to disruption of multiple planetary systems such as rising sea levels and increasing frequency of extreme weather events. Systems of food production release GHG into the atmosphere directly and also drive land use change, releasing additional carbon dioxide when forests are cleared, wetlands drained, and soils tilled.

Food production is the prime source of methane and nitrous oxide, which have 56 and 280 times on a per unit basis the effect on global warming compared to carbon dioxide. Methane is produced during the breakdown of manure from livestock from cows and sheep and anaerobic decomposition of organic material in flooded rice paddies. Nitrous oxide mainly arises from soil microbes and crop plants and pastures and is affected by soil fertility issues such as fertilizer application. Carbon dioxide is released when land is cleared to allow planting of crops and when forests are converted into agricultural fields. For all these reasons, it will be essential to find ways to diminish GHG emissions from food production, particularly if healthy diets for the global population and global warming targets from the Paris Agreement are to be achieved.

33.5 FRESH WATER USE

Food production is the world's largest consumer of fresh water. Most farmland uses fresh water from rain (84%), while 16% uses irrigation water (i.e. water from freshwater lakes, rivers, and aquifers). Seventy percent of all global water withdrawals are used for irrigation [47]. It may be quite difficult to reduce food production's share of water consumption; however, countries that have advanced technologies may be able to limit water withdrawals to 20% of current levels. This finding suggests that substantial reductions may be possible through improved use of existing technologies. Conversely, it is difficult to reduce consumption of water use since plants transpire and grow and water evaporates from the soil.

33.6 NITROGEN AND PHOSPHORUS FLOWS

Nitrogen and phosphorus are crucial to plant growth. They are both nutrient elements, and they are vital to the structure and metabolism of living organisms both on the land and in oceans. The natural availability of these two elements limits plant growth in many ecosystems [2]. Thus, the supply of nitrogen and phosphorus fertilizers to crop lands is essential to maximize crop yields, and this will continue to be necessary for feeding the global population. Excessive application of nitrogen and phosphorus in food production has multiple substantial adverse consequences particularly based on run off into streams and rivers, where it drives eutrophication of fresh water and marine ecosystems. This creates subsequent development of hypoxic conditions which cause fish to die and other environmental harm. Even though fertilizer is the major source of nitrogen and phosphorus, human sewage is also an important source, as is atmospheric nitrogen deposition which is usually carried by rain, snow, or fog to the air's surface.

Nitrogen application can also reduce biodiversity and acidification of water and soils through ammonia emissions [2]. Furthermore, nitrous oxide emissions are a potent GHG and a significant component of ammonia in the atmosphere. All of these issues harm human health. Nitrogen fertilizer is made by an industrial process to convert plentiful nonreactive nitrogen gas to ammonia. Unfortunately, this process is associated with high levels of GHG emissions. Phosphorous fertilizer is a nonrenewable resource mined from phosphate rock deposits. These deposits are estimated to run out within 50–100 years.

The major challenge that interacts with both human nutrition and farming practices is to make the maximum allotted nitrogen and phosphorous loading into the biosphere while maintaining a stable earth system. One potential response is to try to maximize food production per unit of nitrogen and phosphorous input while maintaining loss of nutrients reduced to a minimum. Literature is available that suggests how this can be accomplished. Deposits of phosphorous are deficient in some areas and saturated in others. A closer balance for phosphorous can be achieved by recycling 50% of human waste and reapplying recycled phosphorous to crop lands.

33.7 BIODIVERSITY LOSS

Biodiversity involving the diversity and richness of all living organisms both on land and water is essential to the stability of ecosystems as well as resilience of food production systems. The world is currently losing species at the rate of 100–1,000 times greater than previous eras [2,48,49].

Multiple human actions contribute to biodiversity loss. These include loss of both terrestrial and aquatic habitats, climate change, chemical pollution, invasive species, and unsustainable harvest of wild species. In addition, habitat fragmentation occurs particularly from human appropriation of land for food production and represents a significant driver of biodiversity loss. Since the rate of decline in biodiversity can ultimately trigger irreversible changes to the earth system, the losses through food production should be no greater than the historical background rate. It has been suggested that no more than 1–80 extinctions per million species per year is an appropriate goal to achieve [2].

33.8 LAND SYSTEM CHANGE

In some areas land for food production has remained constant in the 20th century [50–52]. These include temperate regions in Europe, Russia, and North America. Substantial expansion of agricultural land, however, has occurred in the tropics. Food production is the largest driver of land use and land use change mainly through clearing of forests and burning of biomass. Major land loss has occurred in countries such as Brazil, the Democratic Republic of Congo, and Indonesia. Land system change is a major contributor to declines in biodiversity as well as increases in GHG emissions. About 40% of the ice free terrestrial land mass in the world is dedicated to crop lands and grazing lands. Of this 40%, about 23% of land surface is considered for grazing lands, which may be important for biodiversity, conservation, and carbon sequestration. Reforestation may also play a role in reversing some of the adverse effects of expansion of agricultural land.

33.9 ACHIEVING HEALTHY DIETS FROM SUSTAINABLE FOOD SYSTEMS

It is currently estimated that the current food production system is not sustainable for food security for the expanding population of the world moving forward [2,13]. The capacity to produce enough food in the future is limited, potentially by water, soil fertility, land use, and sewage dispersal in seas, and oceans. As already indicated, the current food production system affects a variety of natural resources including greater than 70% use of fresh water, up to 30% of human-generated GHG emissions, and 80% of deforestation. Food production is also the single largest contributor to loss of biodiversity and phosphorous flows, which can lead to degradation of fresh water and salt water.

It has been argued that the most promising methods to meet both present and future food needs involve shifting individual and population food choices and patterns. As indicated in multiple chapters in this book, there is a substantial amount of evidence that dietary patterns that promote human health, including the Dietary Approach to Stop Hypertension (DASH) diet [51], the Mediterranean dietary pattern (MDP) [52], vegetarian diets and their variations, and the Healthy U.S.-Style Dietary Pattern [29]. When these patterns are consumed at appropriate caloric levels, they reduce the risk of preventable chronic diseases such as CVD [53], T2DM, obesity, and some cancers. Most modeling studies have shown that these types of diets result in substantial decreases in GHG emissions and use of resources such as water, energy, and land use for agriculture. In one model, the GHG emissions from self-selected meat eaters were two times as high as those for vegans. In addition, the Mediterranean diet, compared to a carnivorous diet, not only reduced the risk of CVD and T2DM and cancer mortality but also reduced GHG emissions and crop land use compared with the current Western diet [54].

The DASH diet was also associated with lower GHG emissions in several studies while meat consumption was associated with increased GHG emissions [8]. It should be noted, however, that greater adherence to the DASH diet was associated with higher dietary costs, with a mean cost of diets in the top quintile of DASH scores being 18% higher than diets in the lowest quintile. Thus, the cost of diets should also be a consideration. One study from the United Kingdom, however, showed that a sustainable diet that did not eliminate meat or dairy products while still resulting in lower GHG emissions could be accomplished without increased cost to the consumer.

In 2015, the Dietary Guidelines Advisory Committee in the United States concluded "Consistent evidence indicates that in general a dietary pattern that is higher in plant-based food such as vegetables, fruits, whole grains, legumes, nuts and seeds and lower in animal based foods is more heath promoting and is associated with lesser environmental impact (GHG, energy, land and water use) than is the current US diet" [55].

33.10 DIETARY PATTERNS IN RELATION TO HEALTH AND SUSTAINABILITY OUTCOMES

Various dietary patterns have been assessed not only for their individual health benefits but also for their sustainability outcomes and planetary health [57]. These include the following:

- Vegetarian and Omnivorous Diets
  Several studies have explored variations in vegetarian diets, with the range of diets ranging from vegan to omnivorous dietary patterns related to associated health and environmental outcomes. These studies have demonstrated that reduced meat consumption was expected to improve health outcomes and decrease GHG emissions and land energy and water usage [54–56]. In the United States, the average meat-based diet was compared to a lacto-ovo vegetarian diet. This analysis showed that energy, land, and water use was higher for the meat-based diet than the lacto-ovo vegetarian diet. The amount of fossil fuel required to produce one kilocalorie of protein was highest for beef and lamb [18].

  Data from the Adventist Health Study Two characterized differential environmental and health effects of three dietary patterns—vegetarian, semi-vegetarian, and nonvegetarian that varied with foods with respect to animal and plant foods [18]. Compared to nonvegetarian and semi-vegetarian, the vegetarian diets were projected to decrease GHG emissions and mortality rates. Another study compared pescatarian and vegetarian diets with omnivorous diets. This global assessment of the 100 most populus nations demonstrated that pescatarian and vegetarian diets decreased all-cause and ischemic heart disease mortality as well as type 2 diabetes and cancer incidence compared with the omnivorous diet. Furthermore, these diets also resulted in projected reduction in GHG emissions and crop land use [57–59]. Once again, the highest GHG emissions were found between ruminant beefs (beef and lamb) compared to legumes with GHG emissions per gram of protein basis. In studies that assess the Dietary Guidelines–related eating pattern, findings included not only health benefits but improved environmental measures, including GHG emissions and land and water energy, when compared with average consumption patterns.

In England, a number of studies compared various diets in terms of both human and planetary impacts. Overall, GHG emissions were associated with self-selected meat eaters and were approximately two times higher than those of vegans. These research studies have shown that self-selected diets are consistent with results of modeling analyses.

- MDP and DASH

Several studies have compared MDP to other vegetarian and dietary guideline–related patterns. In both of these studies adherence to MDP compared with usual intake reduced the environmental footprint of the diet by decreasing GHG emissions, energy, land use for agriculture, and water [60,61]. In one modeling study using population forecasts, it was found that by 2050 the MDP not only offered reduced CHD mortality, type 2 diabetes, and cancer but also reduced GHG emissions and crop land use when compared to current trends and dietary changes.

The DASH diet has also been studied in relation to environmental outcomes. The human health benefits of the DASH diet are well established. It has been shown to prevent or control hypertension and other chronic diseases. A cross sectional study assessed adherence to the DASH diet with the standard Western diet (WD) with regard to GHG emissions and diet costs. Greater adherence to the DASH dietary pattern was associated with lower GHG emissions. GHG emissions were most strongly and positively associated with meat consumption and negatively associated with whole grain consumption [62–64]. It should be noted that in the highest quintile of DASH scores in this study, the expense was 18% higher than diets in the lowest quintile.

Studies have also been conducted on energy intake GHG. Very high-calorie diets are common in the developed world have demonstrated high total per capita carbon dioxide emissions as a result of the high intake of animal products, whereas low-calorie diets had the lowest total per calorie carbon dioxide emissions [65].

With regard to sustainability, meat-based diets have been compared to plant-based diets with regard to their effects on the environment. In one study, a meat-based food system was compared to a lacto-ovo vegetarian (plant-based) diet with calories consumed constant at 3,533 kcals per person. The meat-based diet required more energy, land, and water resources than the lacto-ovo vegetarian diet. Thus, for planetary health, the lacto-ovo vegetarian diet is more sustainable than the average American meat-based diet [65].

Recent interest has arisen in the type of diet that is called "flexitarian" diet [66]. The word "flexitarian" is a combination of two words: Flexible and vegetarian. There have been a variety of definitions adopted for the flexitarian diet, but it is generally defined as a semi-vegetarian, plant-forward diet that incorporates dairy and eggs and allows room for occasional meat. The concept behind this diet is to approximate the health benefits associated with a vegetarian diet without requiring compliance to the dietary rules of a 100% vegetarian or vegan diet. Calories in a flexitarian diet come from nutrient-rich food such as fruits, legumes, whole grains, and vegetables. In the area of protein, plant-based foods (e.g. soy food and legumes, nuts and seeds) are the primary source. Protein comes also from eggs and dairy in the flexitarian diet with lesser amounts coming from meat, particularly red and processed meat.

It is thought that this type of flexible vegetarian diet will have similar benefits of reducing chronic disease, although the literature on this is still being developed [67,68]. The replacement of animal-sourced foods with plant-based foods has been repeatedly shown to exert less adverse effects on the environment. Plant-based foods can thus help consumers meet functional nutrition requirements while generating fewer GHG emissions compared to omnivorous diets or animal foods.

33.11 THE FUTURE OF FOOD IN THE FACE OF CLIMATE CHANGE

An additional concern about the unsustainability of the current food production relates to how climate change will affect this issue in the future. Most studies that have examined this have suggested that climate change will result in a reduction in future agricultural productivity, particularly in low-latitude regions. One study modeled a predicted 8% reduction in mean yield of all crops across Africa and South Asia by the year 2050 [69]. Climate change will also affect fisheries and agriculture. Increased productivity is estimated in high latitudes and decreased productivity in low and mid latitudes with a great deal of regional variation. For example, migration of fish toward either the North or South Pole alone has been estimated to reduce maximum catch potential in some tropical areas by up to 40%.

The effects of climate change on agriculture are also predicted to substantially impact human health. Reduction in agricultural production due to climate change has been estimated to cause 500,000 climate-related deaths by the year 2050, most of which are a result of reduced fruit and vegetable production and consumption followed by increases in underweight from reduced availability of food. In addition, the overall quality of food and water is predicted to decrease because of elevated carbon dioxide concentration. At elevated carbon dioxide concentrations, protein and amino acid concentrations decrease in spring wheat (a major staple crop), while nonstructural carbohydrates (except starch and lipids) significantly increase.

Diversifying crops has been offered as a potential solution for decreasing yields and nutritional quality caused by climate change. This represents one of the major recommendations from the FAO of the UN, which has placed crop diversity at the forefront of adaptation solutions. Developing crop varieties that can withstand heat, drought, flood, and other extremes of weather might represent an important step to adapt to climate change.

33.12 THE ROLE OF SEAFOOD IN GLOBAL DIETS

Seafood provides 3.1 billion people with about 20% of daily intake of animal protein [2]. Seafood consumption is particularly important for the world's poorest regions, where fish eaten constitutes a critical source of essential micronutrients.

Unfortunately, 90% of global wild fish stocks are currently being overfished or fished at capacity, while seafood extraction potential from the wild has either reached its ceiling or is declining [2]. There is potential for future expansion of seafood from aquaculture, but this carries the negative effect of potentially adverse environmental and social habitat destruction from overfishing and social displacement.

Agricultural production is projected to increase from 60 million tons in 2010 to 100 million tons in 2030 and up to 140 million tons in 2050 [2]. Farmed nonfished dependable animal species such as muscles and oysters might be a sustainable alternative; however, even this may be hampered by deteriorating water quality due to pollution and ocean acidification. While seafood may be a viable source of food in the future, aquaculture alone is insufficient to solve the challenges posed by feeding about 10 billion people healthy diets, although seafood could help strip production away from animal-sourced proteins.

33.13 FRAMEWORK FOR A GREAT FOOD TRANSFORMATION

In order to both achieve healthy diets and a sustainable food system, it will be necessary to move from the current situation to what some experts have called a "great food transformation" [2]. This will require widespread and multilevel actions to change what food is eaten and how it is produced. This, in turn, will require hard work, political will, and many resources.

Data are currently sufficient and strong enough to warrant action, but this transformation will require consensus around the world and political will to accomplish this. There are examples of other transformations in areas such as national controls and historical precedents from various recession, hunger, and famine which have affected countries around the world at various times. Making the dramatic changes necessary in order to balance a healthy diet with sustainable food production will require an enormous commitment and political will from around the globe. The EAT-Lancet Commission [2] recommended five potential strategies to assist in this enormous transformation. They are the following:

- Strategy I: Seek international and national commitment to shift toward healthy diets.
- Strategy 2: Reorient agriculture priorities from producing large quantities of food to producing healthy food.
- Strategy 3: Sustainably intensify food production generating high-quality output.
- Strategy 4: Implement strong and coordinated governments approaches to land and oceans.
- Strategy 5: At least cut in half food loss and waste in line with sustainable dietary goals.

33.14 CONCLUSIONS

There is a strong relationship between the human diet and planetary health. Moreover, there is a very strong relationship between food production and diet.

Unhealthy and unsustainably produced foods pose a global risk for people and the planet. More than 800 million people around the world currently have insufficient food, and many more consume an unhealthy diet, which contributes to premature death and morbidity.

In addition, global food production carries the largest adverse impact caused by humans on earth which threatens ecosystems and stability. Transforming healthy diets and sustainable food systems will be required to guide a great food transformation. Healthy diets not only improve health for individuals and populations but also carry less adverse impact on the planet.

Clinicians should be concerned not only about the diet of their individual patients but also as a community and must play an active role in making the connection between healthy diets and planetary health.

Clinical Applications

- Clinicians should not only counsel their patients on the individual benefits from a healthy diet but also make the link between a healthy diet for individuals and planetary health.
- Healthy diets consist of increased fruits and vegetables and whole grains as opposed to unhealthy diets which feature more red meat, sugar, and tropical oils.
- Healthy diets have less of an adverse impact on the health of the planet than do unhealthy diets.
- Physicians, as opinion leaders, have should advocate strongly for healthy diets, not only for their individual patients but also for the health of the planet.

REFERENCES

1. Willett W, Rockström J, Loken B, et al. Food in the anthropocene: The EAT-lancet commission on healthy diets from sustainable food systems. Lancet. 2019;393(10170):447–492.
2. Springmann M, Wiebe K, Mason-D'Croz D, et al. Health and nutritional aspects of sustainable diet strategies and their association with environmental impacts: A global modelling analysis with country-level detail. Lancet Planet Health. 2018;2(10):e451–e461.
3. Eshel G, Shepon A, Makov T, et al. Land, irrigation water, greenhouse gas, and reactive nitrogen burdens of meat, eggs, and dairy production in the United States. Proc Natl Acad Sci. 2014;111(33):11996–12001.
4. Eisen M, Brown P. Rapid global phaseout of animal agriculture has the potential to stabilize greenhouse gas levels for 30 years and offset 68 percent of CO2 emissions this century. PLOS Climate. 2022;1(2):e0000010.
5. FAOSTAT. Food and Agriculture Organization of the United Nations. www.fao.org/faostat/en/#data (Accessed May 1, 2023).
6. Harwatt H, Sabat J, Eshel G, et al. Substituting beans for beef as a contribution toward US climate change targets. Clim Change. 2017;143(1–2):261–270.
7. Ridoutt B, Hendrie G, Noakes M. Dietary strategies to reduce environmental impact: A critical review of the evidence base. Adv Nutr. 2017;15;8(6):933–946.
8. Thompson H, Brick M. Perspective: closing the dietary fiber gap: An ancient solution for a 21st century problem. Adv Nutr. 2016;7(4):623–626.
9. Marinova D, Bogueva D. Planetary health and reduction in meat consumption. Sustain Earth Reviews. 2019;(2):3.

10. Shah U, Merlo G. Personal and planetary health-the connection with dietary choices. JAMA. 2023;6;329(21):1823–1824.
11. Vermeulen S, Campbell B, Ingram J. Climate change and food systems. Annu Rev Environ Resourc. 2012;37(1):195–222.
12. Whitmee S, Haines A, Beyrer C, et al. Safeguarding human health in the anthropocene epoch: Report of the rockefeller foundation-lancet commission on planetary health. Lancet. 2015;14;386(10007):1973–2028.
13. Meybeck A, Gitz V. Sustainable diets within sustainable food systems. Proc Nutr Soc. 2017;76(1):1–11.
14. Malik VS, Willett WC, Hu FB. Global obesity: Trends, risk factors and policy implications. Nat Rev Endocrinol. 2013;9(1):13–27.
15. World Health Organization. Cardiovascular Diseases. WHO 2017. www.who.int/news-room/fact-sheets/detail/cardiovascular-diseases-(cvds) (Accessed January 24, 2024).
16. World Health Organization. Diabetes. WHO 2017. www.who (Accessed January 24, 2024).
17. Sabaté J, Soret S. Sustainability of plant-based diets: Back to the future. Am J Clin Nutr. 2014;100(Suppl 1):476S–482S.
18. Pimentel D, Pimentel M. Sustainability of meat-based and plant-based diets and the environment. Am J Clin Nutr. 2003;78(Suppl 3):660S–663S.
19. Dietary Guidelines Advisory Committee. Report of the 2015 Dietary Guidelines Advisory Committee. Washington, DC: US Department of Agriculture and US Department of Health and Human Services, 2015.
20. Aune D, Giovannucci E, Boffetta P, et al. Fruit and vegetable intake and the risk of cardiovascular disease, total cancer and all-cause mortality-a systematic review and dose-response meta-analysis of prospective studies. Int J Epidemiol. 2017;1;46(3):1029–1056.
21. Zong G, Gao A, Hu F, et al. Whole grain intake and mortality from all causes, cardiovascular disease, and cancer: A meta-analysis of prospective cohort studies. Circulation. 2016;14;133(24):2370–2380.
22. Tzioumis E, Kay M, Bentley M, et al. Prevalence and trends in the childhood dual burden of malnutrition in low- and middle-income countries, 1990–2012. Public Health Nutr. 2016;19(8):1375–1388.
23. Brent K, Santo R, Scatterday A, et al. Country-specific dietary shifts to mitigate climate and water crises. Global Environ Change. Elsevier. 2020;62:101926.
24. Springmann M, Wiebe K, Mason-D'Croz D, et al. Health and nutritional aspects of sustainable diet strategies and their association with environmental impacts: A global modelling analysis with country-level detail. Lancet Planet Health. 2018;2(10):e451–e461.
25. Sáez-Almendros S, Obrador B, Bach-Faig A, et al. Environmental footprints of Mediterranean versus Western dietary patterns: Beyond the health benefits of the Mediterranean diet. Environ Health. 2013;12:118.
26. Aleksandrowicz L, Green R, Joy E, et al. The impacts of dietary change on greenhouse gas emissions, land use, water use, and health: A systematic review. PLoS One. 2016;11(11):e0165797.
27. FAO/WHO 2015 Second International Conference on Nutrition (ICN2). Report of the Joint FAO/WHO Secretariat on the Conference. The Food and Agricultural Organization of the United States. Rome: FAO.
28. Nelson M, Hamm M, Hu F, et al. Alignment of healthy dietary patterns and environmental sustainability: A systematic review. Adv Nutr. 2016;7(6):1005–1025.
29. U.S. Department of Agriculture and U.S. Department of Health and Human Services. *Dietary Guidelines for Americans, 2020–2025*, 9th edition. December 2020. DietaryGuidelines.gov. 2020. www.dietaryguidelines.gov/resources/2020-2025-dietary-guidelines-online-materials.

30. World Food Summit (1996) Rome Declaration World Food Security Rome: FAO. www.fao.org/3/w3613e/w3613e00.htm (Accessed January 2024).
31. Bechthold A, Boeing H, Tetens I, et al. Perspective: Food-based dietary guidelines in Europe-scientific concepts, current status, and perspectives. Adv Nutr. 2018;1;9(5):544–560.
32. Afshin A, Micha R, Khatibzadeh S, et al. Consumption of nuts and legumes and risk of incident ischemic heart disease, stroke, and diabetes: A systematic review and meta-analysis. Am J Clin Nutr. 2014;100(1):278–288.
33. Anderson J, Major A. Pulses and lipaemia, short- and long-term effect: Potential in the prevention of cardiovascular disease. Br J Nutr. 2002;88(Suppl 3):S263–S271.
34. Wang D, Li Y, Chiuve S, et al. Association of specific dietary fats with total and cause-specific mortality. JAMA Intern Med. 2016;176(8):1134–1145.
35. Li Y, Hruby A, Bernstein A, et al. Saturated fats compared with unsaturated fats and sources of carbohydrates in relation to risk of coronary heart disease: A prospective cohort study. J Am Coll Cardiol. 2015;66(14):1538–1548.
36. Zong G, Li Y, Sampson L, et al. Monounsaturated fats from plant and animal sources in relation to risk of coronary heart disease among US men and women. Am J Clin Nutr. 2018;1;107(3):445–453.
37. Johnson R, Appel L, Brands M, et al. American Heart Association nutrition committee of the council on nutrition, physical activity, and metabolism and the council on epidemiology and prevention. Dietary sugars intake and cardiovascular health: A scientific statement from the American Heart Association. Circulation. 2009;120(11):1011–1020.
38. World Health Organization. WHO calls on countries to reduce sugars intake among adults and children. www.who.int/news/item/04-03-2015-who-calls-on-countries-to-reduce-sugars-intake-among-adults-and-children (Accessed January 26, 2024).
39. Sobal J, Khan LK, Bisogni C. A conceptual model of the food and nutrition system. Soc Sci Med. 1998;47(7):853–863.
40. FAO 2015 Presentation by Alexandre Meybeck at the 12th European Nutrition Conference, FENS 2015, Sustainable Diet III: Future and Matter of Debate, October 2015. Berlin.
41. Alexandratos N, Bruinsma J. World agriculture towards 2030/2050: The 2012 Revision. ESA Working Paper 12-3. 2012.
42. Ericksen P, Stewart B, Dixon J, et al. John. The value of a food system approach. Food security and global environmental change. London: Earthscan, 2010.
43. Ericksen P. What is the vulnerability of a food system to global environmental change? Ecol Soc. 2008;13(2).
44. Ingram J. A food systems approach to researching food security and its interactions with global environmental change. Food Sec. 2011;3:417–431.
45. ICPP. Climate change 2014: Impacts, adaptation, and vulnerability. Cambridge & New York: Cambridge University Press, 2014.
46. HLPE. Food losses and waste in the context of sustainable food systems. A Report by the High Level Panel of Experts on Food Security and Nutrition of the Committee on World Food Security. Rome: FAO, 2014.
47. Xu X, Sharma P, Shu S, et al. Global greenhouse gas emissions from animal-based foods are twice those of plant-based foods. Nat Food. 2021;2(9):724–732.
48. Smith Y, Smith A, Seymour C, et al. Response of avian diversity to habitat modification can be predicted from life-history traits and ecological attributes. Landscape Ecol. 2015;(30):1225–1239.
49. Machovina B, Feeley K, Ripple W, et al. Biodiversity conservation: The key is reducing meat consumption. Sci Total Environ. 2015;(536):419–431.
50. Milà i Canals, Muñoz I, McLaren S, et al. LCA Methodology and modelling considerations for vegetable production and consumption. CES Working Paper 02/07. https://

db.iseki-food.net/sites/default/files/digital_library_attachments/LCA_Methodol_0.pdf (Accessed February 5, 2024).
51. European Commission Joint Research Centre. ILCD Handbook: Recommendations for Life Cycle Impact Assessment in the European Context Based on Existing Environmental Impact Assessment Models and Factors. Vol. 24571. Luxembourg: Publication Office of the European Union, 2011.
52. Ewing B, Moore D, Goldfinger S et al. The Ecological Footprint Atlas 2010. Oakland: Global Footprint Network. Ecological_Footprint_Atlas_2010.pdf (footprintnetwork.org) (Accessed February 15, 2024).
53. Sacks F, Svetkey L, Vollmer W, et al. Effects on blood pressure of reduced dietary sodium and the Dietary Approaches to Stop Hypertension (DASH) diet. DASH-Sodium Collaborative Research Group. N Engl J Med. 2001;344(1):3–10.
54. Estruch R, Ros E, Salas-Salvado J, et al. Primary prevention of cardiovascular disease with a Mediterranean diet. N Engl J Med. 2013;368(14):1279–1290.
55. U.S. Department of Health and Human Services and U.S. Department of Agriculture. 2015–2020 Dietary Guidelines for Americans, 8th edition. http://health.gov/dietaryguidelines/2015/guidelines/ (Accessed December, 2015).
56. Notarnicola B, Tassielli G, Renzulli P et al. Environmental impacts of food consumption in Europe. J Clean Prod. 2017;(140), Part 2:753–765.
57. Springmann M, Godfray HC, Rayner M, et al. Analysis and valuation of the health and climate change co-benefits of dietary change. Proc Natl Acad Sci. 2016;12;113(15):4146–4151.
58. Aston L, Smith J, Powles J. Impact of a reduced red and processed meat dietary pattern on disease risks and greenhouse gas emissions in the UK: A modelling study. BMJ Open. 2012;10;2(5):e001072.
59. Poore J, Nemecek T. Reducing food's environmental impacts through producers and consumers. Science. 2018;1;360(6392):987–992. Erratum in: Science. 2019. 22;363(6429).
60. Meybeck A, Redfern S, Paoletti F, et al. Assessing sustainable diets within the sustainability of food systems. In Mediterranean Diet, Organic Food. New Challenges Rome: FAO, 2015.
61. Monsivais P, Scarborough P, Lloyd T, et al. Greater accordance with the dietary approaches to stop hypertension dietary pattern is associated with lower diet-related greenhouse gas production but higher dietary costs in the United Kingdom. Am J Clin Nutr. 2015; 102(1):138–145.
62. Tukker A, Goldbohm R, de Koning A, et al. Environmental impacts of changes to healthier diets in Europe. Ecological Economics. 2011;70(10):1776–1788.
63. Milner J, Green R, Dangour A, et al. Health effects of adopting low greenhouse gas emission diets in the UK. BMJ Open. 2015;30;5(4):e007364.
64. van Dooren C, Marinussen M, Blonk H, et al. Exploring dietary guidelines based on ecological and nutritional values: A comparison of six dietary patterns. Food Policy. 2014;44:36–46.
65. Tom M, Fischbeck P, Hendrickson C. Energy use, blue water footprint, and greenhouse gas emissions for current food consumption patterns and dietary recommendations in the US. Environ Syst Decis. 2016(36):92–103.
66. Pike A. What is the flexitarian diet? Washington, DC: International Food Information Council, May 17, 2021.
67. Grasso S, Jaworska S. Part meat and part plant: Are hybrid meat products fad or future? Foods. 2020;17;9(12):1888.
68. Derbyshire E. Flexitarian diets and health: A review of the evidence-based literature. Front Nutr. 2016;3:55.
69. Vermeulen S, Campbell B, Ingram J. Climate change and food systems. Annu. Rev. Environ. Resour. 2012;37:195–222.

34 Public Policy Support for Healthy Eating

Key Points

- Public policy significantly impacts nutrition policy.
- The landscape for public policy and nutrition has now changed from the provision of adequate amounts of food to the provision of healthier eating patterns.
- Promoting healthier eating patterns is important, not only for individual patients but also for the health of the entire planet.
- Physicians need to play an expanded role not only in advocating for healthier nutrition for individual patients but also for helping to develop partnerships with communities and policy makers to encourage the shift to healthier plant-based eating.

34.1 INTRODUCTION

The foods that people eat are impacted by a wide variety of external factors [1]. These factors are, in turn, impacted by diverse and complex influences, all of which come together within the framework of nutrition and public policy [1–7]. While many of these factors are beyond the control of individuals and their physicians, it is important to understand the importance of public policy in nutrition and what drives this relationship.

Historically, public policy in the area of nutrition largely dealt with how to provide enough food for individuals [8]. However, in the past several decades emphasis has shifted in the area of nutrition and health. Public policy now must focus on a variety of chronic diseases which are strongly influenced by dietary practices [9–11]. Unfortunately, public policy in the area of nutrition has had a difficult time switching from the provision of food to combat hunger and malnutrition to the more germane issues related to nutrition and health.

While many people draw from their own personal knowledge and preferences when it comes to food choices, the environment that influences what food is available to individuals is exceedingly complex. There are multiple layers including potential targets, barriers, facilitators, and adverse modifiers of food policies which the government must consider when developing nutritional policy.

This chapter is focused on issues related to nutritional policy with an emphasis on how the changing landscape related to nutrition and health can and should impact on various aspects of nutritional policy.

DOI: 10.1201/9781003452607-34

34.2 DEFINITION OF NUTRITION POLICY

Nutrition policy has been defined as follows: "The goal of nutrition policy is to have a safe, wholesome, nutritious, culturally appropriate food supply that is economically accessible and available in adequate amounts to promote health, prevent dietary deficiency and reduce other diet related diseases [4]."

Typically, nutrition policy is framed by a statement from an authoritative body (usually the government) on issues related to the intent to act in order to maintain or alter the food supply, nutritional status, or some other indicator in society [12]. This is distinct and broader than "food policy" since food policy does not explicitly incorporate food and health concerns. Nutrition policy and politics are inextricably bound to each other in most settings, particularly when governmental institutions are involved [12–14].

Other individuals often make broad statements about nutrition policies particularly in the area of their need to address the burden of malnutrition and the prevention of diet-related diseases as well as maintaining a sustainable and safe food supply. The basis for the global development of nutritional policies was provided by the World Declaration of Nutrition and Plan of Action on Nutrition 1992 (FAO 1992).

34.3 THE CHANGING LANDSCAPE OF PUBLIC POLICY AND NUTRITION

As already indicated, throughout most of history, even through most of the 20th century, providing sufficient food was the greatest challenge. In response to this, governments sought to stimulate production and distribution of as much inexpensive food as possible. This resulted typically in starchy (high carbohydrate) staple commodities and shelf-stable products. Throughout most of this time, the concept that there might be a global pandemic of obesity and chronic diseases as a result of the inexpensive, unhealthy food was not even contemplated.

Recently clear scientific data supporting the rise of diet-related chronic diseases such as obesity, type 2 diabetes, cardiovascular disease, and several cancers have resulted in part from this historical approach [9–11]. Moreover, nutrition science over this this period has slowly shifted focus from undernutrition defined by inadequate calories and nutrient deficiencies to food based dietary patterns and overall health effects of the food supply.

As will be discussed in the next few sections, multiple complex factors beyond personal decisions strongly influence dietary choices and patterns. Even among individuals, dietary patterns are determined by a wide variety of factors including personal preference, age, gender, culture, education, income, health status, nutritional knowledge, and cooking skills. Psychological influences also play a prominent role, as do early life exposures. In addition, family and community norms, social pressures, social networks, and race/ethnicity play important roles. Commercial pressures also influence consumer choices. These may include food marketing, packaging, and advertising. Foreign policy, production practices, and national and international trade agreements also play roles.

These many factors are powerful and may create nearly insurmountable barriers to making healthy dietary choices for people around the world. In addition, these factors can play a role in health inequities. All of these issues provide an opportunity for governments to support improvements in diet, health, and equity.

34.4 TYPES OF POLICY INTERVENTIONS

Governments can use a variety of policies extending from voluntary to mandatory. Public health concerns must also play a role [9,13,14]. This chapter will focus largely on policies directly targeting nutrition. However, it should be noted that indirect mechanisms involving farming, trade, food waste, and economic empowerment also play roles which are beyond the scope of this chapter.

Government food policy strategies might include education and point-of-purchase labeling which are widely used [13,14]. These policies place most of the responsibility on the individual consumer. Their effectiveness on behavior change has been variable.

Fiscal incentives and disincentives which are aimed at consumers, food producers, and retailers have generated more consistent evidence of effectiveness. For example, additional incentives such as sales taxes on unhealthy items or removing industry tax benefits on unhealthy products have sometimes been employed.

In addition, quality standards also can make an impact and are typically low-cost strategies for governments to implement. For example, limits on trans fat and sodium have been implemented in many countries. Such standards are also being contemplated for free or added sugars in a number of countries.

Schools and worksites are natural and complementary settings for effective nutrition policy (see later in this chapter) [8–11,15,16]. Interestingly, healthcare systems are one of the least frequently used settings to promote better nutrition. For example, one strategy might include a multidisciplinary lifestyle program for conditions such as prediabetes or medically tailored meals for patients with complex, chronic diseases. This is an approach being explored in the Food Is Medicine initiative. Prescriptions for food or vegetables or health promotion disease prevention and nutrition counseling during pregnancy and early childhood could also be implemented.

34.5 TRANSLATION OF EVIDENCE TO POLICY ACTION

Local and national governments have important roles to play in bringing both healthier food and food security to the populations they serve. This will require the government to have appropriate knowledge to translate evidence into policy actions. This includes understanding the scientific basis for what constitutes a healthy diet. For example, this is a key consideration in the *Dietary Guidelines for Americans 2020–2025* [17]. The government must also have the capacity to intervene and the will to act. Political willingness to act can be undermined by a variety of factors and is particularly influenced by the perception that dietary interventions require long periods to achieve benefits, which will not often coincide with political and budget cycle realities. In addition, public opinion may see such policies as intrusive.

34.6 OTHER STAKEHOLDERS

A variety of other stakeholders besides the government must be engaged to help complement and execute a policy. For example, nutrition research should prioritize optimal dietary targets. Health systems should implement strategies on patient behavior change. Employers, schools, hospitals, and religious congregations should also play roles in implementing healthier eating.

Multinational companies have significant influence in this area and must be engaged in policy decisions. It is only through broad partnerships among all of these stakeholders that a nutrition policy seeking healthier diets can be achieved.

34.7 HEALTHIER EATING VERSUS CALORIE COUNTING

Given the rapidly increasing levels of obesity around the world, many governments and health care organizations have focused on reducing the amount of calories and developing other calorie-focused policies such as calorie menu labeling in an attempt to slow the obesity epidemic [18,19]. These efforts seem to have resulted in only minor shifts toward healthier choices and public health improvements. Many nutrition scientists are now strongly urging that government policies focus more on healthier foods and meals rather than reducing calories. The argument is that benefits for reducing caloric intake typically result in low-calorie foods, which may not result in calorie reduction. These investigators argue that it would be better to consume a given number of calories from high-quality foods than a smaller number of calories from low-calorie foods.

It has been well established that foods are more than just a collection of calories and nutrients. Nutrients interact differently when presented as foods. In addition, different subtypes of macronutrients have the same caloric value but are metabolized and influence health in different ways. A good example of this is the equivalence of calories from trans fats and monounsaturated fats. While trans fats may increase lipogenesis due to raising low-density lipoprotein (LDL) and lowering high-density lipoprotein (HDL), monounsaturated fats have the opposite effect. This argument also includes recommendations to improve food processing and cooking methods, yet all of these efforts recommend future nutrition policy to stop encouraging people to focus on calorie counting to fight noncommunicable diseases and instead focus on nutritional value, ingredients, dietary sources, food processing, and cooking methods.

34.8 NUTRITION POLICY AND HEALTH EQUITY

The disparate responses to the health consequences of the COVID-19 pandemic underscore issues of how health equity and its relationship to nutrition play an enormous role in health around the world [2,3]. Individuals who had obesity, diabetes, or hypertension were three to four times as likely to be hospitalized with severe COVID compared to individuals without these conditions. [20]. Similar but different responses occurred in mortality where individuals with these chronic conditions were three to four times as likely to die from COVID as were individuals who did not have these conditions. All of these conditions have clear nutritional underpinnings and also tended to disproportionately affect Black and Brown communities and individuals of low socioeconomic status.

A component of difference in health equity also involves nutritional security. It has been estimated that over 30 million individuals in the United States are food insecure, and this includes over 9 million children [21]. These numbers expanded greatly during the COVID-19 epidemic when many individuals who had never experienced food insecurity were forced for the first time to rely on food banks and federal assistance to meet their nutritional needs [22,23]. (These issues are discussed in more detail in subsequent sections of this chapter).

Major health care organizations such as the American Heart Association (AHA) [2] and the American College of Physicians (ACP) [3] have become involved and have issued policy statements or position papers related to ways that food policies and programs can work to promote equity and nutritional security. Both of these prestigious healthcare organizations have focused on the fact that nutritionally inadequate dietary intake is a leading contributor to chronic metabolic diseases. These considerations include differences in dietary quality as well as food insecurity. Both of these organizations argue that there is a difference between food security and nutritional security.

The AHA defines nutrition security as "an individual or household condition of having equitable and stable availability, access, affordability and utilization of foods and beverages that promote well-being and prevent and treat disease" [2]. AHA goes on to recommend that these components of nutrition security will require development and implementation of national measures of nutritional security over and above the current U.S. food security measures. As such, a nutritional security plan will require coordinated and sustained efforts at federal, state, and local levels including advocacy and research to expand existing food assistance policies and programs with the goal of developing and implementing new policies and programs to improve cardiovascular health and reduce disparities in chronic disease. (Issues related to current food security programs sponsored by the federal government will be discussed in subsequent sections of this chapter).

34.9 NUTRITION POLICIES AND THE COVID-19 PANDEMIC

A sharp rise in food insecurity occurred during the first several months of the COVID-19 pandemic and exposed both the strengths and weaknesses of existing U.S. nutrition-related policies and programs [22,23]. Starting at the beginning of the pandemic in April 2020, many families experienced food insecurity for the first time and were forced to join millions of other households that had been food insecure before the pandemic. The federal government quickly responded to this crisis with increased benefits and reduced barriers for the Supplemental Nutrition Assistance Program (SNAP) and Women, Infants and Children (WIC) programs and also implemented the Pandemic Electronic Benefits Program, which provided additional funds to states for children to compensate for the loss of school meals [24,25].

When a crisis such as the pandemic occurs, equitable access to any food issue (i.e. food sufficiency) is prioritized. Moving forward, however, as the crisis abates, it is important to continue extending current and new policies to provide availability, access, affordability, and utilization of nutritious food. For example, in October 2020 one strategy was the Thrifty Food Plan. The trial of this initiative, which realistically estimated the cost of a nutritious meal, resulted in a 20% change in benefit levels for SNAP recipients [24].

34.10 U.S. FOOD AND NUTRITION POLICY AND PUBLIC HEALTH FOOD ASSISTANCE PROGRAMS

The federal government has a variety of domestic food programs which are largely focused on reducing hunger and food insecurity and increasing healthy nutrition and related benefits for Americans. The largest of these programs is SNAP, which serves more than 40 million individuals monthly. Its beneficiaries include children and adults all the way from newborns to senior citizens. Enrollment numbers in this program are significantly affected by the strength and state of the U.S. economy as well as policy elements. WIC is the second largest program. It is considered one of the most effective public health programs. Its impact is on a large number of infants and their mothers each year. In addition, WIC has enrolled individuals across the country who qualify under income eligibility guidelines regardless of residency status. WIC and SNAP work in tandem since approximately half of WIC households also qualify for SNAP benefits. In addition, the Healthy Hunger Free Kids Act of 2010 (HHFKA), which has been in existence since 2010 [26], also includes the National School Lunch Program (NSLP), school breakfast program, and several smaller programs.

The NSLP is provided daily in over 100,000 U.S. schools from pre-K to grade 12 [27]. At the urging of then-First Lady Michelle Obama, updated nutritional policies in many standards resulted in demonstratively improved food and nutrition environment in U.S. schools. In addition, the school breakfast program feeds approximately 30 million students each day. It should be noted that not all elements of HHFKA are supported by the food industry or a number of school food service representatives.

When taking into account both the Farm Bill and the childhood nutrition programs and the HHFKA, close to 100 billion dollars is expended each year on federal nutrition programs [28]. Included in the Farm Bill are elements to encourage diversification of crops, conservation principles, and more careful use of water, soil, and chemicals—all of which are designed to improve food's sustainability.

A variety of voices have been heard urging public health communities throughout the world to encourage both healthier nutrition and practices that are more sustainable. Perhaps the most prominent of these is the EAT- Lancet Commission healthy diets for sustainable food systems [29] (This is discussed in more detail in the chapter on planetary health.)

34.11 CHILDREN AND NUTRITIONAL HEALTH AND SCHOOL NUTRITION STANDARDS

Both the SNAP and WIC programs have a particular emphasis on healthy nutrition for children. These were buttressed with the 2010 HHFKA, which altered school lunch regulations increasing fruits and vegetables, whole grains, and fat-free and low-fat milk while decreasing sodium, saturated fat, and trans fat. Initial evidence from this program suggests that these changes have improved the nutrient density in lunches while energy density has declined. In addition, the federal government sponsored the Smart Snack in School nutrition standards, which are designed to apply to all foods and beverages sold outside of school meals in the school building (e.g. vending machines and a la cart offerings). This has caused some controversy since the food industry uses revenues from vending machines for developing curriculum materials and fundraising programs.

Another area of controversy has to do with tomato paste in pizza. While pizza is not typically considered a healthy food, when the U.S. Department of Agriculture (USDA) attempted to close the loophole designating tomato paste as a healthy food, the companies that produce school pizza were able to block progress in this area. Thus, pizza sauce continues to count as a vegetable serving. The USDA has also played a role in this. For example, in 2018, the USDA reintroduced 1% flavored milk and weakened the whole grain requirements. This was done largely on the recommendation of the School Nutrition Association and has remained very controversial, since these positions also resulted in children consuming more sodium.

It must be recognized that schools are politically complicated institutions where at times the industry goals are at cross purposes with healthy nutrition. It should also be noted that during the COVID-19 pandemic when most schools were closed, the federal government stepped in with an expanded school lunch program to help children achieve greater school security [30–32] (The federal government response to food insecurity during COVID-19 is handled in a subsequent section of this chapter).

34.12 FOOD SECURITY AND HEALTHY EATING

Food security and healthy eating are strongly related to each other. Achieving a food-secure home requires adequate quantity, quality, and diversity of foods to be healthy for everyone in the household. Nutrition security is a somewhat broader issue than food security. Nutrition security encompasses a variety of additional factors including availability, affordability, access, acquisition, and consumption of foods that promote well-being and prevent disease [33]. As the prevalence of nutrition-related chronic diseases has increased, shifts in environmental and policy priorities have occurred going beyond caloric sufficiency and food quantity to a more health-promoting, nutrition-security focus, which underlies the adoption of healthy eating behaviors among individuals from diverse communities.

Food insecurity is very prevalent in virtually every community in the United States. In 2020, the USDA estimated that over 10% of households experienced food insecurity. This equates to over 38 million people [23]. These rates of food insecurity decreased from a high of 14.9% in 2011 to 10.5% in 2020; however, the COVID-19 pandemic erased much of this progress.

One type of disparity of food insecurity exists among different racial and ethnic groups. For example, there is a significant difference in food insecurity comparing Blacks, indigenous people, and people of color to White, non-Hispanic/Latinx households. In addition, USDA data showed that households with children had substantially higher rates of food insecurity (14.8%) than those without children (8.8%).

The highest rates of food insecurity existed among households headed by single mothers (27.7%).

There is a strong relationship between food security and chronic disease. While causes of chronic disease are multifactorial, low-income Black, indigenous, and people of color households are disproportionately affected by food insecurity [34,35].

One particular problem is that food insecurity and chronic disease appear to be cyclical in nature. For example, households may adopt unhealthful behaviors in times of food insecurity and may overconsume calories during times of adequate food supply. These unhealthful coping strategies can lead to both adverse physical and mental health outcomes. In addition, individuals of lower socioeconomic status may be forced to choose between healthful eating and paying electric bills or rent.

It may appear counterintuitive, but high rates of overweight and obesity are higher in families that are food insecure. In this setting these individuals face unique challenges in adopting and maintaining healthful eating behaviors and are more likely to be exposed to marketing of unhealthy foods and beverages, which can contribute to poor eating behaviors.

34.13 ENVIRONMENTAL SUPPORTS FOR HEALTHY EATING

A variety of aspects of the environment may interact with policy decisions that impact on healthy eating [33,34]. For example, many individuals who live in impoverished areas do not have an adequate food supply. This might include certain types of restaurants or fresh produce. Food deserts are places lacking access to foods that are nutritious such as fruits, vegetables, whole grains, and low-fat dairy products. Many food deserts exist in the United States [36–38]. There is a considerable scientific literature about how food deserts in the United States adversely impact on health. As defined by the USDA, a food desert contains a variety of components including a low-access community, small number of individuals impacted, and distance the individual lives from the supermarket or grocery store that is not considered a convenience store. In rural areas, to qualify as a food desert the distance must be greater than 10 miles from the supermarket. Policy interventions such as encouraging farmers markets have had some success [38]. In addition, efforts to increase knowledge, skills, and behavior related to consumption of healthy foods are important. Shopping patterns may also impact on food purchasing. These patterns shifted to online purchasing during the COVID-19 pandemic. It was initially thought that this might increase healthy food shopping; however, consumers are often reluctant to buy fresh produce online and thus, online shopping may actually negatively impact on food purchases.

Many food purchases are impacted by what is called "behavioral economics." This may include the fact that individuals may make poor food choices even in a supermarket. Such simple issues as how various food products are placed in a supermarket can significantly impact on food choice.

School vending machines can also impact on healthy eating. There has been a significant effort to ban non-nutritious foods in school vending machines. For example, the Smart Snacks in Schools guidelines mandate that grain products have 50% or more of whole grain and that the first ingredient be a fruit or vegetable or dairy product. In addition, the food must meet nutritional standards for calories, sodium, sugar, and fats [39,40]. These include calories 200 or less, sodium 200 mg or less, total fats 35% of calories or less, saturated fat less than 10% of calories, trans fat zero, and sugar 35% by weight or less. Many of these factors interact with public policy decisions since a number of mandates have required federal, state, or local action.

Healthcare and dietetic professionals should play key roles in helping to make the environment more likely to promote healthy food choices. For example, the Academy of Nutrition and Dietetics (AND) has made a case for a federal nutrition policy that supports healthy eating. Dietitians, nutritionists, and registered dietitian nutritionists (RDNs) can play a key role in how individuals consume healthy diets with the goal of chronic disease prevention.

Another aspect of the environment that can help with healthy food selections are worksite supports for healthy eating. Strategies for healthy worksite food environments include ensuring access to clean water, providing healthful food at onsite cafeterias and vending machines, and reducing prices of fruits and vegetables.

34.14 POLICY SUPPORTS FOR HEALTHY EATING

Both the federal nutrition policy and the Dietary Guidelines for Americans, which are issued every five years, provide useful guidelines for healthy eating patterns. In the current *Dietary Guidelines for Americans 2020–2025*, multiple key messages about healthy eating can be summarized by the goal of improving the nutritional density in the campaign with the slogan "Make Every Bite Count" [17].

34.15 THE ROLE OF FOOD LABELS

The Food and Drug Administration (FDA) requires food labels that promote healthy eating. This must be combined with improved consumer education. An example of the redesigned food labels is found in Chapter 3. All manufacturers were required to update their food labels by July 1, 2021 [41,42]. The updates were intended to help consumers make better-educated choices about foods. Recommendations included making serving sizes that actually reflect what people consume and making the calorie count font size larger and bolder. Added sugars are now listed in grams and a percentage of daily value which is hoped to help individuals achieve the Dietary Guidelines goal of "less than 10% of calories per day from added sugar." Vitamin D and potassium were added to the food label since they are typical nutrients that Americans underconsume. Footnotes have been added to help the consumer better understand what the product provides as a percentage in relationship to total daily consumption.

34.16 RESTAURANT MENU LABELING

Menu labeling in restaurants is now mandated for all restaurant establishments with 20 or more locations [43]. Such restaurants are now required to have calories listed beside the name and price of the item. This mandated menu labeling rule provides another example of how policy can impact on healthy eating.

34.17 BUILDING ALLIANCES FOR HEALTHY EATING

Both environmental and policy changes are best developed by building on community strengths and knowledge of both individuals and their social network as well as community structures, norms, cultures, histories, and values [44,45]. Because of the importance of these strategic alliances, many federal, state, and nongovernment agencies have called for the development of such alliances with the goal of promoting healthy eating. A great example of this was the follow-up to the September 2022 White House Conference on Hunger, Nutrition and Health, which called for the establishment of many of these alliance in collaboration with the federal government. In addition, clinicians who are interested particularly in the area of lifestyle medicine can play an important role in these strategic alliances. There is increasing recognition that physician involvement in these types of efforts constitutes a professional responsibility.

Within the clinical setting, in addition to focusing on individual social and family-level factors to enhance the health of patients, advocacy and participation in alliances for healthy eating have increasingly been seen as a critical responsibility of physicians. Partnering with community members such as school teachers, retired nurses, parents, and children can ensure that goals and activities are feasible. In addition, physicians should play leadership roles in the area of information resources and communication to improve the desired outcome of healthy eating.

34.18 HEALTHY EATING AND PHYSICAL ACTIVITY

While this chapter has focused on public policy initiatives to encourage healthy eating, an analogous set of public policy initiatives are necessary to increase other components of healthy living, including physical activity [18]. Built environments, federal mandates for inclusion of physical activity in clinical medicine, and the very important role of physicians to advocate for not only individual physical activity among patients but also community resources to improve physical activity levels are important. Of course, other lifestyle medicine components such as weight management and avoidance of risky substances including tobacco also play very important roles. Public policy can underscore the important role that physicians play in these areas.

34.19 CONCLUSIONS

Public policy plays a critically important role in the area of nutrition. The landscape in nutrition has changed dramatically in the past 20 years. No longer is the core underlying principle of public policy in nutrition to provide adequate amounts of food. Nutrition policy has now shifted based on scientific understandings that poor diet drives a considerable percentage of chronic disease. Therefore, moving forward it will be vitally important that public policy continue to shift to focus on healthy nutrition. This is particularly true for individuals who are food insecure.

Changing to a healthier diet involving increased consumption of fruits, vegetables, and whole grains and decreased consumption of red meats, tropical oils, and refined grains will require a multilevel commitment and policy changes not only on the national level but also the international level. These changes will also be vitally important to preserving the health of the planet. (These issues are discussed in more detail in the chapter on planetary health.) This represents an expanded responsibility for practitioners of lifestyle medicine to advocate not only for individual patients but also for the health of the environment that we all share.

Clinical Applications

- Multiple factors impact public policy in the area of nutrition.
- The landscape in the area of nutrition has changed based on scientific information that shows that the current diet in the Western world contributes to the ongoing epidemic of chronic diseases such as obesity, diabetes, and cardiovascular disease.
- Lifestyle medicine clinicians should focus not only on encouraging individual patients to follow a healthier, plant-based eating pattern but also in leadership roles in developing alliances that promote this on community, state, and national levels.
- Moving to a healthier eating pattern is important not only for individual patients and communities but also is vitally important to preserve the health of the planet.

REFERENCES

1. Mozaffarian D, Angell S, Lang T, et al. Role of government policy in nutrition-barriers to and opportunities for healthier eating. BMJ. 2018;361:k2426.
2. Thorndike A, Gardner C, Kendrick K, et al. Strengthening US food policies and programs to promote equity in nutrition security: A policy statement from the American Heart Association. Circulation. 2022;145(24):e1077–e1093.
3. Serchen J, Atiq O, Hilden D. Health, public policy committee of the American College of P. strengthening food and nutrition security to promote public health in the United States: A position paper from the American College of Physicians. Ann Intern Med. 2022;175(8):1170–1171.
4. Dwyer J. Nutrition Policy. Reference Module in Food Science. Amsterdam, The Netherlands: Elsevier, 2016.
5. Shannon K, Kim B, McKenzie S, et al. Food system policy, public health, and human rights in the United States. Annu Rev Public Health. 2015;36(1):151–173.
6. Dennison B. Public policy to improve child nutrition and health: Challenges and opportunities. Arch Pediatr Adolesc Med. 2012;166(5):485–487.
7. Gorski M, Roberto C. Public health policies to encourage healthy eating habits: Recent perspectives. J Healthc Leadersh. 2015;7:81–90.
8. Mozaffarian D, Rosenberg I, Uauy R. History of modern nutrition science-implications for current research, dietary guidelines, and food policy. BMJ. 2018;361:k2392.
9. Afshin A, Micha R, Khatibzadeh S, et al. Dietary policies to reduce non-communicable diseases. In Brown GW, Yamey G, and Wamala S (eds). The Handbook of Global Health Policy. Hoboken, NJ: John Wiley & Sons, Ltd., 2014: 175–193.
10. Afshin A, Penalvo J, Del Gobbo L, et al. CVD prevention through policy: A review of mass media, food/menu labeling, taxation/subsidies, built environment, school procurement, worksite wellness, and marketing standards to improve diet. Curr Cardiol Rep. 2015;17(11):98.

11. World Cancer Research Fund International. NOURISHING framework. NOURISHING Framework | World Cancer Research Fund International (wcrf.org) (Accessed December 29, 2023).
12. Mozaffarian D, Afshin A, Benowitz N; American Heart Association Council on Epidemiology and Prevention, Council on Nutrition, Physical Activity and Metabolism, Council on Clinical Cardiology, Council on Cardiovascular Disease in the Young, Council on the Kidney in Cardiovasc. Population approaches to improve diet, physical activity, and smoking habits: A scientific statement from the American Heart Association. Circulation. 2012;18;126(12):1514–1563.
13. Informas. The Healthy Food Environment Policy Index (Food-EPI). 2017. www.imformas.org/food-epi/Food-PRICE. Food Policy Review and Intervention Cost-Effectiveness (Food-PRICE). 2018. https//www.food-price.org.
14. Brug J. Determinants of healthy eating: Motivation, abilities and environmental opportunities. Fam Pract. 2008;(Suppl 1):i50–i55.
15. U.S. Food and Drug Administration. Menu and vending machine labeling. Menu and Vending Machine Labeling | FDA (Accessed December 29, 2023).
16. Dodson E, Hipp J, Gao M, et al. The impact of worksite supports for healthy eating on dietary behaviors. J Occup Environ Med. 2016;58(8):e287–e293.
17. U.S. Department of Agriculture and U.S. Department of Health and Human Services. *Dietary Guidelines for Americans, 2020–2025*, 9th edition. December 2020. DietaryGuidelines.gov. 2020. www.dietaryguidelines.gov/resources/2020-2025-dietary-guidelines-online-materials.
18. Public Policies Promoting Healthy Eating and Exercise. Evaluating the Relationship Among Income, Obesity and Life Expectancy. The Center for American Progress. Public Policies Promoting Healthy Eating and Exercise—Center for American Progress. (Accessed December 29, 2023).
19. Fernandes A, Rieger D, Proenca R. Perspective: Public health nutrition policies should focus on healthy eating, not on calorie counting, even to decrease obesity. Adv Nutr. 2019;10(4):549–556.
20. Blumenthal D, Fowler E, Abrams M, et al. Covid-19—Implications for the health care system. N Engl J Med. 2020;383(15):1483–1488.
21. Feeding America. Our Work | Feeding America. (Accessed December 29, 2023).
22. Coleman-Jensen A, Rabbit M, Gregory C, et al. Household food security in the United States in 2020, ERR-298 55 pp. U. S. Department of Agriculture, Economic Research Service. Household Food Security in the United States in 2020 (usda.gov) (Accessed December 29, 2023).
23. Feeding America. 2021. The Impact of Coronavirus on Food Insecurity. Available from Food Insecurity and Poverty in the US—Feeding America. (Accessed December 29, 2023).
24. Ralston K, Treen K, Coleman-Jensen A, et al. Children's food security and USDA child nutrition programs. U.S. Department of Agriculture, Economic Research Service. 2017. Children's Food Security and USDA Child Nutrition Programs (Accessed December 29, 2023).
25. Gleason S, Wolford B, Wilkin M, et al. Analysis of Supplemental Nutrition Assistance Program Education (SNAP-Ed) Data for All States Study: Final Report. Prepared by Altarum Institute for the U.S. Department of Agriculture, Food and Nutrition Service, August 2018. Analysis of SNAP-Ed Data for All States | Food and Nutrition Service (usda.gov) (Accessed December 29, 2023).
26. Mansfield J, Savaiano D. Effect of school wellness policies and the healthy, hunger-free kids act on food-consumption behaviors of students, 2006–2016: A systematic review. Nutr Rev. 2017;75(7):533–552.
27. USDA Economic Research Service. National School Lunch Program. USDA ERS—National School Lunch Program. (Accessed December 29, 2023).

28. USDA Economic Research Service. Farm Bill Spending. USDA ERS—Farm Bill Spending. (Accessed December 29, 2023).
29. The EAT-Lancet Commission on Food, Planet, Health. The EAT-Lancet Commission on Food, Planet, Health—EAT Knowledge (eatforum.org) (Accessed December 29, 2023).
30. Bleich S, Moran A, Vercammen K, et al. Strengthening the public health impacts of the supplemental nutrition assistance program through policy. Annu Rev Public Health. 2020;41:453–480.
31. Sanjeevi N, Freeland-Graves J, Sachdev P. Association of loss of supplemental nutrition assistance program benefits with food insecurity and dietary intake of adults and children. Am J Clin Nutr. 2021;114(2):683–689.
32. Huang J, Barnidge E, Kim Y. Children receiving free or reduced-price school lunch have higher food insufficiency rates in summer. J Nutr. 2015;145(9):2161–2168.
33. Story M, Kaphingst K, Robinson-O'Brien R, et al. Creating healthy food and eating environments: Policy and environmental approaches. Ann Rev Public Health. 2008;29(1):253–272.
34. Grier S, Kumanyika S. The context for choice: Health implications of targeted food and beverage marketing to African Americans. Am J Public Health. 2008;98(9):1616–1629.
35. Seligman H, Laraia B, Kushel M. Food insecurity is associated with chronic disease among low-income NHANES participants12. J Nutr. 2010;140(2):304–310.
36. Gateway to Health Communication & Social Marketing Practice. Centers for disease control and prevention. Tools & Templates | Gateway to Health Communication | CDC (iiab.me) (Accessed December 29, 2023).
37. Michimi A, Wimberly M. Associations of supermarket accessibility with obesity and fruit and vegetable consumption in the conterminous United States. Int J Health Geogr. 2010;9:49.
38. USDA. Economic research service. Mapping food deserts in the United States. USDA ERS—Data Feature: Mapping Food Deserts in the U.S. (Accessed December 29, 2023).
39. Anderson E, Wei R, Liu B, et al. Improving healthy food choices in low-income settings in the United States using behavioral economic-based adaptations to choice architecture. Front Nutr. 2021;8:734991.
40. U.S. Food and Drug Administration. A Guide to Smart Snacks in Schools. www.fns.usda.gov/tn/guide-smart-snacks-school (Accessed January 18, 2024).
41. FDA. U.S. Food and Drug Administration. Changes to the nutrition facts label. Changes to the Nutrition Facts Label | FDA. (Accessed December 29, 2023).
42. FDA. U.S. Food and Drug Administration. How to understand and use the nutrition facts label. How to Understand and Use the Nutrition Facts Label | FDA (Accessed December 29, 2023).
43. FDA. U.S. Food and Drug Administration. Menu labeling requirements. Menu Labeling Requirements | FDA. (Accessed December 29, 2023).
44. Hancock T. People, partnerships and human progress: Building community capital. Health Promot Int. 2001;16(3):275–280.
45. Harnack L, Block G, Subar A, et al. Association of cancer prevention-related nutrition knowledge, beliefs, and attitudes to cancer prevention dietary behavior. J Am Diet Assoc. 1997;97(9):957–965.

35 Eating for Nutrition for Good Health and to Protect the Planet

Key Points

- Modern nutrition science has identified characteristics of healthy diets.
- These diets are very consistent with each other and include abundant fruits and vegetables, whole grains, and nontropical oils, while minimizing red and processed meat, salt, and sugar.
- Physicians currently are not adequately trained in the area of nutrition.
- The current "Western" diet promotes many chronic diseases and underlies increased caloric consumption as well as chronic inflammation.
- Healthy diets have less inflammatory potential and are important not only for individual health but also for the health of the entire planet.

35.1 INTRODUCTION

This book has two specific goals. The first is to provide an evidence-based overview of modern nutrition science and its relationship to good health. The second goal is to bring this information forth in a user-friendly manner that will encourage more physicians and other healthcare workers to adopt healthier nutrition in their own lives and also counsel patients on the benefits of sound nutrition for good health and reduction of chronic disease reduction.

It is also apparent that nutrition is not only critically important for good health and chronic disease reduction but also mandatory to protect the environment and the planet (see Chapter 33 for more details). Moreover, healthy nutrition also underpins the vast and unfortunate inequities in the modern healthcare system in the United States (see Chapter 6 for more details).

It is important to remember that healthy nutrition is only one of many habits and actions that impact on the daily lives of individuals which can either promote or impair health. These habits and actions are the basis for the rapidly growing field of lifestyle medicine [1].

In the area of nutrition, while there has been enormous progress, there are still enormous challenges. The two major challenges are interrelated. The first is that the vast majority of physicians feel that they lack adequate knowledge in the area of nutrition [2]. This leads to a distinct minority counseling their patients in this area. The second major challenge is that people are not following sound nutrition in their daily lives. For example, only 12% of individuals consume the recommended

DOI: 10.1201/9781003452607-35

number of fruits, and less than 10% consume the recommended number of servings of vegetables [3]. The amount of fiber in the American diet is less than half of what is recommended.

In addition, there are profound linkages between the type of diet that is currently being followed by the overwhelming majority of Americans and others around the world and planetary health. While most physicians are deeply concerned about greenhouse gases and planet warming, only a distinct minority understand that agricultural practices are a leading cause of the looming environmental catastrophe that is in progress unless the type of diet that people consume around the world changes dramatically [4]. Thus, there is great synergy between following healthy nutrition practices for good health and how these practices impact on protecting the health of the planet.

35.2 LIFESTYLE NUTRITION FOR PHYSICIANS AND OTHER HEALTHCARE WORKERS

In cardiology for many years, the mantra was that people should consume a low-fat diet to lower their risk of heart disease and other diseases caused by atherosclerosis. The theory was that cholesterol and saturated fat accumulated in the coronary arteries and arteries in other locations in the body and ultimately caused them to occlude causing heart attack, stroke, or other manifestations of atherosclerosis (see Chapter 12).

Modern nutrition science has clearly shown that low-fat diets are not superior to placebo when it comes to risk factors for coronary heart disease (CHD) [5]. The modern understanding of healthy diets involves diets that are high in fruits and vegetables and whole grains [3,6]. Larger amounts of fats, particularly monounsaturated and polyunsaturated fats, can be included in these diets and have been clearly shown to lower the risk of CHD. Perhaps most prominently the Mediterranean diet (MedDiet) [7] and the Dietary Approach to Stop Hypertension (DASH) [8] as well as the Healthy U.S.-Style Dietary all follow these precepts [3]. These will be discussed in a separate section of this chapter. The theory is that these diets lower inflammation in the body. For this reason, these are the diets that are recommended not only by the *Dietary Guidelines for Americans 2020–2025* but also the 2021 Nutrition Update from the American Heart Association [6]. These were the diets that are featured in multiple chapters throughout this book.

Even in my subspecialty of cardiology, 90% of cardiologists feel that they do not have adequate training in the area of nutrition [9]. The good news is that a similar number of cardiologists feel that it is imperative that they discuss nutrition with their patients.

Other subspecialties of medicine have similarly low knowledge bases in nutrition. This is not surprising, given that only 17% of medical schools have significant courses in nutrition [10]. It is also very telling that over 60% of patients feel that they do not get adequate nutritional counseling from their physicians. This is clearly a missed opportunity since over 70% of individuals see their primary care physician at least once a year.

35.3 NUTRITION IN THE CONTEXT OF OTHER HEALTHY LIFESTYLE HABITS AND PRACTICES

The goal of the emerging literature in lifestyle medicine is to bring the components of positive lifestyle habits and practices together so that physicians and other healthcare workers can have efficient access to this literature. I had the privilege of editing the first multiauthored academic textbook in lifestyle medicine. This first academic textbook in the field published in 1999 actually coined the term "lifestyle medicine," which was defined as "the discipline of studying how daily habits and practices impact both on the prevention and treatment of disease, often in conjunction with pharmaceutical or surgical therapy, to provide an important adjunct to overall health" [11]. Now, 24 years later, these initial sentiments have proven to be prescient. The field of lifestyle medicine has grown dramatically in the past 24 years. In addition to sound nutrition, lifestyle medicine incorporates other habits and actions which have been shown to improve both short- and long-term health. These have been summarized in the "six pillars of lifestyle medicine" [12]. They include healthy nutrition, regular physical activity, weight management, avoiding tobacco and other harmful substances, stress reduction, and healthy sleep. While this book has focused on the area of nutrition, it is important for physicians and other healthcare workers to put healthy nutrition in the context of multiple other healthy habits and actions which can act synergistically, along with nutrition, to lower the risk of chronic disease and improve people's health. There are multiple resources available that describe the key components of lifestyle medicine. Some are single-topic books published in the *Lifestyle Medicine Series*. Additional resources are available in in multiple authoritative documents generated by the American College of Lifestyle Medicine (ACLM). These resources are listed in the references to this chapter.

35.4 THE WESTERN DIET

The typical diet consumed in the United States has been called the "Western Diet" (WD). It also has been called the standard American diet (see Chapter 2). The acronym for this diet is SAD, which seems highly appropriate since this diet contributes to significant adverse consequences because of its association with multiple chronic diseases.

The WD is characterized by considerable amounts of red and processed meat, refined grains, processed foods, tropical oils, saturated fats, salt, and refined sugar. It minimizes consumption of fruits and vegetables and whole grains. There are multiple negative effects of consuming this diet. It has been clearly shown to increase the risk of CHD, type 2 diabetes mellitus (T2DM), obesity, metabolic syndrome, and even many cancers.

Multiple underlying reasons exist for why the WD is associated with so many chronic diseases. The leading hypothesis now in nutrition research is that this diet, in and of itself, is highly inflammatory. This nutritional pattern creates a situation where chronic diseases, which are also inflammatory, can thrive (see also Chapter 9). In addition, the WD is very low in fiber, which contributes to multiple adverse effects on the microbiome. It also is high in calories and has contributed to the pandemic of overweight and obesity experienced in the United States and around the world. Unfortunately, as various countries around the world have become more affluent, many of them have switched to a more "Western" style of eating. For example, in China, obesity rose from 3–4% to over 20% in the past two decades. The same type of rapidly accelerating prevalence of chronic disease has occurred in many other countries where a WD has increasingly been consumed. It has been estimated that over 85% of calories in the United States are consumed from packaged and processed foods. While the actual role of processed foods in this diet remains under debate, it is clear that processing of grains results in the loss of much of the fiber, further exacerbating metabolic problems associated with the WD.

35.5 HEALTHY PLANT-BASED DIET

Modern nutrition science has clearly demonstrated that diets high in fruits and vegetables, whole grains, nontropical oils, and fish (preferably oily fish) are associated with decreased risk of CHD and T2DM as well as obesity. Multiple diets qualify as "healthy" plant-based diets. These include the Mediterranean diet, the DASH diet, the Healthy U.S.-Style Dietary, the Nordic diet, and many vegetarian diets.

Perhaps the most compelling information available in this area comes from the large PREDIMED Study of the MedDiet conducted in Spain, which showed significant decreases in CHD. This diet is named after the type of eating pattern followed in most countries around the Mediterranean Sea. The MedDiet is high in fruits and vegetables, whole grains, nuts, and nontropical oils. It minimizes packaged foods and also minimizes red meat or processed meat, salt, and sugar. Adding extra-virgin olive oil to this diet further reduces the risk of CVD.

It has been hypothesized that the various healthy plant-based diets derive much of their benefit from lowering inflammation in the body. These diets themselves are much lower in inflammatory properties than the WD.

35.6 NUTRITION, LIFESTYLE MEDICINE, AND CHRONIC DISEASE

As discussed in multiple chapters in this book, numerous nutrition science studies have shown over the past 20 years that the SAD is associated with a wide variety of chronic diseases. These include hypertension, stroke, CHD, cancer, decreased cognition, peripheral artery disease, chronic kidney disease, erectile dysfunction, prediabetes and diabetes, and overweight and obesity. Separate chapters in this book are devoted to each of these chronic diseases.

The underlying pathophysiology that appears to link all of these chronic diseases has to do with the association of the WD with increased inflammation and decreased immune function in the body. In contrast, as already indicated, healthy plant-based diets are anti-inflammatory. It is hypothesized that this is the key attribute for why these diets have been demonstrated to lower the risk of the chronic diseases enumerated here.

35.7 NUTRITION AND HEALTH EQUITY

Multiple significant disparities exist in health in the United States. Many of the disparities have to do with nutrition. For example, individuals who are below 130% of the U.S. poverty line have generally lower scores on the Healthy Eating Index than do more affluent individuals. In addition, these individuals are much more likely to consume low-quality food, which often has significant amounts of sugar and salt in it. In addition, these individuals often live in environments that have been called "food deserts" since they lack full-service grocery stores which would provide sources of fruits and vegetables and other produce.

It is clear that individuals of color, including both Brown and Black individuals, are more susceptible to decreased health equity than are Caucasians. In addition, these individuals often have less access to healthcare than do more affluent individuals. This issue is so important that both the American Heart Association [13] and the American College of Physicians [14] have issued position statements describing the problem and outlining steps that they intend to take within the medical community to help address the enormous disparities in health that currently exist in the United States. The disparities in health equity were underscored during the recent COVID-19 pandemic where people who had underlying poor nutrition were much more likely to develop severe illness, require hospitalization, and die as a result of COVID-19. These issues will be discussed in more detail in a subsequent section of this chapter [15].

35.8 HUNGER, FOOD INSECURITY, AND MALNUTRITION

Hunger, food insecurity, and malnutrition are interrelated, particularly in the United States. Malnutrition in the United States is a very significant problem, although all of these concerns are also very significant problems in underdeveloped countries (see also Chapter 7). Of these three concepts the broadest one is malnutrition, which is typically defined as not consuming an adequate amount of foods that carry sufficient nutritional value. This can result in both undernutrition and overnutrition. Malnutrition is thought to significantly contribute to the rapidly increasing prevalence of overweight and obesity throughout the world.

In the United States, significant increases have occurred in both overweight and obesity in the past 30 years. Currently, over 70% of adults in the United States are either overweight or obese, 40% of individuals are obese (body mass index [BMI] ≥ 30 kg/m^2) [16].

Over 38 million individuals in the United States are food insecure, meaning that they do not have enough food to eat. This includes over 12 million children [17]. These individuals often experience hunger and are forced into situations of skipping meals or consuming inadequate amounts of food or meals with poor nutritional value.

Obviously, these high levels of hunger and food insecurity are unacceptable in the most affluent country in the world. This was one of the key issues discussed in the September 2022, White House Conference on Hunger, Nutrition and Health [18]. Multiple follow-ups were articulated from this conference. While there are numerous public policy supports that attempt to ameliorate this problem (see a subsequent section of this chapter), the problems of hunger, food insecurity, and malnutrition will require multiple concentrated efforts from both the public and private sector.

The issue of malnutrition is a worldwide problem and one of the key issues addressed in the World Health Organization (WHO) initiative on noncommunicable diseases (NCDs) [19]. In the United States, malnutrition is often a problem experienced for individuals under 3 years of age and increasingly for individuals over the age of 65 years. While there are multiple underlying causes of malnutrition, the tragic fact is that the medical community tends to not adequately diagnose this issue. It is incumbent on all physicians to be aware of the issues of malnutrition and help combat the health problems that result from this condition that should be preventable in an affluent country such as the United States.

35.9 *DIETARY GUIDELINES FOR AMERICANS 2020–2025*

If clinicians wish to have only one document in their toolchest to summarize modern, evidence-based understandings of nutrition science, the Executive Summary of the *Dietary Guidelines for Americans 2020–2025* (DGA 2020–2025) is the essential document to have [3]. The DGAs are federally mandated to be published every five years and provide up-to-date nutrition science (for more details see Chapter 8). Many other federal programs are based on the information found in the DGAs.

The most recent DGAs focused on several issues. First of all, the document focuses on the difference between energy density and nutrient density. The phrase coined in the DGA 2020–2025 to emphasize nutrient density is "make every bite count." In other words, the DGA recommended that without exceeding calories, it is possible to have healthy nutrition as long as individuals pay attention to the nutrient density of the foods that they do eat.

In addition, the 2020–2025 DGAs firmly focused on the concept of overall eating patterns. Previous DGAs initially focused on nutrients and then subsequently on individual foods. It has now become clear in nutrition science that it is the overall quality of the diet that matters. Thus, most nutrition science is based now on overall dietary quality, as is the DGA 2020–2025. For individuals who want to delve more deeply into nutrition science, the entire DGA 2020–2025 is a worthwhile read. The document focuses on healthy nutrition for infants, children, adults, and older adults. There are also important sections on nutrition for women and nutrition for a healthy pregnancy.

35.10 NUTRITION AND METABOLIC HEALTH

Metabolism is the basic process that converts foods consumed into the various energy-producing and -utilizing processes in the body. These are summarized in the concept of metabolic health (see Chapter 10 for more detail). Recently, a concept has arisen making a distinction, particularly in obese individuals, between "metabolically healthy" and "metabolically unhealthy" individuals. This concept also applies to individuals who are not overweight or obese.

The most reliable way to ensure metabolic health is to consume an overall healthy diet. This is emphasized in multiple chapters throughout this book. Metabolically unhealthy individuals are at a much higher risk for CHD, T2DM, metabolic syndrome, and even some cancers. This is a useful concept for all clinicians and other healthcare workers to emphasize to their patients for how to achieve an overall metabolically healthy life through the foods they consume.

35.11 NUTRITION AND ATHEROSCLEROSIS

Atherosclerosis is a systemic underlying process through which coronary arteries and, indeed, arteries throughout the body can become compromised, ultimately leading to a wide variety of significant diseases and problems including heart attacks, stroke, hypertension, metabolic syndrome, chronic kidney disease, and erectile dysfunction (see Chapter 19).

In the past 20 years understanding of the process of atherosclerosis has changed dramatically. It used to be thought that atherosclerotic plaque was built up when individuals consumed increased dietary cholesterol and saturated fats. Modern understandings of atherosclerosis, however, are much more complex.

It is now known that this process starts with an inflammatory component that disrupts the fragile endothelial lining of arteries throughout the body. Once the endothelium is compromised, a number of immune cells are attracted to the area, inciting a process where plaque is built up, which includes cholesterol and other fats as well as a variety of immune cells and processes. Ultimately, these plaques may become fragile and rupture. This is the process that occurs in most myocardial infarctions (heart attacks).

It is clear that nutritional practices impact on the entire process of atherosclerosis. This is the fundamental underlying principle that has been largely established through the PREDIMED study which evaluated the MedDiet. It has also been demonstrated in multiple studies on the DASH diet and other plant-based healthy diets. The leading hypothesis now is that these diets which contain abundant fruits and vegetables, whole grains, nontropical oils, and, in some instances, several servings of fish per week, are anti-inflammatory. Thus, these diets, which have been demonstrated to lower the risk of CHD and other atherosclerotic diseases, are important to understand and promote for all patients.

35.12 NUTRITION AND COVID-19

The COVID-19 pandemic clearly underscored the relationship between nutrition and health. Individuals who had chronic diseases such as hypertension, obesity, diabetes, and heart disease were three to four times as likely to be hospitalized and die from complications of COVID-19 compared to individuals who did not have any of these chronic diseases [15]. The underlying linkage between these conditions and diseases is typically nutritional practices. COVID-19 exerts profound effects on the body's immune system, so issues related to inflammation and decreased immune function played a prominent role in individuals who were likely to become extremely sick and even die from COVID-19. These factors also disproportionately affected Hispanic and Black individuals as well as individuals living in crowded urban environments who also typically followed less healthy nutritional practices.

35.13 NUTRITION FOR VARIOUS POPULATIONS

The fundamental nutrition principles which underlie healthy nutrition such as increased consumption of fruits and vegetables, whole grains, etc., and avoidance of red and processed meat, salt, and sugar apply to the vast majority of adults in the United States. They also apply equally well to children and individuals over the age of 65. The best single source of information concerning nutrition and its effects on these various populations is contained in the DGAs 2020–2025. This evidence-based compendium of modern nutritional science has specific chapters on various population groups and represents an important foundation to develop a knowledge base on healthy nutrition.

35.14 NUTRITION AND THE MICROBIOTA

An enormous upsurge has occurred in research and understanding of the microbiota in the last decade (see Chapter 24). The human gut houses literally trillions of bacteria, fungi, and viruses, which profoundly interact with human physiology and may either enhance or diminish human health. It has been clearly demonstrated in recent research that following healthy nutritional practices can improve the diversity and the type of organisms in the microbiome. For example, fiber can be converted to butyrate and other short-chain fatty acids, which can have a significant effect on lowering the risk of heart disease and other atherosclerotic-based diseases. Conversely, the WD may promote dysbiosis in the microbiome and lead to such condition as "leaky gut" syndrome and a number of immune and inflammatory processes, which can increase the risk of chronic disease. The study of the microbiome is in its infancy, but it is destined to lead to important new understandings of nutrition and human health in the decades to come.

35.15 GENETICS, EPIGENETICS, AND PRECISION NUTRITION

One of the most rapidly advancing fields in nutrition research has to do with genetics, epigenetics, and precision nutrition (see Chapter 32). It is well known that overweight and obesity have greatly increased in the United States and around the world in the last 40 years. The human genetic pool changes only minimally over millennia and cannot be responsible for the rapid increase in obesity and other chronic obesity-related conditions. Thus, the way the genetic code is transcribed must play an important role. Therefore, the field of epigenetics has grown rapidly and has offered multiple important insights into how nutrition interacts with the development of various chronic diseases such as obesity. A particular process involving methylation of cytosine, which is one of the four DNA base pairs, often contributes to chronic diseases. Methylation impacts on whether or not various sequences of DNA are either read or suppressed. Epigenetic changes are thought to contribute in significant ways to various metabolic diseases such as heart disease, diabetes, and cancer.

The ability to rapidly read the DNA has allowed advances to be made in the area of precision prevention. Different individuals clearly respond differently to different foods and dietary practices. This has led to a number of research laboratories around the United States and elsewhere to look at ways to provide more precise nutritional recommendations based on genetic and epigenetic profiles. The National Institutes of Health (NIH) has also become involved in this area and has launched a $150 million five-year campaign to encourage nutrition researchers to develop more precise nutrition recommendations [20]. While this field is in its infancy, it carries great promise for the future. Individuals should be cautioned, however, that a number of the commercially available systems that propose to help individuals precisely determine their nutritional patterns are often guilty of "overpromising." These available products should be approached with caution.

35.16 HEALTHY NUTRITION AND PLANETARY HEALTH

There is no longer any serious question that current nutritional patterns, particularly in the United States and around the world that have been characterized as the "Western diet," exert enormous adverse effects on the planet (see Chapter 33). For example, the U.S. food production system is responsible for about 50% of total U.S. land area, 80% of fresh water, and 17% of fossil fuel used in the country.

It has been estimated that 19–29% of greenhouse gases are a result of current agricultural practices to support a Western-style diet. Methane produced by cattle and goat waste products bred to meet demands for meat consumption is associated with both environmental degradation and generation of approximately 9% of greenhouse gases in the United States.

A number of prestigious organizations have issued stern warnings that unless major changes are made in the area of human nutrition, irreparable damage will be done to the environment. This, indeed, has already started. The EAT-Lancet Commission warns that as population continues to grow, agricultural resources will no longer be sufficient in the next 10–15 years to meet the increased demands from this expanding population.

In addition, agricultural practices, including deforestation and runoff of phosphorous and nitrogen from fertilizers, are causing enormous adverse environmental impacts. Thus, it is imperative for members of the medical community to sound the alarm both to individual patients and also to broader audiences such as the agriculture and food industry and the federal government to underscore that healthy nutrition is essential not only for individual health but also for protecting the planet. The EAT-Lancet Commission warned that unless significant changes were made in the way human beings consume food, irreparable planetary damage will ultimately ensue.

35.17 PUBLIC POLICY SUPPORT FOR HEALTHY EATING

Governments around the world have become increasingly engaged in the area of healthy eating (see Chapter 34). In the past, food policies in the United States and around the world were largely focused on ensuring an adequate supply of calories. Nutritional science has now warned indicated that the shift must occur to focus on the *quality* of foods over and above the *quantity* of food available.

The recently completed White House Conference on Hunger, Nutrition and Health underscored that multiple federal and private resources will be required to address currently existing problems including not only environmental impacts but also food insecurity and food and health inequities. Programs such as the Supplemental Nutrition Assistance Program (SNAP) and the Women, Infants and Children Nutrition Program (WIC) have been enormously important to the least affluent segments of the U.S. population. The Farm Bill has recently increased funding for environmentally sustainable programs in healthy nutrition. It will require an enormous effort for both public and private sectors around the world to address current nutritional practices and promote healthier nutrition.

This is the underlying principle also from the WHO initiative on NCDs. Many of the underlying factors that contribute to the chronic NCD diseases are based on poor nutritional practices. The WHO estimates that 71% of all mortality each year comes from NCDs [19].

35.18 PHYSICIAN HEAL THYSELF

It is critically important that physicians become not only more knowledgeable in the area of nutrition but also to adopt these practices in their own lives. There are good data to show that physicians who pay attention to nutrition, physical activity, and other positive lifestyle factors in their own lives are more likely to counsel their patients in these areas than physicians who do not [21].

In addition, physicians are subject to a high-stress environment, which can contribute to a variety of chronic diseases as well as decreased mental health and burnout [22]. Paying more attention to healthy nutrition, physical activity, and other lifestyle practices can potentially make a huge impact on the health of medical professionals throughout the United States and, indeed, throughout the world. As it has been said, and it is certainly true in this area, physicians need to both "walk the walk" and "talk the talk."

35.19 CONCLUSIONS

The area of healthy nutrition is of unsurpassed importance for the health of the American population and, indeed, the population around the world. Modern nutrition science has made enormous strides in this area and has developed incontrovertible evidence that diets that consist of abundant fruits and vegetables, whole grains, nontropical oils, and whole plant-based foods while diminishing red and processed meat, salt, and sugar lead to enormous health benefits.

The current WD has been clearly shown to contribute to multiple ongoing chronic diseases that are extremely common in the United States and around the world. In addition, current agricultural processes that promote a meat-based WD have already begun to create enormous adverse health and sustainability consequences for the entire planet. It is time for physicians to become knowledgeable about healthy nutrition and practice it both in their own lives and recommend it for their patients as well as a way to protect the health of the plant. The stakes could not be higher!

Clinical Applications

- Modern nutrition science has clearly defined healthy nutritional practices that lower the risk of heart disease, diabetes, weight gain and obesity, and even some cancers.

- Healthy diets are consistent with each other and are the ones recommended by the DGA 2020–2025 and the recent nutrition guidelines put out by the American Heart Association.
- These diets are high in fruits and vegetables and whole grains and low in tropical oils, red meat and processed meat, salt, and refined sugar.
- Modern nutrition science focuses on overall dietary practices.
- Healthy diets include the MedDiet, the DASH diet, and the Healthy U.S.-Style Dietary contained in the Dietary Guidelines for 2020–2025.

REFERENCES

1. Rippe J. Lifestyle Medicine, 4th edition. Boca Raton: CRC Press, 2024.
2. Aggarwal M, Ospina N, Kazory A, et al. The mismatch of nutrition and lifestyle beliefs and actions among physicians: A wake-up call. Am J Lifestyle Med. 2020;14(3):304–315.
3. U.S. Department of Agriculture and U.S. Department of Health and Human Services. *Dietary Guidelines for Americans, 2020–2025*, 9th edition. December 2020. DietaryGuidelines.gov. 2020. www.dietaryguidelines.gov/resources/2020-2025-dietary-guidelines-online-materials.
4. EAT-Lancet Commission Summary Report. EAT-Lancet Commission Summary Report—EAT. eatforum.org (Accessed January 5, 2024).
5. Mozaffarian D. Mediterranean diet for primary prevention of cardiovascular disease. N Engl J Med. 2013;369:673–674.
6. Lichtenstein A, Appel L, Vadiveloo M, et al. 2021 Dietary guidance to improve cardiovascular health: A scientific statement from the American Heart Association. Circulation. 2021;144(23):e472–e87.
7. Estruch R, Ros E, Salas-Salvado J, et al. Primary prevention of cardiovascular disease with a Mediterranean diet. N Engl J Med. 2013;368(14):1279–1290.
8. Appel L, Moore T, Obarzanek E, et al. A clinical trial of the effects of dietary patterns on blood pressure. DASH Collaborative Research Group. N Engl J Med. 1997;336(16):1117–1124.
9. Devries S, Agatston A, Aggarwal M, et al. A deficiency of nutrition education and practice in cardiology. Am J Med. 2017;130(11):1298–1305.
10. Frates B. The evolving state of nutrition education. Am J Lifestyle Med. 2023;17(6): 759–761.
11. Rippe J. Lifestyle Medicine, 1st edition. London: Blackwell Science, Inc., 1999.
12. American College of Lifestyle Medicine. ACLM. Home—American College of Lifestyle Medicine. (Accessed January 5, 2024).
13. American Heart Association. Championing Health Equity for All. 2024 Health Equity Impact Goal—Professional Heart Daily | American Heart Association. (Accessed January 5, 2024).
14. American College of Physicians. Promoting Health Equity Through Excellence in Diagnostic Decision Making. Promoting Health Equity Through Excellence in Diagnostic Decision Making | ACP Online. (Accessed January 31, 2024).
15. Price-Haywood E, Burton J, Fort D, et al. Hospitalization and mortality among black patients and white patients with Covid-19. N Engl J Med. 2020;382(26):2534–2543.
16. Fryar C, Carroll M, Afful J. Prevalence of overweight, obesity, and severe obesity among Adults aged 20 and over: United States, 1960–1962 through 2017–2018. NCHS Health E-Stats. 2020. Products—Health E Stats—Prevalence of Overweight, Obesity, and Extreme Obesity Among Adults Aged 20 and Over: United States, 1960–1962 Through 2017–2018. cdc.gov (Accessed January 5, 2024).

17. Feeding America. Hunger in America. Hunger in America | Feeding America. (Accessed January 5, 2024).
18. The White House. White House Announces Conference on Hunger, Nutrition and Health in September. White House Announces Conference on Hunger, Nutrition and Health in September | The White House. (Accessed January 5, 2024).
19. World Health Organization. Noncommunicable diseases. (who.int) (Accessed January 5, 2024).
20. National Institutes of Health. NIH awards $170 million for precision nutrition study. NIH Awards $170 Million for Precision Nutrition Study | National Institutes of Health (NIH). (Accessed January 5, 2024).
21. Frank E, Holmes D. Physician health practices and lifestyle medicine. In Rippe J (ed). Lifestyle Medicine, 3rd edition. Boca Raton: CRC Press, 2019.
22. Merlo G, Rippe J. Physician burnout: A lifestyle medicine perspective. Am J Lifestyle Med. 2021;15(2):148–157.

Index

Note: Page numbers in *italics* indicate a figure and page numbers in **bold** indicate a table on the corresponding page.

B

D

E

F

G

I

J

K

L

N

O

P

T

U

V

W

Y

Z

For Product Safety Concerns and Information please contact our EU representative GPSR@taylorandfrancis.com Taylor & Francis Verlag GmbH, Kaufingerstraße 24, 80331 München, Germany